BASIC & APPLIED CONCEPTS *of*
BLOOD BANKING and TRANSFUSION PRACTICES

Fourth Edition

Paula R. Howard, MS, MPH, MT(ASCP)SBB
Professional Education and Corporate Training
Training Program Design and eLearning Course Development
Hobe Sound, Florida
http://paularhoward.com/

ELSEVIER

ELSEVIER

3251 Riverport Lane
St. Louis, Missouri 63043

BASIC & APPLIED CONCEPTS OF BLOOD BANKING AND
TRANSFUSION PRACTICES, FOURTH EDITION   ISBN: 978-0-323-37478-1

Notices

Library of Congress Cataloging-in-Publication Data

Names: Howard, Paula R., author.
Title: Basic & applied concepts of blood banking and transfusion practices /
    Paula R. Howard, MS, MPH, MT(ASCP)SBB, Hobe Sound, Florida.
Other titles: Basic and applied concepts of immunohematology
Description: Fourth edition. | St. Louis, Missouri : Elsevier, [2017] |
    Revision of: Basic & applied concepts of immunohematology / Kathy D.
    Blaney, Paula R. Howard. c2013. 3rd. | Includes bibliographical references
    and index.
Identifiers: LCCN 2016027802 | ISBN 9780323374781 (pbk.)
Subjects: LCSH: Blood banks. | Immunohematology. | Blood--Transfusion.
Classification: LCC RM172 .B54 2017 | DDC 615.3/9--dc23 LC record available at
https://lccn.loc.gov/2016027802

Executive Content Strategist: Kellie White
Content Development Manager: Lisa P. Newton
Senior Content Development Specialist: Tina Kaemmerer
Publishing Services Manager: Hemamalini Rajendrababu
Project Manager: Minerva Irene Viloria-Reyes
Designer: Brian Salisbury

Printed in the United States of America

Last digit is the print number: 9   8   7   6   5   4   3   2   1

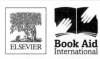

Working together
to grow libraries in
developing countries

www.elsevier.com • www.bookaid.org

Reviewers

Charlotte Bates, MEd, MLS(ASCP)
Interim Program Director
Medical Laboratory Science Department
Armstrong Atlantic State University
Savannah, Georgia

Jimmy L. Boyd, MLS(ASCP), MS/MHS
Department Head/Program Director
Medical Laboratory Technology Program
Arkansas State University-Beebe
Beebe, Arkansas

Cara Calvo, MS, MT(ASCP)SH
Assistant Professor
Oregon Tech & Oregon Health Science University
Portland, Oregon

Linda A. Collins, MS, MLS(ASCP)
Medical Laboratory Technician Program Director
Delaware Technical Community College
Georgetown, Delaware

Nibal Maher Harb, MT, ASCP(BB)
Medical Technologist
OneBlood, Inc.
Tampa, Florida

Kathleen A. Park, MA, MT(ASCP)
Professor
Medical Laboratory Technology Program
Austin Community College
Austin, Texas

Nicole S. Pekarek, MAT, MT(ASCP)
Instructor and Clinical Coordinator
Winston-Salem State University
Winston-Salem, North Carolina

Jayanna Slayton
Indianapolis, Indiana

Deborah Wagner, MS, MT(ASCP)
Adjunct Faculty
Medical Laboratory Technician Program
De Anza College
Cupertino, California

Stacy E. Walz, PhD, MS, MT(ASCP)
Department Chair, Assistant Professor
Clinical Laboratory Sciences Department
Arkansas State University
Jonesboro, Arkansas

Preface

Basic & Applied Concepts of Blood Banking and Transfusion Practices was developed for students in 2- or 4-year medical laboratory science programs, laboratory professionals undergoing retraining, and other health care professionals who desire knowledge in routine blood banking practices. Basic concepts are introduced accompanied by many illustrative figures, and the practical application of these theories to modern transfusion and blood bank settings is emphasized.

The fourth edition includes updates to the ever-changing field of blood banking and introduces QR codes to enrich the student experience beyond the pages of this text. Additional case studies and critical thinking exercises will provide more student interactions. Donor criteria and testing, including the current donor restrictions, infectious disease testing methods, and current requirements for viral marker testing, are updated to the status quo. New and expanded topics in this fourth edition include patient blood management, molecular techniques applying to blood banking, and pathogen inactivation methods and blood products.

This textbook provides important features to assist both the student and the instructor. Each chapter features:

- Chapter outlines listing the important elements in the chapter
- Learning objectives for use by both the student and the instructor
- Study questions for self-assessment
- Key words with definitions on the same page
- Margin notes that enhance information in the text
- Chapter summaries to provide a succinct overview of the chapter's important points
- Critical thinking exercises to illustrate the practical applications to the clinical environment
- Illustrations and tables designed to reinforce and summarize the most important information found in the chapter
- QR codes to provide enhancement of student learning beyond the boundaries of this edition

The fourth edition's Evolve website is updated with more content. For students, the ancillaries include additional case studies, review questions, and access to the laboratory manual. The instructor ancillaries include an image collection that features figures found in the text, an extensive collection of test bank questions, as well as answers to the critical thinking exercises, and PowerPoint presentations for each chapter that include illustrations appearing in this text.

I am very appreciative of Elsevier's editors for their efforts in the manuscript review and publication process. Thank you to all subject matter experts for their outstanding critique of the manuscript. I am proud of the fourth edition of this textbook, which meets the original goal of a user-friendly textbook for students and instructors.

Paula R. Howard

Contents

QUALITY ASSURANCE AND REGULATION OF THE BLOOD INDUSTRY AND SAFETY ISSUES IN THE BLOOD BANK

1

CHAPTER OUTLINE

LEARNING OBJECTIVES

On completion of this chapter, the reader should be able to:

1. Define and list the elements of good manufacturing practices.
2. Describe regulatory agencies that govern activities in the blood bank and apply their regulations.
3. Apply voluntary agency compliance guidelines to the workplace.
4. Differentiate quality assurance (QA) from quality control (QC).
5. Identify the responsibilities of the QA department.
6. Discuss the importance of job descriptions and personnel qualifications.
7. Compare and contrast proficiency and competency testing.
8. List the elements of and explain the importance of a well-written standard operating procedure (SOP).
9. Compare and contrast good record keeping with poor record keeping.
10. Describe the elements of a good training program.
11. Give examples of methods used to evaluate competency.
12. Define calibration, preventive maintenance, and QC requirements; discuss the importance to each in reporting accurate results.
13. Define and describe the purpose behind root-cause analysis in error management.
14. Define and apply universal and standard precautions.
15. Dispose of laboratory waste material properly.
16. List safety equipment and protective devices.
17. Recognize the need for accident reporting.
18. Encourage employee education in safety.
19. Conduct testing using safety principles.

This edition begins with an introduction to quality assurance and regulation of the blood industry in conjunction with an overview of safety practices. Blood banking and transfusion medicine ascribe to high standards of quality and safety in the process that begins with the collection of blood to the final step of transfusion to the patient (Fig. 1.1). For this reason, this chapter lays the foundation for all other topics that follow.

Food and Drug Administration: U.S. agency responsible for the regulation of the blood bank industry and other manufacturers of products consumed by humans

The **Food and Drug Administration** (FDA) classifies blood as a drug. This classification requires all **blood banks** and **transfusion services** to follow its legally required standards. The FDA describes standards for quality and safety for transfusion services and blood banks through quality assurance (QA) programs and current good manufacturing practices (cGMPs). Quality efforts and activities enhance efficiency and customer relations, satisfy regulatory requirements, and ultimately provide a safe blood product for transfusion. This chapter discusses the elements of a QA program as it applies to blood banks and transfusion services. The cGMPs that guide these efforts are also described.

Blood bank: collects, processes, stores, and transports human blood intended for transfusion

Transfusion service: performs testing and issues blood and blood components for transfusion

This chapter provides an overview of a blood bank safety program. Safety is a concern for everyone. Employer and employee must understand their respective roles in the issues of compliance in blood banking safety. This understanding focuses on efforts to decrease infection risk and physical and chemical hazards in the workplace. The responsibility by law for employee safety ultimately resides with the employer or director of the laboratory. The employer has an obligation to provide a safe work environment by following the imposed standards of care. However, the individual employee must also assume responsibility for his or her health and safety and the safety of coworkers by following laboratory safety policies and procedures. When everyone practices and endorses safety, fewer errors and accidents occur.

Because blood is classified as a drug, blood banks and transfusion services must comply with the FDA's regulations.

SECTION 1
REGULATORY AND ACCREDITING AGENCIES FOR QUALITY AND SAFETY

The blood industry is monitored by many regulatory and accrediting agencies. Compliance with industry, federal, state, and local requirements is reviewed by these agencies. Although the rules are presented in different formats, they focus on ensuring product quality and blood donor and patient safety. Regulatory and accrediting agencies address similar issues regarding QA and quality improvement. The agencies differ in the degree of authority they have to enforce the standards. Compliance with standards set by governmental agencies, such as the FDA, Centers for Medicare and Medicaid Services (CMS), and state agencies, is enforceable by law. Accrediting agencies, such as the **AABB,** are considered industry associations, and compliance with their requirements is voluntary and evaluated by peer review.

AABB: professional organization that accredits and provides educational and technical guidance to blood banks and transfusion services

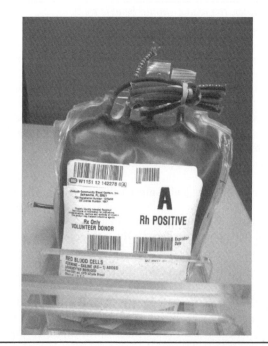

Fig. 1.1 Unit of red blood cells for transfusion to a patient.

FOOD AND DRUG ADMINISTRATION

The FDA enforces regulations to ensure the safety and efficacy of biologics, drugs, and devices, including blood and blood components and diagnostic reagents used or manufactured by blood establishments. The regulation of biologics products in the United States began when Congress passed the Biologics Control Act of 1902.[1] Provisions of the act include requirements for the licensing of manufacturers and products, labeling, facility inspections, suspension or revocation of licenses, and penalties for violation. Current implementation of the law is placed under the Public Health Service (PHS) Act 42 USC §262.[2]

The FDA is the agency that enforces the regulations of the PHS Act and the federal Food, Drug and Cosmetic Service Act.[3] The FDA inspects blood establishments and transfusion services to ensure the enforcement. Each inspection is designed to follow a unit of blood or a blood product from blood donor to patient. The inspection includes many elements of quality and safety: errors, accidents and fatalities, facilities, equipment, personnel, and disposal of infectious waste. The FDA publishes its legal requirements in a book called the *Code of Federal Regulations* (CFR).

The FDA falls under the jurisdiction of the Department of Health and Human Services. Many industries fall within the jurisdiction of the FDA, including drugs, cosmetics, food, and blood. The agency is involved in three areas:

- Surveillance of facilities (inspections)
- Policy enforcement
- Establishment and issue of regulations

The FDA uses several tools to enforce its policy: regular unannounced inspections, warning letters, license suspension, license revocation, and injunction (consent decree). The last four tools are used only when the violations identified during an establishment inspection are considered serious enough to compromise public safety or when a persistent history of noncompliance with the organization exists. Scan the QR code for more information.

Code of Federal Regulations: publication from the Food and Drug Administration outlining the legal requirements of blood banking facilities

CENTERS FOR MEDICARE AND MEDICAID SERVICES

The CMS is a federal agency with the following administrative responsibilities:

- Medicare
- Medicaid
- Health Insurance Portability and Accountability Act (HIPAA)
- **Clinical Laboratory Improvement Amendments (CLIA)**

The CMS regulates all laboratory testing (except research) performed on humans in the United States. The Clinical Laboratory Improvement Amendments of 1988 were enacted to provide safe and accurate laboratory work. CMS issues a certification to laboratories or other test sites performing clinical tests on human samples. CLIA has regulations for accurate and reliable laboratory tests in the *Code of Federal Regulations*, 42 CFR Part 493. CLIA also conducts routine inspections and may impose **sanctions** to laboratories not meeting the requirements. Scan the QR code for more information on the CLIA program.

Clinical Laboratory Improvement Amendments (CLIA): act to ensure that laboratory tests are consistently reliable and of high quality

CLIA applies to physician office laboratories, hospital laboratories, areas within the hospital such as the operating room and emergency room, and independent testing laboratories.

AABB

The AABB, formerly known as the American Association of Blood Banks, is a voluntary accrediting agency. Its publications serve as guidelines for members seeking accreditation; these include the *Standards for Blood Banks and Transfusion Services*, the *Technical Manual,* and others. The AABB *Standards for Blood Banks and Transfusion Services* provides the basis for the inspection and accreditation of blood banks by a private, professional organization. Blood banks and transfusion services voluntarily comply with AABB inspection and accreditation. Accreditation is a high recognition of standards. AABB publications have served as principal guidelines for blood banks and transfusion services since 1958.

Sanctions: penalties or other means of enforcement to provide incentive for obedience with rules and regulations

TABLE 1.1	Elements of Quality Assurance

- Records and SOPs
- Personnel selection and training
- Validation, calibration, preventive maintenance, proficiency testing
- Supplier qualification
- Error management
- Process improvement
- Process control
- Label control
- Internal auditing

SOPs, Standard operating procedures.

Standards for Blood Banks and Transfusion Services: AABB publication that outlines minimal standards of practice in areas relating to transfusion medicine

Technical Manual: AABB publication that provides a reference to current acceptable practices in blood banking

In recent years, the AABB has increased the emphasis on quality principles. The AABB has supported its members by designing documents that facilitate the implementation of QA programs, such as the *Quality Essentials.* Compliance with the AABB *Quality Essentials* became mandatory as of January 1, 1998, for organizations seeking accreditation. The *Quality Essentials* itemizes all the elements of QA appropriate for blood banks or transfusion services. The AABB *Quality Essentials* defined elements for the maintenance of a quality system within the blood bank or transfusion service. These quality essentials are listed in Table 1.1.

INTERNATIONAL SOCIETY OF BLOOD TRANSFUSION

The International Society of Blood Transfusion (ISBT) was founded in 1935 as a scientific society, which grew into an international society for transfusion medicine professionals. Although ISBT is not a regulatory or accrediting agency, the goal of the society is to improve the safety of blood transfusion worldwide.[4] The ISBT supports working parties focusing on specific topics. One working party, Red Cell Immunogenetics and Blood Group Terminology, is dedicated to the classification of human blood group systems under a common nomenclature. This common nomenclature is especially critical when searching for rare blood donors on an international basis. The ISBT provided a global standard for worldwide terminology, identification, and labeling of medical products of human origin (ie, blood, cell, tissue, and organ products). Known as ISBT 128, the standard provides international consistency to support the transfer, traceability, and transfusion/transplantation of blood, cells, tissues, and organs.

OTHER SAFETY REGULATIONS

Occupational Safety and Health Act

The Occupational Safety and Health Act was passed by Congress in 1970. The act's goal was "to assure safe and healthful working conditions for working men and women; by authorizing enforcement of the standards developed under the act; by assisting and encouraging the states in their efforts to assure safe and healthful working conditions; by providing for research, information, education, and training in the field of occupational safety and health; and for other purposes."[5] The act is enforced by the **Occupational Safety and Health Administration** (OSHA).

Occupational Safety and Health Administration: agency responsible for ensuring safe and healthful working conditions

Each year, updated regulations are published in the *Code of Federal Regulations* (CFR), and standards are enforced under OSHA by workplace inspections. Most clinical facility inspections follow employee or consumer complaints. However, OSHA may choose, under authority of the Occupational Safety and Health Act, to inspect any facility at any time. Employers are responsible for informing employees of the OSHA standards and must post OSHA literature that informs employees of their rights and responsibilities.

States and territories operate their own job safety and health plans under OSHA. These standards are identical to, or as stringent as, the federal OSHA standards and must cover state and local government employees. State and local governments may impose additional requirements for safety.

Environmental Protection Agency

The Environmental Protection Agency (EPA) is involved in the assessment of medical waste as specified in the Medical Waste Tracking Act of 1988.[6] This act requires the EPA to determine types, numbers, and sizes of generators of medical waste in the United States. The EPA examines the present or potential threat of medical waste to human health and the environment. Most medical waste regulations emanate from the individual states or local authorities and are variable because no national policy exists for the handling of medical waste.

SECTION 2
QUALITY ASSURANCE AND GOOD MANUFACTURING PRACTICES

QUALITY ASSURANCE

QA comprises the combined activities performed by an organization to ensure the quality of products and services they offer, which must include good manufacturing practices (cGMPs). Quality assurance is part of the organization's goal to maintain an atmosphere of continuous quality improvement. The basic components of a QA program are listed in Table 1.1. These activities are planned and documented by written policies and procedures.

Quality Assurance Department

Responsibilities

Blood banks are required to establish QA departments that are separate from manufacturing and report to upper management. QA responsibilities include the following:
- Compliance with cGMPs
- Review and approval of all standard operating procedures (SOPs)
- Specifications and validation protocols
- Development, review, and approval of training programs
- Investigation of product recalls, errors, and complaints
- Coordination of internal quality auditing programs

> Quality is the responsibility of everyone in the organization.

> Internal quality audits evaluate the effectiveness of the quality system in the organization. Audits are systematic investigations to confirm the level of compliance with established SOPs.

GOOD MANUFACTURING PRACTICES

Good manufacturing practices are performed in blood banks and transfusion services as part of QA and are legal requirements established by the FDA. These regulations itemize "what" needs to be done without necessarily specifying "how." In other words, each organization must determine the best way to implement all these practices. Table 1.2 describes the elements of cGMPs. cGMPs applicable to the blood industry are found in the CFR, specifically Title 21, Part 606, and in the 200 series.[7] The cGMPs are only a part of the overall QA program in any given facility.

> QA is a comprehensive documentation practices program monitoring the entire testing process. Quality control (QC) monitors the test system's components, such as reagents and instrumentation. QC is part of the QA system.

> The CFR 200 series contains cGMPs applicable to drug manufacturers; the CFR 600 series contains cGMPs applicable to biologics; the CFR 800 series are the quality system regulations.

TABLE 1.2	Elements of Good Manufacturing Practices
<ul><li>Write SOPs</li><li>Follow SOPs</li><li>Record and document all work performed</li><li>Qualify personnel by training and education</li><li>Design and build proper facilities and equipment</li><li>Clean by following a housekeeping schedule</li><li>Validate equipment, personnel, and processes</li><li>Perform preventive maintenance on facilities and equipment</li><li>Control for quality</li><li>Audit for compliance with all of the above</li></ul>	

SOPs, Standard operating procedures.

COMPONENTS OF A QUALITY ASSURANCE PROGRAM

Records and Documents

According to the AABB *Standards for Blood Banks and Transfusion Services*, the facility shall have policies, processes, and procedures to ensure document identification, review, approval, and retention.[8] Records are created and stored in accordance with the record retention policies. Examples of records include manual logs, worksheets, computer printouts, temperature charts, CD-ROMs, DVDs, and photographs.

Document Control

Document control: plan for the management of all documents in an organization that addresses the design, responsibility, storage, removal, and revision of all records, forms, and procedures

Regulatory and accrediting agencies' documentation expectations include:
- Comprehensive and well-organized documents
- Appropriate storage of documents
- Document access in a reasonable amount of time
- Protection from unauthorized access, modification, and destruction[9]

Document control programs should specify and describe acceptable media to be used, types of documents to be kept, and record-retention intervals.[8] Alternative methods should be in place to handle situations when the automated systems become unavailable. Finally, all record systems, including control, handling, and disposal, must be described thoroughly in the facility's **standard operating procedures (SOPs)**.

Standard operating procedures (SOPs): written procedures to ensure the complete understanding of a process and to achieve consistency in performance from one individual to another

Facility record-retention times are documented in the AABB *Standards for Blood Banks and Transfusion Services*, ed 29, Section 6, Reference Standards 6.2A–6.2E.[8] Tables 1.3 and 1.4 describe some of the recommended retention times for blood donor and blood unit records and patient records.

TABLE 1.3   Retention of Donor and Blood Unit Records
Indefinite
Donors placed on permanent deferral and indefinite deferral lists for protection of the recipient
Minimum of 10 Years of Retention
Identification of individuals performing each significant step in collection, processing, compatibility testing, and transportation of blood and blood components
Source to final disposition of each unit of blood or blood component and, if issued by facility for transportation, identification of the recipient
Unique identification of each unit
Consent of donors
Notification to donor of significant abnormal findings
Donor information, including address, medical history, physical examination, health history, or other conditions thought to compromise suitability of blood or blood component
Donor acknowledgment that educational materials have been read
ABO group and Rh type for all collections
Donor identification number and collecting facility for each unit in pooled components
Preparation of specific components
Allogeneic donor testing to detect unexpected antibodies to red cell antigens
Interpretations of disease marker testing for allogeneic testing
Quarantine of units from prior collections when a repeat donor has a reactive disease marker screening test
Final review of records relating to testing and acceptability criteria
Review of donor records to ensure any units from an ineligible donor are quarantined
Collection facility's investigation of transmissible diseases
Distribution or issue of units before completion of tests
Serologic confirmation of donor blood ABO/Rh typing
A signed statement from the requesting physician indicating that the clinical situation was sufficiently urgent to require release of blood before completion of compatibility testing or infectious disease testing

From Levitt J: *Standards for blood banks and transfusion services*, ed 29, Bethesda, MD, 2014, AABB.

Record Keeping

If it was not recorded, it never happened. The concept seems simple; however, poor record keeping is the most common violation identified by regulatory and accrediting agencies. Good documentation practices (GDP), whether manual or computerized, allow tracing of all products collected or transfused by an organization. A thorough record-keeping system recreates every step related to the production and distribution of a unit of blood and all its components. This concept is known as an **audit trail** and is important when investigating errors and accidents, as discussed later in this chapter.

Audit trail: record-keeping system that recreates every step in the manufacturing process

Manual Record Guidelines

Good documentation practices for manual inputs are outlined in Table 1.5. Common record-keeping errors often encountered in laboratories are also listed. For example, error correction is a critical issue. The original data must not be obliterated or deleted when making a correction (Fig. 1.2). The identity of the person making the change also needs to be recorded. A standard practice is to cross off with a single line the item that is incorrect and write the correct data or information next to it, followed by the date and initials of the person making the correction. An additional recommendation is to state why the record was changed.

Computerized Record Guidelines

A mechanism to trace back the original entry and the person making the correction is also necessary in computer systems.[9] Processes and procedures exist to support the management of computer systems and routine backup of all critical data. Corrections to computer records must include the following information: the previous result, the new result, the date and time, and the name of the person changing the result. In the event of a system failure, a backup method for retrieval of computer records must be available. Backup data should be stored at an off-site location.

Never provide password information to another staff member. Never use another person's password to enter information into the computer.

TABLE 1.4	Retention of Patient Records

Indefinite

Difficulty in blood typing, clinically significant antibodies, significant adverse events to transfusions, and special transfusion requirements

Minimum of 10 Years of Retention

Source to final disposition of each unit of blood or blood component and, if issued by the facility for transfusion, identification of recipient
Test results and interpretation of patient's ABO group and Rh type
Patient testing for unexpected antibodies to red cell antigens
Additional testing to detect clinically significant antibodies
Pretransfusion testing for autologous transfusion
Test results and interpretations of serologic crossmatch
Detection of ABO incompatibility when no clinically significant antibodies are detected
Two determinations of recipient's ABO group
Look-back to identify recipients who may have been infected with HCV or HIV
Irradiation of cellular components, if applicable
A signed statement from the requesting physician indicating that the clinical situation was sufficiently urgent to require release of blood before completion of compatibility testing or infectious disease testing
Immediate evaluation of suspected transfusion reactions

Minimum of 5 Years of Retention

Requests for blood and blood components
Orders for blood, blood components, tests, and derivatives
Recipient consent
Verification of patient identification before transfusion

HIV, Human immunodeficiency virus; *HCV,* hepatitis C virus.
From Levitt J: *Standards for blood banks and transfusion services,* ed 29, Bethesda, MD, 2014, AABB.

TABLE 1.5	Good Record Keeping Versus Bad Record Keeping
GOOD RECORD KEEPING	**BAD RECORD KEEPING**
Use of indelible (permanent) blue or black ink	Use of correction fluid or white tape when making a correction
Blue ink is preferred	Use of pencil or nonpermanent ink
Recording data on appropriate form or log	Recording data on a piece of scratch paper or sticky notes
Recording date and initials of person making a correction	*Not* recording date or initials of person making a correction
	Recording data for someone else
Recording data immediately after performance of task	Recording data later or not immediately after performance of task
Not obliterating or deleting the original entry when making a correction	Obliterating or deleting original entry when making a correction
Indicating "broken," "closed," or "not in use" when appropriate	*Not* recording "broken," "closed," or "not in use" when appropriate
Not using "dittos"	Use of "dittos"

NOT ACCEPTABLE

Anti-A	Anti-B	Anti-D	A1 Cells	B Cells	Interpretation
0	0	3+	4+	4+	AB positive / O positive

ACCEPTABLE

Anti-A	Anti-B	Anti-D	A1 Cells	B Cells	Interpretation
0	0	3+	4+	4+	AB positive O / Rm 9/1/99

Fig. 1.2 Correcting a manual record. A record is corrected by placing a single line through the error, recording the correct information next to the error, and placing the initials of the person making the correction along with the date. A statement describing the reason for the correction is also recommended.

Standard Operating Procedures

SOPs describe how a particular task is to be accomplished. Established methods for performing and administering processes ensure the consistent quality of the final product or result. Internal and external auditors carefully assess noncompliance with written SOPs, one of the most serious violations that can be identified during an inspection.

SOPs are important training tools for new employees. These documents should be written using a standard format, as illustrated in Fig. 1.3. The Clinical and Laboratory Standards Institute publishes guidelines for the development of SOPs in document GP2-A5, *Laboratory Documents: Development and Control; Approved Guideline,* ed 5.1.[10] They need to be written following recommendations of reagent and equipment manufacturers and in compliance with other cGMPs and industry standards as appropriate. Effective procedures do not need to be wordy. If the documents are user friendly, they are more likely to be used by staff. Well-written procedures include all the steps that ensure process control and contribute to the safety, purity, and potency of the blood product.

Facilities need to say what they do (write SOPs) and do what they say (follow SOPs).

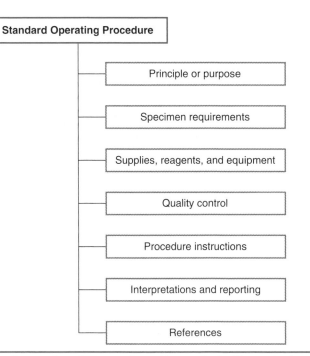

Fig. 1.3 Elements of a procedure. SOPs are written with a standardized format that is user friendly.

Change Control

Change control is a general element of process control. Because the blood industry is in a constant state of change, blood banks and transfusion services need a process, known as change control, to develop or change existing processes or procedures. Blood banks and transfusion services are being challenged routinely by new technologies and new regulatory and accrediting requirements. In addition, facilities have to keep up with internal trends and business issues, such as mergers, acquisitions, employee turnover, expansion, and downsizing. These changes need to be controlled to prevent oversights that could affect multiple aspects of the organization. Manufacturing changes especially need to be well developed and planned *before* implementation to guarantee their success and effectiveness. Similar to validation (discussed later in this chapter), change control needs the allocation of time, money, and labor. However, the many benefits outweigh the cost.

Change control programs are used by manufacturing firms to ensure that nothing "falls through the cracks." For example, the addition of a new blood storage refrigerator would seem straightforward; however, the installation goes beyond the purchase and plug-in steps. Fig. 1.4 illustrates a change protocol for a new refrigerator that addresses critical steps in equipment installation to prevent potential problems.

Change control: system to plan and implement changes in procedures, equipment, policies, and methods to increase effectiveness and prevent problems

The key in change control is the anticipation and prevention of problems.

Personnel Qualifications

Selection Criteria and Job Descriptions

Good employees are essential to the success of any organization. Hiring unqualified individuals can add significant expense to the organization and create a demoralizing environment for coworkers who have to accommodate poor performance. The selection process must be thorough, and minimal preestablished criteria should be identified. These criteria must be identified for each type of position in the organization and address the experience, background, skills, and credentials (eg, degrees, licensure, and certification) deemed necessary to perform the job. The selection criteria are not stagnant. They should be revised as changes in job duties or tasks occur.

Job description documents should be developed for each type of position in the organization. These documents describe the tasks for which the employee is responsible and outline the areas of knowledge and skills needed during training to perform the job. These documents also necessitate updating as appropriate to reflect all employee duties.

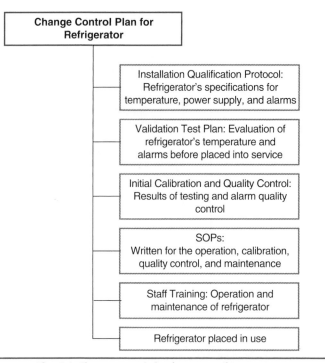

Fig. 1.4 Change control plan for a new refrigerator.

Training

Training is a critical aspect of compliance with cGMPs that necessitates a significant organization-wide commitment for success. Facilities that allocate time and resources for training and education benefit by reducing rework and inconsistency. In the development of a training program, the designation of trainers is important. Individuals selected as trainers should be able to convey information clearly, are respected by their peers, enjoy sharing expertise, and have a positive attitude toward building teams.

Training is provided during new employee orientation and is necessary whenever there are procedure changes or evidence of poor performance. Training activities usually include, but are not limited to, the following activities:

- Employee's review of SOP documents and associated materials
- Trainer's demonstration of task or procedure
- Employee's performance of task or procedure with the trainer's assistance
- Employee's demonstration of knowledge and application of the learned skill without the trainer's assistance

Good training programs allow the trainer to explain all functions and demonstrate the task before employee performance. Repetition of tasks in a "test" environment or with supervision is necessary before the trainee is allowed to perform the procedure independently. Throughout the training process, the employee must have ample opportunities to ask questions and receive explanations. Finally, training is not complete until it is documented, which typically takes place in the form of a checklist signed by the trainee, trainer, and supervisor.

Competency Assessment

Competency assessment: evaluation of the employee's ability and knowledge to perform a procedure or skill

Training is concluded only when documented evidence exists that the employee is able to demonstrate knowledge and application of the new skill. This demonstration is the purpose of **competency assessment.**

Initial competency assessment refers to the evaluation of the level of knowledge and skill an employee has gained during training to determine whether the individual is ready to perform a procedure. In addition, periodic competency assessment is used to determine whether the employee has maintained the level of knowledge and skill necessary to perform the job or task as described in the facility's SOP. The CMS and AABB, through the

Clinical Laboratory Improvement Amendments of 1988, have established requirements of proof of competency for testing personnel twice during the first year of employment and annually thereafter.[9] Most regulatory and accrediting agencies require retraining for employees who fail to prove competency. The employee must not be allowed to perform the procedure (or procedures) until retraining is provided and subsequent competency assessment proves to be satisfactory.

In the case of unacceptable performance, corrective actions should be taken. Actions include retraining and documenting performance and competency assessment. The employee may not perform the tasks in which unacceptable performance was demonstrated.

> Competency assessment may be performed in many formats: direct observation of performance, written tests, simulations, review of results and records, or using unknown samples.

Supplier Qualification

The quality of any given product is as good as the quality of the raw materials that go into its production. Supplier qualification has become a standard practice among many blood banks and transfusion services.[8] The AABB *Standards for Blood Banks and Transfusion Services* provides guidance on supplier qualification. Facilities have established procedures to evaluate whether the quality of critical products and services received from suppliers meets preestablished criteria. Written agreements between blood banks and their suppliers are common practice. These documents, among many things, usually specify terms, including expectations between the involved parties. In some instances, facilities choose to audit their suppliers on an ongoing basis to determine the level of compliance with product specifications. This practice also should be included in written agreements. In addition, facilities should have procedures for inspecting and testing incoming materials (when applicable). These procedures should specify acceptable criteria and the course of action to be taken when they are not met.

> Blood products, test reagents, blood bags, and labels are examples of critical products.

> Size, color, type of container, temperature, purity, and potency are examples of product specifications.

Error Management

Root-Cause Analysis and Problem Solving

As part of a QA plan, facilities must have in place mechanisms for the detection and management of errors and their consequences. Errors, incidents, variances, and any nonconformance should be thoroughly documented and investigated. Employees must be actively involved in the problem-solving stages for the process to be successful. Once a problem is identified, an immediate response follows to correct the problem. The facility should initiate a **root-cause analysis** to identify what factors contributed to the occurrence of the problem. Once the cause is identified, a proposed plan for prevention should be drafted. After changes are made and the process is fine-tuned or adjusted, a subsequent review should be made to evaluate the effectiveness of the preventive corrective action. If the error recurs, another root-cause analysis is indicated. The adoption of this strategy ensures continuous quality improvement of all processes. Errors should be viewed as opportunities for improvement, and employees should be encouraged to report errors without concern for reprisal.

Errors can be identified internally by employees or externally by customers. Errors must be logged, and their frequencies must be tracked and monitored. Graphing incidences of occurrence and subsequent recurrences can provide QA departments with a comprehensive understanding of the reliability of a given process or individual and the effectiveness of a corrective action taken. Tracking can also help identify where quality efforts should be focused and which areas need to be addressed and corrected first.

> **Root-cause analysis:** investigation and subsequent identification of the factors that contributed to an error

> Errors are classified as incidents, deviations, complaints, and nonconformances.

> Any error or accident that compromises the safety of a donor or patient requires reporting to the FDA.

Biological Product Deviations

After the release of blood products, blood banks may discover that a product was in violation of its specifications, standards, or cGMP regulations. The blood bank must report the problem to the FDA and the buyer. In this event, the QA department must issue a biological product deviation (BPD). BPDs provide information on how a blood product's safety, purity, or potency may be affected.

Recalls

Recalls are usually issued by manufacturers in an attempt to remove products from the market that might compromise the safety of the recipient. They can be initiated voluntarily by the organization or at the request of the FDA. In some instances, recalls are issued months or years after the product has been transfused or has expired. In this case the objective of the recall notification is to alert the client of possible hazards or adverse consequences the recipient might have incurred by receiving the product. Recalls are classified based on the degree of danger or hazard they impose.

Validation

Validation is a process that establishes documented evidence providing a high degree of assurance that a specific process consistently produces a product that meets its preestablished quality and performance specifications. Even if regulatory and accrediting agencies did not make it necessary, validation is a good business practice. Procedures, equipment, personnel, new methods, and computer information systems must be proven reliable before being put into use. The best way to prove reliability is by stressing and challenging the process or system *before* it is implemented.

Facilities and Equipment

The blood bank and transfusion service need to address the adequacy of the facility and equipment used in the facility for compliance to cGMPs. Fig. 1.5 summarizes these activities.

Proficiency Testing

Proficiency testing is a required component of the QA program for testing laboratories. It is used to ensure that test methods and equipment are working as expected and that staff members are following procedures.[9] Proficiency surveys are prepared by accredited agencies that distribute samples for testing to requesting laboratories.

A common proficiency test is the CAP Survey, issued by the College of American Pathologists.[11] Tests are run by routine testing personnel, using routine test equipment, during regular test runs, and in conformance with the facility's SOP. The results are recorded on standard forms and submitted to the agency within a given period. The test results are evaluated and scored, and a report is returned to the institution for review. Corrective action is implemented and monitored for improvement when results are not acceptable. Proficiency tests can be used to prove competency; however, competency tests cannot replace proficiency testing.

Label Control

Many blood product recalls are due to mislabeling. If the incorrect label is placed on a unit of blood, the product is called misbranded. Similar to other recalls, mislabeling errors are not

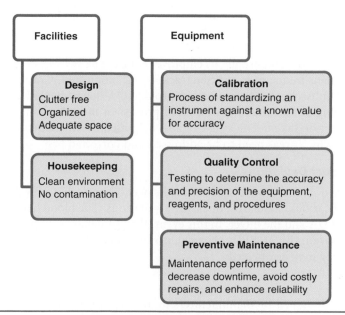

Fig. 1.5 QA essentials for facilities and equipment.

only time consuming but also embarrassing. For this reason, blood banks, similar to pharmaceutical firms, have instituted label control programs. In many facilities, it is the responsibility of the QA department to inspect and approve all labels on receipt and before they are put into use, ensuring that all labels are in compliance with requirements. Labeling is a critical step in manufacturing and should be done in areas designed only for that purpose.

SECTION 3
SAFETY

STANDARD VERSUS UNIVERSAL PRECAUTIONS

The concept of **standard precautions** was first introduced in 1987 by the Centers for Disease Control and Prevention (CDC) to decrease the occupational risks of bloodborne diseases, such as acquired immunodeficiency syndrome and hepatitis B virus (HBV), to health care workers.[12] In 1991 OSHA issued its final standard on occupational exposure to bloodborne pathogens, which mandated the use of **universal precautions.** Current universal precautions focus on treating all body substances as potentially harmful and applying appropriate safety measures to decrease possible exposure and infection. The use of protective measures is now based on the health care worker's contact with body fluids rather than on a patient's diagnosis. Standard precautions apply when there is a risk of exposure to blood, all body fluids, secretions, excretions (except sweat), nonintact skin (including rashes), or mucous membranes.[13]

Standard precautions: CDC term defining policies of treating all body substances as potentially infectious and applying safety measures to reduce possible exposure. Standard precautions incorporate universal precautions and body substance isolation together.

Universal precautions: OSHA term defining policies of treating all body substances as potentially infectious and applying safety measures to reduce possible exposure

Blood Bank Safety Program

The blood bank safety program must be a comprehensive program that includes policies and procedures of all regulatory bodies and any voluntary-compliance accrediting agencies. In addition, any state and local laws must be taken into consideration. Most important, the safety program must be one that employees and employers endorse. Adherence to the safety program reduces any occupational hazards of the workplace and maintains a safe environment. The program should incorporate the OSHA regulations as outlined in Table 1.6.

The blood bank's director or administrator must appoint an individual or individuals responsible for the program. A written safety program that itemizes the requirements must be available to all blood bank personnel. The document should enumerate current safety policies, which need to be cross-referenced in each preanalytical, analytical, and postanalytical procedure in the laboratory. Safety program administrators need to consider not only the technical staff but also potential risks for donors, ancillary personnel, volunteers, and visitors.

Physical Space, Safety Equipment, Protective Devices, and Warning Signs
Physical Space

The physical design of the blood bank and organization of tasks can reduce many potential hazards. Ready access to eyewashes, showers, and hand washing is essential.

TABLE 1.6	Occupational Safety and Health Administration Regulations for Protection from Bloodborne Pathogens Requirements

Employers must:
* Provide a hazard-free workplace
* Educate and train staff
* Evaluate all procedures for potential exposure risks
* Evaluate each employment position for potential exposure risks
* Implement labeling procedures and post signs
* Apply universal precautions for handling all body substances
* Provide personal protective equipment, such as gloves or other barriers, without cost to the employee
* Make HBV vaccine prophylaxis available to all staff who have occupational exposure, unless previously vaccinated or immune, and provide hepatitis B immune globulin treatment for percutaneous injury at no cost to the employee

HBV, Hepatitis B virus.

Laboratory Attire

Most tasks in the blood bank can be safely performed while wearing laboratory attire that protects the worker from common infectious hazards. A fluid-resistant laboratory coat, gown, or apron, whether disposable or made of cotton material, is recommended. Laboratory coats should be large enough to close completely in front, or aprons may be worn over long-sleeved uniforms. These personal barrier protection garments should be changed immediately if they are contaminated with blood or toxic substances. All outerwear worn during the performance of blood banking tasks should be considered contaminated. Such garments should not be worn outside the laboratory into public areas. If nondisposable protective garments are used, they must be removed and stored in a suitable container and laundered in a manner that ensures decontamination. To contain the risk of infectious materials, home laundering is prohibited because unpredictable methods of transportation and handling can spread contamination, and laundering techniques might not be effective.

Personal Protective Equipment, Eyewashes, and Showers

Safety glasses, face shields or masks, splash barriers, and goggles are devices categorized as personal protective equipment (Fig. 1.6). Safety glasses or goggles should be worn when splashes are likely to occur during a task. Masks are better because they protect the mouth, nose, and eyes. Face shields are made of shatterproof plastic and wrap around the face, offering greater protection. Permanently mounted splash barriers over the bench area are preferred when task performance risks splashing or aerosol contamination. Opening tubes of blood and using corrosive liquids warrant this protection for the employee. The shields should be cleansed and decontaminated on a regular basis.

If a splash does occur, the blood bank should have the availability of a shower and an eyewash device. An eyewash device should be capable of providing a gentle stream or spray of aerated water for an extended period. Safety showers treat immediate first-aid needs of personnel contaminated with hazardous materials and for extinguishing clothing fires. Procedures and indications for use must be posted, and routine maintenance checks must be performed.

Biological Safety Cabinets

Biological safety cabinets (BSCs) are containment devices that facilitate safe handling of infectious materials and reduce the risk to personnel and the laboratory environment. Procedures that expose opened tubes of blood or units known to be positive for hepatitis B surface antigen or human immunodeficiency virus (HIV) are examples of blood bank procedures in which a BSC may be useful.

Employees need training in the operation of the BSC for maximum protection. The effectiveness of the BSC is a function of directional airflow inward and downward through

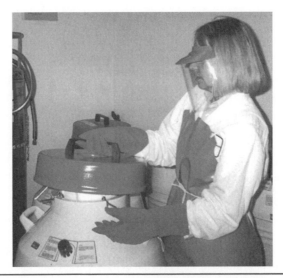

Fig. 1.6 Personal protective equipment. Gloves, gown, and face shield used while working with liquid nitrogen frozen red blood cell samples. (Courtesy Micro Typing Systems, Inc., Pompano Beach, FL.)

a high-efficiency filter. Disruption of the airflow prevents maximum efficiency and usefulness of the cabinet.

Gloves and Hand Washing

Blood bank personnel should wear gloves as a protective barrier when handling any blood or blood products. OSHA does not require the routine use of gloves by phlebotomists working with healthy prescreened donors or, if gloves are worn, the changing of unsoiled gloves between donors. Guidelines recommend the use of gloves for the phlebotomy of autologous donors or patients (eg, therapeutic apheresis procedures). However, all employees likely to be exposed to blood should follow good practice by wearing gloves as another measure of precaution because even prescreened "healthy" donors may have had contact with an infectious agent and may be unaware of the contact. A prudent part of the safety procedure of the blood bank includes the policy that all employees must wear gloves when tasks are likely to involve exposure to blood. Gloves used in a contaminated area should not be worn to a "clean" area or when using or touching telephones, doorknobs, or computer terminals.

Even when gloves are worn, hand washing remains the most effective defense in infection control and safety. Bloodborne pathogens generally do not penetrate intact skin, and hand washing prevents their transfer to mucous membranes, such as nasal passages or broken skin areas. Hand washing also reduces the transmission of infectious agents to others. Hands should be washed after the removal of gloves in the following situations: after task completion; before leaving a work area; before, between, and after seeing patients; and immediately after contact with blood.

Warning Signs

Many regulatory agencies have designed warning signs and posted them in the laboratory for identification of hazardous materials or areas. OSHA emphasizes the importance of alerting personnel to potential danger with labels and signs. Biohazard warning labels, signs, and containers are fluorescent orange or red with lettering or symbols in a contrasting color (Fig. 1.7). Signs are intended to alert workers and others to take necessary precautions.

Decontamination

All laboratory surfaces and reusable equipment should routinely be cleaned and decontaminated daily and as needed while performing tasks and as spills occur. A list of EPA-approved disinfectant solutions is published by the agency.[14] OSHA allows the use of EPA-registered disinfectants effective against HIV and HBV, a diluted bleach solution, or a combination of these disinfectants for decontamination of work surfaces. A fresh solution of 1:10 dilution of sodium hypochlorite (bleach) can be used for general disinfection or for spills.

Safety Fact:
• Blood bank personnel should wear gloves as a protective barrier when handling any blood or blood products.

Safety Fact:
• All laboratory surfaces and reusable equipment should routinely be cleaned and decontaminated daily and as needed while performing tasks and as spills occur.

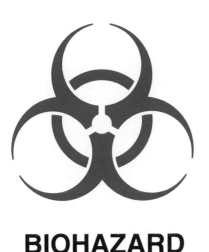

BIOHAZARD

Fig. 1.7 Biohazard symbol.

Chemical Storage and Hazards

The blood bank houses chemicals that may be of significant hazard. Chemical hazards are most often classified by their corrosiveness, ignitability, reactivity, and toxicity. Containment of chemicals is based on the nature of these hazards. The Hazard Communications Standard (29 CFR 1910.1200) created a "right to know" procedure for the worker who handles or is exposed to hazardous chemicals.[15] Manufacturers, importers, or distributors of all toxic substances are required to supply material safety data sheets (MSDS). MSDS forms, required by OSHA, contain information including the chemical names, hazards, required personal protective equipment, and the spill clean-up details. MSDS must be readily available in the workplace to all employees.

Radiation Safety

Few laboratory tests incorporate radionuclides. However, the blood bank uses gamma irradiators for the irradiation of blood components. Employee safety needs to be emphasized with proper training in the use of the equipment, personal protective equipment, and exposure monitoring.

Blood irradiators vary in the amount of radiation scatter and leakage. The Nuclear Regulatory Commission requires training for all personnel using irradiators and records indicating exposure. Although monitors may not be required for some equipment, leak detection is necessary.

Biohazardous Wastes

Blood bank safety programs must include policies for handling all waste materials from areas where waste is contaminated with blood or body fluids. This medical waste is known as biohazardous waste. All laboratory personnel should be trained in a waste management program that protects staff members and meets federal, state, and local regulatory requirements. Untrained personnel should not come in contact with or be responsible for biohazardous waste materials.

Correct identification of material is important to segregate potentially infectious waste from mainstream waste and to control cost and volume of infectious waste. Proper handling ensures that medical waste marked as biohazardous materials is placed in designated containers. Containers should be leak proof. Incineration and decontamination by autoclaving are currently recommended for disposing of blood samples and blood products.

Storage and Transportation of Blood and Blood Components

Storage

Storage of blood and blood components for transfusion should be separate from reagents, specimens, and any other unrelated materials. Ideally, a separate refrigerator should be used; however, if one is not available, areas within the refrigerator must be segregated to reduce spills or accidents. Refrigerators should be large enough to accommodate the anticipated blood storage need.

> Safety Fact:
> • Food or drink should not be allowed in the blood storage or testing areas.

Transportation

Blood and blood components transferred within an institution for transfusion purposes do not require packaging and labeling as for shipping. Specimens should be transported in a plastic bag to prevent spills or leakage. To avoid contamination, paperwork should not be placed in the bag.

Any shipping of diagnostic materials or etiologic agents to or from the laboratory must follow the regulations of the Department of Transportation and the U.S. Postal Service. Blood banks should contact the carrier for correct packaging and label identification requirements.

Personal Injury and Reporting

In the event an employee or other person is injured or possible injury or infection exists, an accident report should be initiated. Worker's compensation, OSHA, and other regulatory and accrediting bodies require these reports. An accident report should be initiated in *all* accidents and injuries involving employees or other persons. Routine investigation of a minor incident and follow-up to correct the risk may thwart a major accident later. Personnel should be encouraged to report all incidents no matter how insignificant they may seem because accident reporting is an essential part of maintaining a safe working environment. Each incident should be treated with a thorough investigation in a non-threatening manner to the employee.

Employee Education

Employee education not only makes good sense, but it is a mandate of OSHA and other regulatory and accrediting agencies. The blood bank safety program should be reviewed with new employees during their orientation and training before independent work is permitted. All employees whose tasks carry risk of infectious exposure should annually review the safety program as a condition of OSHA. The supervisor or responsible safety officer should document all employee participation in this education, and performance evaluations should include the employee's adherence to the safety policies and procedures of the blood bank.

CHAPTER SUMMARY

Regulatory and Accrediting Agencies

- The blood industry is regulated by multiple regulatory and accrediting agencies. All these entities require compliance with QA and quality improvement concepts. However, only regulatory agencies have the lawful authority to enforce their requirements.
- The FDA regulates the manufacture of blood and blood components and publishes these requirements in the *Code of Federal Regulations*.
- cGMPs are the minimum federal requirements that guarantee the safety, potency, purity, and quality of blood products. They include SOPs, record keeping, training, facilities, maintenance, equipment, validation, quality control, change control, and audits.

Quality Assurance Program

- cGMPs are only a part of the QA program.
- QA encompasses all other planned activities that, when executed, ensure the quality of the products or services offered. These include record keeping and SOPs, personnel selection and training, validation, supplier qualification, calibration, preventive maintenance, proficiency testing, error management, process improvement, process control, label control, and internal auditing.

Safety Program

- Safety concerns everyone. Employer and employee must understand their respective roles in the issues of compliance in blood banking safety. This understanding centers on the need to decrease infection risk and physical and chemical hazards in the workplace.
- Safety programs should address fire, electrical, biological, chemical, and radioactive hazards in the workplace.
- The responsibility by law for employee safety ultimately resides with the employer or director of the laboratory. The employer has an obligation to provide a safe work environment by following the imposed standards of care.
- Individual employees must assume responsibility for their own health and safety and the safety of coworkers by following laboratory safety policies and procedures.
- Fewer errors and accidents occur when safety is endorsed and practiced by everyone in the blood bank.

CRITICAL THINKING EXERCISES

Exercise 1.1

PEC is a successful and modern blood donor center located in the northeastern region of the United States. Its management style has always stood out among other blood centers in the United States because of its modern and progressive views. The blood center is known for embracing changes in manufacturing with a positive approach by appropriately planning and allocating resources to ensure things are done the right way. However, in the last few years, both employees and customers have noticed a steady decline in control and quality. The number of manufacturing errors and product and service complaints reported by customers has drastically increased. PEC has tripled in size in the last 3 years, after the acquisition of several small blood banks in the state. Changes have occurred quickly to accommodate this growth, and thorough planning before the implementation of these changes has not always been possible. Among many of its growing pains, PEC employees finally realized that their blood bank computer system was outdated and unable to handle the workload volume increase in the last few years.

Management at PEC selected EJO, Inc., as the new software vendor. Although EJO's experience, reputation, expertise, and client support were well known, its new blood banking software was not. However, the cost of implementing this new software fit well within the approved fiscal budget. With full management support, validation and training efforts began early in the year with a proposed "live" date for September of that year. By June, multiple "bugs" had been identified during system testing. EJO's technical support was excellent, but with so many problems to be addressed and corrected, management was getting anxious. They wanted the new system to go "live" before their next FDA inspection. September came and went, and the system was not ready for implementation. Finally, in March of the following year, parallel testing was completed. Because of time constraints, not all functions were tested, in particular, functions pertaining to the issue of products. Management was aware but decided to go ahead with implementation of the system.

In April, the new system at PEC was implemented with no major problems. Everything was okay until 3 months later, when the distribution supervisor noticed that the system had allowed the release of human T-cell lymphotropic virus (HTLV) I/II repeatedly reactive donor units. The PEC QA department was immediately notified, and recall procedures were initiated. By that time, 35 donor units and all their parts had been released.

1. What did PEC fail to do? What were the consequences?
2. What are some of the factors that contributed to the release of unacceptable units?
3. What steps could have been taken to prevent this situation?

Exercise 1.2

AKC Blood Center collects more than 600 platelet apheresis products each month. Platelet counts for donors and these products are determined using KB1, a state-of-the-art automated hematology instrument. This piece of equipment, similar to many others, requires extensive QC and preventive maintenance by the manufacturer. During the last 4 days, Fred, the medical technologist assigned to run the instrument, has failed to notice that the low-level control has consistently fallen below the mean. Fred has been too busy trying to train new personnel in the department and has had no time to plot his results on the QC chart, which is a departmental procedure requirement. If he performed this task, he would have noticed the obvious shift.

Today the new trainee, Fran, is running platelet counts with Fred's assistance. Once again, the low-level control falls below the mean. On this run, the control falls outside the manufacturer's range altogether. Fran notices the value is flagged by KB1 and notifies Fred of the problem. Fred is too busy on the phone handling an irate call from a client hospital and tells Fran to "keep running it until it falls in. You know, sometimes it takes a while for controls to come in."

1. If you were Fred's supervisor, what would you do?
2. What is the root cause of the problem?
3. What steps can be taken to prevent this situation?
4. What is your opinion of Fred's results since he started using the instrument?

Exercise 1.3

The transfusion services department at PSB Medical Center has always been happy with the level of service offered by YR Blood Center. However, during the last 3 months, they have noticed quite a few platelet units with visible clumps. If you worked for the QA unit at YR Blood Center and were asked to investigate this problem, what areas would you investigate to identify the root cause of the problem?

Exercise 1.4

Patient PC needed a transfusion of an irradiated red blood cell (RBC) unit. ABC Blood Center shipped the unit to the hospital. The unit was labeled as irradiated but did not complete the irradiation process. The RBC unit was issued to the nursing unit for transfusion to Patient PC. The unit was not transfused and was returned to the laboratory. The laboratory was notified by ABC Blood Center of the labeling error later that day. Is this a reportable deviation to the FDA? State your reasons for your decision.

Exercise 1.5

Identify the consequences of the following cGMP violations:
1. *Not* taking daily temperature reading for a blood refrigerator
2. Extending test incubation times beyond what the SOP states
3. Overloading a refrigerator beyond its capacity
4. Cutting an employee's training short
5. Running proficiency samples repeatedly until the samples are depleted
6. Using expired reagents
7. Reporting test results when controls are out of range
8. Not performing preventive maintenance on an instrument as required by the manufacturer

STUDY QUESTIONS

1. Which of the following is *not* a basic component of a QA program?
   a. calibration
   b. preventive maintenance
   c. viral marker testing
   d. record keeping

2. What criteria apply to the correction of manual records?
   a. the original entry is neither obliterated nor deleted
   b. the person making the correction dates and initials the change
   c. the item to be corrected is crossed off with a single line
   d. all of the above

3. What statement does not apply to the definition of an SOP?
   a. step-by-step instructions
   b. used to monitor accuracy and precision
   c. written in compliance with cGMPs
   d. written in compliance with manufacturer's recommendations

4. What is the purpose of competency assessment?
   a. identify employees in need of retraining
   b. evaluate an individual's level of knowledge during a job interview
   c. identify employees who need to be fired
   d. all of the above

5. What statement does not apply to the performance of internal audits?
   a. help identify problems early
   b. ensure continuous quality improvement efforts
   c. are used solely for the purpose of identifying "troublemakers"
   d. are one of the many responsibilities of the QA unit

6. Employees are the core of an organization. What item reinforces this statement?
   a. employees must be trained
   b. employees must report errors without fear of reprisal
   c. employees are a key part of problem solving
   d. all of the above

7. Where can cGMPs applicable to the blood industry be located?
   a. AABB *Standards for Blood Banks and Transfusion Services*
   b. SOP manual
   c. FDA *Code of Federal Regulations*
   d. QA manual

8. What term describes the process to identify what factors contributed to the occurrence of a nonconformance?
   a. root-cause analysis
   b. accident reports
   c. internal audits
   d. FDA inspections

For questions 9 through 11, match the following descriptions with the appropriate organization:

Description	Organization
9. government agency that regulates blood banks	a. AABB
10. voluntary peer review organization	b. FDA
11. agency responsible for safety	c. OSHA

12. Who is ultimately responsible for a safety program in the laboratory?
    a. CDC
    b. the employer or laboratory director
    c. OSHA
    d. the employee

13. What organization publishes the *Technical Manual*, which is often used for principal guidelines in the blood bank?
    a. CAP
    b. ISBT
    c. AABB
    d. OSHA

14. Which of the following items is mandated by law for all blood banks?
    a. blood bank refrigerator
    b. written laboratory safety program
    c. BSC
    d. foot-operated hand wash

15. What designation is given to goggles, face shields, and splash barriers?
    a. personal protective equipment
    b. not necessary unless working with HIV-positive or HBV-positive specimens
    c. mandated at all times when working with blood specimens and blood products
    d. provided by the employee if needed

16. What is the name of the policy of treating all body substances as potentially harmful, regardless of the patient diagnosis?
    a. OSHA Exposure Program
    b. isolation guidelines
    c. AABB safety policy
    d. universal precautions

17. In addition to wearing gloves, what is the most effective defense for infection control and safety?
    a. goggles
    b. laboratory coats
    c. posting warning signs
    d. hand washing

18. Select the most economical disinfectant to use for decontamination.
    a. 1:10 fresh solution of sodium hypochlorite (bleach)
    b. 1:5 solution of household Lysol
    c. 1:15 solution of sodium hydroxide
    d. detergent and water mixture

19. When should an accident or injury be reported?
    a. injury may result in a fatality
    b. injury involves possible infection with HIV or HBV
    c. accident involves nonemployees or jeopardizes a patient
    d. at the time the accident or injury occurs

20. Select one of the best ways to protect employees and keep a safe laboratory environment.
    a. health insurance
    b. safety education
    c. rest breaks
    d. fluid-repellent laboratory coats

Answers to Study Questions can be found on page 387.

(e) Additional student resources, including review questions, a laboratory manual, and case studies, can be found on the Evolve website.

REFERENCES

1. The St. Louis Tragedy and Enactment of the 1902 Biologics Control Act. http://www.fda.gov/AboutFDA/WhatWeDo/History/ProductRegulation/100YearsofBiologicsRegulation/ucm070022.htm. Accessed April 2016.
2. Public Health Service Act of 1944, Public Law 42 *USC 262*, 1944.
3. Food, Drug and Cosmetic Act of 1938, Public Law 21 *USC 321*, 1938.
4. International Society of Blood Transfusion. http://www.isbtweb.org/. Accessed March 2015.
5. Occupational Safety and Health Act of 1970, Public Law 29 *USC 651*, 1970.
6. U.S. Environmental Protection Agency: *Medical waste tracking act*, Washington, DC, 1988, U.S. Government Printing Office. 40 USC 6992.
7. Food and Drug Administration: *Code of federal regulations*, 21 CFR 600–799. Washington, DC, 2011, U.S. Government Printing Office. Revised annually.
8. Levitt J: *Standards for blood banks and transfusion services*, ed 29, Bethesda, MD, 2014, AABB.
9. Fung MK, editor: *Technical manual*, ed 18, Bethesda, MD, 2014, AABB.
10. Clinical and Laboratory Standards Institute: *Quality management system: development and management of laboratory documents; approved guideline*, ed 6, Wayne, PA, 2015, CLSI. QMS02-A6.
11. College of American Pathologists: Proficiency testing. http://www.cap.org/web/lab/proficiency-testing? Accessed March 2015.
12. Centers for Disease Control and Prevention: Recommendations for preventing HIV transmission in healthcare settings, *MMWR Morb Mortal Wkly Rep* 36(2S):1, 1987.
13. Centers for Disease Control and Prevention: http://www.cdc.gov/HAI/settings/outpatient/basic-infection-control-prevention-plan-2011/standard-precautions.html. Accessed March 2015.
14. Centers for Disease Control and Prevention: Regulatory framework for disinfectants and sterilants, *MMWR Morb Mortal Wkly Rep* 52:62, 2003.
15. Occupational Safety and Health Administration: Hazard Communication. https://www.osha.gov/dsg/hazcom/. Accessed March 2015.

2

IMMUNOLOGY: Basic Principles and Applications in the Blood Bank

CHAPTER OUTLINE

LEARNING OBJECTIVES

On completion of this chapter, the reader should be able to:

1. Define the following terms in relation to red cells and transfusion: antigen, immunogen, epitopes, and antigenic determinants.
2. Describe the characteristics of antigens that are located on red cells, white cells, and platelets.
3. Diagram the basic structure of an IgG molecule and label the following components: heavy and light chains, Fab, and Fc regions, variable region, hinge region, antigen-binding site, and macrophage-binding site.
4. Compare and contrast IgM and IgG antibodies with regard to structure, function, and detection by agglutination reactions.
5. Distinguish the primary and secondary immune response with regard to immunoglobulin class, immune cells involved, level of response, response time, and antibody affinity.
6. Apply the properties that influence the binding of an antigen and antibody to agglutination tests to achieve optimal results.
7. List the variables in the agglutination test that affect sensitization and lattice formation.

8. Accurately grade and interpret observed agglutination reactions using the agglutination grading scale for antigen–antibody reactions performed in test tubes.
9. Compare the classical and alternative pathways of complement activation.
10. Outline the biological effects mediated by complement proteins in the clearance of red cells.
11. Recognize hemolysis in an agglutination reaction and explain the significance.
12. Outline how the immune system responds to antigen stimulation through transfusion and pregnancy. Explain the factors that cause variations in these in vivo responses.
13. Apply the principles of antigen–antibody reactions to immunohematology testing.
14. Describe the basic principles of routine testing in the immunohematology laboratory.
15. Describe several routine tests performed in the immunohematology laboratory.
16. Interpret red cell antigen and antibody reactions in routine tests.

The science of **immunohematology** embodies the study of blood group antigens and antibodies. Immunohematology is closely related to the field of immunology because it involves the immune response to the transfusion of cellular elements. Red cells (erythrocytes), white cells (leukocytes), and platelets are cellular components that can potentially initiate immune responses after transfusion. To enhance the reader's understanding of the physiology involved in this immune response, this text presents an overview of the immune system with an emphasis on the clinical and serologic nature of antibodies and antigens. This chapter provides concepts of immunology as it relates to transfusion medicine.

Immunohematology: study of blood group antigens and antibodies

SECTION 1
CHARACTERISTICS ASSOCIATED WITH ANTIGEN–ANTIBODY REACTIONS

GENERAL PROPERTIES OF ANTIGENS

An **antigen** is a molecule that binds to an antibody or T-cell receptor. This binding can occur within the body (**in vivo**) or in a laboratory test (**in vitro**). In chemical terms, antigens are large-molecular-weight proteins (including conjugated proteins such as glycoproteins, lipoproteins, and nucleoproteins) and polysaccharides (including lipopolysaccharides). These protein and polysaccharide antigens may be located on the surfaces of cell membranes or may be an integral portion of the cell membrane. Antigens are located on viruses, bacteria, fungi, protozoa, blood cells, organs, and tissues.

Antigen: foreign molecules that bind specifically to an antibody or a T-cell receptor

In vivo: reaction within the body

Transfused red cells contain antigens that may be recognized as foreign to the individual receiving the blood. These antigens are called **allogeneic** because they do not originate from the individual being transfused but are derived from the same species. These foreign antigens may elicit an immune response in the recipient. The body's immune system normally recognizes and tolerates self-antigens. These antigens are termed **autologous** because they originate from the individual. However, the failure to tolerate self-antigens may cause an immune response against cells or tissue from self. This immune response to self may result in various forms of autoimmune disease. In terms of transfusion, an allogeneic transfusion involves the exposure to antigens that are different from the individual receiving a transfusion, whereas an autologous transfusion involves antigens that originated in the recipient.

In vitro: reaction in an artificial environment, such as in a test tube, microplate, or column

Allogeneic: cells or tissue from a genetically different individual

Autologous: cells or tissue from self

Hapten: small-molecular-weight particle that requires a carrier molecule's recognition by the immune system

The concept of an antigen having sufficient size to induce an immune response contrasts with a **hapten,** which is a small-molecular-weight particle that requires a carrier molecule to initiate the immune response. Haptens may include medications such as penicillin. They are sometimes referred to as partial antigens.

Antigens that exhibit the greatest degree of foreignness from the host elicit the strongest immune response.

The immune response to foreign or potentially pathogenic antigens involves a complex interaction between several types of leukocytes. In the transfusion setting, immune response is primarily humoral, involving mainly **B lymphocytes (B cells).** After a transfusion, the recipient's B cells may "recognize" these foreign red cell antigens through B-cell receptors (Fig. 2.1). This recognition causes the B cells to present the antigen to the **T lymphocytes (T cells).** After presentation, the T-cell **cytokines** signal the B-cell transformation into **plasma cells,** which produce antibodies with the same specificity as the original B-cell receptors. These antibodies are glycoprotein molecules that continue to circulate and specifically recognize and bind to the foreign antigen that originally created the response. **Memory B cells** are also made at this time. If there is another exposure, the memory B cells can respond quickly and change into plasma cells; memory B cells do not require presentation to the T cell for activation. Memory B cells allow a fast response to an antigen, an important principle used in vaccination.[1]

B lymphocytes (B cells): lymphocytes that mature in the bone marrow, differentiate into plasma cells when stimulated by an antigen, and produce antibodies

T lymphocytes (T cells): lymphocytes that mature in the thymus and produce cytokines to activate the immune cells, including the B cell

Cytokines: secreted proteins that regulate the activity of other cells by binding to specific receptors; they can increase or decrease cell proliferation, antibody production, and inflammation reactions

Many different antibodies to foreign antigens are produced in the immune response, each binding to the surface of a different antigen. For example, red cells have many different antigens on their surface. When red cells from one donor are transfused to a patient, several different antibodies may be produced in the immune response to the transfused red cells. The different **antigenic determinants,** also called **epitopes,** on a red cell can elicit the production of different antibodies. Each B cell has a unique receptor that interacts with a specific epitope. This interaction causes the B cell to transform into plasma cells. Each plasma cell is a **clone** that makes antibodies with the same specificity as the original B-cell receptor.

Plasma cell: antibody-producing B cell that has reached the end of its differentiating pathway

Memory B cells: B cells produced after the first exposure that remain in the circulation and can recognize and respond to an antigen faster

Antigenic determinants: sites on an antigen that are recognized and bound by a particular antibody or T-cell receptor (also called epitopes)

Epitopes: single antigenic determinants; functionally, parts of the antigen that combine with the antibody

Clone: family of cells or organisms having genetically identical constitution

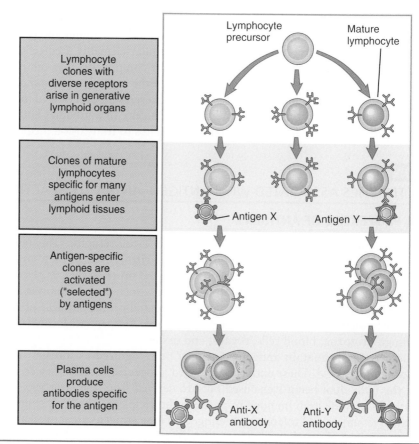

Fig. 2.1 B-cell response to an antigen. Mature lymphocytes develop receptors for antigens before they encounter the antigen. The antigen stimulates the lymphocyte that has the receptor with the best fit. These lymphocytes are signaled to produce a B-cell clone, which differentiates into plasma cells that produce an antibody with a single specificity. (From Abbas AK, Lichtman AH, Pillai S: *Basic immunology,* ed 5, Philadelphia, 2016, Elsevier.)

Immunogen: antigen in its role of eliciting an immune response

Carbohydrates: simple sugars, such as monosaccharides and starches (polysaccharides)

Lipids: fatty acids and glycerol compounds

An immunogen is an antigen that provokes the immune response. Not all antigens are immunogens.

Foreign molecules that can stimulate an immune response are called immunogens. An **immunogen** is distinguishable from an antigen. An antigen is a foreign molecule that can specifically bind to components of immune response such as lymphocytes and antibodies. An immunogen is an antigen that is capable of binding antigen and eliciting an immune response in the body. Not all antigens are immunogenic.[2] The immune system's ability to recognize an antigen and respond to it varies among individuals and can even vary within an individual at a given time. Several important characteristics of a molecule contribute to its degree of immunogenicity (Table 2.1). For example, different biological materials have varying degrees of immunogenicity. Protein molecules are the most immunogenic, followed by **carbohydrates** and **lipids,** which tend to be immunologically inert. In addition, complex compounds, such as a protein–carbohydrate combination, are more immunogenic than simpler molecules. Antigens on red cells, white cells, and platelets vary in their ability to elicit an immune response.

GENERAL PROPERTIES OF ANTIBODIES

Molecular Structure

Antibody: glycoprotein (immunoglobulin) that recognizes a particular epitope on an antigen and facilitates clearance of that antigen

Immunoglobulin: antibody; glycoprotein secreted by plasma cells that binds to specific epitopes on antigenic substances

Antibodies belong to a family of proteins called immunoglobulins. They are structurally related with two common functions: combine with antigen and mediate various biological effects.[3] Antibody molecules are glycoproteins composed of four polypeptide chains joined together by disulfide bonds (Fig. 2.2). The terms **antibody** and **immunoglobulin** (Ig) are often used synonymously. Five classifications of antibodies exist with the designations of IgG, IgA, IgM, IgD, and IgE. The five classes are differentiated based on certain physical, chemical, and biological characteristics. Each antibody molecule has two identical **heavy chains** and two identical **light chains** joined by disulfide bond (S-S) bridges. These molecular bridges provide flexibility to the molecule to change its three-dimensional shape.

The five distinctive heavy-chain molecules distinguish the class, or **isotype.** Each heavy chain imparts characteristic features, which permit them to have unique biological functions. For example, the IgA family, which possesses alpha heavy chains, is the only antibody class capable of residing in mucosal linings. IgE antibodies can activate mast cells, causing immediate hypersensitivity reactions. IgD is an antigen receptor on the naive B

Heavy chains: larger polypeptides of an antibody molecule composed of a variable and constant region; five major classes of heavy chains determine the isotype of an antibody

Light chains: smaller polypeptides of an antibody molecule composed of a variable and constant region; two major types of light chains exist in humans (kappa and lambda)

Isotype: one of five types of immunoglobulins determined by the heavy chain: IgM, IgG, IgA, IgE, and IgD

TABLE 2.1	Factors Contributing to Immunogenicity: Properties of the Antigen
Chemical composition and complexity of the antigen	Proteins are the best immunogens, followed by complex carbohydrates
Degree of foreignness	Immunogen must be identified as nonself; the greater the difference from self, the greater the likelihood of eliciting an immune response
Size	Molecules with a molecular weight >10,000 D are better immunogens
Dosage and antigen density	Number of red cells introduced and the amount of antigen that they carry contribute to the likelihood of an immune response
Route of administration	Manner in which the antigenic stimulus is introduced; intramuscular or intravenous injections are generally better routes for eliciting an immune response

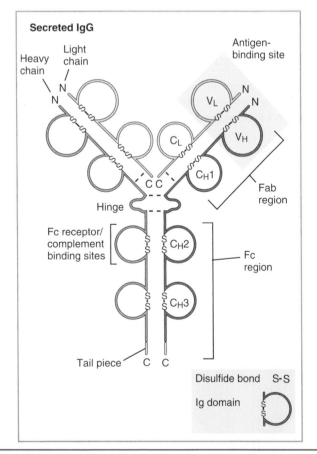

Fig. 2.2 Basic structure of an IgG molecule. Antigen binds to the variable region of the heavy and light chains. The variable region (VL and VH) is part of Fab (fragment antigen binding). The opposite end, composed of the heavy chain, is constant for each type of immunoglobulin and called the Fc (fragment crystallizable) region, which determines the antibody function. The Fc region contains the complement-binding region and the cell activation region. (Modified from Abbas AK, Lichtman AH, Pillai S: *Basic immunology,* ed 5, Philadelphia, 2016, Elsevier.)

Kappa chains: one of the two types of light chains that makes up an immunoglobulin

Lambda chains: one of the two types of light chains that makes up an immunoglobulin

Variable regions: amino-terminal portions of immunoglobulins and T-cell receptor chains that are highly variable and responsible for the antigenic specificity of these molecules

Constant regions: nonvariable portions of the heavy and light chains of an immunoglobulin

Idiotope: variable part of an antibody or T-cell receptor; the antigen-binding site

Hinge region: portion of the immunoglobulin heavy chains between the Fc and Fab region; provides flexibility to the molecule to allow two antigen-binding sites to function independently

Extravascular hemolysis: red cell destruction by phagocytes residing in the liver and spleen, usually facilitated by IgG opsonization

Valency: the number of antigen-binding sites for any given antibody, or the number of antibody-binding sites for any given antigen

cell.[4] The immunoglobulins most involved in transfusion medicine are IgM and IgG, and these are discussed in more detail later in this chapter. There are two types of light chains: **kappa chains** and **lambda chains**. Antibodies possess either two kappa or two lambda chains but never one of each.

Each heavy-chain and light-chain molecule also contains **variable regions** and **constant regions** (or domains). The constant regions of the heavy-chain domain impart the unique antibody class functions, such as the activation of complement or the attachment to certain cells. The variable regions of both the heavy chains and the light chains are concerned with antigen binding and constitute the area of the antibody that contains the **idiotope**. This area is the binding site or pocket into which the antigen fits (Fig. 2.3). The **hinge region** of the antibody molecule imparts flexibility to the molecule for combination with the antigen.

Fab and Fc Regions

Early experiments to identify antibody structure and function used enzymes to cleave the immunoglobulin molecule. Enzymes such as pepsin and papain can divide the immunoglobulin molecule to produce two fragments known as Fab (fragment antigen binding) and Fc (fragment crystallizable). Fab contains the portion of the molecule that binds to the antigenic determinant. Fc consists of the remainder of the constant domains of the two heavy chains linked by disulfide bonds (see Fig. 2.2). Certain immune cells, such as macrophages and neutrophils, possess receptors for the Fc region of an immunoglobulin. These immune cells are able to bind the Fc portion of antibodies attached to red cells or pathogens and assist in their removal by phagocytosis. This mechanism is one way that antibodies facilitate the removal of potential harmful antigens (Fig. 2.4). In transfusion medicine, the antibodies attached to red cell antigens can signal clearance in the liver and spleen, a process called **extravascular hemolysis**.

COMPARISON OF IgM AND IgG ANTIBODIES

Because IgM and IgG antibodies have the most significance in immunohematology, the following discussion focuses on these two immunoglobulins. Table 2.2 summarizes important features of IgM and IgG antibodies. Scan the QR code for molecular images of IgG and IgM.

IgM Antibodies

When the B cells initially respond to a foreign antigen, they produce IgM antibodies first. The IgM molecule consists of five basic immunoglobulin units containing two mu heavy chains and two light chains held together by a joining chain (J chain) (Fig. 2.5). Structurally classified as a large pentamer, one IgM molecule contains 10 potential antigen-combining sites, or has a **valency** of 10. Because of their large structure and high valency,

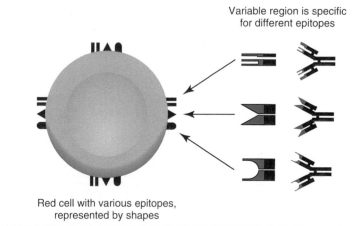

Variable region is specific for different epitopes

Red cell with various epitopes, represented by shapes

Fig. 2.3 Variable region of an immunoglobulin. The specificity of an antibody is determined by the unique variable region that "fits" antigenic determinants or epitopes.

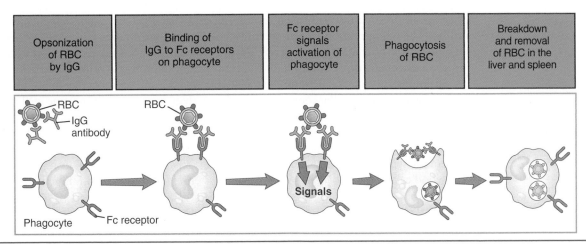

| Opsonization of RBC by IgG | Binding of IgG to Fc receptors on phagocyte | Fc receptor signals activation of phagocyte | Phagocytosis of RBC | Breakdown and removal of RBC in the liver and spleen |

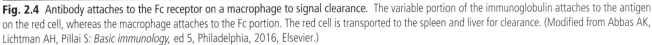

Fig. 2.4 Antibody attaches to the Fc receptor on a macrophage to signal clearance. The variable portion of the immunoglobulin attaches to the antigen on the red cell, whereas the macrophage attaches to the Fc portion. The red cell is transported to the spleen and liver for clearance. (Modified from Abbas AK, Lichtman AH, Pillai S: *Basic immunology,* ed 5, Philadelphia, 2016, Elsevier.)

TABLE 2.2	Comparison of IgM and IgG	
CHARACTERISTIC	**IgM**	**IgG**
Heavy-chain composition	Mu (μ)	Gamma (γ)
Light-chain composition	Kappa (κ) or lambda (λ)	Kappa (κ) or lambda (λ)
J chain	Yes	No
Molecular weight (D)	900,000	150,000
Valence	10	2
Total serum concentration (%)	10	70-75
Serum half-life (days)	5	23
Crosses the placenta	No	Yes
Activation of classical pathway of complement	Yes; very efficient	Yes; not as efficient
Clearance of red cells	Intravascular	Extravascular
Detection in laboratory tests	Immediate-spin	Antiglobulin test

From Abbas AK, Lichtman AH: *Basic immunology,* ed 3, Philadelphia, 2011, Saunders.

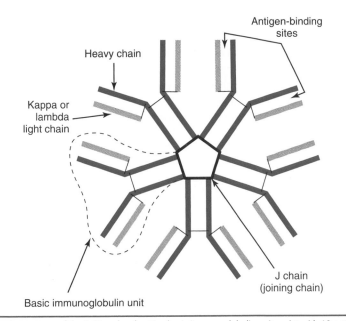

Fig. 2.5 Pentameric structure of the IgM molecule. Five basic immunoglobulin units exist with 10 antigen-binding sites.

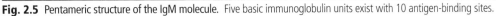

these molecules cause visible agglutination of antigen-positive red cells suspended in saline. The agglutination of red cell antigens by IgM antibodies is referred to as direct agglutination and may be observed during the **immediate-spin** phase of testing. IgM antibodies constitute about 10% of the total serum immunoglobulin concentration.[4]

An important functional feature associated with IgM antibodies is the ability to activate the classical pathway of the **complement system** with great efficiency. Only one IgM molecule is required for the initiation of the classical pathway in complement activation. The complete activation of the classical pathway of complement system results in **hemolysis** of the red cells and intravascular destruction (**intravascular hemolysis**). Antibodies of the ABO blood group system are typically IgM and can cause rapid hemolysis of red cells if an incompatible unit of red blood cells is transfused. The complement system is discussed later in this chapter.

IgG Antibodies

The IgG antibody molecule consists of a four-chain unit with two gamma heavy chains and two light chains, either kappa or lambda in structure. This form of an immunoglobulin molecule is a monomer. IgG antibodies constitute about 70% to 75% of the total immunoglobulin concentration in serum.[4] The molecule is **bivalent;** it possesses two antigen-combining sites. Because of the relatively small size and bivalent structure of the molecule, most IgG antibodies are not effective in producing visible agglutination with antigen-positive red cells suspended in saline. These antigen-antibody complexes are seen with the use of the antiglobulin test discussed in Chapter 3.

IgG is the only immunoglobulin that can be transferred across the placenta from mother to fetus. Fc receptors on placental cells allow the transfer of IgG antibodies across the placenta during pregnancy. This transfer of IgG antibodies from the mother to the fetus protects newborns from infections. The mother's IgG antibodies may also cause destruction of fetal red cells in a condition called **hemolytic disease of the fetus and newborn** (HDFN). This condition occurs if the mother makes an antibody to red cell antigens from exposure through transfusions or prior pregnancies. If the fetus has the corresponding antigen, the IgG antibodies target the red cells for destruction. Laboratory testing to detect this process is discussed in subsequent chapters.

Four IgG subclasses (IgG1, IgG2, IgG3, and IgG4) exist because of minor variations in the gamma heavy chains. The amino acid differences in these heavy chains affect the biological activity of the molecule. For example, subclasses IgG1 and IgG3 are most effective in activating the complement system.[5] Because of their immunoglobulin structure, two molecules of IgG are necessary to initiate the classical pathway of complement activation.

PRIMARY AND SECONDARY IMMUNE RESPONSE

Immunologic response after exposure to an antigen is influenced by the host's previous history with the foreign material. There are two types of immune responses: primary and secondary. The **primary immune response** is stimulated on first exposure to the foreign antigen. The primary response is characterized by a lag phase of approximately 5 to 10 days and is influenced by the characteristics of the antigen and immune system of the host. Host properties that can contribute to the antigen response include the following:

- Age
- Route of administration
- Genetic makeup
- Overall health—stress, fatigue, disease
- Medications (immunosuppressive)

Lag phases may extend for longer periods. During this period, no detectable circulating antibody levels exist within the host. After this lag period, antibody concentrations increase and sustain a plateau before a decline in detectable antibody levels. IgM antibodies are produced first, followed by the production of IgG antibodies. The specificity of the original IgM molecule (determined by the variable region) is the same as the specificity of the IgG molecule seen later in the immune response. Because of a process of gene rearrangement in the B cell, the affinity of the antibody produced after each exposure increases. This process is called **affinity maturation** and is the reason why antibodies often produce a stronger reaction in laboratory tests if the patient has had repeated exposure to the antigen.

The second contact with the identical antigen initiates a **secondary immune response,** or **anamnestic response,** within 1 to 3 days of exposure. Because of the significant production of memory B cells from the initial exposure, the concentrations of circulating antibody are much higher and sustained for a much longer period. Antibody levels are many times higher because of the larger number of plasma cells. IgM antibodies are also generated in the secondary immune response. However, the principal antibody produced is of the IgG class (Fig. 2.6). In the clinical setting, detecting a higher level of the IgM form of an antibody may indicate an acute or early exposure to an immunogen, whereas finding an increase in the IgG form of an antibody of the same specificity may indicate a chronic or previous exposure.

Secondary immune response: immune response induced after a second exposure to the antigen, which activates the memory lymphocytes for a quicker response

Anamnestic response: secondary immune response

Multiple stimulations of the immune system with the same antigen produce antibodies with increased binding strength because of affinity maturation.

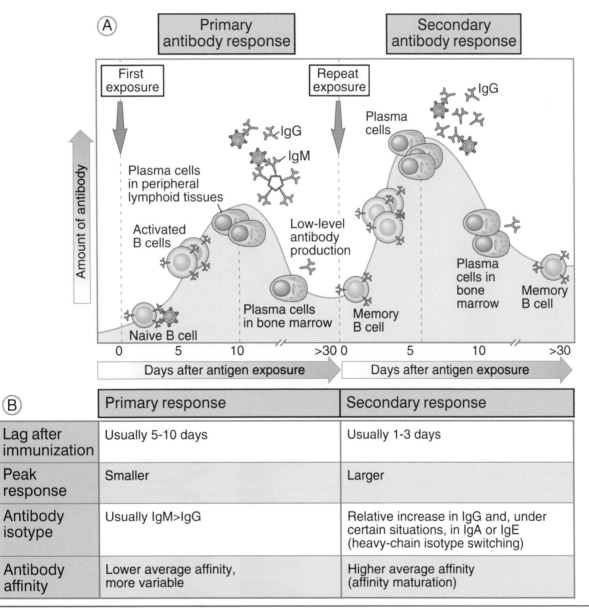

(B)	Primary response	Secondary response
Lag after immunization	Usually 5-10 days	Usually 1-3 days
Peak response	Smaller	Larger
Antibody isotype	Usually IgM>IgG	Relative increase in IgG and, under certain situations, in IgA or IgE (heavy-chain isotype switching)
Antibody affinity	Lower average affinity, more variable	Higher average affinity (affinity maturation)

Fig. 2.6 Primary and secondary immune responses. The initial exposure to an antigen elicits the formation of IgM, followed by IgG antibodies and memory B cells. The second response to the same antigen causes much greater production of IgG antibodies and less IgM antibody secretion. (From Abbas AK, Lichtman AH, Pillai S: *Basic immunology,* ed 5, Philadelphia, 2016, Elsevier.)

ANTIGEN–ANTIBODY REACTIONS

Properties That Influence Binding

The binding of an antigen and antibody follows the law of mass action and is a reversible process. This union complies with the principles of a chemical reaction that has reached equilibrium. When the antigen and antibody combine, an antigen–antibody complex, or **immune complex,** is produced. The amount of antigen–antibody complex formation is determined by the association constant of the reaction. The association constant drives the forward reaction rate, whereas the reverse reaction rate is influenced by the dissociation constant. When the forward reaction rate is faster than the reverse reaction rate, antigen–antibody complex formation is favored. A higher association constant influences greater immune complex formation at equilibrium (Fig. 2.7). When the equilibrium constant is high, the bond between the antigen and antibody is not easily broken.[3]

Several properties influence the binding of antigen and antibody. They are the goodness of fit and the overall strength of binding known as **avidity.** The goodness of fit and the complementary nature of the antibody for its specific epitope contribute to the strength and rate of the reaction. Factors such as the size, shape, and charge of an antigen determine the binding of the antigen to the complementary antibody. The concept of goodness of fit is best explained by viewing the antigen–antibody binding as a lock-and-key fit (Fig. 2.8). If the shape of the antigen is altered, the fit of the antigen for the antibody is changed. Likewise, if the charge of the antigen is altered, the binding properties of the antigen and antibody are affected. The strength of binding between a *single* combining site of an antibody and the epitope of an antigen is called the **affinity.**

Immune complex: complex of one or more antibody molecules bound to an antigen

Avidity: overall strength of reaction between several epitopes and antibodies; depends on the affinity of the antibody, valency, and noncovalent attractive forces

Affinity: strength of the binding between a single antibody and an epitope of an antigen

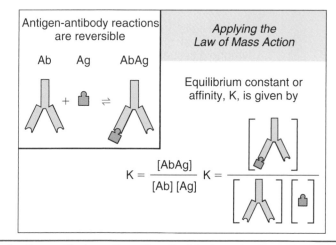
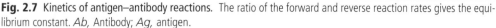

Fig. 2.7 Kinetics of antigen–antibody reactions. The ratio of the forward and reverse reaction rates gives the equilibrium constant. *Ab,* Antibody; *Ag,* antigen.

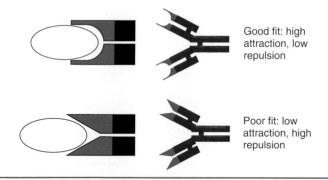

Fig. 2.8 Good fit. A good fit between the antigenic determinant and the binding site of the antibody molecule results in high attraction. In a poor fit, the forces of attraction are low.

No covalent bonding occurs between the antigen and antibody.[3] When the immune complex has been generated, noncovalent attractive forces, including electrostatic forces (ionic bonding), hydrogen bonding, hydrophobic bonding, and van der Waals forces, hold the complex together. The influence of these forces on immune complex stability is described in Table 2.3. The cumulative effect of these forces maintains the union between the antigen and antibody molecules. Avidity is the overall strength of attachment of *several* antigen–antibody reactions and depends on the affinity of the antibody, valency of the antigen, and noncovalent attractive forces. The goal of laboratory testing procedures in the blood bank is to create optimal conditions for antigen–antibody binding to facilitate the detection and identification of antibodies and antigens.

SECTION 2
CHARACTERISTICS ASSOCIATED WITH RED CELL ANTIGEN–ANTIBODY REACTIONS

When a blood sample undergoes centrifugation, the denser red cells travel to the bottom of the tube. The liquid portion of the sample is known as plasma (if an anticoagulant was added) or serum (no anticoagulant added and sample is allowed to clot) and is seen in the top portion of the tube. Scan the QR code to see a colored picture of a centrifuged blood sample showing plasma and red cells.

- Red cell *antigens* are located on the red cells. They are part of the cell membrane or protrude from the cell membrane.
- Red cell *antibodies* are molecules in the plasma or serum (Fig. 2.9).

TABLE 2.3	Forces Binding Antigen to Antibody
Electrostatic forces (ionic bonding)	Attraction between two molecules on the basis of opposite charge; a positively charged region of a molecule is attracted to the negatively charged region of another molecule
Hydrogen bonding	Attraction of two negatively charged groups (X−) for an H+ atom
Hydrophobic bonding	Weak bonds formed as a result of the exclusion of water from the antigen–antibody complex
van der Waals forces	Attraction between the electron cloud (−) of one atom and the protons (+) within the nucleus of another atom

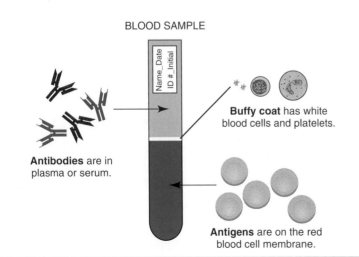

BLOOD SAMPLE

Name_Date
ID #_Initial

Buffy coat has white blood cells and platelets.

Antibodies are in plasma or serum.

Antigens are on the red blood cell membrane.

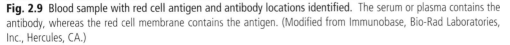

Fig. 2.9 Blood sample with red cell antigen and antibody locations identified. The serum or plasma contains the antibody, whereas the red cell membrane contains the antigen. (Modified from Immunobase, Bio-Rad Laboratories, Inc., Hercules, CA.)

The International Society of Blood Transfusion's (ISBT's) Working Party on Red Cell Immunogenetics and Blood Group Terminology assign the blood group systems.

Glycoproteins: compounds containing carbohydrate and protein molecules

Glycolipids: compounds containing carbohydrate and lipid molecules

Agglutination: visible clumping of particulate antigens caused by interaction with a specific antibody

In addition to red cell antigens, white cells and platelets contain antigens that are important in transfusion medicine. Human leukocyte antigens (HLA) and human platelet antigens (HPA) are discussed later in the book.

RED CELL ANTIGENS

Researchers have defined 36 blood group systems with more than 250 unique red cell antigens.[6] A blood group system is composed of antigens that have been grouped according to the inheritance patterns of many blood group genes. Every individual possesses a unique set of red cell antigens. Because of a diversity of blood group gene inheritance patterns, certain racial populations may possess a greater prevalence of specific red cell antigens.

Scientific research has determined the biochemical characteristics of many red cell antigens and their relationship to the red cell membrane. In biochemical terms, these antigens may take the form of proteins, proteins coupled with carbohydrate molecules (glycoproteins), or carbohydrates coupled with lipids (glycolipids). Antigenic determinants may be sequential, as in linear proteins, or may have a structure involving molecules brought in close proximity by folding.[3] Generally, the red cell antigens protrude from the surface of the red cell membrane in three-dimensional configurations (Fig. 2.10). Because of this orientation on the surface of the red cell, the antigens are accessible to and may interact with antibody molecules, resulting in agglutination reactions. Agglutination using red cells is called hemagglutination. Determination of the specificity of the red cell antigen or antibody in most routine blood banking procedures is performed by hemagglutination tests that can be done in a tube, in a microplate, or in a microtube filled with gel particles (the gel test). Solid-phase testing is an alternative method that uses red cell adherence to a solid support rather than hemagglutination. More information on these methods and the reagents used in these laboratory tests is located in Chapters 3 and 10.

Scan the QR code for the ISBT classification of the 36 blood group systems.

Some red cell antigens are more immunogenic than other red cell antigens and must be matched to the patient receiving a transfusion. For example, the D antigen within the Rh blood group system is highly immunogenic compared with other red cell antigens. There is the possibility of stimulating anti-D antibody production in an individual lacking D antigens, who is transfused with red cells possessing D antigens. Patients who lack the D antigen should receive blood components containing red cells that lack the D antigen. Scan the QR code for a picture of agglutination.

RED CELL ANTIBODIES

The most significant immunoglobulins in transfusion medicine are IgG and IgM. Most clinically important antibodies react at body temperature (37° C), are IgG, and can

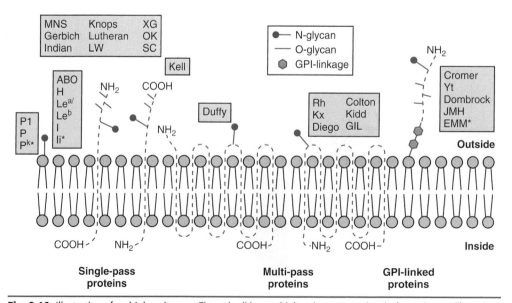

Fig. 2.10 Illustration of multiple epitopes. The red cell has multiple epitopes or antigenic determinants. The unique configuration of the antigenic determinant allows recognition by a corresponding antibody molecule. (From Reid ME, Lomas-Francis C: *The blood group antigen facts book,* ed 2, San Diego, 2004, Elsevier Academic Press.)

cause immune destruction of transfused red cells possessing the corresponding antigen. The destruction of the red cells can cause transfusion reactions, anemia, and HDFN.

IgM antibodies react best at room temperature (20° C to 22° C) or lower (to 4° C) and are usually not implicated in the destruction of transfused red cells. The antibodies to ABO antigens are an important exception to this rule. Antibodies to ABO antigens are of the IgM class and react in vitro at room temperature and in vivo at body temperature. A transfusion of the wrong ABO blood group (antigen) would effectively activate the complement system and cause hemolysis of the transfused cells.

> IgG antibodies react best at 37° C, and IgM antibodies react best at room temperature or lower (in vitro).

> Most IgM antibodies agglutinate red cells suspended in physiologic saline.

IMMUNOHEMATOLOGY: ANTIGEN–ANTIBODY REACTIONS IN VIVO

Transfusion, Pregnancy, and the Immune Response

During transfusion and pregnancy, a patient is exposed to many potentially foreign antigens on red cells, white cells, and platelets that possess varying degrees of immunogenicity. Because of this exposure to foreign antigens, a patient's immune system may become activated, or "sensitized," with the resultant production of circulating antibodies. The antibodies produced in response to transfusion and pregnancies are classified as **alloantibodies.**

The **antibody screen test** is performed on the patient before transfusion to detect any existing red cell alloantibodies. If a red cell alloantibody is detected, a test is performed to identify the specificity of the antibody. Once the specificity is identified, donor units lacking the red cell antigen are selected for transfusion. Detecting and identifying antibodies in the patient before transfusion are important to avoid the formation of antigen–antibody complexes in vivo (within the patient's body), which would lessen the survival of the transfused cells.

> **Alloantibodies:** antibodies with specificities other than self; stimulated by transfusion or pregnancy

> **Antibody screen test:** test to determine the presence of alloantibodies

Immunization may also occur during pregnancy because fetal blood cells may enter the maternal circulation at delivery. Alloantibody production may be observed as an immune response to red blood cell, white blood cell, or platelet antigens of fetal origin. Women are routinely screened during the first trimester of pregnancy for the presence of red cell alloantibodies that can destroy fetal red cells before or after delivery. The red cell destruction may lead to clinical complications of anemia and high levels of bilirubin in the fetus or newborn.

Complement Proteins

The complement system is a group of serum proteins that have numerous biological roles related to antigen clearance, cell lysis, and vasodilation (Fig. 2.11). These proteins normally circulate in an inactive or proenzyme state. On activation, they are converted into active enzymes that enhance the immunologic processes.

Nine components of the complement family are designated C1 through C9.[3] When an antibody activates the **classical pathway**, the complex C1q, C1r, C1 splits the C4 and C2 proteins into two parts. Each protein is converted into protein fragments and given the distinction *a* or *b* (eg, C4 is converted into C4a and C4b). The smaller fragment is designated *a*, and the larger one is designated *b*. Typically, the larger *b* fragment binds to the cell, and the smaller *a* fragment enhances the inflammatory response. From the splitting of C4 and C2, C4b and C2a fragments join to form C3 convertase, which splits C3 into C3a and C3b. The C3 convertase joins with C3b to form C5 convertase, which splits C5. The final formation of a **membrane attack complex** causes lysis of various cells (hemolysis of red cells), bacteria, and viruses by disrupting the cell membrane. The direct attachment of the membrane attack complex, consisting of the complement proteins C5 to C9, to the cell surface produces holes in the cell membrane and osmotic lysis. If the membrane attack complex becomes attached to transfused red cells, hemolysis occurs with a subsequent release of free hemoglobin into the circulation.

> **Classical pathway:** activation of complement that is initiated by antigen–antibody complexes

> **Membrane attack complex:** C5 to C9 proteins of the complement system that mediate cell lysis in the target cell

> Ca^{2+} and Mg^{2+} are needed for activation of the classical pathway.[3]

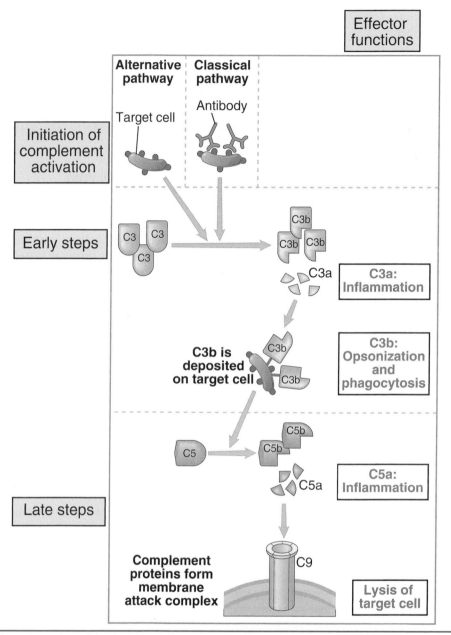

Fig. 2.11 Comparison of the classical and alternative complement pathways. The classical pathway is initiated by an antigen–antibody reaction. The alternative pathway is initiated by the membrane property of a microorganism. After the split of the C3 component, the two pathways are identical. Three major biological activities of the complement system are opsonization, lysis of target cells, and stimulation of inflammatory mediators. (Modified from Abbas AK, Lichtman AH, Pillai S: *Basic immunology*, ed 5, Philadelphia, 2016, Elsevier.)

The early steps in the activation of the complement proteins can occur in either of two pathways:

- The classical pathway is activated by the presence of an antibody bound to an antigen. Red cell destruction that may result from antibody-coated red cells is caused by the activation of this pathway.
- The **alternative pathway** does not require a specific antibody for activation. Foreign cell-surface constituents, such as bacterial or viral proteins or carbohydrates, initiate it.

Regardless of the activation mode, the final steps involved in cell lysis are common to both pathways. In addition, the consequences of complement activation, which serves as an important amplifier of the immune system, are common to both pathways. The

Alternative pathway:
activation of complement that is initiated by foreign cell-surface constituents

TABLE 2.4	Biological Effects Mediated by Complement Proteins
Opsonization	Clear immune complexes
	Enhance phagocytosis
	Promote release of enzymes from neutrophils
Anaphylaxis	Increase smooth muscle contraction and inflammation
Lysis	Kill foreign antigens by membrane lysis
Chemotactic	Recruit platelets and phagocytes

peptides generated during the formation of the membrane attack unit have the following additional functions (Table 2.4):

- **Anaphylatoxins** C3a, C4a, and C5a assist in the recruitment of phagocytic cells and the promotion of inflammation. These complement proteins attach to mast cells and promote the release of **vasoactive amines,** which help make blood vessels permeable for fluid and cells to enter the area.
- The C5a protein is **chemotactic** for neutrophils and attracts these cells to the site of injury.
- Complement also functions as an **opsonin,** which is a molecule that binds to an antigen to promote phagocytosis. **Phagocytic cells** are generally inefficient. If complement binds to an antigen, the process of phagocytosis becomes extremely efficient. **Receptors** on the surface of the phagocytic cell have a higher affinity for opsonins. C3b and antibodies are opsonins, which promote the clearance of bacteria and other cells to which the opsonins are attached. In the blood bank, a test to determine whether the red cell is coated with complement components is a useful serologic tool when red cell destruction is being investigated. C3b and C4b proteins are made up of a "c" and "d" complex. The C4d and C3d breakdown products can also be detected on red cells.

Clearance of Antigen–Antibody Complexes

Antigen–antibody complexes are removed from the body's circulation through the **mononuclear phagocyte system.**[4] This system acts as a filter to remove microbes and old cells. The system is present in secondary lymphoid organs such as the spleen, lymph nodes, liver, and lungs. The largest lymphoid organ, the spleen, is particularly effective for removing old and damaged red cells from the blood and clearing the body of antigen–antibody complexes. The spleen removes red cells opsonized by IgG or complement components.

IMMUNOHEMATOLOGY: ANTIGEN–ANTIBODY REACTIONS IN VITRO

Overview of Agglutination

Antigen–antibody reactions occurring in vitro (in laboratory testing) are detected by visible agglutination of red cells or evidence of hemolysis at the completion of testing (a positive result). The absence of hemagglutination in immunohematologic testing (a negative result) implies the lack of antigen–antibody complex formation. A negative result is interpreted to mean that the antibody in the test system is not specific for the antigen. A positive result indicates that an antigen–antibody immune complex was formed, and the specificity of the antibody matched the antigen in the test system. The agglutination test must be performed correctly to reach the correct conclusion regarding the presence or absence of the antigen or antibody.

The next section describes the factors affecting the hemagglutination reaction, which occurs in two stages, referred to as the **sensitization** step and the **lattice formation** step.[1] These concepts are summarized in Table 2.5.

Sensitization Stage or Antibody Binding to Red Cells

In the first stage of red cell agglutination, the antibody binds to an antigen on the red cell membrane. This stage requires an immunologic recognition between the antigen and

Anaphylatoxins: complement split products (C3a, C4a, and C5a) that mediate degranulation of mast cells and basophils, which results in smooth muscle contraction and increased vascular permeability

Vasoactive amines: products such as histamines released by basophils, mast cells, and platelets that act on the endothelium and smooth muscle of the local vasculature

Chemotactic: movement of cells in the direction of the antigenic stimulus

Opsonin: substance (antibody or complement protein) that binds to an antigen and enhances phagocytosis

Phagocytic cells: cells that engulf microorganisms, other cells, and foreign particles; include neutrophils, macrophages, and monocytes

Receptors: molecules on the cell surface that have a high affinity for a particular molecule such as antibody, hormone, or drug

Mononuclear phagocyte system: system of mononuclear phagocytic cells, associated with the liver, spleen, and lymph nodes that clears microbes and damaged cells

A positive reaction is indicated by agglutination. A negative reaction is indicated by no agglutination.

Sensitization: binding of antibody or complement components to a red cell

Lattice formation: combination of antibody and a multivalent antigen to form cross-links and result in visible agglutination

TABLE 2.5	Factors Affecting Agglutination	
STAGE	**FACTOR**	**DESCRIPTION**
Sensitization	Temperature	IgG, 37°C; IgM, ≤22° C
	Incubation time	Immediate-spin or after a specific time at 1-8° C, room temperature, or 37° C
	pH	7.0 (physiologic is ideal)
	Ionic strength	Can be adjusted with reagents
Lattice formation	Zeta potential	Distance between cells caused by charged ions
	Zone of equivalence	Antigen and antibody concentrations
	Centrifugation	Time and speed of centrifugation to bring cells close together

antibody. During this recognition stage, antigenic determinants on the red cell combine with the antigen-binding site of the antibody molecule. No visible agglutination is observable at this stage.

The physical joining of an antigen and antibody is essentially a random pairing of the two structures determined largely by chance. Antibody concentration and antigen receptor accessibility and quantity may influence the probability for this collision. An increase in antibody concentration increases the probability of collision events with the corresponding antigen. Accordingly, this probability of antigen–antibody interaction relies upon the overall effect of the **serum-to-cell ratio,** or concentration of antigen and antibody, in immunohematologic tests.

Increasing the amount of serum placed in the test tube increases the concentration of antibodies available for binding to red cell antigens. When a patient's serum demonstrates weak reactions in agglutination testing, this simple technique may be used to enhance the first stage of the agglutination reaction. Increasing the amount of antigen or red cell concentration does *not* increase the reaction probability.

Serum-to-cell ratio: ratio of antigen on the red cell to antibody in the serum

Factors Influencing the First Stage of Agglutination

In addition to the serum-to-cell ratio, certain environmental factors may influence the sensitization and lattice formation in the two stages of agglutination reaction.

Temperature of the Reaction

Temperature acts by increasing the rate of the reaction. A temperature of 37° C is recommended for antibody detection because the antibody will combine more rapidly at this temperature.[3] Most antibodies of clinical relevance in transfusion are IgG antibodies reacting at approximately 37° C.[5] By combining the sources of antigen and antibody and incubating them at this temperature, the first stage of the agglutination reaction is enhanced. In contrast, IgM antibodies are more reactive at lower temperatures, generally at room temperature (ambient temperature) or lower.

Incubation Time

Allowing adequate time for the combination of antigen and antibody to attain equilibrium also enhances the first stage of the agglutination reaction. The length of time recommended for optimal antigen–antibody reactivity varies with the test procedure and the reagents used in testing. Some test procedures may indicate a predetermined incubation period performed at variable temperatures, such as 37° C, room temperature, or 1° C to 8° C. Additionally, the test procedures may indicate an immediate-spin step that indicates a combination of test reagents and sample with no period of incubation.

Increasing the incubation time may help in weak antibody investigations.

pH

The optimal pH for hemagglutination is around 7.0, which is the physiologic pH range. This pH range is adequate for most of the important red cell antibodies. Several red cell antibodies are readily detectable when the pH is reduced (eg, anti-I, anti-M).[3]

Ionic Strength

In an isotonic environment, such as **physiologic saline**, Na$^+$ and Cl$^-$ ions are attracted to the oppositely charged groups on antigen and antibody molecules. Because of this attraction, the combination of antigen and antibody is hindered. If the ionic environment is reduced, this shielding effect is reduced, and the amount of antibody uptake onto the red cell is increased. Low-ionic-strength reagents act by increasing the rate of antibody uptake on the cells.

Physiologic saline: NaCl prepared in water to a concentration of 0.9%

Lattice-Formation Stage or Cell–Cell Interactions

After the red cells have been sensitized with antibody molecules, random collisions between the antibody-coated red cells are necessary to develop cross-linkages for the visualization of red cell clumping or agglutination within the test tube (Fig. 2.12). Visible agglutinates form when red cells are in close proximity to promote the lattice formation of antibody-binding sites to antigenic determinants on adjacent red cells.

Factors Influencing the Second Stage of Agglutination

Distance Between Red Cells

The **zeta potential,** or the force of repulsion between red cells in a physiologic saline solution, exerts an influence on the agglutination reaction. Red cells possess a net negative charge on the cell surface in a saline suspension. Cations (positively charged ions) from the saline environment are attracted to these negative charges. A stable cationic cloud surrounds each cell and contributes a force of repulsion between molecules of similar charge. Because of this repulsive force, the red cells remain at a distance from each other. This distance between the red cells is proportional to the zeta potential (Fig. 2.13). Because of

Zeta potential: electrostatic potential measured between the red cell membrane and the slipping plane of the same cell

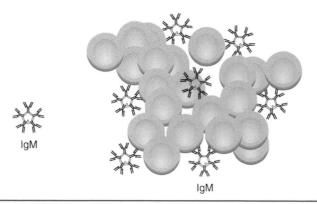
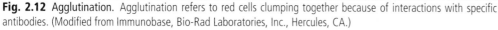

IgM

IgM

Fig. 2.12 Agglutination. Agglutination refers to red cells clumping together because of interactions with specific antibodies. (Modified from Immunobase, Bio-Rad Laboratories, Inc., Hercules, CA.)

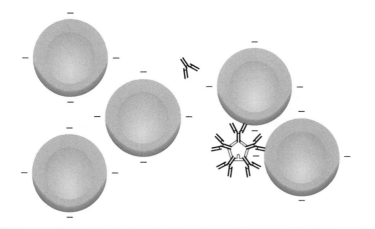

Fig. 2.13 Effect of the zeta potential on the second stage of agglutination. The zeta potential keeps red cells apart and does not promote agglutination by IgG antibodies. IgM antibodies are more likely to cause direct agglutination. (Modified from Immunobase, Bio-Rad Laboratories, Inc., Hercules, CA.)

the larger size, pentamer shape, and multivalent properties of IgM molecules, agglutination is facilitated between adjacent red cells that have IgM attached to them. In contrast, IgG antibody molecules are smaller and less able to span the distance between adjacent red cells generated by the zeta potential. IgG molecules may attach, but visible agglutination might not occur.

Optimal Concentrations of Antigen and Antibody

Zone of equivalence: number of binding sites of multivalent antigen and antibody are approximately equal

Prozone: excess antibody causing a false-negative reaction

Postzone: excess antigen causing a false-negative reaction

Maximum amounts of agglutination are observed when the concentrations of antigens (red cells) and antibody (serum) fall within the **zone of equivalence** (Fig. 2.14). When the concentration of antibody exceeds the concentration of antigen, antibody excess (or **prozone**) exists, which decreases the amount of agglutinated red cells. In contrast, **postzone** occurs when the concentration of antigen exceeds the number of antibodies present. The amount of agglutinates formed under these circumstances is also suboptimal and diminished.

Immunohematologic testing is designed to obtain reactions within the zone of equivalence. Commercial antibody preparations are diluted to optimal antibody concentrations for testing. Red cell preparations are diluted to a 2% to 5% suspension in saline for optimal antigen concentrations. The use of red cell suspensions greater than 5% may affect the ability of the test reaction to fall within the zone of equivalence and cause a **false-negative** reaction because of postzone.

Effect of Centrifugation

False-negative: test result that incorrectly indicates a negative reaction (the lack of agglutination); an antigen–antibody reaction has occurred but is not detected

The time and speed of centrifugation are important factors for the detection of agglutinated red cells. Centrifugation helps to facilitate the formation of a latticed network by forcing the red cells closer together in the test environment. Centrifuges are calibrated to define the optimal speed and time for the best reaction. Overcentrifugation or undercentrifugation and too-high or too-low speeds can cause **false-positive** or false-negative reactions.

Grading Agglutination Reactions

False-positive: test result that incorrectly indicates a positive reaction (the presence of agglutination or hemolysis); no agglutination reaction occurred

In immunohematology, antigen–antibody reactions are measured qualitatively. The presence of an antigen–antibody reaction is detected with red cell agglutination, but the concentration of the immune complex is not determined in a quantitative manner. Red cell antigen and antibody reactions may be performed in test tubes, in microplate wells, and in

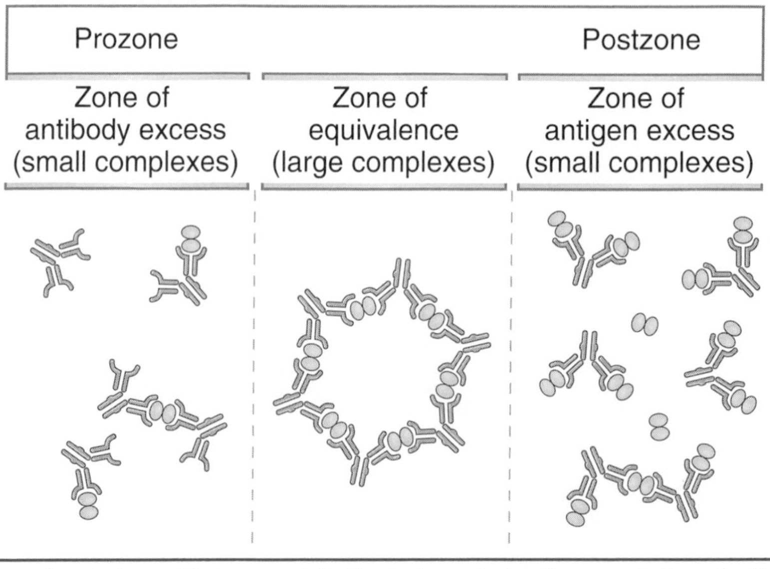

Prozone	Postzone
Zone of antibody excess (small complexes)	Zone of equivalence (large complexes)	Zone of antigen excess (small complexes)

Fig. 2.14 Zone of equivalence. Maximum agglutination is observed when the concentrations of antigens and antibodies fall within the zone of equivalence. (Modified from Abbas AK, Lichtman AH, Pillai S: *Cellular and molecular immunology*, ed 7, Philadelphia, 2011, Saunders.)

microtubes filled with gel particles. Because of the qualitative nature of the measurement, the reading and grading of agglutination reactions are subjective.

To standardize this element of subjectivity among personnel performing the testing, a grading system for agglutination reactions has been established. The conventional grading system for tube testing uses a 0 to 4+ scale (Fig. 2.15).

Slight variations in this conventional grading system may be established in individual institutions. Agglutination reactions are read by shaking and tilting the test tubes until the red cell button has been removed from the bottom of the tube. Negative agglutination reactions are interpreted after the red cell button has been completely resuspended. An agglutination viewer lamp with a magnifying mirror is usually used to evaluate the agglutination reactions. Laboratories using a microscopic reading in some testing have criteria established for grading these reactions. Scan the QR code for pictures of graded agglutination reactions.

Hemolysis as an Indicator of Antigen–Antibody Reactions

In addition to agglutination as an indicator of an antigen–antibody reaction in the immunohematology laboratory, red cell hemolysis observed in the tube is also an indicator of the reactivity of an antigen and antibody in vitro. If activated by an immune complex, the complement system may demonstrate hemolysis of the red cells along with agglutination. The final steps in the process of complement activation initiate the membrane attack complex, causing membrane damage. Because of this damage, intracellular fluid is released to the reaction environment. The red cell button is often smaller compared with the red cell button present in other tubes. A pinkish to reddish **supernatant** is observed after the tubes have been centrifuged. For grading a tube with hemolysis, an *H* is traditionally used when this phenomenon is observed. Some red cell antibodies characteristically display hemolysis in vitro, such as antibodies to the Lewis system antigens and anti-Vel, which are discussed in later chapters.[7] It is important to recognize hemolysis as an antigen–antibody reaction. Hemolysis is detected in vitro using fresh serum samples because serum has active complement proteins. Because anticoagulants bind calcium, which is necessary for complement activation, plasma samples do not demonstrate complement activation.

Credit for QR code image: Feldman, B.F. and Sink, C.A. Methods. In: Feldman B.F. and Sink C.A. (Eds.), Practical Transfusion Medicine. Ithaca: International Veterinary Information Service (www.ivis.org), 2008; Document No. A4805.0708. (Accessed: 31 Mar 2016)

Supernatant: fluid above cells or particles after centrifugation

A hemolyzed patient sample is not acceptable for serologic testing in the blood bank because hemolysis is interpreted as a positive reaction.

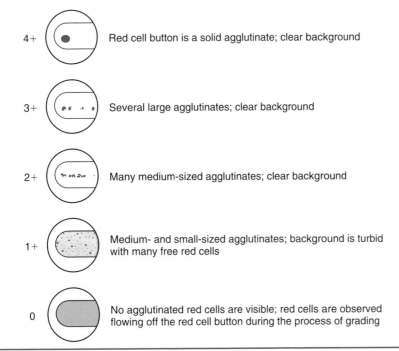

Fig. 2.15 Grading antigen–antibody reactions. Consistency in grading reactions allows for correct interpretation of results in the immunohematology laboratory. (Modified from Gamma Biologicals, Houston, TX.)

SECTION 3

SECTION 3

APPLICATION OF RED CELL ANTIGEN–ANTIBODY REACTIONS FOR ROUTINE TESTING IN IMMUNOHEMATOLOGY

INTRODUCTION TO ROUTINE TESTING IN IMMUNOHEMATOLOGY

This section describes how the basic principles of antigen–antibody (Ag-Ab) reactions in vitro are applied in the immunohematology laboratory. The basic procedures in immunohematology are derived from the principle of placing a source of antigen and a source of antibody into a testing environment to detect an Ag-Ab reaction (Fig. 2.16). The evidence for the formation of an Ag-Ab reaction in vitro has traditionally been the visualization of agglutinates or the presence of hemolysis within the test tube. Alternative techniques for the detection of Ag-Ab reactions are available based on detection systems using gel and solid-phase adherence technology. These methods all share common denominators: a source of antigen and a source of antibody added to a testing environment.

Selection of the appropriate source of either antigen or antibody for inclusion in the procedure depends on the purpose or intent of the test. Is testing directed toward detecting the presence or absence of a particular red cell antigen? Alternatively, is testing directed toward detecting the presence or absence of a particular red cell antibody? In either situation, no matter what variable is unknown in testing, a known source is used for the other variable. If the unknown variable is the antigen, the unknown antigen source combines with a known source of antibody to enable Ag-Ab reactions. For example, in the procedure to detect the presence of the B antigen on a patient's red cells, the red cells are combined with a commercial source of antibody, anti-B reagent. If the B antigen is present on the red cells, agglutination is observed in the test tube. If the B antigen is absent on the red cells, no agglutination is observed in the test tube (Fig. 2.17).

> For antigen testing, antigens are on the red cell; antibodies are in the antisera (commercial antibodies).

SOURCES OF ANTIGEN FOR TESTING

Sources of antigen for immunohematology testing include reagent red cells or red cells from patient or donor blood samples. Reagent red cells are commercially prepared cell suspensions. The manufacturer of reagent red cells has previously identified many of the red cell antigens. Therefore these reagent red cells provide known sources of red cell antigens. By using a known antigen, an unknown antibody can be detected or identified based on a positive or negative agglutination reaction.

When using red cell suspensions from a patient's sample, the red cell antigens are the unknown factor. Red cell suspensions are prepared in physiologic saline to a 2% to 5% suspension. The patient's red cells are tested with a known antibody to determine the

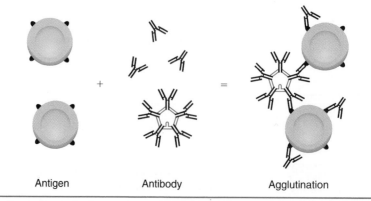

Antigen   Antibody   Agglutination

Fig. 2.16 Routine testing in the immunohematology laboratory. Sources of antigen from red cells and sources of antibody from serum are added together. The Ag-Ab reaction shows agglutination, which is a positive test result. (Modified from Immunobase, Bio-Rad Laboratories, Inc., Hercules, CA.)

Testing patient RBCs for B antigen with reagent anti-B

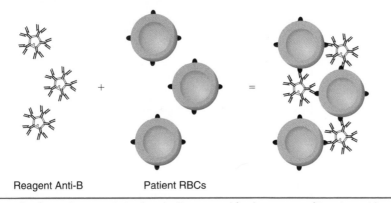

Reagent Anti-B   Patient RBCs

Fig. 2.17 Example of a routine test. Patient's red cells are tested for the presence of B antigen with a commercial antibody reagent, anti-B. The presence of agglutination indicates that the patient's red cells possess B antigens. The patient's type is interpreted as group B. (Modified from Immunobase, Bio-Rad Laboratories, Inc., Hercules, CA.)

TABLE 2.6	Sources of Antigen and Antibody in Agglutination Reactions for Blood Bank Tests	
TESTING FOR	**KNOWN SOURCE**	**UNKNOWN SOURCE**
Antigen	Reagent red cells	Patient or donor red cells
Antibody	Commercial antisera (anti-A, anti-B)	Patient or donor serum/plasma

antigen identity. When a known antibody is used, the unknown antigens on the patient's red cells can be detected, based on agglutination reaction. If antigen is present, agglutination is visible. If antigen is absent, no agglutination is visible (see Fig. 2.17).

SOURCES OF ANTIBODY FOR TESTING

Sources of antibody for immunohematology testing include commercial antisera, serum, or plasma from the patient. Commercial antisera are manufactured with known red cell antibodies and are used to identify unknown antigens.

Antibodies may also be present in the serum or plasma of blood samples from patients or donors. Similar to patient antigens, the antibodies made by patients are usually unknown. Patient serum or plasma samples are tested for the presence of red cell antibodies using a known antigen source for identification or detection (Table 2.6).

ROUTINE TESTING PROCEDURES IN THE IMMUNOHEMATOLOGY LABORATORY

Several universal procedures in immunohematology apply these principles in the testing of patient samples before transfusion with blood products containing red cells or in the testing of donor samples. Table 2.7 lists the sources of antigen and antibody in these procedures.
- ABO and D typing for the detection of the A, B, and D antigens
- ABO serum/plasma testing for the detection of ABO antibodies, anti-A and anti-B
- Determination of the presence or absence of red cell antigens from other blood group systems in patient and donor samples (eg, testing a donor unit for the E antigen of the Rh blood group system)
- Antibody screen (antibody detection) for the detection of preformed antibodies to red cell antigens as a result of previous exposure to red cells through transfusion and pregnancy
- **Antibody identification** for determination of the red cell antibody **specificity** after detection with the antibody screen
- **Crossmatch** for the serologic check of the donor unit and patient compatibility before transfusion

Antibody identification: procedure that determines the identity of a red cell antibody detected in the antibody screen by reacting serum with commercial panel cells

Specificity: unique recognition of an antigenic determinant and its corresponding antibody molecule

Crossmatch: procedure that combines donor's red cells and patient's serum to determine the serologic compatibility between donor and patient

Antibody screen testing detects any red cell antibodies that may be present in patient or donor samples. Antibody identification will tell what antibody or antibodies are present (eg, anti-D, anti-E, etc.).

TABLE 2.7	Routine Procedures in the Immunohematology Laboratory			
PROCEDURE	**PURPOSE**	**SOURCE OF ANTIGEN**	**SOURCE OF ANTIBODY**
ABO/D typing (forward grouping)	Detects A, B, and D antigens	Patient's red cells	Commercial anti-A, anti-B, and anti-D
ABO serum testing (reverse grouping)	Detects ABO antibodies	Reverse grouping cells (A_1 and B)	Patient's serum or plasma
Antibody screen	Detects antibodies with specificity to red cell antigens	Screening cells	Patient's serum or plasma
Antibody identification	Identifies specificity of red cell antibodies	Panel cells	Patient's serum or plasma
Crossmatch	Determines serologic compatibility between donor and patient before transfusion	Donor's red cells	Patient's serum or plasma

CHAPTER SUMMARY

Characteristics of Antigens
- Antigens are foreign molecules that combine with an antibody or immunoglobulin. The part of the antigen that combines with the antibody is the epitope or antigenic determinant.
- Red cells, white cells, and platelets have numerous antigens that can elicit an immune response after exposure from transfusions, pregnancy, and transplantation.

Characteristics of Antibodies
- The structural components of immunoglobulins consist of heavy chains and light chains, constant regions and variable regions, disulfide bonds, and a hinge region.
- The five types of immunoglobulins—IgM, IgG, IgA, IgD, and IgE—differ in their heavy chain, function, and role in the immune response.
- IgM molecules are pentameric with 10 antigen-binding sites and are most efficient in the activation of complement proteins. IgM is produced first. IgM antibodies are usually detectable by direct or immediate-spin agglutination in tube testing.
- IgG molecules possess two antigen-binding sites and constitute the greatest percentage of the total immunoglobulin concentration in serum. The antiglobulin test is required to detect IgG.

Antigen–Antibody Interactions
- An immune complex is an antibody bound to an antigen. Immune complexes are formed in vivo and are eventually cleared by the body.
- In laboratory testing, immune complexes are formed in vitro to determine the identity of an antigen or antibody or to predict the reaction after transfusion of a blood product. Typically, the antigen is on the red cell, and the antibody is in the patient's serum or plasma or in the reagent.
- Hemagglutination is a two-step process involving the antibody binding to red cells and the formation of lattices between sensitized red cells.
- The fit or the complementary nature of the antibody for its specific epitope determines the strength and rate of the reaction, also called the affinity of the bond.
- Attractive forces, including electrostatic forces, hydrogen bonding, hydrophobic bonding, and van der Waals forces, hold the immune complex together.
- Hemagglutination and hemolysis are indicators of a red cell antigen–antibody reaction.

Application of Red Cell Antigen–Antibody Reactions for Routine Testing in Immunohematology
- The reagents used in the immunohematology laboratory provide the tools to detect Ag-Ab reactions.
- Principles of routine testing are based on the combination of a source of antigen and a source of antibody in a test environment.

- Sources of antigen and antibody are derived from commercially available reagents and patient or donor samples.
- Agglutination or hemolysis is indicative of Ag-Ab recognition.
- The purposes of reagents used in the immunohematology laboratory are to:
  - Determine the ABO/Rh type of donors and patients
  - Detect antibodies produced by patients or donors who have been exposed to red cells through transfusion or pregnancy
  - Identify the specificity of antibodies detected in the antibody screen procedure
  - Determine the presence or absence of additional antigens on the red cells in addition to the A, B, and D antigens
  - Perform crossmatches to evaluate serologic compatibility of donor and patient before transfusion

CRITICAL THINKING EXERCISES

Exercise 2.1
Draw an IgG molecule and identify the following parts:
a. Antigen-binding site
b. Complement-binding region
c. Macrophage-binding site
d. Variable region
e. Hinge region

Exercise 2.2
Two different patients received red cell units during surgery. One patient developed an IgG antibody after transfusion; the other patient did not develop an IgG antibody. What factors contribute to an immune response to transfusion?

Exercise 2.3
A patient's blood sample was received at the blood bank for antibody identification. What part of the patient's blood sample is used to perform the antibody identification test?

Exercise 2.4
A technologist failed to notice that the centrifuge had not properly centrifuged the test tubes prepared for antibody identification. The time of centrifugation was 15 seconds instead of 30 seconds. What would be the potential error in the interpretation of this test?

Exercise 2.5
A technologist added extra drops of commercial red cells to the test tube for antibody identification because he observed a weak reaction in the initial antibody screen. Would you recommend this action? What could be the potential impact on the antibody identification test?

Exercise 2.6
What is the difference between physiologic saline and low-ionic-strength saline in the detection of antigen–antibody reactions?

Exercise 2.7
A technologist prepared 2% to 5% red cell suspensions for testing with anti-A and anti-B reagents. After adding the patient's red cells and antisera to tubes, the tubes were centrifuged. All tubes demonstrated hemolysis, and no red cells remained. The technologist looked at the patient's 2% to 5% red cell suspensions and noted hemolysis in these tubes. What situation(s) could explain these results?

Exercise 2.8
In the investigation of a patient's serum showing a weak IgM antibody (1+ agglutination reactions), what variables could you change to make the antigen–antibody reactions stronger in vitro?

Exercise 2.9
Why do IgM antibodies activate the classical pathway of complement more efficiently than IgG antibodies?

Exercise 2.10
Two students performed agglutination tests using the same antigen and antibody. One student observed a 1+ reaction after the immediate-spin reading, whereas the other student observed a 2+ reaction. What variables could cause the differences between these results? When would these differences have a significant impact on testing?

STUDY QUESTIONS

1. What cells can produce antibodies?
   a. natural killer cells
   b. T cells
   c. macrophages
   d. plasma cells

2. What term describes the number of antigen-binding sites per molecule of antibody?
   a. valency
   b. bivalent
   c. isotype
   d. idiotype

3. Select the term that describes the unique part of the antigen that is recognized by a corresponding antibody.
   a. immunogen
   b. epitope
   c. avidity
   d. clone

4. What classification of molecules does not make a good immunogenic substance?
   a. protein
   b. carbohydrate
   c. lipid
   d. glycoprotein

5. What is the chemical composition of an antibody?
   a. protein
   b. lipid
   c. carbohydrate
   d. glycoprotein

6. Where is the antigen located in a hemagglutination test?
   a. on the red cell membrane
   b. secreted by the red cell
   c. in the red cell nucleus
   d. in the plasma or serum

7. Which of the following situations can enhance hemagglutination reactions?
    a. testing at a temperature higher than 37° C
    b. increasing the incubation time
    c. increasing the antigen concentration
    d. making the pH greater than 7

8. What term describes molecules that bind to an antigen to increase phagocytosis?
    a. opsonins
    b. cytokines
    c. haptens
    d. isotypes

9. After performing a tube test, the supernatant of the test was pinkish and the red cell button was small. How do you interpret the result of this test?
    a. false-positive
    b. false-negative
    c. positive
    d. negative

10. How would you grade an agglutination reaction if you observe many small agglutinates in a background of free cells in tube testing?
    a. 1+
    b. 2+
    c. 3+
    d. 4+

11. To determine the presence of a red cell antibody in a patient's sample, what is the source of antigen?
    a. commercial reagent red cells
    b. commercial antisera
    c. patient serum
    d. patient red cells

12. How does complement activation demonstrate within the body?
    a. cell lysis
    b. enhanced cell clearance
    c. neutrophil activation
    d. generation of vasoactive amines
    e. all of the above

13. After addition of anti-A reagent to a patient's red cell suspension, agglutination was observed. The result with anti-B reagent was negative. What is the interpretation of this patient's ABO typing?
    a. patient is group B
    b. patient is group A
    c. cannot interpret this test
    d. false-positive result

For questions 14 through 25, match the characteristic with the correct immuno-globulin class.

Characteristic	Class
14. contains 10 antigen-binding sites	a. IgA
15. produced early in an immune response	b. IgG
16. found in mucosal linings	c. IgM
17. able to cross the placenta	d. IgE
18. highest plasma/serum concentration	
19. shape is a pentamer	
20. activates the complement cascade most efficiently	
21. can initiate allergic reactions	
22. associated with intravascular cell destruction	
23. detected with the antiglobulin test	
24. detected in the immediate-spin phase of the agglutination test	
25. reacts best at room temperature	

Answers to Study Questions can be found on page 387.

Ⓔ Additional student resources, including review questions, a laboratory manual, and case studies, can be found on the Evolve website.

REFERENCES

1. Abbas AK, Lichtman AH: *Basic immunology*, ed 3, Philadelphia, 2011, Saunders.
2. Murphy K: *Janeway's immunobiology*, ed 8, New York, 2012, Garland Science.
3. Klein HG, Anstee DJ: *Mollison's blood transfusion in clinical medicine*, ed 12, West Sussex, 2014, Wiley Blackwell.
4. Stevens CD: *Clinical immunology and serology*, ed 2, Philadelphia, 2003, FA Davis.
5. Fung MK: *Technical manual*, ed 18, Bethesda, 2011, AABB.
6. ISBT. http://www.isbtweb.org/fileadmin/user_upload/files-2015/red%20cells/links%20tables%20in%20introduction%20text/Table%20blood%20group%20antigens%20within%20systems%20v4.0%20141124.pdf. Accessed March 2015.
7. Reid ME, Lomas-Francis C, Olsson ML: *The blood group antigen facts book*, ed 3, San Diego, 2012, Academic Press.

BLOOD BANKING REAGENTS: Overview and Applications

3

CHAPTER OUTLINE

LEARNING OBJECTIVES

On completion of this chapter, the reader should be able to:

1. Describe the relationship of potency and specificity to blood banking reagents.
2. Compare and contrast polyclonal and monoclonal antibodies.
3. Describe the reagents available for ABO typing.
4. Describe the reagents available for D typing.
5. Define the low-protein reagent control and describe its purpose.
6. Describe the different types and purposes of reagent red cells.
7. Describe the basic principles of antiglobulin testing.
8. Distinguish between direct and indirect antiglobulin tests.
9. Identify the indications for implementing direct and indirect antiglobulin tests.
10. Discuss the different sources of possible errors in the performance of antiglobulin testing.
11. Compare and contrast the composition and appropriate uses of polyspecific and monospecific antiglobulin reagents.
12. Discuss the role of potentiators in routine testing.
13. Describe and differentiate the mechanism of action for the following potentiators: low-ionic-strength saline, bovine serum albumin, polyethylene glycol, and proteolytic enzymes.
14. Define and identify common lectins used in blood banking.
15. Compare and contrast the principles of gel technology, microplate techniques, and solid-phase red cell adherence techniques.
16. Analyze quality control data for performance criteria and acceptability.
17. Research product inserts and quality control procedures for product requirements.
18. Apply critical thinking skills to solve issues associated with reagent performance.

SECTION 1

INTRODUCTION TO BLOOD BANKING REAGENTS

As introduced in the previous chapter, reagent red cells and commercial antibodies are routinely used in the blood bank to detect antigen–antibody (Ag-Ab) reactions. These reagents are the tools of blood banking, allowing the provision of safe and viable blood products. Technologists using these tools require a technical knowledge of correct reagent use and the limitations of each reagent to interpret the results from patient and donor testing rapidly and accurately. A discussion of the composition, sources, uses, and limitations of reagents is presented after an overview of the regulatory aspects of reagent manufacturing. This chapter's goal is to introduce the reagents used in blood banking tests and discussed in subsequent chapters. The first part of this chapter will review blood bank reagents used in testing to detect agglutination in test tubes. The final section will introduce alternative methods that do not use the tube test.

There are several categories of reagents with differing functions:

- Reagent red cells: known red cell antigens
- Antisera: known red cell antibodies
- Antiglobulin reagents: anti-IgG or anti-C3d or a combination of anti-IgG and anti-C3d
- Potentiators to enhance antibodies

There are many manufacturers of blood bank reagents. Fig. 3.1 depicts routine blood bank reagents available commercially.

REGULATION OF REAGENT MANUFACTURE

As described in Chapter 1, the U.S. Food and Drug Administration (FDA) provides the regulations for the blood bank industry. These regulations touch all aspects of the industry, including the licensing of blood bank reagents: commercial antisera and reagent red cell products. The Center for Biologics Evaluation and Research (CBER) of the FDA certifies the reagents and provides licensure. The publication, *Code of Federal Regulations* (CFR), outlines the FDA criteria for the licensure of reagents in conjunction with other regulations for the manufacture of blood and blood components.[1]

The FDA has established minimum standards relating to product specificity and **potency** for use in blood banks and transfusion services before assignment of license to a commercial reagent. Specificity reflects the unique recognition of the antigenic determinant and

Potency: strength of an Ag-Ab reaction

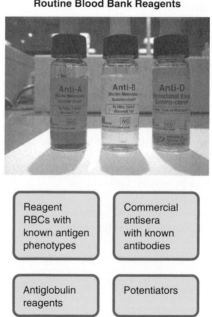

Routine Blood Bank Reagents

Reagent RBCs with known antigen phenotypes

Commercial antisera with known antibodies

Antiglobulin reagents

Potentiators

Fig. 3.1 Routine blood bank testing reagents.

its corresponding antibody molecule. For example, commercial anti-D reacts with red cells possessing D antigens and does not react with red cells lacking D antigens. Potency addresses the strength of the Ag-Ab reaction. For example, commercial anti-A reagents are manufactured to agglutinate strongly (3+ to 4+) with red cells possessing the A antigen.

When a manufacturer has shown that a product has met the FDA specificity and potency requirements, the reagent is assigned a product license number that is displayed on the product's label. Each product possesses a manufacturer's expiration date. According to FDA regulations, routine blood banking reagents cannot be used in testing after the expiration date. Exceptions to this rule can be made for rare antisera and red cells if the reagent has acceptable quality control results. If reagents are produced for in-house use (within the facility), a license is not required. In this situation, the FDA requirements for specificity and potency must be met and documented.

> Potency can also be related in the manufacture of blood components. Components are required to meet FDA-specified potency specifications.

Each manufacturer provides a package or product insert to the consumer that describes in detail the reagent, intended use, summary, principle, procedure for proper use, the specific performance characteristics, and the limitations of the reagent. Laboratory standard operating procedures (SOPs) are written to reflect the procedures outlined in these product inserts. As new reagent lots are received in the blood bank, the product inserts must be reviewed for any procedural changes. Any revisions must be incorporated into the SOPs before introduction of the reagent in routine testing. The total compliance with the manufacturer's directions cannot be overemphasized because that document details the appropriate procedures and recommends the appropriate reagent controls for accurate interpretation of test results (Box 3.1).

> Proper use of blood bank reagents requires a thorough understanding of the product inserts.

REAGENT QUALITY CONTROL

As introduced in Chapter 1, quality control is the term assigned to technical procedures to determine whether the analytical testing phase is working properly. Quality control includes checks on blood banking reagents and equipment before their use in tests on patient or donor samples. Requirements for quality control are obtained from regulations, accreditation standards, manufacturers' product inserts, and state and local requirements. Using these requirements, each laboratory establishes quality control protocols for the validation and documentation of reagent and equipment function. The quality control of reagents is performed daily on commercial reagent red cells and antisera. These reagents are tested to determine whether they meet preset acceptable performance criteria.[2]

Requirements for the acceptable performance of a reagent are outlined in the facility's SOP. Typically, the potency of the agglutination reaction defines the acceptability of the reagent's performance when challenged with the corresponding red cell antigen. For example, anti-A is tested against reagent red cells known to possess the A antigen. When the anti-A reagent and group A red cells are combined, a 3+ to 4+ reaction is expected for optimal reagent performance. When anti-A is reacted with group B red cells, no agglutination is expected. If agglutination results are less than 3+ in strength with group A red cells (eg, 2+ or less), the potency of the anti-A reagent may be deteriorating. The loss of agglutination strength over time is an indicator of a loss of potency, and the ability to detect A antigens in patient samples is potentially compromised.

BOX 3.1	Reagent Product Insert

The product insert must include the following:

- Description
- Procedure for proper use
- Interpretations
- Performance characteristics
- Limitations
- Quality control

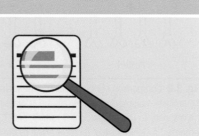

Antisera are visually inspected for any evidence of bacterial contamination. Any turbidity or cloudiness in the reagent bottles raises suspicion of a contaminated product. Reagent red cells are visually inspected for any evidence of hemolysis.

Reagents are tested daily for performance, and the results of quality control testing are recorded and reviewed. Records of quality control testing must be maintained, including results, interpretations, date of testing, and identity of personnel performing the testing. If reagents do not meet performance criteria, appropriate corrective actions are implemented.

SECTION 2
COMMERCIAL ANTIBODY REAGENTS

POLYCLONAL VERSUS MONOCLONAL ANTIBODY PRODUCTS

An ideal reagent antibody product contains a concentrated suspension of highly specific, well-characterized, uniformly reactive immunoglobulin molecules. Commercially prepared antibody reagents can be polyclonal antibody–based or monoclonal antibody–based products. If multiple clones of B cells secrete antibodies in an immunologic response to a foreign antigen, the antiserum produced is called polyclonal. If the antibody is the product of a single clone of B cells, the reagent produced is called monoclonal.

Polyclonal Antibody Reagents

Until the introduction of monoclonal antibody–based blood banking reagents in the early 1990s, commercial antisera were derived from polyclonal sources. The immunization of animals and humans with purified antigens was performed to obtain these reagents. Time-consuming separation techniques were used to produce the polyclonal antisera.

In the polyclonal immune response, B cells secrete antibodies that are specific for the multiple epitopes of the injected antigen. A heterogeneous population of antibodies is made, recognizing different epitopes on a single antigen. Examples of **polyclonal antiserum** produced for blood bank testing are known as antihuman globulin (AHG) reagents. These products contain multiple antibody specificities directed toward different antigens in the immunization injection or toward different parts of a purified antigen injected for an immune response.

Polyclonal antihuman IgG serum is produced by immunizing rabbits with purified human IgG molecules. The rabbits respond by activating multiple B-cell clones. Each B-cell clone produces an antibody directed at a specific epitope of the IgG molecule. The combination of the multiple B-cell clones secreting many antibodies in the rabbit serum makes a polyclonal antibody reagent (Fig. 3.2).

Polyclonal antiserum: made from several different clones of B cells that secrete antibodies of different specificities

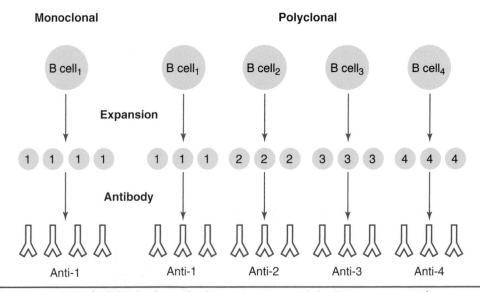

Fig. 3.2 Comparison of polyclonal and monoclonal immune responses. Polyclonal immune responses: After exposure to the antigen, multiple clones of B cells are activated by the immune response to secrete antibodies of different specificities. In this response to the antigen, anti-1, anti-2, anti-3, and anti-4 were secreted by different B-cell clones. Monoclonal immune responses: A single clone of B cells is active by the immune response and secretes an antibody with one specificity (anti-1).

Monoclonal Antibody Reagents

In contrast to polyclonal antisera, **monoclonal antibody** production creates an immortal clone that manufactures antibodies of a defined specificity (see Fig. 3.3). Monoclonal antibodies are manufactured in vitro using hybridoma technology. Monoclonal antibodies are the products of a single clone of B cells. Mice are immunized with antigen; cells from the spleens are harvested and fused with an abnormal cell from a mouse that has myeloma. The fused hybrid cells (**hybridomas**) are cultured, grow rapidly, and are screened for the production of antibody. Each hybridoma is descended from a single B-cell clone. All cells of the hybridoma cell line make the same antibody molecule, called a monoclonal antibody. In contrast to polyclonal antibodies, monoclonal antibodies recognize one specific epitope of the antigen. Murine (mouse) monoclonal antibodies have replaced polyclonal reagents in routine blood typing for A and B antigens and complement proteins.

In addition, human monoclonal antibodies are produced with blood group specificity. For their production, human B lymphocytes are transformed with **Epstein-Barr virus (EBV)**. These transformed cells can grow in tissue culture and secrete antibodies.[3] The first example of human monoclonal antibodies was derived by taking lymphocytes from D-immunized donors. Both IgG and IgM anti-D were obtained from the EBV-transformed cells.[4,5] Another method for the production of stable lines of human monoclonal antibodies is to fuse human lymphocytes with murine myelomas to form **heterohybridomas**.[3] A number of human monoclonal antibodies are now available for use in blood typing.

Monoclonal antibody–based reagents were introduced into the blood bank to replace polyclonal-based reagents because of necessity and desirability. Their introduction transformed the accuracy and cost of blood typing and shifted the procedure away from a dependence on reagents made from human blood donated by volunteers.[6] Examples of FDA-approved monoclonal antibodies include anti-A, anti-B, anti-A,B, anti-D, anti-C, anti-E, anti-c, anti-e, anti-IgG, anti-C3b, anti-C3d, and other blood group system antibodies. Monoclonal antibody reagents have the advantage of producing large quantities of the desired antibody with lot-to-lot consistency of a single specificity.[7] There are also some

Monoclonal antibody: made from single clones of B cells that secrete antibodies of the same specificity

Hybridomas: hybrid cells formed by the fusion of myeloma cells and antibody-producing cells; used in the production of monoclonal antibodies

Epstein-Barr virus (EBV): also called human herpesvirus 4 (HHV-4) and is one of eight viruses in the herpes family

Heterohybridomas: hybrid cells formed by the fusion of lymphocyte of one species with the myeloma cell of a different species

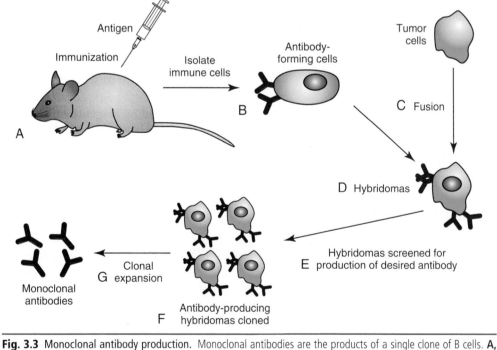

Fig. 3.3 Monoclonal antibody production. Monoclonal antibodies are the products of a single clone of B cells. **A,** Mice are immunized with antigen. **B,** The spleens are harvested for immune cells. **C,** The antibody-forming cells are fused with a tumor cell from a mouse in a process called fusion. **D,** Hybrid cells (hybridomas) are formed, cultured, and grow rapidly. **E,** The hybridomas are screened for the production of desired antibody. **F,** Each hybridoma is descended from a single B-cell clone. **G,** The hybridoma cell line is expanded and makes the same antibody molecule. (Modified from Immucor, Norcross, GA.)

BOX 3.2	Monoclonal Antibody Use Guidelines

Questions
- What clones are used in the formulation?
- What antigens do the antibodies detect?
- What are the typical reaction strengths?
- What antigens don't the antibodies detect?

Tech Tips
- Know characteristics of the clones
- Identify if single or blended clone product
- Read product inserts
- Know limitations for each reagent
- Remember that discrepant reactions are possible depending upon clone formulation

disadvantages to the use of monoclonal antibody reagents. When introduced into routine testing, discrepant reactions were noted between human- or animal-source reagents and the monoclonal antibody reagents. Confirmations of discrepant results with other manufacturers of monoclonal antibodies also produced different results.[8] A classic example of discrepant results due to the use of different monoclonal antibody reagents is D antigen typing.

Monoclonal antibody–based reagents are correctly used in serologic testing by following these guidelines:
- Careful review of the manufacturers' product inserts for proper use and product limitations
- Adherence to the manufacturer's directions for testing
- Recognition of the relevant characteristics of the hybridoma clone
  - Monoclonal antibodies may vary in the recognition of a red cell antigen because red cells might not express every antigenic determinant. Some monoclonal antibody reagents are blends of more than one monoclonal antibody to allow for better antigen recognition.
- Review of the manufacturer's formulation
  - Protein concentrations in the formulation of products produced by different manufacturers may vary. Most of these monoclonal antibody reagents possess a low concentration (3% to 8%) of protein.

These important considerations are summarized in Box 3.2. Scan the QR code for more information on monoclonal antibody reagents.

Monoclonal and Polyclonal Antibody Reagents

Monoclonal and polyclonal antibodies are also blended to produce reagents with specific advantages in blood bank testing. Antiglobulin reagents, discussed later in this chapter, can be a combination of rabbit polyclonal antibodies and a murine (mouse) monoclonal antibody.

The differences between monoclonal and polyclonal antibody–based reagents are summarized in Table 3.1.

REAGENTS FOR ABO ANTIGEN TYPING

Anti-A and anti-B commercial reagents are used to determine whether an individual's red cells possess the A and B antigens of the ABO blood group system. Donor or patient red cells (unknown antigen) are combined with commercial antisera (known antibodies) and observed for the presence or absence of agglutination. Agglutination indicates the presence of antigen; no agglutination indicates the absence of antigen on the red cells tested (Table 3.2).

Based on the testing results, an ABO blood type is assigned to the patient or donor. Four major blood **phenotypes** in the ABO blood group system exist: A, B, AB, and O. Group A individuals possess the A antigen and lack the B antigen. Group B individuals possess the B antigen and lack the A antigen. Group AB individuals possess both the A and B antigens. Group O individuals lack both the A and B antigens. The procedure to determine ABO blood group system assignment has been referred to as ABO grouping, ABO

Phenotype: observable expression of inherited traits

TABLE 3.1   Summary of Monoclonal and Polyclonal Antibody Products

MONOCLONAL ANTIBODY	POLYCLONAL ANTIBODY
Secreted by a single clone of antibody-producing B cells	Secreted by several different clones of antibody-producing B cells
One immunoglobulin class (IgG or IgM)	Mixture of IgM and IgG antibodies
Unique specificity for a particular epitope	Mixture of antibodies that may be directed at different epitopes of the same antigen

TABLE 3.2   ABO Red Cell Testing (ABO Forward Grouping)

ABO BLOOD GROUP ANTIGENS	REACTION WITH ANTI-A	REACTION WITH ANTI-B	ABO PHENOTYPE DEFINED
A	+	0	A
B	0	+	B
AB	+	+	AB
O	0	0	O

+, Agglutination; 0, no agglutination.

forward grouping, front typing, and ABO red cell testing. The *Technical Manual* of the AABB refers to the act of typing, or determining the ABO of an individual's red cells, as a type rather than a group.[9] This textbook adopts the AABB terminology and refers to the determination of an individual's ABO *type (phenotype)*, not an ABO *group*. Many other references retain the terminology of ABO grouping. The FDA name for these reagents remains ABO grouping reagents.

The first ABO red cell typing reagents were derived from pooled human plasma sources. The polyclonal antibodies were obtained from individuals who were stimulated with A or B blood group substances to produce antibodies of high titer. Blood bank reagent manufacturers use monoclonal antibodies to formulate ABO typing reagents. These ABO monoclonal antibody reagents are prepared to produce strong reactions with antigen-positive cells and detect weak expressions of the A and B antigens.[9]

The murine monoclonal antibody ABO typing reagents are tested to meet FDA potency and specificity requirements before licensure. The antibodies are suspended in a diluent that usually does not exceed a 6% bovine albumin concentration and is considered a low-protein medium. The commercial anti-A and anti-B red cell typing reagents demonstrate strong agglutination reactions (3+ to 4+) for most antigen-positive red cells. Testing is performed in **immediate-spin phases.** Manufacturers recommend that testing be confirmed by checking for expected **ABO antibodies** using reagent red cells. Anti-A always contains a blue dye, whereas anti-B contains a yellow dye. These dyes were added to reduce potential errors in testing. Anti-A,B is a blending of clones for A and B antigen recognition and is clear. ABO typing reagents are labeled with the antibody specificity and a phrase that specifies how the product can be used. For instance, a bottle of anti-A may contain the phrase "for slide, tube, and microplate testing." This statement specifies the test method in which the product may be used according to its FDA licensure. The detailed methods are provided in the product insert, along with the unique characteristics of each product. Scan the QR code for more information on monoclonal antibodies used in the manufacture of ABO commercial reagents.

Immediate-spin phases: source antigen and source antibody used in immunohematologic testing are combined, immediately centrifuged, and observed for agglutination

ABO antibodies: anti-A, anti-B, and anti-A,B; patients possess the ABO antibody to the ABO antigen lacking on their red cells (eg, group A individuals possess anti-B)

REAGENTS FOR D ANTIGEN TYPING

Of the antigens within the Rh blood group system, the D antigen is the most important in routine blood banking. The D antigen has been linked to adverse consequences in patients, including hemolytic transfusion reactions and hemolytic disease of the fetus and newborn (HDFN). Because of its increased immunogenicity as a blood group antigen, D antigen typing of all patient and donor samples is required by the AABB *Standards for Blood*

TABLE 3.3	Typing for D Antigen With Patient or Donor Red Cells	
D ANTIGEN	**REACTION WITH ANTI-D**	**REACTION WITH REAGENT CONTROL**
D-positive	+	0
D-negative	0	0
Cannot interpret typing	+	+

+, Agglutination; 0, no agglutination.

Banks and Transfusion Services.[10] This requirement enables the distinction of D-positive and D-negative individuals.

In the D typing procedure, commercial anti-D is combined with patient or donor red cells. Agglutination indicates the presence of the D antigen on the red cells tested (eg, D-positive), and no agglutination in these tests indicates absence of the D antigen (eg, D-negative). A negative reagent control ensures that a false-positive result is not present (Table 3.3).

Historically, reagents for D typing were obtained from various sources. The reagents were divided into two categories: high-protein and low-protein reagents. High-protein reagents of human polyclonal origin were first used for routine D typing. Low-protein reagents formulated with monoclonal anti-D antibodies or monoclonal and polyclonal antibody blends have replaced these high-protein reagents. Similar to ABO typing reagents, D typing reagents are labeled with the antibody specificity and a phrase that specifies how it can be used. This statement specifies the test method in which the product may be used according to its FDA licensure. The detailed methods and the unique characteristics of each product are provided in the product insert. In addition to D typing, similar products are available for the phenotyping of other antigens within the Rh blood group system, such as C, E, c, and e.

Monoclonal anti-D reagents possess a low-protein diluent formulation similar in protein concentration to the diluent of the ABO reagents (approximately 6% bovine albumin). Monoclonal anti-D reagents are derived from human-murine heterohybridoma sources, are IgM, and are often formulated with several different clones to ensure reactivity with the D antigen. Some manufacturers blend monoclonal (IgM) and polyclonal antibodies (IgG) to allow the detection of weak D antigen with the same reagent. The low-protein diluent does not promote the false-positive agglutination associated with the use of high-protein D typing reagents. These reagents do not require a separate Rh control test.

Discrepancies in D antigen phenotyping have occurred in patients because of different monoclonal antibody clone anti-D formulations used in reagent manufacture. Monoclonal antibody formulations for anti-D can vary in the ability to detect partial D antigen and weak D phenotypes. Transfusion service laboratories and blood banks may use different anti-D monoclonal antibody reagents. D typing discrepancies can be observed depending on the commercial source of anti-D. An understanding of the manufacturer's clone formulations and reagent limitations is important in the resolution of these discrepancies. A summary of the ABO and D phenotyping reagents is provided in Fig. 3.4. Scan the QR code for a picture of commercial Rh monoclonal antibody reagents.

LOW-PROTEIN REAGENT CONTROL

A reagent control is used to ensure that the typing results were interpreted correctly. The control should show no agglutination (a negative result). The ABO and D typing reagents are formulated with protein concentrations similar to human serum (approximately 6% bovine albumin). At this low-protein concentration, spontaneous agglutination of red cells occurs less frequently than with reagents formulated using higher concentrations of protein. Spontaneous agglutination of red cells can cause a false-positive result in typing. False-positive test results can also occur if strong cold **autoantibodies** or protein abnormalities are present in the blood specimen. A negative result using ABO low-protein

Autoantibodies: antibodies to self-antigens

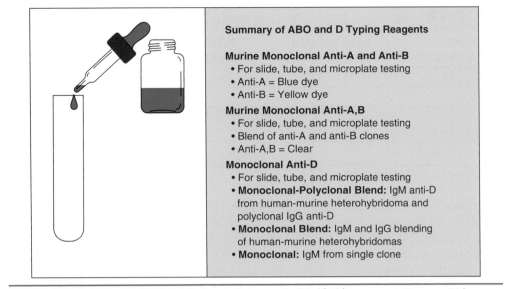

Summary of ABO and D Typing Reagents

Murine Monoclonal Anti-A and Anti-B
- For slide, tube, and microplate testing
- Anti-A = Blue dye
- Anti-B = Yellow dye

Murine Monoclonal Anti-A,B
- For slide, tube, and microplate testing
- Blend of anti-A and anti-B clones
- Anti-A,B = Clear

Monoclonal Anti-D
- For slide, tube, and microplate testing
- **Monoclonal-Polyclonal Blend:** IgM anti-D from human-murine heterohybridoma and polyclonal IgG anti-D
- **Monoclonal Blend:** IgM and IgG blending of human-murine heterohybridomas
- **Monoclonal:** IgM from single clone

Fig. 3.4 Summary of ABO and D phenotyping reagents. (Modified from Immucor, Norcross, GA.)

TABLE 3.4   Examples of Low-Protein Reagent Controls in ABO and D Typing

REACTION WITH ANTI-A	REACTION WITH ANTI-B	REACTION WITH ANTI-D	RED CELL ANTIGENS PRESENT	REAGENT CONTROL PRESENT?
+	0	+	A and D	Yes; no agglutination with anti-B
0	+	0	B	Yes; no agglutination with anti-A
0	+	+	B and D	Yes; no agglutination with anti-A
+	+	0	A and B	Yes; no agglutination with anti-D
+	+	+	Cannot interpret typing	No; reagent control must be tested to determine ABO and D typing results

+, Agglutination; 0, no agglutination.

reagents can serve as a reagent control. An additional reagent control in ABO and D typing is not essential if the patient or donor red cells show no agglutination with anti-A, anti-B, or anti-D in red cell testing. If red cells are agglutinated with anti-A, anti-B, and anti-D, a reagent control is required to interpret the results. The reagent control should be performed as described by the reagent manufacturer (Table 3.4).

> A control is required in tests with an antiglobulin phase, such as the weak D test, to prevent false-positive results in a patient with a positive direct antiglobulin test.

SECTION 3
REAGENT RED CELLS

A₁ AND B RED CELLS FOR ABO SERUM TESTING

Testing a patient's serum or plasma with commercial group A_1 and group B red cells confirms the ABO typing performed on the patient's red cells. Known as ABO reverse grouping or ABO serum testing, this procedure detects ABO antibodies. Patients possess the antibody directed against the antigen of the ABO system that is lacking on their red cells. Patients with A antigen on their red cells (eg, group A) possess the A antigen and lack the B antigen. These patients possess anti-B antibodies in their plasma. Serum or plasma samples from group A individuals agglutinate with reagent B red cells but not with reagent A_1 red cells. Patients with the B antigen on their red cells (eg, group B) possess the B antigen and lack the A antigen. These patients possess anti-A antibodies in their plasma. Serum or plasma samples from group B individuals agglutinate with reagent A_1 red cells but not with reagent B red cells. Compared with red cell testing with commercial anti-A and anti-B reagents, the ABO antibody results provide an additional confirmation or check of the assigned ABO typing (Table 3.5).

TABLE 3.5	ABO Serum Testing (Reverse Grouping)		
ABO BLOOD GROUP ANTIGENS	REACTION WITH REAGENT A_1 CELLS	REACTION WITH REAGENT B CELLS	ABO ANTIBODY DEFINED
A	0	+	Anti-B
B	+	0	Anti-A
AB	0	0	No anti-A or anti-B present
O	+	+	Anti-A and anti-B

+, Agglutination; 0, no agglutination.

Reagent red cells for serum testing are obtained from selected human donors and are manufactured in several optional packages. The most commonly used package consists of a two-vial set of A_1 and B red cells. Depending on the manufacturer, the red cell source may be obtained from either a single donor or a pool of several donors.

During the manufacturing process, all reagent red cells are washed to remove blood group antibodies and are resuspended to a 2% to 5% concentration in a buffered preservative solution to minimize hemolysis and loss of antigenicity during the dating period. These red cell preparations are usually negative for the Rh antigens D, C, and E. Each reagent lot is tested to meet the FDA standards of specificity; however, no potency standard requirement exists for this reagent. Reagent red cells should not be used if the red cells darken, spontaneously agglutinate in the reagent vial, or exhibit significant hemolysis. Scan the QR code for the ABO and D phenotyping procedure.

SCREENING CELLS

Screening cells are used in antibody screen (antibody detection) tests. This procedure looks for antibodies with specificity to red cell antigens in patient and donor samples. Patients and donors may have preformed antibodies to red cell antigens because of exposure to foreign red cell antigens from previous transfusions or pregnancies. For transfusion purposes, detection of these preformed red cell antibodies in a patient or donor sample is an important step in the provision of red cell products.

The reagent red cells are obtained from group O donor sources and are commercially available as two-vial or three-vial sets. Group O donors are selected because the group O phenotype lacks A and B antigens, and so these red cells do not react with ABO antibodies present in patient or donor serum or plasma. Serum or plasma from any ABO type may be used in the antibody screen test without interference from the ABO antibodies. Each vial in these sets represents the red cells harvested from a single donor. In addition, a product with pooled screening cells is commercially available and contains group O red cells derived from two donors in equal proportions.

According to the AABB *Standards for Blood Banks and Transfusion Services*, tests for antibodies performed on **recipient** specimens (eg, specimens of a patient who may be receiving a transfusion) require unpooled screening cells.[10] Recipient testing must maximize sensitivity to detect the presence of weakly reactive antibodies. Because a pooled red cell reagent decreases the ability to detect a weakly reactive antibody, this reagent is not recommended for recipient samples. Pooled screening cells are acceptable in screening donors for red cell antibodies.

Each lot of reagent screening cells arrives with an accompanying antigenic profile, or **antigram,** of each donor (Fig. 3.5). Screening cells licensed by the FDA require an antigenic profile capable of detecting most clinically significant red cell antibodies. Blood group antigens required on the screening cells include D, C, E, c, e, M, N, S, s, P_1, Le^a, Le^b, K, k, Fy^a, Fy^b, Jk^a, and Jk^b.[9] Diminished reagent reactivity may be observed as the screening cells approach the end of their dating period. Because of the danger of antigen deterioration, these screening cells should not be used beyond their expiration date. Any signs of significant hemolysis, discoloration, or agglutination might indicate contamination. Scan the QR code for the antibody screen test procedure.

Recipient: patient receiving the transfusion

Antigram: profile of antigen phenotypes for each donor used in the manufacture of commercially supplied screening and panel cells

	Rh							MNSs				P$_1$	Lewis		Lutheran		Kell		Duffy		Kidd					
Cell	D	C	E	c	e	f	Cw	M	N	S	s	P$_1$	Le^a	Le^b	Lu^a	Lu^b	K	k	Fy^a	Fy^b	Jk^a	Jk^b				
I R1R1 (56)	+	+	0	0	+	0	0	+	+	0	+	0	+	0	0	+	+	+	+	0	+	+				
II R2R2 (89)	+	0	+	+	0	0	0	0	+	+	0	+	0	+	0	+	0	+	0	+	+	0				

Fig. 3.5 Example of an antigram for commercial screening cells. The antigram is a profile of antigen phenotypes of each donor used in the screening cells. +, The antigen is present on the screening cell; 0, the antigen is absent on the screening cell.

ANTIBODY IDENTIFICATION PANEL CELLS

Reagent red cell antibody identification panels are required to determine the specificity of a red cell antibody in a blood banking procedure called antibody identification. Patient or donor serum/plasma is tested with the reagent panel cells to identify an antibody to red cell antigens. The antibody identification panel cells are individual group O donors packaged in sets of 10 or more, depending on the individual manufacturer. The selected donors for the identification panels possess the majority of the most frequently inherited red cell antigens. An antigenic profile of each donor is provided with each lot number of panel cells. A laboratory often has several in-dated panels to help resolve antibody problems. It is important to use the correct antigram according to the panel lot number when selecting the panel used for antibody identification. Scan the QR code for a picture of commercial panel cells.

SECTION 4
ANTIGLOBULIN TEST AND REAGENTS

PRINCIPLES OF ANTIGLOBULIN TEST

In 1945 Coombs, Mourant, and Race[11] showed that red cells may combine with antibodies without producing agglutination. These investigators prepared an antibody that reacted with human globulins (eg, a family of human proteins) and used this reagent to agglutinate antibody-coated red cells. The reagent was called AHG; the procedure is referred to as the antiglobulin test. This test is applied to many blood banking testing protocols and provides important information. The antiglobulin test is important because it detects IgG antibodies and complement proteins that have attached to red cells either in vitro or in vivo but do not produce visible agglutination.

The principle of the antiglobulin test is not complicated. The test uses a reagent that has been prepared by injecting animals (eg, rabbits) with human antibody molecules (human IgG) and complement proteins. In these animals, the injected proteins are recognized as foreign antigens, stimulating the animal's immune system to produce antibodies to human antibody molecules and complement proteins. The reagent, polyspecific AHG, contains antibodies to IgG molecules (anti-IgG) and complement proteins (anti-C3d, anti-C3b). This AHG reagent reacts with human IgG antibody and complement proteins, whether freely present in serum or bound to antigens on the red cells. It is essential that red cells be washed with physiologic saline to remove any unbound molecules before the addition of the AHG reagent. The washing step of an antiglobulin test requires the filling of test tubes with saline to mix with the red cells already present in the tube. The saline-suspended red cells are centrifuged. The saline wash is decanted, and this process is repeated for two to three additional cycles. On completion of the third or fourth wash, the saline is removed, and the tube is blotted dry to remove most traces of the saline.

Red cell washing is an important technical aspect in the performance of an antiglobulin test. If the test red cells are inadequately washed, any unbound antibody or complement present in the test can potentially bind to the AHG reagent and inhibit its reaction with antibody or complement molecules attached to the red cells. This effect is known as **neutralization** of the AHG reagent. Neutralization of the AHG reagent is a source of error in antiglobulin testing because it can mask a positive antiglobulin test.[9] To detect potential neutralization, IgG-sensitized cells are added to tubes with negative reactions. After centrifugation, a positive reaction should be observed to confirm that washing was adequate.

An antibody identification panel is performed when the antibody screen test is positive.

Three types of reagent red cells for routine testing include:
- A$_1$ and B cells in ABO serum testing
- Screening cells to detect red cell antibodies
- Panel cells to identify red cell antibodies

Neutralization: blocking antibody sites, causing a negative reaction

Neutralization causes false-negative AHG test results.

Sensitized: immunoglobulin or complement attached to the cells from the immune system (in vivo) or from a test procedure (in vitro)

Direct antiglobulin test: test used to detect antibody bound to red cells in vivo

Indirect antiglobulin test: test used to detect antibody bound to red cells in vitro

Autoimmune hemolytic anemia: immune destruction of autologous (self) red cells

After adequate red cell washing, the AHG reagent is added to the test. If the red cells in the test are **sensitized** with IgG or complement, the AHG reagent crosslinks the sensitized cells and causes agglutination. The anti-IgG in the AHG reagent attaches to the Fc portion of the IgG molecule that is bound to the red cell; the anti-C3 in the AHG reagent attaches to C3 molecules bound to the red cell as the consequence of complement activation. The formation of agglutinated red cells after the addition of AHG shows that IgG or complement proteins were attached to the red cells (Fig. 3.6). Agglutination is interpreted as a positive antiglobulin test. No agglutination at the completion of the antiglobulin test is interpreted as a negative antiglobulin test and indicates that no IgG or complement proteins were attached to the red cells.

Two types of antiglobulin tests are performed in the immunohematology laboratory: **direct antiglobulin test** (DAT) and **indirect antiglobulin test** (IAT). The distinction between these tests is often difficult for individuals entering this field because both tests use the AHG reagents. The DAT is a test in immunohematology to detect antibody bound to red cells in vivo or within the body. In contrast, the IAT is used in immunohematology testing to detect antibody bound to red cells in vitro or within a test tube.

Direct Antiglobulin Test

Under normal circumstances, red cells are not sensitized with either IgG or complement in vivo. The DAT is ordered to detect IgG or complement proteins bound to patient cells, which is a consequence of certain clinical events, including **autoimmune hemolytic anemia**, HDFN, a drug-related mechanism, or an antibody reaction to transfused red cells. A positive DAT is an important indicator of potential immune-mediated red cell destruction in the body. Because of IgG or complement attachment to red cells, macrophages are signaled to clear them using the mononuclear phagocytic system, particularly in the spleen. This event can signal immune destruction of red cells and often leads to anemia.

In the DAT procedure, the patient's red cells are first washed three or four times with physiologic saline to remove unbound proteins. The AHG reagent is added after the

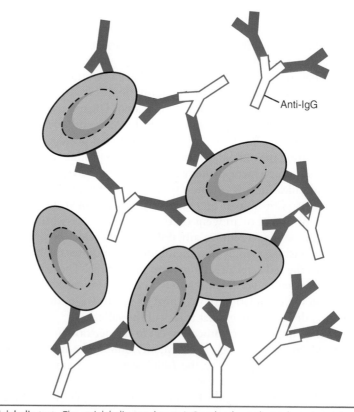

Anti-IgG

Fig. 3.6 Antiglobulin test. The antiglobulin test detects IgG molecules and complement protein molecules that have attached (sensitized) to red cells but have not resulted in a visible agglutination reaction. (Modified from Stroup MT, Treacy M: *Blood group antigens and antibodies,* Raritan, NJ, 1982, Ortho Diagnostic Systems, Inc.)

washing process. Agglutination with AHG reagent indicates that IgG antibodies, complement molecules, or both are bound to the patient's red cells. Agglutination after the addition of the AHG reagent is interpreted as a positive DAT (Fig. 3.7). If **polyspecific AHG reagent** is used, it can detect both IgG and complement molecules on the red cell. If the test result is positive, the test is repeated using **monospecific AHG reagents** that are specific for IgG and complement separately to determine which molecule was on the red cell. No agglutination after the addition of polyspecific AHG reagent is interpreted as a negative DAT. Retesting with monospecific AHG is unnecessary.

As noted earlier, a positive DAT detects attached antibody or complement from a clinical process or event (Table 3.6). Incubation is not necessary because the antibody was attached in vivo. The significance of a positive DAT should be assessed in relation to the patient's medical history and clinical condition.

The sample of choice for a DAT is collected in an ethylenediaminetetraacetic acid (EDTA) tube. Because complement can attach nonspecifically to red cells when samples are stored, it is important to use an anticoagulated EDTA sample when performing this test. Because EDTA negates the in vitro activation of the complement pathway, the test detects only complement proteins that have been bound to the red cells in vivo.[9] Complement proteins, attaching to red cells due to red cell storage, will not be detected when plasma is used. In addition, complement-dependent antibodies will not be detected when plasma is used. Scan the QR code for more information on the DAT procedure.

Polyspecific AHG reagent: contains both anti-IgG and anti-C3d antibodies and detects both IgG and C3d molecules on red cells

Monospecific AHG reagents: reagents prepared by separating the specificities of the polyspecific AHG reagents into individual sources of anti-IgG and anti-C3d/anti-C3b

Indirect Antiglobulin Test

The IAT is designed to detect in vitro sensitization of red cells. This test is a two-stage procedure. Antibodies first must combine with red cell antigens in vitro during an incubation step. In this first stage, a plasma source is incubated at body temperature with a red cell source to allow the attachment of IgG antibodies to specific red cell antigens. The red cell suspension is washed with physiologic saline to remove unbound antibody or complement proteins. After red cell washing, the AHG reagent is added to the test and centrifuged. Any agglutination at this step is interpreted as a positive IAT. A positive IAT indicates a specific reaction between an antibody in the serum/plasma and an antigen present on the red cells (Fig. 3.8). No agglutination at this step is interpreted as a negative IAT.

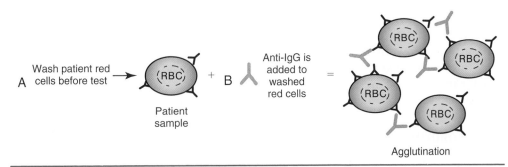

Fig. 3.7 Direct antiglobulin test. **A,** In the DAT, patient red cells are washed to remove unbound immunoglobulins. **B,** AHG reagent, either polyspecific or monospecific, is added. If either IgG or C3d molecules are present on the patient's red cells, agglutination is observed. The patient has a positive DAT result. (Modified from Immucor, Norcross, GA.)

TABLE 3.6 Clinical Examples Causing a Positive Direct Antiglobulin Test

CLINICAL CONDITION	CAUSED BY	SOURCE OF IgG
Transfusion reaction	Donor cells coated with IgG	Recipient (patient) antibody
Hemolytic disease of the fetus and newborn	Fetal red cells coated with IgG	Maternal antibody crossing the placenta
Autoimmune hemolytic anemia	IgG or C3 on patient red cells	Patient autoantibody
Drug-related mechanism	IgG-drug complex attached to cells	Immune complex formed with drug

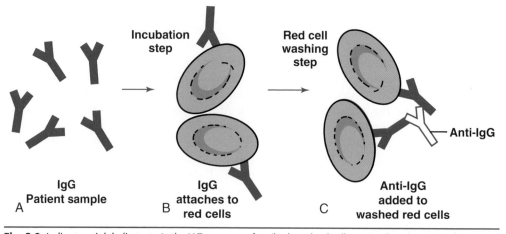

Fig. 3.8 Indirect antiglobulin test. In the IAT, a source of antibody and red cells are incubated at 37° C for a specified time to allow Ag-Ab reactions to occur. After incubation, the red cells are washed to remove unbound molecules. AHG reagent, monospecific anti-IgG is added. If IgG is present on the red cells, agglutination is observed. The result is a positive IAT. (Modified from Stroup MT, Treacy M: *Blood group antigens and antibodies,* Raritan, NJ, 1982, Ortho Diagnostic Systems, Inc.)

Reaction phase: observation of agglutination at certain temperatures, after incubation, or after addition of AHG

The IAT is routinely used in immunohematology in testing both patient and donor samples. Several immunohematologic tests incorporate an indirect antiglobulin **reaction phase** in their procedures. These procedures include antibody screening, antibody identification, crossmatching, and antigen typing (Table 3.7). All of these procedures are important in the immunohematology laboratory and are discussed in subsequent chapters. Table 3.8 compares the DAT and IAT procedures. Scan the QR code for more information on the IAT procedure.

SOURCES OF ERROR IN ANTIGLOBULIN TESTING

Sources of error in antiglobulin testing can lead to either false-negative or false-positive results. A false-negative result is a test result that incorrectly indicates a negative reaction. In the antiglobulin test, no agglutination is observed, yet the red cells in the test are sensitized with IgG or complement. An Ag-Ab reaction has occurred but is not shown in testing. Conversely, a false-positive result is a test result that incorrectly indicates a positive reaction. In antiglobulin testing, agglutination is observed, but the red cells in the test are not sensitized with IgG or complement. No Ag-Ab reaction has occurred in testing. With careful attention to the test procedures, individuals who perform the AHG tests can avoid many of these false-positive and false-negative results. Common sources of error in antiglobulin testing are summarized in Tables 3.9 and 3.10.[5]

ANTIGLOBULIN REAGENTS

The antiglobulin test is important for the detection of IgG antibodies and complement proteins that have attached to the red cells but have not resulted in visible agglutination. Two categories of antiglobulin reagents exist: polyspecific and monospecific. The AHG reagents can be either monoclonal antibody products or polyclonal antiserum products.

Polyspecific Antihuman Globulin Reagents

Polyspecific AHG reagents are used primarily in the DAT to determine that either IgG or complement molecules have attached to the red cells in vivo. This reagent contains both anti-IgG and anti-C3d antibodies and detects both IgG and C3d molecules on red cells. The detection of either IgG or C3d is a positive DAT result indicating the red cells were sensitized in vivo as a result of a clinical event (ie, an immune response to a foreign antigen). Several reagent preparations are commercially available for polyspecific products derived from either polyclonal or monoclonal antibody sources. Other complement antibodies may also be present, including anti-C3b. All these products meet the FDA requirements for licensure.

TABLE 3.7 Applications of Indirect Antiglobulin Test in the Immunohematology Laboratory

PROCEDURE	PURPOSE
Antibody screening	Detects antibodies with specificity to red cell antigens
Antibody identification	Identifies specificity of red cell antibodies
Crossmatch	Determines serologic compatibility between donor and patient before transfusion
Antigen typing	Identifies a specific red cell antigen in a patient or donor

TABLE 3.8 Comparison of Direct Antiglobulin Test and Indirect Antiglobulin Test Procedures

DIRECT ANTIGLOBULIN TEST	INDIRECT ANTIGLOBULIN TEST
Detects IgG- and complement-coated red cells	Detects IgG- and complement-coated red cells
IgG attachment to red cells has occurred within the patient's body	IgG attachment to red cells occurred during the incubation step
One-stage procedure	Two-stage procedure
Patient's red cells are tested with antiglobulin reagent without an incubation step	Test requires an incubation step before the addition of antiglobulin reagent
Test for certain clinical conditions: hemolytic disease of the fetus and newborn, hemolytic transfusion reaction, and autoimmune hemolytic anemia	Used as a reaction phase of several tests in immunohematology: antibody screen and antibody identification panel

TABLE 3.9 Common Sources of False-Positive Error in Antiglobulin Testing

FALSE-POSITIVE	POSSIBLE EXPLANATIONS
Red cells are agglutinated before washing step and addition of antihuman globulin reagent	Potent cold reactive antibody of patient origin
Use of dirty glassware	Particles or contaminants
Improper centrifugation—overcentrifugation	Red cell button packed so tightly on centrifugation that nonspecific clumping cannot be dispersed

TABLE 3.10 Common Sources of False-Negative Error in Antiglobulin Testing

FALSE-NEGATIVE	POSSIBLE EXPLANATIONS
Failure to wash cells adequately during the test procedure before the addition of AHG reagent	Unbound human serum globulins neutralize AHG reagent
Testing is interrupted or delayed; AHG reagent is not added immediately after washing	Bound IgG or complement molecules may detach from the coated red cells
Failure to identify weak positive reactions	Technical error in testing
Loss of reagent activity	Improper reagent storage, bacterial contamination, or contamination with human serum
Failure to add AHG reagent	Technical error in testing
Improper centrifugation: undercentrifugation	Conditions for promoting agglutination are not optimal
Inappropriate red cell concentrations—red cell suspensions fall outside the optimal 2%-5%	Concentration of red cells influences the agglutination reaction

AHG, Antihuman globulin.

Monospecific Antihuman Globulin Reagents

Monospecific AHG reagents are used in the investigation of a positive DAT to determine the nature of the molecules attached to the red cells. Are the patient's red cells sensitized with IgG, complement, or both proteins? To answer this question, a **differential DAT** is performed with monospecific AHG reagents using individual sources of anti-IgG and anti-C3d/anti-C3b (Table 3.11). Monospecific AHG reagents are prepared by separating the specificities of the polyspecific AHG reagents.

Anti-IgG monospecific AHG products contain antibodies to human gamma chains. They are commercially available as either polyclonal or monoclonal antibody products. Often these products are labeled heavy-chain specific, meaning that the antiserum contains antibodies specific for the gamma heavy chains of the IgG molecule. Products without this label may contain antibodies that react with immunoglobulin light chains. Recall from the immunology discussion that immunoglobulin light chains (kappa and lambda) are common to all immunoglobulin classes (eg, IgG, IgM, IgA). In addition to their use in the investigation of a positive DAT, anti-IgG reagents are used in many laboratories for antibody detection, antibody identification, and crossmatching procedures.

Anti-C3b and anti-C3d monospecific reagents contain no reactivity to human immunoglobulin molecules. These reagents specifically detect complement proteins that attach to the red cell surface because of the activation of the complement's classical pathway. Activation of the complement pathway can lead to red cell destruction in vivo through either intravascular hemolysis or extravascular hemolysis. For the detection of any complement proteins bound in vivo, a product requires specificity for the C3d fragment. This fragment of complement is usually the only protein that remains attached to the patient's red cells. Anti-C3d is commercially available as either polyclonal or monoclonal antibody products. The antiglobulin reagents are summarized in Fig. 3.9.

IgG-Sensitized Red Cells

The AABB *Standards for Blood Banks and Transfusion Services*[10] requires a control system for antiglobulin tests interpreted as negative. The control system consists of red cells that have been commercially prepared with IgG antibodies attached. The addition of IgG-sensitized red cells to negative AHG tests is required for antibody detection and crossmatch procedures. This control is often referred to as check cells or Coombs control cells. Because antiglobulin testing has its own set of test limitations that might affect interpretation of results, IgG-sensitized red cells were designed as an additive system for negative antiglobulin tests to control the possibility of false-negative results. On addition to a negative AHG test, the IgG-sensitized red cells should react with the AHG reagent and show agglutination (Fig. 3.10).

IgG-sensitized red cells cannot provide assurance that all causes of false-negative results are controlled. Following are three potential reasons for a false-negative result detected by the use of IgG-sensitized red cells in an antiglobulin test:
• Failure to add the antiglobulin reagent to the test
• Failure of the added antiglobulin reagent to react
• Failure to wash red cells adequately

TABLE 3.11	Differential Direct Antiglobulin Test Procedure	
INTERPRETATION	**MONOSPECIFIC ANTI-IgG**	**MONOSPECIFIC ANTI-C3d**
Patient red cells sensitized with IgG only	+	0
Patient red cells sensitized with IgG and C3d	+	+
Patient red cells sensitized with C3d only	0	+

+, Agglutination; *0*, no agglutination.

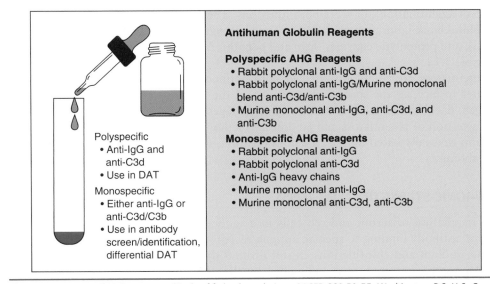

Antihuman Globulin Reagents

Polyspecific AHG Reagents
• Rabbit polyclonal anti-IgG and anti-C3d
• Rabbit polyclonal anti-IgG/Murine monoclonal blend anti-C3d/anti-C3b
• Murine monoclonal anti-IgG, anti-C3d, and anti-C3b

Monospecific AHG Reagents
• Rabbit polyclonal anti-IgG
• Rabbit polyclonal anti-C3d
• Anti-IgG heavy chains
• Murine monoclonal anti-IgG
• Murine monoclonal anti-C3d, anti-C3b

Polyspecific
• Anti-IgG and anti-C3d
• Use in DAT

Monospecific
• Either anti-IgG or anti-C3d/C3b
• Use in antibody screen/identification, differential DAT

Fig. 3.9 Summary of AHG reagents. (*Code of federal regulations*, 21CFR 660.50-55, Washington, DC, U.S. Government Printing Office, revised annually. Illustration modified from Immucor, Norcross, GA.)

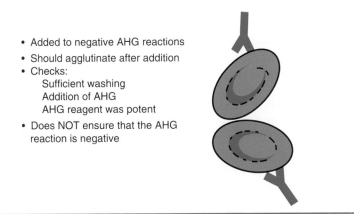

• Added to negative AHG reactions
• Should agglutinate after addition
• Checks:
  Sufficient washing
  Addition of AHG
  AHG reagent was potent
• Does NOT ensure that the AHG reaction is negative

Fig. 3.10 IgG sensitized red cells.

SECTION 5
PRINCIPLES OF ANTIBODY POTENTIATORS AND LECTINS

As discussed in Chapter 2, the zeta potential, or the force of repulsion between red cells in a physiologic saline solution, exerts an influence on the agglutination reaction. Because of the larger size, pentameric shape, and multivalent properties of IgM molecules, agglutination is facilitated between adjacent red cells that have IgM attached to them. IgM antibodies can easily react in a saline medium. In contrast, IgG antibody molecules are smaller and less able to span the distance between adjacent red cells generated by the zeta potential. IgG molecules may attach, but visible agglutination might not occur.

Antibody potentiators, or **enhancement media,** are commercially available reagents that enhance the detection of IgG antibodies by increasing their reactivity. Enhancement media can reduce the zeta potential of the red cell membrane by adjusting the in vitro test environment to promote agglutination. Potentiators enhance the detection of Ag-Ab complex formation in routine tests. In this role, potentiators may enhance antibody uptake (first stage of agglutination), promote direct agglutination (second

Antibody potentiators: reagents or methods that enhance or speed up the antibody–antigen reaction

Enhancement media: reagents that enhance or speed up the antibody–antigen reaction

Proteolytic enzymes: enzymes that denature certain proteins

stage of agglutination), or serve both functions. The major types of potentiators used in the blood bank laboratory include low-ionic-strength saline (LISS), polyethylene glycol (PEG), and **proteolytic enzymes** (ficin and papain). A summary of these reagents is found in Table 3.12.

Potentiators are commonly used in both antibody screening and identification procedures to increase the speed and sensitivity of the antibody attachment to the red cell antigen. Each method has limitations and advantages, which are explained in this section. The selection of potentiators and laboratory methods for antibody detection and identification is usually based on the patient population, workload, and degree of expertise in the laboratory.

LOW-IONIC-STRENGTH SALINE (LISS)

The incubation of serum and red cells in a reduced ionic environment increases the rate of antibody binding to specific antigen receptor sites on red cells.[12] In physiologic saline, sodium and chloride ions cluster around the antigen and antibody molecules. Ag-Ab complex formation is influenced by the attraction of opposite charges, and the clustering of these free sodium and chloride ions hinders the complex formation. When the ionic strength is reduced, the antigen and antibody molecules are capable of combining at a faster rate.[13] In 1974 Löw and Messeter[14] applied this principle in routine testing to detect unknown red cell antibodies by using LISS as the suspending medium for red cells (the source of known antigens in the test). Other investigators confirmed that LISS enhanced antibody reactions, especially in the indirect antiglobulin phases of testing.[15]

The low-ionic environment may happen in two ways:
* Suspending red cells of the test in LISS reagent
* Using additive LISS reagent in conjunction with saline-suspended red cells

The LISS reagent contains sodium chloride, glycine, and salt-poor albumin (approximately 0.03 M) ionic strength compared with saline (approximately 0.17 M) and is formulated to prevent hemolysis of red cells, which is a concern when using LISS.[16] In addition, some low-ionic–saline solution reagents may contain macromolecular additives to potentiate the direct agglutination of antigen-positive red cells by some antibodies. The reagent supplies a low-ionic environment to enhance antibody uptake and improve detection at antiglobulin phases of testing. The result is sensitization or the potentiation of the first stage in the agglutination reaction. The advantage of the increased antibody uptake is the reduction of incubation time and time to a result.

LISS is a commonly used potentiator with the antibody screen because it speeds the agglutination, is economical, and provides good sensitivity. However, LISS testing also has several disadvantages. Increasing serum in the test alters the ionic strength of a LISS procedure, decreasing the sensitivity of the test system. LISS also has been observed to enhance cold autoantibodies, especially if the tubes are centrifuged at immediate-spin and microscopic evaluations are performed.

TABLE 3.12 Summary of Antibody Potentiators	
POTENTIATOR	**MECHANISM OF ACTION**
Low-ionic-strength saline (LISS)	Increases rate of antibody uptake
Polyethylene glycol (PEG)	Concentrates the antibody in the test environment in LISS
Proteolytic enzymes (papain and ficin)	Removes negative charges from the red cell membrane, which reduces the zeta potential; denatures some red cell antigens
Bovine serum albumin (BSA)	Reduces the repulsion between cells but does not shorten the incubation time

POLYETHYLENE GLYCOL (PEG)

PEG additive in a low-ionic-saline medium effectively concentrates antibody in the test mixture, while creating a low-ionic environment that enhances the rate of antibody uptake. The enhancement medium is a water-soluble polymer, which has been reported to increase the sensitivity of the IAT.[16] The PEG reagent removes water molecules in the test environment to allow a greater probability of collision between antigen and antibody molecules.[17,18] Because PEG can directly affect the aggregation of red cells, the reagent can be used only in indirect antiglobulin testing. Tubes should not be centrifuged and read before washing. Only monospecific anti-IgG AHG reagent is suitable for use with PEG because of reports of nonspecific agglutination with polyspecific AHG reagents.

PEG increases the sensitivity of antibody detection and identification and often detects the presence of antibodies not found with bovine serum albumin or LISS. Antibodies generally considered of little clinical significance (IgM in nature) do not react well or at all with this potentiator. PEG has been observed to enhance warm autoantibodies, which is an important consideration when using this potentiator.

> LISS and PEG are commonly used as potentiators in routine blood bank testing.

ENZYMES

Proteolytic enzymes commonly used in the immunohematology laboratory include papain, ficin, and bromelin, all of which are commercially available. The term proteolytic refers to the breakdown of protein molecules. These enzymes possess the property to modify red cell membranes by removing the negatively charged molecules from the red cell membrane and denaturing certain antigenic determinants. The loss of these negatively charged molecules reduces the zeta potential and enhances the agglutination of some antigens to their corresponding antibodies. If the antibody specificity is in the Rh, Kidd, and Lewis blood group systems, there is an enhanced reaction using enzymes. Certain other red cell antigens are denatured when exposed to these proteolytic enzymes. These red cell antigens include M, N, S, Xg^a, Fy^a, and Fy^b. Depending on the red cell antibody, the use of enzymes in testing may enhance, depress, or inhibit entirely the Ag-Ab complex formation. A good knowledge of the blood group systems aids in the interpretation of these enzyme tests.

Proteolytic enzymes (ficin or papain) are not usually used as potentiators in the screen because they eliminate some antigens from the red cells. Enzymes can be used as additional tools for investigating complex antibody problems, but they should never be the sole method. Enzymes may enhance the reactions of one antibody in a mixture of antibodies or abolish the reactions, which lends important information in the solution of the problem. Enzymes enhance cold and warm autoantibodies.

> Proteolytic enzymes originate from plants: Ficin comes from figs, bromelin from pineapple, and papain from papaya.

BOVINE SERUM ALBUMIN (BSA)

BSA is prepared from bovine serum or plasma and is commercially available in either a 22% or a 30% concentration. This reagent's use as a potentiator is less common than other enhancement media. In contrast to LISS, BSA does not promote the antibody uptake stage of agglutination, but it influences the second stage by allowing antibody-sensitized cells to become closer together than is possible in a saline medium without additives. The addition of BSA to reaction tubes favors the direct agglutination of Rh antibodies and enhances the sensitivity of the IAT for a wide range of antibody specificities. For optimal results, increased incubation time is necessary. BSA does not enhance warm autoantibodies, which is beneficial in working with samples from patients with autoantibodies in their serum.

BSA reduces the repulsion between cells but does not shorten the incubation time. The enhancement properties of BSA are explained with several theories. Pollack et al[19] suggested that albumin reduces the zeta potential by dispersing some of the positively charged ions surrounding each negatively charged red cell. In this theory, albumin increases the dielectric constant of the medium, defined as a measure of the ability to dissipate a charge.

TABLE 3.13	Summary of Common Lectins in the Blood Bank
LECTIN	**ANTIGEN SPECIFICITY**
Dolichos biflorus	A_1
Ulex europaeus	H
Vicia graminea	N
Iberis amara	M

Other investigators believe that albumin bound to the cell membrane affects the degree of water hydration of the red cell membrane itself.[20]

LECTINS

Lectins: plant extracts useful as blood banking reagents; they bind to carbohydrate portions of certain red cell antigens and agglutinate the red cells

Lectins are useful alternatives to antisera for blood typing purposes in blood group serology. They were first discovered in plants but have also been found in bacteria to mammals.[3] Extracts of seeds have specificity toward certain red cell antigens. These extracts contain proteins that behave in a manner identical to that of antibodies but are not immunoglobulin in nature. Lectins bind specifically to the carbohydrate determinants of certain red cell antigens with resultant agglutination. Although no antibodies exist in these reagents, lectins can be useful in identifying antigens present on patient or donor red cells. Table 3.13 reviews the major lectins used in blood group serology.

Lectins are not antibodies. Lectins are sugar-binding proteins of nonimmune origin. For example, a lectin from the eel *Anguilla anguilla* is a useful anti-H reagent.

SECTION 6
ALTERNATIVE METHODS TO THE TUBE TEST

Blood bank reagents were designed to detect agglutination in the classic tube test. Other commercially available methods for detecting Ag-Ab reactions use different techniques. This section presents a brief overview of these techniques. Chapter 10 will provide more details on these methods.

GEL TECHNOLOGY METHOD

The FDA licensed gel technology by Micro Typing Systems, Inc. (Pompano Beach, Florida) as the ID-MTS Gel Card in 1994. Developed by Lapierre et al[21] in 1985, the technology uses dextran acrylamide gel particles to trap agglutinated red cells. Lapierre et al developed gel technology to standardize traditional tube testing methods. Tube-shaking techniques to resuspend the red cell button in tube testing vary among technologists. This technical variation affects the grading and interpretation of the test results. Gel technology provides stable and defined endpoints of hemagglutination, providing a method where objective and consistent interpretations of agglutination are possible. Refer to Fig. 3.11 for a picture of a gel card and gel reactions.

MICROPLATE TESTING METHODS

Since the late 1960s, microplate methods have been used for routine processing in blood donor centers. A microtiter plate with 96 wells serves as the substituted test tubes to which the principles of blood banking are applied. Each well is considered a short test tube. The microplate technique can be adapted to red cell antigen testing or serum testing for antibody detection. The principles that apply to agglutination in test tubes also apply to testing in microplate methods. The microplate may have either a U-shaped or a V-shaped bottom in the microtiter plate well; the U-bottom well is more widely used (Fig. 3.12). Small quantities of red cells and antisera are added to the microtiter wells, followed by centrifugation of the microtiter plates. The cell buttons are resuspended

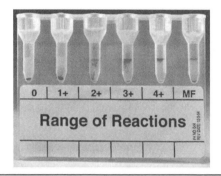

Fig. 3.11 Gel test. Range of reactions in gel testing. The agglutination reaction is graded from 4+ to 0. The assigned grade is dependent on the position of the red cells in the gel microtube. (Courtesy Ortho Clinical Diagnostics, Raritan, NJ, and Micro Typing Systems, Pompano Beach, FL.)

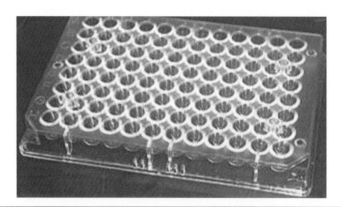

Fig. 3.12 Microtiter plate method. Microtiter plate wells are used to add reagents and samples for hemagglutination tests. (Courtesy Thermo Fisher Scientific, Rochester, NY.)

by manually tapping the plate or with the aid of a mechanical shaker. A concentrated button of red cells is indicative of Ag-Ab reactions, whereas the red cells in a negative result are dispersed throughout the well. Automated photometric devices are available to read and interpret the reactions on the plates. Alternatively, the microtiter plates may be observed for a streaming pattern of red cells when the plate is placed on an angle[9] (Fig. 3.13).

SOLID-PHASE RED CELL ADHERENCE METHODS

Another method used in blood bank testing is solid-phase red cell adherence.[22] Commercial solid-phase test procedures have been available for the detection of both red cell and platelet antibodies since the late 1980s (Capture; Immucor, Norcross, Georgia). This technology uses microplate test wells with immobilized reagent red cells. Solid-phase technology is licensed for antibody screening, antibody identification, and compatibility testing. As previously identified with gel technology, the major advantages of solid-phase technology include standardization and stable, defined endpoints, leading to more objective and consistent interpretations of agglutination reactions. This technology is also suitable for automation, and blood bank instrumentation is available.

The antigen or antibody is immobilized to the bottom and sides of the microplate wells. In a direct test, the antibody is fixed to the wells. Antigen-positive red cells from donor or patient sources adhere to the sides and bottom of the wells. Antigen-negative red cells from donor or patient sources settle to the bottom of the well and form a red cell button after centrifugation. In an indirect test, red cell membranes are bound to the wells.

Microtiter Plate Assay

- 1 drop of anti-A and 1 drop of anti-B are placed in separate wells of a U-bottom microplate.
- 1 drop of a 2% to 5% saline suspension of red cells is added to each well.
- Wells are mixed by gently tapping them.
- The plate is centrifuged at an appropriate time and speed.
- The cell button is resuspended by manually tapping the plate or using a mechanical shaker or placed at an angle for the tilt and stream method.
- Reactions are read, interpreted, and recorded.

A

Reactions of Microplate Testing

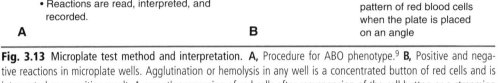

Negative reaction well

Positive reaction well

Positive Reaction: A concentrated button of red blood cells

Negative Reaction: Smooth suspension of red blood cells or a streaming pattern of red blood cells when the plate is placed on an angle

B

Fig. 3.13 Microplate test method and interpretation. **A,** Procedure for ABO phenotype.[9] **B,** Positive and negative reactions in microplate wells. Agglutination or hemolysis in any well is a concentrated button of red cells and is interpreted as a positive result. A smooth suspension of red cells after resuspension of the cell button or a streaming pattern of red cells when the plate is placed on an angle is interpreted as no agglutination and a negative test result.

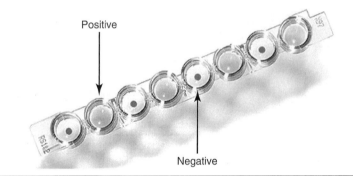

Positive

Negative

Fig. 3.14 Solid-phase red cell adherence reactions. (Courtesy Immucor, Norcross, GA.)

Microplate techniques apply the same principle of hemagglutination as the tube test. In contrast, solid-phase technology reactions are opposite. A positive reaction is adherence to the wells; a negative reaction is a red cell button.

Unknown patient or donor serum is added and allowed to react. This step allows for the capture of IgG antibodies from the patient or donor serum to the red cell membranes. A washing step removes unbound IgG antibodies followed by the addition of anti-IgG–coated indicator red cells. In a positive indirect test, the indicator cells adhere to the sides and bottom of the well. In a negative indirect test, the indicator cells settle to the bottom of the wells and form a red cell button after centrifugation (Fig. 3.14).

CHAPTER SUMMARY

- The reagents used in the immunohematology laboratory provide the tools to detect Ag-Ab reactions.

Regulation of Reagent Manufacture

- The FDA provides the regulations for the licensing of blood bank reagents: commercial antisera and reagent red cell products.
- The FDA has established minimum standards relating to product specificity and potency.
- Potency in blood banking reagents refers to the strength of an Ag-Ab reaction.
- Specificity in blood banking reagents refers to recognition of antigen and antibody to make the Ag-Ab reaction.
- A package or product insert describes in detail the reagent, intended use, summary, principle, procedure for proper use, the specific performance characteristics, and the limitations of the reagent.

Reagent Quality Control

- The quality control of reagents is performed daily on commercial reagent red cells and antisera.
- Reagents are tested to determine whether they meet preset acceptable performance criteria.
- Records of quality control testing must be maintained, including results, interpretations, date of testing, and identity of personnel performing the testing.

Commercial Antibody Reagents

- Polyclonal antibodies are made from several different clones of B cells that secrete antibodies of different specificities.
- Monoclonal antibodies are made from a single clone of B cells that secretes antibodies of the same specificity.
- Reagents for ABO typing are derived from monoclonal antibody sources and may be blended to create reagents that recognize the corresponding A or B antigen. These reagents contain IgM antibodies in a low-protein environment.
- Reagents for D typing are derived from monoclonal antibody sources and may be monoclonal antibody blends or monoclonal-polyclonal antibody blends. The reagents can contain either IgM or IgG antibodies in a low-protein environment.
- The low-protein control reagent checks for the presence of spontaneous agglutination of patient or donor red cells in testing. The control should always show no agglutination.

Reagent Red Cells

- Reagent red cells are used as sources of antigen in antibody screens, ABO reverse grouping, and antibody identification tests.

Antiglobulin Test and Reagents

- The antiglobulin test detects IgG molecules and complement protein molecules that have attached (sensitized) to red cells but have not resulted in a visible agglutination reaction.
- The DAT detects antibody or complement molecules that have sensitized red cells because of a clinical event within the body.
- The IAT requires an incubation step for sensitization and is an in vitro test. The IAT is commonly used in antibody screens, antibody identification, and testing of donor and recipient compatibility.
- The AHG test can possess sources of error that cause false-positive or false-negative AHG test results. Recognition and prevention of these sources of error aid the correct interpretation of the AHG test result.
- Polyspecific AHG reagents are used primarily in direct antiglobulin testing to determine whether IgG or complement molecules have attached to the red cells in vivo. This reagent contains both anti-IgG and anti-C3d antibodies and detects both IgG and C3d molecules on red cells.
- Monospecific AHG reagents are used in the investigation of a positive DAT to determine the nature of the molecules attached to the red cells. Monospecific AHG reagents are prepared by separating the specificities of the polyspecific AHG reagents into individual sources of anti-IgG and anti-C3d/anti-C3b.

Antibody Potentiators and Lectins

- Antibody potentiators, or enhancement media, are commercially available reagents that enhance the detection of IgG antibodies by increasing their reactivity. Examples of enhancement media include LISS, PEG, BSA, and enzymes.
- Enhancement media can reduce the zeta potential of the red cell membrane by adjusting the in vitro test environment to promote agglutination.
- Enhancement media improve the detection of Ag-Ab complex formation. In this role, potentiators may enhance antibody uptake (first stage of agglutination), promote direct agglutination (second stage of agglutination), or serve both functions.
- Lectins are plant or other extracts that bind to carbohydrate portions of certain red cell antigens and agglutinate the red cells. Although no antibodies exist in these reagents, lectins can be useful in identifying antigens present on patient or donor red cells.

Alternative Methods to the Tube Test

- Gel technology uses gel particles combined with diluent or reagents to trap agglutination reactions within the gel matrix.
- Microplate techniques use a microtiter plate with 96 wells to serve as the substituted test tubes. The microplate technique can be adapted to red cell antigen testing or serum testing for antibody detection. The principles that apply to agglutination in test tubes also apply to testing in microplate methods.
- In solid-phase red cell adherence testing, the antigen or antibody is immobilized to the bottom and sides of the microplate wells. IgG antibodies or red cell antigens adhere to the microplate wells if an Ag-Ab reaction is observed.
- An awareness of the proper use and limitations of reagents enhances the ability of laboratory personnel to provide accurate interpretations of results generated in testing and ultimately affects overall transfusion safety.

CRITICAL THINKING EXERCISES

Exercise 3.1
The quality control procedure for commercial anti-A and anti-B reagents is performed using A_1 and B reagent red cells. The results of the daily quality control for ABO reagents for your facility are presented in the following chart. Do the quality control results meet acceptable performance criteria, or are they unacceptable for the commercial ABO typing reagents? Discuss your answer.

ABO Typing Reagent	Reactions with Reagent Red Cells	
	A_1 Cells	B Cells
Anti-A	4+	0
Anti-B	0	4+

Exercise 3.2
The results of anti-D reagent quality control for the past week are presented in the following chart. What are the implications of these results regarding reagent potency and specificity?

	Anti-D Quality Control	
	Reactions of Anti-D Reagent with D-Positive and D-Negative Red Cells	
Days	D-Positive	D-Negative
1	3+	0
2	3+	0
3	2+	0
4	2+	0
5	1+	0

Exercise 3.3
Using several product inserts as resources, determine the visible signs of possible reagent deterioration in both reagent red cells and antisera as outlined by the manufacturers.

Exercise 3.4
Using a product insert for a commercial source of antisera, identify the product limitations as described by the manufacturer.

Exercise 3.5
Read a reagent quality control procedure from a transfusion service, and identify the criteria for acceptable performance for each reagent.

Exercise 3.6
The saline in an automated red cell washer did not fill the test tubes consistently when the instrument was evaluated during a routine quality control check. Would this situation affect the results of the AHG test? How would you detect this problem in testing?

Exercise 3.7
You have added IgG-sensitized red cells to the negative indirect antiglobulin test result of the antibody screen procedure. You observe agglutination in the tube. Is the antibody screen interpretation positive or negative? Explain your answer.

Exercise 3.8
A donor unit obtained from the central blood bank was labeled as group O, D-positive. When the hospital transfusion service confirmed the donor's type, the result was group O, D-negative. Investigation of the label issued at the blood bank was performed with verification of correct labeling. How can you explain the discrepancy in the D typing of this donor unit?

STUDY QUESTIONS

1. What is the purpose of including a reagent control when interpreting group AB, D-positive red cells after testing with a low-protein anti-D reagent?
   a. to detect false-positive agglutination reactions
   b. to detect false-negative agglutination reactions
   c. to identify a mix-up with a patient's sample
   d. to confirm ABO typing results

2. What characteristic is associated with monospecific AHG reagents?
   a. increase the dielectric constant in vitro
   b. contain either anti-IgG or anti-C3d antibody specificities
   c. are not useful in identifying the molecule causing a positive DAT
   d. contain human IgG or complement molecules

3. You have added IgG-sensitized red cells to a negative indirect antiglobulin test. You observe agglutination in the tube. What situation was *not* controlled for in testing by adding these control cells?
   a. the addition of patient serum
   b. the addition of AHG reagent
   c. adequate washing of cell suspension
   d. adequate potency of AHG reagent

4. Part of the daily quality control in the blood bank laboratory is the testing of reagent antisera with corresponding antigen-positive and antigen-negative red cells. What does this procedure ensure?
   a. antibody class
   b. antibody titer
   c. antibody specificity
   d. antibody sensitivity

5. Why are group O red cells used as a source for commercial screening cells?
   a. anti-A is detected using group O cells
   b. anti-D reacts with most group O cells
   c. weak subgroups of A react with group O cells
   d. ABO antibodies do not react with group O cells

6. Where can you locate information regarding reagent limitations?
   a. SOPs
   b. blood bank computer system
   c. product inserts
   d. product catalogs

7. What regulatory agency provides licensure for blood banking reagents?
   a. AABB
   b. FDA
   c. American Red Cross
   d. College of American Pathologists

8. What antibodies are present in polyspecific AHG reagent?
   a. anti-IgG
   b. anti-IgM and anti-IgG
   c. anti-IgG and anti-C3d
   d. anti-C3d

9. In which source are the regulations regarding the manufacturing of blood banking reagents published?
   a. *Code of Federal Regulations*
   b. AABB *Standards for Blood Banks and Transfusion Services*
   c. AABB *Technical Manual*
   d. AABB *Accreditation Requirements Manual*

10. After the addition of anti-D reagent to a patient's red cell suspension, agglutination was observed. The result with anti-A reagent was negative. What is the interpretation of this patient's D typing?
    a. patient is D-negative
    b. patient is D-positive
    c. cannot interpret the test
    d. invalid result

11. Select the reagent to use for detection of unexpected red cell antibodies in a patient's serum sample.
    a. A_1 and B cells
    b. panel cells
    c. IgG-sensitized cells
    d. screening cells

12. Select the method that uses the principle of sieving to separate larger agglutinates from smaller agglutinates in Ag-Ab reactions.
    a. gel technology
    b. solid-phase adherence
    c. microplate
    d. none of the above

13. What source of antibody is selected to determine the specificity of a red cell antigen in a patient sample?
    a. commercial reagent red cells
    b. commercial antisera
    c. patient serum
    d. patient plasma

14. What source of antigen is selected to determine the presence of a red cell antibody in a patient sample?
    a. commercial reagent red cells
    b. commercial antisera

   c. patient serum
   d. patient's red cells

15. What reagents are derived from plant extracts?
   a. panel cells
   b. commercial anti-B
   c. lectins
   d. antiglobulin reagents

Answers to Study Questions can be found on page 387.

ⓔ Additional student resources, including review questions, a laboratory manual, and case studies, can be found on the Evolve website.

REFERENCES

 1. Food and Drug Administration: *Code of federal regulations*, 21 CFR 211-800, Washington, DC, U.S. Government Printing Office, revised annually.
 2. Commendable Practices, 5.0 Process Controls, Quality Control: *Quality control summary blood bank*, AABB. http://www.aabb.org/sa/tools/commendable/Documents/Quality%20Control%20Summary%20-%20Blood%20Bank.pdf. Accessed April 2015.
 3. Klein HG, Anstee DJ: *Mollison's blood transfusion in clinical medicine*, ed 12, West Sussex, UK, 2014, Wiley Blackwell.
 4. Koskimies S: Human lymphoblastoid cell line producing specific antibody against Rh antigen D, *Scand J Immunol* 11:73–77, 1980.
 5. Boylston AW, Gardner B, Anderson RL, et al.: Production of human IgM anti-D in tissue culture by EB virus transformed lymphocytes, *Scand J Immunol* 12:355–358, 1980.
 6. Marks L: Monoclonal antibodies and the transformation of blood typing, *mAbs* 6:1362–1367, 2014.
 7. Walker PS: *Using FDA-approved monoclonal reagents: the compendium*, Arlington, 1997, AABB.
 8. Moulds MK: Review: monoclonal reagents and detection of unusual or rare phenotypes or antibodies, *Immunohematology* 22:52–63, 2006.
 9. Fung MK: *Technical manual*, ed 18, Bethesda, 2014, AABB.
10. Levitt J, editor: *Standards for blood banks and transfusion services*, ed 29, Bethesda, 2014, AABB.
11. Coombs RRA, Mourant AE, Race RR: A new test for the detection of weak and "incomplete" Rh agglutinins, *Br J Exp Pathol* 26:255, 1945.
12. Hughes-Jones NC, Polley MJ, Telford R: Optimal conditions for detecting blood group antibodies by the antiglobulin test, *Vox Sang* 9:385, 1964.
13. Elliot M, Bossom E, Dupuy ME, et al.: Effect of ionic strength on the serologic behavior of red cell isoantibodies, *Vox Sang* 9:396, 1964.
14. Löw B, Messeter L: Antiglobulin test in low ionic strength salt solution for rapid antibody screening and crossmatching, *Vox Sang* 26:53, 1974.
15. Wicker B, Wallas CH: A comparison of a low ionic strength saline medium with routine methods for antibody detection, *Transfusion* 16:469, 1976.
16. Issitt PD, Anstee DJ: *Applied blood group serology*, ed 4, Durham, 1988, Montgomery Scientific.
17. Nance SJ, Garratty G: A new potentiator of red cell antigen-antibody reactions, *Am J Clin Pathol* 87:633, 1987.
18. de Man AJ, Overbeeke MA: Evaluation of the polyethylene glycol antiglobulin test for detection of red cell antibodies, *Vox Sang* 58:207, 1990.
19. Pollack W, Hager HJ, Reckel R, et al.: A study of forces involved in the second stage of hemagglutination, *Transfusion* 5:158, 1965.
20. Steane EA: Red cell agglutination: a current perspective. In Bell CA, editor: *Seminar on antigen-antibody reactions revisited*, Arlington, 1982, AABB.
21. Lapierre Y, Rigal D, Adam J, et al.: The gel test: a new way to detect red cell antigen-antibody reactions, *Transfusion* 30:109, 1990.
22. Plapp FV, Rachel JM, Beck ML, et al.: Blood antigens and antibodies: solid phase adherence assays, *Lab Med* 22:39, 1984.

4 GENETIC PRINCIPLES IN BLOOD BANKING

CHAPTER OUTLINE

LEARNING OBJECTIVES

On completion of this chapter, the reader should be able to:

1. Define the term blood group system with regard to serologic and genetic classifications.
2. Distinguish the term phenotype from genotype using the ABO system as an example.
3. Using a Punnett square, illustrate the potential offspring from group A and group B parents.
4. Contrast the terms allele and antithetical with regard to genes and antigens.
5. Predict the potential phenotypes of the offspring of a trait with an X-linked inheritance pattern.
6. Illustrate the genetic and serologic characteristics of the terms homozygous and heterozygous and dosage using the M and N blood group antigens.
7. Draw a diagram to illustrate the difference between *cis* and *trans* and their effect on gene interactions.
8. Apply the terms codominant, recessive, and dominant to the possible inheritance patterns in the ABO blood group system.
9. Calculate the probability of finding compatible red blood cell (RBC) units for a recipient with multiple antibodies.
10. Apply the Hardy–Weinberg law to calculate the percentage of homozygous and heterozygous expressions in

a select population given the frequency of a certain phenotype.
11. Evaluate examples of paternity results to determine if direct or indirect exclusions are present.
12. Demonstrate the principles of Mendelian laws of independent assortment and independent segregation by describing how they apply to blood group antigen inheritance.
13. Evaluate the results of a family study to predict the potential phenotype of untested family members.
14. List the applications of molecular testing methods to the field of blood banking.
15. Compare and contrast molecular techniques used to identify HLA antigens: SSP, SSOP, and SBT.
16. Describe the theory of STR testing and its application to the evaluation of hematopoietic progenitor cell engraftment.
17. Outline the principle of molecular techniques used to identify red cell antigens and the applications to patient care.

Blood group systems: groups of antigens on the red cell membrane that share related serologic properties and genetic patterns of inheritance

The concept of an antigen as a molecule that can elicit an immune response was introduced in Chapter 2. In the study of immunohematology, the antigens of interest are part of the red cell membranes. These antigens are inherited characteristics or traits categorized into **blood group systems** based on their genetic and serologic properties. Similarly, human leukocyte antigens (HLAs) are defined and named based on serologic and genetic information.

The study of blood group systems requires an understanding of certain genetic principles and terminology. The characteristics that make each blood group system unique are the structure and location of the antigens present on the red cells, the antibodies they elicit, and the genetic control of antigen expression. Because these properties may be demonstrated in serologic and molecular methods, each blood group system is said to be serologically and genetically defined. Classification of some blood group systems was modified because of enhanced knowledge regarding the molecular structure of the genes producing the antigens.[1]

In subsequent chapters describing the blood group systems, the reader is introduced to the specific genetic pathways that create each antigen. In some systems, such as the Rh blood group system, the gene directly encodes a protein on the red cell, which is recognized by the immune system as an Rh antigen. With other blood group systems, several interacting genes encode a particular antigen on the red cell. For example, expression of the ABO antigens requires the interaction of the *ABO, Hh,* and *Se* genes. Appreciating that each blood group system is the product of a gene or a group of genes assists in their classification and further enhances the understanding of their related serologic properties.

This chapter's final section reviews molecular genetics as it applies to the field of immunohematology. Molecular genetics has enhanced the understanding of the molecular basis of blood group antigens, provided sensitive methods for viral antigen testing, and contributed more accurate methods for "relationship testing" (previously called paternity tests). Methods for detecting viral nuclear material by nucleic amplification tests for viral markers in donors have reduced the exposure window for hepatitis C virus and human immunodeficiency virus (HIV). The identity of the antigens in the HLA system, described in Chapter 7, has greater accuracy using the molecular methods outlined in this chapter.

SECTION 1
BLOOD GROUP GENETICS

GENETIC TERMINOLOGY

A **gene** is a unit of inheritance that encodes a particular protein and is the basic unit for inheritance of a trait. Genetic information is carried on double strands of DNA known as **chromosomes** (Fig. 4.1). Humans have 23 pairs of chromosomes: 22 pairs of **autosomes** and 1 pair of sex chromosomes. Cell division allows the genetic material in cells to be replicated so that identical chromosomes can be transmitted to the daughter cells. This cell division occurs through a process called **mitosis** in somatic cells and through **meiosis** in gametes.

Before knowledge of genes and DNA was established, the inheritance patterns of certain detectable traits were observed, and theories of inheritance were established. These theories are applicable to the study of blood group genetics. In this section, the genetic terms are described as they pertain to red cell antigen inheritance patterns and as products of specific genes.

Phenotype Versus Genotype

Serologic testing determines the presence or absence of antigens on the red cells. The phenotype, or the physical expression of inherited traits, is determined by reacting red

Gene: segment of DNA that encodes a particular protein

Chromosomes: structures within the nucleus that contain DNA

Autosomes: chromosomes other than the sex chromosomes

Mitosis: cell division in somatic cells that results in the same number of chromosomes

Meiosis: cell division in gametes that results in half the number of chromosomes present in somatic cells

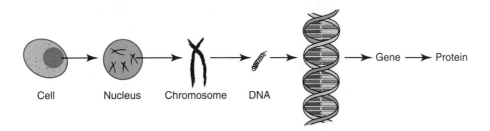

Fig. 4.1 Chromosomes. Chromosomes are found in the cell's nucleus and contain double-stranded DNA that has specific areas called genes that code for proteins.

The patient's red cell phenotype is determined by hemagglutination of red cell antigens using specific antisera.

Genotype: actual genetic makeup; determined by family studies or molecular typing

Hemagglutination does not detect a genotype such as *AO*. DNA-based assays or family studies are needed to determine the genotype.

Punnett square: square used to display the frequencies of different genotypes and phenotypes among the offspring of a cross

Genetic loci: sites of a gene on a chromosome

Alleles: alternate forms of a gene at a given locus

Antithetical: opposite antigens encoded at the same locus

When writing the identity of a gene, use italics. Red cell antigen phenotypes do not require italics.

Polymorphic: genetic system that expresses two or more alleles at one locus

cells with known antisera and observing for the presence or absence of hemagglutination. Reagents used for this purpose were described in Chapter 3. For example, testing red cells with anti-A or anti-B reagents can determine whether a person has the A or B antigen. If neither anti-A nor anti-B shows agglutination, the red cells are classified as group O. This determination is called the phenotype.

The **genotype,** or the actual genes inherited from each parent, may be inferred from the phenotype. Family studies or molecular tests are required to determine the actual genotype. If an individual's phenotype is A, the genotype may be *A/A* or *A/O*. *A/A* indicates that both parents contributed the *A* gene. The *A/O* genotype indicates that one parent contributed the *A* gene, and the other contributed the *O* gene. Because the *O* gene has no detectable product, only the A antigen is expressed when the *A/O* genotype is inherited. If the *A/O* individual has a group O child, it becomes evident that the individual carried the *O* gene. Two people with group A red cells have the same phenotype but can have different genotypes.

Punnett Square

Examination of family history is an important component in the investigation of inheritance patterns. Fig. 4.2 is an example of genotypes and phenotypes for the ABO blood group system.

A **Punnett square** illustrates the probabilities of phenotypes from known or inferred genotypes. It visually portrays the genotypes of the potential offspring or the probable genotypes of the parents. Fig. 4.3 shows possible ABO blood group system gene combinations with Punnett squares. From this figure, it would be easy to determine that two group A parents can have a group O child. It could also be illustrated that the parents of a group AB child can be group A, B, or AB but not group O.

Genes, Alleles, and Polymorphism

Genes, the basic units of inheritance on a chromosome, are located in specific places called **genetic loci.** Several different forms of a gene, called **alleles,** may exist for each locus (Fig. 4.4). For example, *A, B,* and *O* are alleles on the *ABO* gene locus. The term **antithetical,** meaning opposite, refers to the antigens produced by allelic genes. For example, the Kp^a antigen is antithetical to the Kp^b antigen. *Kp^a* and *Kp^b* are examples of alleles in the Kell blood group system. Scan the QR code for more information from the National Human Genome Research Institute.

The term **polymorphic** refers to having two or more alleles at a given locus, as with the ABO blood group system. Some blood group systems are more polymorphic than other blood group systems (ie, many more alleles exist at a given locus). The Rh blood group system is highly polymorphic compared with the ABO blood group system because of the greater number of alleles. The frequency of a particular phenotype in a population depends upon the degree of polymorphism within a blood group system. A highly polymorphic system makes it less likely to find two identical individuals. An example

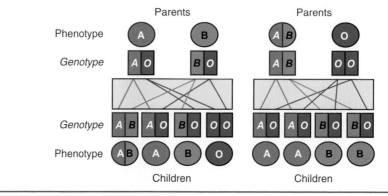

Fig. 4.2 Difference between phenotype and genotype. The difference between the genotype and phenotype is illustrated in this diagram of ABO system inheritance patterns.

	A	B
O	AO	BO
O	AO	BO

	A	B
A	AA	AB
B	AB	BB

	A	O
O	AO	OO
O	AO	OO

	B	B
O	BO	BO
O	BO	BO

	A	A
B	AB	AB
B	AB	AB

	A	O
A	AA	AO
O	AO	OO

Fig. 4.3 Punnett squares showing ABO inheritance.

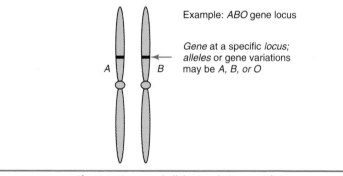

Example: *ABO* gene locus

Gene at a specific *locus;*
alleles or gene variations
may be *A, B, or O*

A   B

Fig. 4.4 Genes and alleles in relation to a chromosome.

of a highly polymorphic system is one involving the genes that encode HLA antigens. Because bone marrow and organ transplants require HLA matching, HLA polymorphism contributes to the challenge of finding suitable donors. If several polymorphic systems are used to determine a phenotype of an individual, finding two identical individuals becomes increasingly difficult.

Inheritance Patterns

In most cases, blood group antigens are inherited in an autosomal **codominant** pattern, or with equal expression of both inherited alleles found on autosomes. In other words, the product of each allele is expressed when inherited as a codominant trait. If one parent passed on an *A* gene and the other parent passed on a *B* gene, both the A and the B antigens are expressed equally on the red cells. **Recessive** inheritance requires that the same allele from both parents be inherited to show the trait. An example is a group O phenotype that requires both parents to pass on an O gene (O/O). In blood group genetics, a recessive trait can express a null phenotype such as Lu(a–b–), Rh$_{null}$, or O phenotypes because of homozygosity for a silent or amorphic gene.[2]

A **dominant** expression would require only one form of the allele to express the trait, such as a group A phenotype that inherits an *A* gene from one parent and an O gene from the other parent (*A/O*). The alleles of the ABO blood group system display dominant, recessive, and codominant patterns of inheritance.

Silent Genes

In some blood group systems, genes do not produce a detectable antigen product. These silent genes, known as **amorphs,** produce phenotypes often called null types. The

Codominant: equal expression of two different inherited alleles

Recessive: trait expressed only when inherited by both parents

Dominant: gene product expressed over another gene

Null phenotypes mean that when certain recessive alleles are inherited, there is no expression of the expected red cell antigens.

Inheritance of the group O phenotype is an example of a recessive trait. Group O is the most common ABO phenotype in many populations.

TABLE 4.1	Amorph and Suppressor Genes in Blood Groups		
BLOOD GROUP SYSTEM	**AMORPH GENE**	**SUPPRESSOR GENE**	**RESULTING PHENOTYPE**
ABO	*O*		O
H	*H*		Bombay
Kell	*K⁰*		Kell_null
Lutheran	*Lu*	*In(Lu)*	Lu(a–b–)
Kidd	*Jk*	*In(Jk)*	Jk(a–b–)
Duffy	*Fy*		Fy(a–b–)

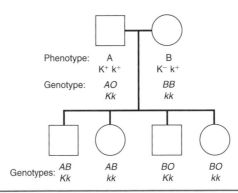

Fig. 4.5 Independent assortment. ABO system genes are sorted independently from Kell system genes because they are inherited on different chromosomes.

Amorphic: describes a gene that does not express a detectable product

Suppressor genes: genes that suppress the expression of another gene

Independent segregation: passing of one gene from each parent to the offspring

Independent assortment: random behavior of genes on separate chromosomes during meiosis that results in a mixture of genetic material in the offspring

expressions of the blood group system antigens are not apparent in null phenotypes. For example, an Rh_null individual lacks the presence of all Rh system antigens. The amorphic gene must be inherited from both parents (homozygous) to produce a null phenotype. If the gene is rare, this phenomenon is uncommon. Because the O allele has a high frequency in the population, the O phenotype is common. Examples of null phenotypes include Rh_null, O, and Lu(a–b–).[2]

Unusual phenotypes may also result from the action of **suppressor genes.** These genes act to inhibit the expression of another gene to produce a null expression. The occurrence of suppressor genes that affect blood group antigen expression is rare. An example of a suppressor gene is *In(Jk)*, which affects the Kidd blood group system expression, causing the Jk(a–b–) phenotype. In addition to the silent gene, *Lu*, the *In(Lu)* gene suppresses Lutheran blood group system antigens, resulting in the Lu(a–b–) phenotype. Null phenotypes can be a result of either an amorphic or a suppressor gene. Table 4.1 includes examples of suppressor and amorphic genes.

Mendelian Principles

Mendel observed certain hereditary patterns in his early genetic experiments that subsequently applied to the study of blood group system genetics. Mendel's law of **independent segregation** refers to the transmission of a trait in a predictable fashion from one generation to the next.[2] This concept was described previously with the Punnett square using the ABO blood group system genes (refer to Fig. 4.3). Independent segregation illustrates that each parent has a pair of genes for a particular trait, either of which can be transmitted to the next generation. The genes "segregate" and allow only one gene from each parent to be passed on to each child. Another important law, **independent assortment,** is demonstrated by the fact that blood group antigens, inherited on different chromosomes, are expressed separately and discretely. Fig. 4.5 illustrates that the ABO blood group system genes, located on chromosome 1, and the Kell blood group system genes, located on chromosome 7, are inherited independent of each other.

TABLE 4.2	Chromosomal Assignment of Genes for Common Blood Group Systems
BLOOD GROUP SYSTEM	**CHROMOSOME**
Rh	1
Duffy	1
MNS	4
Chido/Rodgers	6
Kell	7
ABO	9
Kidd	18
Lewis	19
Landsteiner–Wiener	19
Lutheran	19
H	19
P1PK	22

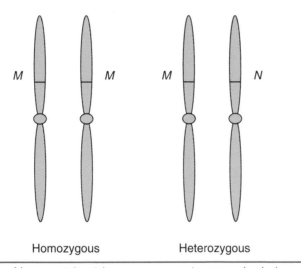

Fig. 4.6 Homozygosity and heterozygosity. A homozygous expression means that both parents contributed the same gene, giving a "double dose" of antigen expression. In some blood group systems, the antigen may appear to have stronger expression.

Chromosomal Assignment

The genetic loci of most of the blood group system genes have been determined. Table 4.2 shows the chromosomal assignment for common blood group systems.[1] Most of the blood group–associated genes are on autosomes. Inheritance patterns are the same, regardless of gender. The Xg blood group system is an exception. Genes coding for this system are found on the X chromosome. In this system, if the Xg^a allele is carried on the father's X chromosome, he would pass it on to all of his daughters but none of his sons. Conversely, if the father lacked the Xg^a gene and the mother carried the gene, both the sons and the daughters would express the Xg^a antigen.

Heterozygosity and Homozygosity

An individual whose genotype is made up of identical genes, such as *AA*, *BB*, or *OO*, is called a homozygote and is homozygous for the gene. An individual who has inherited different alleles from each parent, such as *AO*, *AB*, or *BO*, is called a heterozygote and is **heterozygous** for the genes (Fig. 4.6).

In serologic testing, the concept of homozygous and heterozygous inheritance is important with some blood group antigens. As discussed in the previous chapters, agglutination

Homozygous: two alleles for a given trait are identical

Heterozygous: two alleles for a given trait are different

Cell	Rh							MNSs				P₁	Lewis		Lutheran		Kell		Duffy		Kidd		Antibody reaction
	D	C	E	c	e	f	Cʷ	M	N	S	s	P₁	Leᵃ	Leᵇ	Luᵃ	Luᵇ	K	k	Fyᵃ	Fyᵇ	Jkᵃ	Jkᵇ	
1 R1R1	+	+	0	0	+	0	0	+	0	+	0	+	0	+	0	+	+	+	+	+	+	0	3+
2 R2R2	+	0	+	+	0	0	0	+	+	+	+	+	+	0	0	+	0	+	+	0	+	+	1+

Fig. 4.7 **Dosage effect.** Homozygous expressions of some red cell antigens react more strongly than heterozygous expressions. This antibody screen result shows that the antibody reacts more strongly (3+) with the red cell #1 homozygous (M+N−) expression than with the red cell #2 heterozygous (M+N+) expression of the antigen.

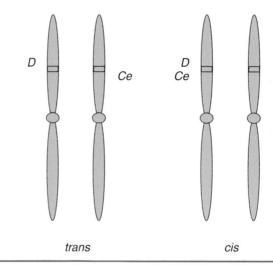

trans   *cis*

Fig. 4.8 *Cis* and *trans* position genes. When the *Ce* gene is inherited on opposite chromosomes or in *trans* to the D gene, the D antigen expression is weaker than when the *Ce* gene is inherited in *cis*, or on the same chromosome.

Dosage effect: stronger agglutination when a red cell antigen is expressed from homozygous genes

The concept of dosage will be important when we are identifying red cell antibodies in antibody identification procedures.

cis: two or more genes on the same chromosome of a homologous pair

trans: genes inherited on opposite chromosomes of a homologous pair

Linked: when two genes are inherited together because they are very close on a chromosome

Haplotype: linked set of genes inherited together because of their close proximity on a chromosome

reactions vary in strength. This variation can be due to the strength of the antibody or the density of the antigens on the red cells. When antigen density varies between red cells of different individuals, it is often due to the inheritance of the antigen expression. An individual who inherits different blood group system alleles from each parent (*MN*) has a "single dose" of that antigen on the red cells (one M and one N). The agglutination reaction may demonstrate a weaker antigenic expression, or lower antigen density, on the red cell. When the same allele is inherited from both parents (*MM* or *NN*), a stronger red cell antigen is apparent because a "double dose" of the M or N antigen is present on the red cells. The variation in antigen expression because of the number of alleles present is called the **dosage effect** (Fig. 4.7). The dosage effect is not observed with all blood group antigens or with all antibodies of a given specificity.

Genetic Interaction

Sometimes genes can interact with each other, depending on whether they are inherited on the same chromosome (*cis*) or on the opposite chromosome (*trans*). This interaction may weaken the expression of one of the antigens encoded by the genes. For example, the *Ce* and *D* genes of the Rh blood group system are inherited on different genetic loci. The *Ce* gene encodes the C and e antigens, and the *D* gene encodes the D antigen. When *Ce* is inherited in *trans* to *D*, it weakens the D antigen expression on the red cell (Fig. 4.8).[2]

Linkage and Haplotypes

In some blood group systems, antigens are encoded by two or more genes close together on the same chromosome and are inherited from each parent as a unit. Genes that are so close together on a chromosome that they are inherited as a unit are **linked.** Independent assortment does not occur when genes are linked. These gene units are called **haplotypes.** For example, in the MNS blood group system, *M* and *N* are alleles on one gene, and *S* and

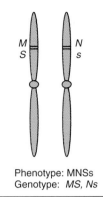

Phenotype: MNSs
Genotype: *MS, Ns*

Fig. 4.9 Haplotypes. Haplotypes are genes that are very close on a chromosome and often inherited together.

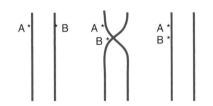

Fig. 4.10 Unequal crossing over meiosis. Crossing over causes the predicted inheritance patterns to be changed.

s are alleles on another gene. Because the genes are close, they are inherited as haplotypes: *MS, Ms, NS,* or *Ns* (Fig. 4.9). Haplotypes occur in the population at a different frequency than would be expected if the genes were not linked. **Linkage disequilibrium** refers to the phenomenon of antigens occurring at a different frequency in the population, depending on whether they were inherited by linked or unlinked genes. In other words, if the *M* and *S* genes were not linked, the expected frequency of the M and S antigen in the population would be 17% according to calculated frequency probabilities.[2] Because of linkage disequilibrium, the observed frequency of the MS haplotype is actually 24%.

Crossing Over

Another exception to the law of independent assortment occurs if two genes on the same chromosome recombine. **Crossing over** is the exchange of genetic material during meiosis after the chromosome pairs have replicated (Fig. 4.10). The resulting genes are exchanged during this process but are not lost. The recombination results in two new and different chromosomes. Crossing over can be observed with genes on the same chromosome but does not usually occur when the genes are close together. Because the genes expressing blood group systems are close (linked) or on different chromosomes, crossing over rarely affects the inheritance of the blood group system. Crossover frequencies are used to map the relative locations of genes on a chromosome because the closer the genes, the rarer the possibility for the genes to be separated.

SECTION 2
POPULATION GENETICS

Population genetics is the statistical application of genetic principles to determine genotype and phenotype occurrence, which is dependent on the gene frequency.[2] Two types of calculations are applicable in the study of blood group population genetics. The first calculation involves combined phenotype frequencies, and the second involves gene or allele frequency estimates.

COMBINED PHENOTYPE CALCULATIONS

Determining the frequency of a particular phenotype in the population enables finding a donor unit of red blood cells (RBCs) with certain antigen characteristics. For example, patients with multiple antibodies may require RBC units that are negative for several

Linkage disequilibrium: occurrence of a set of genes inherited together more often than would be expected by chance

Linkage disequilibrium also occurs in the HLA system because these genetic loci are very close. The major histocompatibility (MHC) genes that encode HLA antigens are inherited as haplotypes.

Crossing over: exchange of genetic material during meiosis between paired chromosomes

Problem: Patient needs one (1) RBC unit that lacks C, E, and S antigens. How frequent is a unit in the population?

Frequency Antigen-positive	Frequency Antigen-negative	Percentage of Donors Negative for Antigen
68% C+ (C-positive)	32% C– (C-negative)	0.32 C–
29% E+ (E-positive)	71% E– (E-negative)	0.71 E–
52% S+ (S-positive)	48% S– (S-negative)	0.48 S–

Calculate the combined phenotype frequencies for a donor unit that lacks C, E, and S antigens for transfusion: 0.32 x 0.71 x 0.48 = 0.109, rounded to 0.11 x 100 = 11%

For this patient, 11% of the population has a probability of being negative for all three antigens. This means that approximately 1 in 10 units of RBCs is likely to be negative for the combined antigens for transfusion to this patient.

Fig. 4.11 Example of combined phenotype calculations.

different antigens. The calculation of combined phenotype frequencies provides an estimate of the number of units that may need testing to find the unit with the desired antigens.

The frequency of multiple traits inherited independently is calculated by multiplying the frequency of each trait. If a patient produced red cell antibodies from exposure during previous transfusions or pregnancies, red cells that were negative for the corresponding antigens would be required for transfusion. For example, if a patient produced antibodies such as anti-C, anti-E, and anti-S, RBC units that are negative for the antigens C, E, and S would be required for transfusion. The frequency of donors negative for the individual antigens is expressed as a decimal point and then multiplied (Fig. 4.11).

The percentages used are established antigen frequencies and can be found in the AABB *Technical Manual,* package inserts for the corresponding antisera, and *The Blood Group Antigen Facts Book*.[1] Antigen frequencies vary with race. The predominant race found in the donor population for the area should be used when calculating antigen frequencies. The frequency of an antigen in the population is the occurrence of the positive phenotype. Subtracting the frequency from 100 yields the antigen-negative percentage.

For example, if a patient has an anti-Fy^a, an anti-Jk^b, and an anti-K, how many units should be tested to find two RBC units of the appropriate phenotype? Remember that the patient needs RBC units that are negative for Fy^a, Jk^b, and K antigens.

Step 1. Determine the frequency of antigen-negative units for Fya, Jkb, and K antigens.
    Look up the frequency for antigens.

68% Fy(a+)	32% Fy(a–)
74% Jk(b+)	26% Jk(b–)
9% K$^+$	91% K$^-$

Step 2. Multiply the combined antigen-negative frequencies.

$$0.32 \times 0.26 \times 0.91 = 0.076, \text{ rounded to 0.08 or 8\%}$$

The calculation shows the probability of finding a unit of RBCs negative for all three antigens to be 8 of 100 units.

Step 3. The patient requires 2 RBC units for transfusion.
    If 2 units are needed, solve for X:

$$\frac{8}{100} = \frac{2}{X}$$

$$X = 25$$

Solving for X shows that antigen typing 25 units may be required to find 2 units that are negative for all three antigens.

GENE FREQUENCIES

The concept of genetic equilibrium was developed independently in 1908 by the English mathematician Hardy and the German physician Weinberg.[3] Their theories led to the formulation of the Hardy–Weinberg law. The statistical formulas derived from these principles estimate the frequency of genetic diseases or observed traits. The formula is based on the principle that the sum of the gene frequencies, when expressed as a decimal, is equal to 1.0. This formula is used for predictions of populations at equilibrium, meaning that there is no migration, mutations, or natural selection. In addition, random mating must occur. By observing phenotypes or traits in a large number of individuals, the percentage of trait occurrences is established. The Hardy–Weinberg formula can calculate a determination of the gene frequencies that produced that trait. The probability of heterozygous and homozygous expression for each of the genes in a system is predicted. With the ability to characterize genes and determine the zygosity through molecular methods, this formula is less frequently used.

For example:

p is the frequency of allele A

q is the frequency of allele a

Genotype proportions are: $p + q = 1.0$

$p^2(AA) + 2\,pq\,(Aa) + q^2(aa) = 1.0$

Step 1. If the frequency of p is 0.3, what is the value of q? Subtract 0.3 from 1.

$$1 - p = q$$

$$1 - 0.3 = 0.7$$

Step 2. What part of the population is homozygous for A *(AA)*, *heterozygous (Aa)*, and homozygous for a *(aa)*?

$$p^2\,(AA) + 2pq\,(Aa) + q^2\,(aa) = 1.0$$

$$AA = p^2 = 0.3 \times 0.3 = 0.09$$

$$Aa = 2pq = 2\,(0.3 \times 0.7) = 0.42$$

$$aa = q^2 = (0.7 \times 0.7) = 0.49$$

RELATIONSHIP TESTING

The high degree of polymorphism of the human leukocyte antigens (HLA) and blood group systems has made them valuable tools in cases of disputed paternity. Although paternity, or relationship, testing is typically performed by molecular methods, recognizing inheritance patterns of blood group and HLA using family studies helps reinforce the genetic concepts important in understanding blood groups.

If maternity is assumed, paternity can be excluded by either indirect or direct exclusion. In a **direct exclusion,** the child has inherited a genetic marker that is not found in the mother or **alleged father** (the B gene in the following example). This gene is the **obligatory gene,** the gene that is passed by the father to establish probability of paternity. The alleged father could not be father to this child, because the child inherited the B gene.

Direct exclusion: exclusion of paternity when a child has a trait that neither parent shows

Alleged father: man accused of being the biological father; the putative father

Obligatory gene: gene that should be inherited from the father to prove paternity

	Mother	Alleged Father	Child
Phenotype	Group O	Group A	Group B
Genotype	O/O	A/A or A/O	B/O

In an **indirect exclusion,** the child lacks a genetic marker that the father should have transmitted to all of his offspring. Refer to the allele in the following example. Because a silent gene can cause an indirect exclusion, it is not used as the only marker to exclude paternity. In the following case, the child lacks the Jk^b, which should have been transmitted to the offspring.

Indirect exclusion: failure to find an expected marker in a child when the alleged father is apparently homozygous for the gene

	Mother	**Alleged Father**	**Child**
Phenotype	Jk(a+b−)	Jk(a−b+)	Jk(a+b−)
Genotype	*Jkᵃ/Jkᵃ*	*Jkᵇ/Jkᵇ*	*Jkᵃ/Jkᵃ*

If an alleged father cannot be excluded, the probability of paternity can be calculated based on the gene frequency of the obligatory gene in the population with the same race or ethnic group as the alleged father. The result is expressed as a likelihood ratio (paternity index) or as a percentage.[2]

SECTION 3
MOLECULAR GENETICS

APPLICATION OF MOLECULAR GENETICS TO BLOOD BANKING

Procedures based on the detection or analysis of DNA and RNA are important contributions to biological science. Applications of molecular technology in the field of blood banking and transplantation include HLA typing, red cell typing, viral marker testing, and determination of engraftment in **hematopoietic progenitor cell (HPC)** transplantation (Table 4.3).[4] Nucleic acid testing (NAT) is a general term used for molecular-based methods of screening for infectious agents. This methodology further reduces the "window period" in viral testing when antibodies may be below detectable levels. NAT is discussed later in the textbook. DNA-based assays have also largely replaced red cell and HLA typing for identity (relationship) testing, also referred to as DNA fingerprinting.[2] The next section outlines the concept of the polymerase chain reaction (PCR) and its application in transplantation and transfusion medicine.

POLYMERASE CHAIN REACTION

The genes encoding many of the red cell and HLA antigens are sequenced and cloned, providing "maps" for the specific **nucleotide** differences that define each allele. Most HLA and red cell antigen differences are the result of single nucleotide substitutions in the coding sequence of each unique allele. DNA-based assays identify single-nucleotide polymorphisms (SNPs) by amplifying the part of the DNA where the SNPs are located.[5] This amplification is performed by PCR, which allows specific DNA sequences to be multiplied rapidly and precisely (Fig. 4.12). PCR is an in vitro technique used to amplify specific DNA sequences of interest through cycles of denaturation, annealing of primers

Hematopoietic progenitor cell (HPC): type of stem cell committed to a blood cell lineage collected from marrow, peripheral blood, and cord blood and used to treat certain malignant diseases and congenital immune deficiencies

Nucleotide: phosphate, sugar, and base that constitute the basic monomer of the nucleic acids DNA and RNA

TABLE 4.3	Applications of Molecular Testing in the Blood Bank
Transplantation	HLA antigen-level and allele-level typing for HPC and organ transplants
	Engraftment studies for HPC transplants
Transfusion	Red cell typing in multiply transfused patients
	Determine blood type when the DAT is positive
	Complex Rh genotypes, weak D expression
	Screen for antigen-negative donor units when antisera are unavailable
	Donor antigen screening for prevention of alloimmunization
HDFN	Determine parental RhD zygosity
	Type fetal blood
Donor testing	Detect virus in donors that may be below detectable levels by antibody detection methods
Relationship testing	Establish paternity and legal relationships for immigration

DAT, Direct antiglobulin test; *HDFN*, hemolytic disease of the fetus and newborn; *HLA*, human leukocyte antigen; *HPC*, hematopoietic progenitor cell.
From Alexander L: Personalized therapy reaches transfusion medicine, *AABB News* 13:10, 2011.

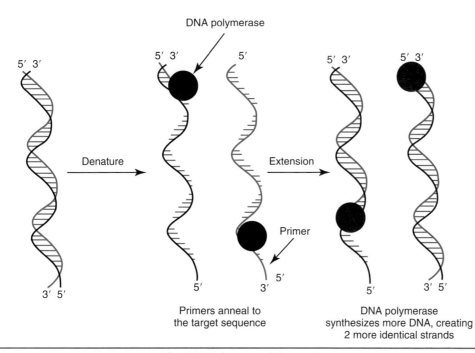

Fig. 4.12 Polymerase chain reaction.

TABLE 4.4	Polymerase Chain Reaction Components
COMPONENT	**DESCRIPTION**
Target DNA	DNA that contains the region of the DNA fragment to be amplified
Taq polymerase	Thermostable enzyme that catalyzes the replication of template DNA into copies
Primers	Short pieces of single-stranded DNA that are complementary to the opposite strands that flank the target DNA. Primers mark the sequence to be amplified and provide the initiation site on each DNA
Nucleotides	dNTPs, which are the building blocks for the newly synthesized DNA
MgCl$_2$ and buffer	Allows proper pH and divalent cations for the enzyme to function

dNTPs, Deoxynucleotide triphosphates.

that select the area of the DNA for amplification and replication that result in a millionfold copies of a specific area of DNA. Components of the PCR reaction are listed in Table 4.4.

Polymerase Chain Reaction–Based Human Leukocyte Antigen Typing Procedures

HLA typing procedures are based on the amplification by PCR of one or more alleles. The test methods vary in the techniques used to detect and identify the amplified products.[6] This section describes the principles and application of several methods used in HLA typing.

Sequence-Specific Primers

In the sequence-specific primers (SSP) test method, primers that are specific for a particular sequence select the area of the DNA to be evaluated during the PCR reaction.[7] As described previously, the specificity of the genetic material being amplified is determined by the primer. Each primer pair can amplify one or several alleles. Primers can be either low or high resolution, resulting in either antigen-level or allele-level results. Low-resolution results are similar to identification by serologic testing, whereas high-resolution

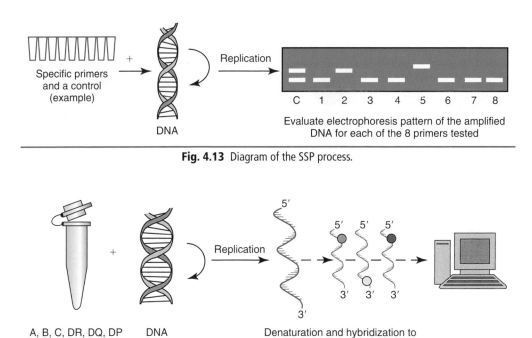

Fig. 4.13 Diagram of the SSP process.

A, B, C, DR, DQ, DP   DNA   Denaturation and hybridization to
primers   labeled probes. Followed by reading
                              and analysis by a flow cytometer

Fig. 4.14 Diagram of the SSOP process.

Amplicon: short sequence of amplified DNA flanked on either end by the primer

Hybridize: to attach a complementary sequence of DNA using the properties of complementary base pair sequencing

DNA probe: short sequence of DNA complementary to the area being identified and attached to a marker (usually fluorescent) that can be read by an instrument such as a flow cytometer

primers define alleles that are more specific. The primers are purchased in PCR trays in various configurations for most common HLA antigen specificities. The test DNA is added to the tray wells and amplified by a thermal cycler according to the manufacturer's recommended protocol.[8]

After PCR, the specificity of the amplified DNA, or **amplicons**, is assessed using gel electrophoresis. The amplified DNA from each well is transferred to an agarose gel prepared with ethidium bromide to allow for DNA detection under ultraviolet light after electrophoresis of the gel. Low-molecular-weight amplicons migrate faster than high-molecular-weight amplicons. A blank well indicates that the primer did not detect the portion of DNA in question. The identity of the allele that defines the antigen is determined by comparing the migration pattern of the gel with the primer specificities and patterns provided by the manufacturer (Fig. 4.13).

Sequence-Specific Oligonucleotide Probes

In the sequence-specific oligonucleotide probes (SSOP) technique, the target DNA is amplified using a group-specific primer in separate wells (eg, A, B, C, DR, DQ, DP specific for HLA loci).[9] After amplification by PCR, the DNA is denatured and **hybridized** to a mixture of complementary **DNA probes** conjugated to fluorescently coded microspheres (Fig. 4.14). There can be 30 to 70 probes per locus to characterize the various alleles. The hybridized solution is evaluated with a flow analyzer such as the Luminex. The fluorescent intensity is measured, the instrument software analyzes the reaction pattern, and the pattern is compared with patterns associated with published HLA gene sequences. An assignment of the HLA typing is then determined. The SSOP typing test provides serologic and allele-level evaluations.

Sequence-Based Typing

Donor and recipient typing for HPC transplants require high-resolution typing at the allele level.[2] This resolution is most accurately performed by sequence-based typing (SBT). In SBT, the amplified DNA is purified after the PCR reaction, and a fluorescent locus-specific sequencing mix is added.[10] After a sequencing step on the thermal cycler, the DNA is washed and denatured. The actual nucleotide sequence and predicted amino acid sequence, corresponding to the allele, can be read and analyzed by a capillary array instrument. The allele identification is not limited to available primers, but rather the nucleotide sequences define the allele.[11] Instrument software helps to facilitate the analysis and the assignment of alleles.

Short Tandem Repeats

Most of our DNA is identical to the DNA of others. However, inherited regions of DNA can vary from person to person. Variations in DNA sequence between individuals are termed polymorphisms.[2] Sequences with the highest degree of polymorphism are very useful for relationship testing, forensics, and determining engraftment after HPC transplants. Engraftment evaluations, also called **chimerism** studies, determine the percentage of hematopoietic and lymphoid cells from the donor that have engrafted into the recipient at several intervals after transplant. This test can determine the success of the transplant and if further treatment is necessary. Because the HLA alleles of the donor and recipient have been closely matched, testing HLA alleles would be of little value to differentiate the donor and recipient cells in a sample.

Chimerism: mixture of donor and recipient cell populations after hematopoietic stem cell transplants

Short tandem repeats (STRs) are short sequences of DNA, normally two to five base pairs in length, that are repeated 4 to more than 50 times. The number of times the repeats occur varies between individuals and is genetically determined. STR identification is useful to establish genetic relationships between individuals. If six to twelve STR loci are used, the ability to discriminate between individuals has a high degree of accuracy.

STR testing first amplifies DNA from the donor, the recipient, and the posttransplant samples. Locus-specific primers for the STR are added to the DNA that has been isolated from donor, pretransplant, and posttransplant recipient samples. After amplification by PCR, the amplicons are denatured and labeled with fluorescent dyes that are analyzed on a sequencing instrument such as the capillary array used for SBT. Pretransplant STRs from the donor and recipient samples are identified and compared with the posttransplant sample. A calculation of the percent of donor-to-recipient STRs is made. In 100% engraftment, the only STRs detected are those from the donor. In chimerism studies where less than 100% engraftment is determined, early relapses or graft failures can be detected and treated with this knowledge.

MOLECULAR TESTING APPLICATIONS IN RED CELL TYPING

Classic hemagglutination testing is a simple and quick method for blood bank testing. Automated platforms are designed around this fundamental principle. However, several limitations are associated with hemagglutination. First, an accurate antigen phenotype is difficult in recently transfused patients. When a patient presents with a positive direct antiglobulin test (DAT) due to anti-IgG, accurate phenotype results are challenging. Second, some antigen typing reagents are short in supply or are not available. Third, hemagglutination methods cannot determine the zygosity of the tested red cells. DNA-based methods for genotyping have become more available in recent years to supplement traditional hemagglutination methods. There are several situations where molecular testing yields more accurate results and can be a more cost-effective method for donor red cell antigen typing. Table 4.3 lists molecular applications for red cell typing.

Molecular typing methods are valuable tools when serologic typing cannot be completed due to limitations in the sample or reagent.

Polymerase Chain Reaction–Based Red Cell Typing Procedures

Bead-Chip Technology

After the genes encoding the major blood group antigens have been sequenced and cloned, the correlation of the differences in DNA sequences with red cell antigen expression can be applied to the development and standardization of laboratory tests.[6] In many of the blood group systems, single-nucleotide substitutions, described earlier, code for the unique blood group allele.

The antigen-defining SNPs are identified through PCR methods combined with bead-chip technology.[12] The principle of human erythrocyte antigen (HEA) bead-chip technology uses oligonucleotide primers attached to silica beads of various colors. The beads are attached to a substrate (eg, a glass slide). A "map" identifying the color and the specific oligonucleotide (primer) is made. When the chip is used, the PCR is amplified, and digested DNA in question is exposed to the surface of the chip, allowing the primers to

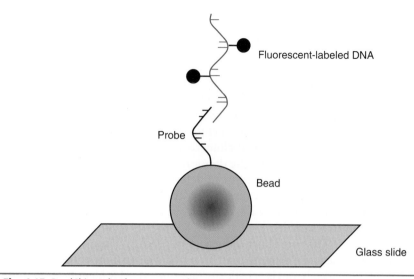

Fig. 4.15 BeadChip technology concept. (Courtesy BioArray Solutions, An Immucor Company, Warren, NJ.)

TABLE 4.1	Advantages and Limitations of Molecular Tests for Red Cell Antigens

Advantages
- Not require special reagents or rare antisera
- Serologic confirmation
- Can type patients with positive DAT without extra efforts
- Can be used in massive screening for rare antigen-negative donors

Limitations
- Discrepancies between molecular and serologic confirmation are documented
- Cannot analyze all polymorphisms
- Results can be challenging if patient or donor has altered alleles

bind to the matches in the single-stranded DNA. Unbound DNA is washed away, and the bound DNA is labeled with fluorescent-labeled deoxynucleotide triphosphates (dNTPs). Computer analysis determines which beads fluoresced and which primers attached (Fig. 4.15). Advantages and limitations of RBC molecular testing are presented in Box 4.1.

Clinical Applications of Molecular Testing for Blood Groups

Prediction of Red Cell Phenotype

In situations where patients receive large amounts of blood, such as massive or chronic transfusions, the donor red cells create a problem when trying to phenotype the patient's red cells. There are cell separation techniques to obtain autologous red cells; however, they are time consuming and often not successful. PCR-based methods provide an alternative technique to derive red cell phenotype. An extended red cell phenotype can predict additional blood group antigens that may cause alloantibody formation in future transfusions.[13]

Autoimmune hemolytic anemia is a condition in which the patient's red cells are sensitized with autoantibody. The bound immunoglobulin makes red cell typing difficult using serologic methods. The red cells must be chemically treated to remove the IgG antibodies. Typing can then proceed on the patient's red cells. Several methods are used to remove these autoantibodies from the red cells: **chloroquine diphosphate** or **EDTA-glycine acid**. These methods also have their limitations and may denature an antigen with the chemical treatment. PCR-based methods provide an alternative technique to derive red cell phenotype.[13]

Applications in Prenatal Practice

Molecular techniques can help identify a fetus who is not at risk for the development of hemolytic disease of the fetus and newborn (HDFN).[2] If the mother has an alloantibody, fetal red cells can be tested for the antigen. If antigen-negative, the fetus is not at risk for

Chloroquine diphosphate: a reagent that removes IgG antibody from red cells; used when patient has a positive DAT to obtain autologous red cells for phenotype determination

EDTA-glycine acid: a reagent that removes IgG antibody from red cells; similar function as chloroquine diphosphate

HDFN, and the mother does not require extensive monitoring. Fetal DNA testing is useful if the mother has an IgG alloantibody implicated in HDFN and the father is heterozygous or not available for testing. If the father is positive for the antigen, DNA testing can determine if he is homozygous or heterozygous for the gene. This result can establish the probability of HDFN occurrence.

Testing for Antigen-Negative Blood Donors

DNA assays applied as mass screening aids can determine phenotype of donor red cells for those red cell antigens where typing is difficult due to lack of commercially available antisera. Examples of these antigens include Hy, Jo^a, Js^a, Js^b, C^w, V, VS, S, and Fy^b.[2]

Confirm the D Type of Blood Donors

Some donors have very weak expressions of D antigens. Commercially available antisera may not detect the D antigen, and the unit label would be D-negative. The use of DNA assays to confirm D-negative phenotypes is a potential future use of molecular testing. Currently there is no testing platform that supports a high throughput and cost-effective method for confirming D-negative units.[2]

CHAPTER SUMMARY

Blood Group Genetics
- Blood group systems are serologically and genetically defined because they can be categorized by molecular and serologic properties.
- Various forms of genes at the same gene locus are called alleles and encode the blood group antigens.
- The testing of red cell antigens determines the phenotype. Inferences regarding the genotype or genetic makeup are often made; however, molecular methods or family studies are necessary to determine the genotype.
- When identical alleles for a given locus are present on both chromosomes, a person is homozygous for the allele; nonidentical alleles are heterozygous. Inheriting homozygous blood group system alleles can code for a greater antigen density, causing agglutination reactions to be stronger.
- Two or more closely linked genes can be inherited as a haplotype.
- Genes with two or more possible alleles are termed polymorphic; the HLA system is the most polymorphic.

Population Genetics
- Combined phenotype calculations are needed when a patient has multiple red cell antibodies and requires transfusion with RBC units negative for the corresponding antigens.
- Gene frequencies can be predicted using the Hardy–Weinberg equation.
- Relationship testing through direct exclusion and indirect exclusion of the alleged father is now better resolved through molecular techniques.

Molecular Genetics
- Techniques of molecular genetics, such as PCR, have made possible significant improvements in HLA tissue typing and viral marker testing on donated blood products.
- PCR is the basis of most molecular tests used in blood banking; variations in the identification of the DNA products of this technique are what distinguish SSOP, SSP, SBT, STR, and bead-chip technology.

CRITICAL THINKING EXERCISES

Exercise 4.1
Given the following pedigree for a family study involving the ABO system, determine the probable phenotype and probable genotype of the father:

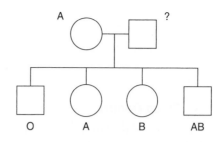

Exercise 4.2

While working in the blood bank, the laboratory staff receive a call from a father asking if his group O son could possibly belong to him. He knows that he is group B and the mother is group A. Provide an explanation in terms understandable to someone without a background in basic genetics.

Exercise 4.3

Is a person whose phenotype is M+N− homozygous or heterozygous for the M gene? Would you expect reactions with this person's red cells to be stronger or weaker than red cells that phenotyped as M+N+?

Exercise 4.4

The following pedigree represents a family study of the Xg blood group system. What are the phenotypes of the sons?

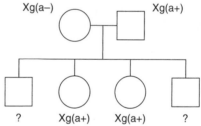

Exercise 4.5

Following antibody identification, your patient possesses anti-K, anti-Jkᵃ, and anti-E. How many RBC units do you need to screen to find two antigen-negative RBC units? The antigens occur in the population with the following frequencies: E+ = 30%; K+ = 9%; Jk(a+) = 77%.

Exercise 4.6

You performed a population study on your class and found that 84% are D-positive. Using the Hardy–Weinberg calculation, determine the percentage of your classmates who are heterozygous for D antigen.

Exercise 4.7

A pregnant woman has a positive antibody screen. Antibody identification revealed anti-K as the antibody specificity. The father's red cells were tested for the K antigen. The father's phenotype is K+ (K-positive). A molecular red cell phenotype was ordered on the father to determine the probability of HDFN due to anti-K. What information would be available through the molecular testing of the father?

Exercise 4.8

Relationship testing assumes maternity and excludes paternity by either indirect or direct exclusion. Given the following results, can you exclude paternity? If so, is the exclusion indirect or direct? Give a reason for your interpretation.

	Mother	Alleged Father	Child
Phenotype	E+e+	e+	E+
Genotype	*E/e*	*e/e*	*E/E*

STUDY QUESTIONS

1. Which of the following describes the expression of most blood group inheritance?
   a. dominant
   b. recessive
   c. sex-linked
   d. codominant

2. With which of the following red cell phenotypes would anti-Jk^a react most strongly?
   a. Jk(a–b+)
   b. Jk(a+b–)
   c. Jk(a+b+)
   d. Jk(a–b–)

3. In relationship testing, what is the criterion for a direct exclusion?
   a. genetic marker is absent in the child but present in the mother and alleged father
   b. genetic marker is absent in the child, present in the mother, and absent in the alleged father
   c. genetic marker is present in the child, absent in the mother, and present in the alleged father
   d. genetic marker is present in the child but absent in both the mother and the alleged father

4. Which of the following items is a useful genetic marker for relationship testing?
   a. all races have the same gene frequencies
   b. the genetic system is polymorphic
   c. there are no amorphic genes
   d. recombination is common

5. What term describes the inheritance of two of the same alleles from each parent?
   a. homozygous
   b. allele
   c. heterozygous
   d. syntenic

6. What term describes alternate forms of a gene at given genetic loci?
   a. alleles
   b. amplicons
   c. nucleotides
   d. amorphs

7. What is the name of the technique that uses a small amount of DNA and amplifies it for identification?
   a. RFLP
   b. DNA probe
   c. PCR
   d. gene mapping

8. What is the term for a gene that does not express a detectable product?
   a. an amorph
   b. a *cis* gene
   c. a *trans* gene
   d. a regulator gene

9. What is the name of synthetic single-stranded DNA that determines the sequence of DNA for amplification in the PCR reaction?
   a. amplicons
   b. nucleotides
   c. DNA primer
   d. *Taq* polymerases

10. What is the mode of inheritance when the genes are located close together on the same chromosome?
    a. inherited as a haplotype
    b. crossover
    c. show independent assortment
    d. suppress each other

11. In molecular techniques for HLA typing, which high-resolution method analyzes the nucleotide sequence to define the allele?
    a. SSP
    b. SSO
    c. STR
    d. SBT

12. Where is a gene inherited in a *cis* position to another gene located?
    a. on an opposite chromosome
    b. on a different chromosome number
    c. on the same chromosome
    d. antithetical

13. In PCR testing, the initial step involves adding the DNA in question to a mixture of *Taq* polymerase, excess nucleotides, $MgCl_2$, and primers. Where does the amplification process take place?
    a. flow cytometer
    b. capillary array sequencer
    c. thermal cycler
    d. electrophoresis chamber

14. Patient RJ types as group O with anti-D and anti-K alloantibodies and requires one unit of RBCs. What percentage of the white population would be compatible with her serum (group O = 0.45; D– = 0.15; K– = 0.91)?
    a. 3%
    b. 6%
    c. 20%
    d. 50%

15. Molecular tests on samples from hematopoietic progenitor cell transplant recipients are used to determine if engraftment is successful. What is the name of this method?
    a. sequence-specific primers (SSPs)
    b. sequence-based typing (SBT)
    c. short tandem repeats (STRs)
    d. sequence-specific oligonucleotide probes (SSOPs)

16. Select the phrase that defines the term antithetical.
    a. similar gene
    b. opposite allele
    c. opposite antigen
    d. heterozygous gene

17. What term is used when red cells with the genotype *MM* react stronger with anti-M than red cells with genotype *MN?*
    a. *trans* effect
    b. dosage effect
    c. *cis* effect
    d. suppressor effect

18. Which term defines a group of antigens on the red cell membrane that share related serologic properties and genetic patterns of inheritance?
    a. meiosis
    b. regulator system
    c. blood group system
    d. molecular classification

19. What genetic information is provided by hemagglutination testing for red cell antigens?
    a. genotype
    b. phenotype
    c. zygosity
    d. polymorphism

20. What genetic information is provided by DNA assays for red cell antigens?
    a. loci location
    b. phenotype
    c. polymorphism
    d. genotype

Answers to Study Questions can be found on page 387.

Additional student resources, including review questions, a laboratory manual, and case studies, can be found on the Evolve website.

REFERENCES

1. Reid ME, Lomas-Francis C, Olsson ML: *The blood group antigen facts book*, ed 3, San Diego, 2012, Academic Press.
2. Fung MK: *Technical manual*, ed 18, Bethesda, 2014, AABB.
3. Watson JD, Baker TA, Bell SP: *Molecular biology of the gene*, ed 5, San Francisco, 2004, Pearson.
4. Alexander L: Personalized therapy reaches transfusion medicine, *AABB News* 13:10, 2011.
5. Anstee DJ: Goodbye to agglutination and all that? *Transfusion* 45(5):652–653, 2005.
6. Reid ME: Applications of DNA-based assays on blood group antigen and antibody identification, *Transfusion* 43:1748, 2003.
7. Rodey GE: *HLA beyond tears*, ed 2, Durango, 2000, DeNovo, Inc.
8. *Olerup package insert*, SSP. Stockholm, Sweden, Olerup SSP AB, Franzengatan 5, 112 51.
9. *LABType SSO Typing Tests package insert*, Canoga Park, One Lambda, Inc. http://www.onelambda.com/en/product/labtype-sso-hd.html. Accessed September 2016.
10. *Invitrogen SeCore Locus Sequencing Kit instructions for use, rev 009*, Brown Deer, 2011, Invitrogen Corporation.
11. Hillyer CD, Silberstein LE: *Blood banking and transfusion medicine, basic principles and practice*, ed 2, Philadelphia, 2007, Churchill-Livingstone.
12. BioArray HEA BeadChip. http://www.immucor.com/en-us/Products/Documents/BioArray_HEA_SalesSheet.pdf. Accessed May 2015.
13. Sapatnekar S, Figueroa P: How do we use molecular red blood cell antigen typing to supplement pretransfusion testing? *Transfusion* 54:1452–1458, 2014.

5

ABO AND H BLOOD GROUP SYSTEMS AND SECRETOR STATUS

CHAPTER OUTLINE

LEARNING OBJECTIVES

On completion of this chapter, the reader should be able to:

1. Define a blood group system with regard to blood group antigens and their inheritance.
2. Explain Landsteiner's rule.
3. List the cells, body fluids, and secretions where ABO antigens can be located.
4. Describe the relationships among the *ABO, H,* and *Se* genes.
5. Differentiate between type 1 and type 2 oligosaccharide structures and state where each one is located.
6. Describe the formation of the H antigen from the gene product and its relationship to ABO antigen expression.
7. List the glycosyltransferases and the immunodominant sugars for the *A, B, O,* and *H* alleles.
8. Compare and contrast the A₁ and A₂ phenotypes regarding antigen structure and serologic testing.
9. Compare and contrast serologic testing among A₃, Aₓ, and A_el subgroups.
10. Predict the possible ABO genotypes with an ABO phenotype.
11. Describe the ABO blood group system antibodies with regard to immunoglobulin class, clinical significance, and in vitro serologic reactions.
12. Discuss the selection of whole blood, red blood cell (RBC), and plasma products for transfusions.
13. Define the terms universal donor and universal recipient as they apply to RBC and plasma products.
14. Apply concepts of ABO compatibility in the selection of blood products for recipients.
15. List the technical errors that may result in an ABO discrepancy.
16. Define the acquired B antigen and the B(A) phenotypes; interpret the ABO discrepancies that would result from these phenotypes and methods used in resolving these discrepancies.
17. List reasons for missing or weakly expressed ABO antigens; identify the test methods used to resolve these discrepancies.
18. Describe ABO discrepancies due to extra reactions in serum testing and their resolution.
19. Illustrate the Bombay phenotype with regard to genetic pathway, serologic reactions, and transfusion implications.
20. Define the terms secretor and nonsecretor.
21. Identify and resolve ABO typing discrepancies from ABO typing results.
22. Apply concepts to solve case studies with ABO-discrepant information.

This chapter begins a section of the textbook dedicated to the basic understanding of blood group systems and their significance in the practice of transfusion medicine. A blood group system is composed of antigens that are produced by alleles at a single genetic locus or at loci so closely linked that genetic crossing over rarely occurs.[1] Blood group antigens are molecules located primarily on the red cell membrane. These molecules can be classified biochemically as proteins and as carbohydrates linked to either a lipid (glycolipid) or a protein (glycoprotein) as shown in Fig. 5.1. With adequate immunologic exposure, a blood group antigen may elicit the production of its corresponding antibody in individuals who lack the antigen. During transfusions, the recipient is exposed to many blood group antigens. Patients receiving transfusions may produce alloantibodies in response to the exposure to blood group antigens not present on their own red cells.

Because the terminology for red cell antigens is inconsistent, the International Society of Blood Transfusion (ISBT) created a Working Party on Terminology for Red Cell Antigens in 1980 to standardize blood group systems and antigen names. The committee's goal was not to create replacement terminology but rather to provide additional terminology suitable for use with computer software. The ISBT Working Party, now called Red Cell Immunogenetics and Blood Group Terminology, has assigned genetically based numeric designations for red cell antigens and presently has defined 36 blood group systems (Table 5.1).[2,3] According to ISBT criteria, genetic studies and serologic data are required before an antigen is assigned to a blood group system. The ABO blood group system has been assigned the ISBT number 001 with four antigens. The H blood group system is ISBT number 018 with one antigen. This textbook addresses blood group systems with commonly used names and includes ISBT symbols and numbers.

> Blood group antigens form part of the red cell membranes. Antigens differ depending on inheritance of blood group genes as described in Chapter 4.

SECTION 1
HISTORICAL OVERVIEW OF ABO BLOOD GROUP SYSTEM

The discovery of the ABO blood group system by Landsteiner[4] in 1900 marked the beginning of modern blood banking and transfusion medicine. In a series of experiments

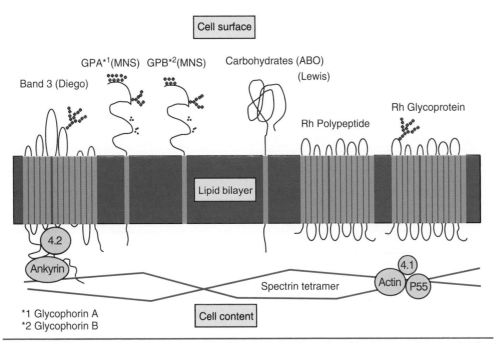

Fig. 5.1 Model of red cell membrane that carries blood group antigens from blood group systems and collections. The red cell antigens are molecules that form part of the red cell membrane's lipid bilayer or extend from the surface of the red cell. (Redrawn from Reid ME, Lomas-Francis C: *The blood group antigen facts book,* ed 2, San Diego, CA, 2004, Elsevier Academic Press.)

TABLE 5.1   ISBT Blood Group System Assignments*

BLOOD SYSTEM NAME	ISBT GENE NAME	ISBT NUMBER
ABO	ABO	001
MNS	MNS	002
P1PK	P1	003
Rh	RH	004
Lutheran	LU	005
Kell	KEL	006
Lewis	LE	007
Duffy	FY	008
Kidd	JK	009
Diego	DI	010
Cartwright (Yt)	YT	011
Xg	XG	012
Scianna	SC	013
Dombrock	DO	014
Colton	CO	015
Landsteiner–Wiener	LW	016
Chido/Rodgers	CH/RG	017
Hh	H	018
Kx	XK	019
Gerbich	GE	020
Cromer	CROM	021
Knops	KN	022
Indian	IN	023
Ok	OK	024
Raph	RAPH	025
JMH	JMH	026
I	IGNT	027
Globoside	GLOB	028
Gil	GIL	029
Rh-associated glycoprotein	RHAG	030
FORS	FORS	031
JR	JR	032
LAN	LAN	033
VEL	VEL	034
CD59	CD59	035
AUG	AUG	036

ISBT, International Society of Blood Transfusion.
*Current as of April 2016.

designed to show serologic incompatibilities between humans, Landsteiner recognized different patterns of agglutination when human blood samples were mixed in random pairings. He described the blood groups as A, B, and O. Several years later, Landsteiner's associates, von Decastello and Sturli, added group AB to the original observations.[5] In his investigations, Landsteiner noted the presence of agglutinating antibodies in the serum of individuals who lacked the corresponding ABO antigen. He observed that

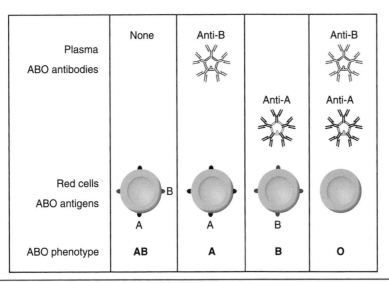

Fig. 5.2 Relationship between ABO antigens and antibodies. ABO antigens are located on the red cells. Group AB possesses both A and B antigens; group A possesses A antigens; group B possesses B antigens; group O lacks both A and B antigens. ABO antibodies are located in plasma. Group AB lacks ABO antibodies; group A possesses anti-B; group B possesses anti-A; group O possesses anti-A and anti-B. (Modified from Immunobase, Bio-Rad Laboratories, Inc., Hercules, CA.)

group A red cells agglutinated with the serum from group B individuals. This observation has been termed **Landsteiner's rule** (or Landsteiner's law). Landsteiner's rule established that normal, healthy individuals possess ABO antibodies to the ABO blood group antigens lacking on their red cells. Individuals with group A red cells possess the A antigen and lack the B antigen. Therefore these individuals possess anti-B antibodies. Individuals with group B red cells possess the B antigen and lack the A antigen. Therefore these individuals possess anti-A antibodies. Antigens and antibodies associated with each ABO phenotype are illustrated in Fig. 5.2. Four major phenotypes are derived from the two major antigens (A and B) of the system. These phenotypes are group A, group B, group AB, and group O. Scan the QR code for more information about Karl Landsteiner.

The first blood group system described, the ABO blood group system, remains the most important blood group system for transfusion purposes. Accurate donor and recipient ABO phenotypes are fundamental to transfusion safety because of the presence of ABO antibodies in individuals with no previous exposure to human red cells. The transfusion of ABO-incompatible blood to a recipient can result in intravascular hemolysis and other serious consequences of an **acute hemolytic transfusion reaction.**

Landsteiner's rule: rule stating that normal, healthy individuals possess ABO antibodies to the ABO blood group antigens absent from their red cells

Acute hemolytic transfusion reaction: complication of transfusion associated with intravascular hemolysis, characterized by rapid onset with symptoms of fever, chills, hemoglobinemia, and hypotension; major complications include irreversible shock, renal failure, and disseminated intravascular coagulation

SECTION 2

ABO AND H BLOOD GROUP SYSTEM ANTIGENS

GENERAL CHARACTERISTICS OF ABO ANTIGENS

ABO antigens are widely distributed and are located on red cells, lymphocytes (adsorbed from plasma), platelets (adsorbed from plasma), most epithelial and endothelial cells, and organs such as the kidneys.[3] Soluble forms of the ABO blood group system antigens can also be synthesized and secreted by tissue cells. As a result, ABO blood group system antigens are found in association with cellular membranes and as soluble forms. Soluble antigens are detected in secretions and all body fluids except cerebrospinal fluid.[3] ABO blood group system antigens, which are intrinsic to the red cell membrane, exist as either glycolipid or glycoprotein molecules, whereas the soluble forms are primarily glycoproteins.

Cord blood: whole blood obtained from the umbilical vein or artery of the fetus

When phenotyping cord blood samples, blood grouping reagents anti-A and anti-B may show weaker agglutination reactions.

The ABO locus is located on chromosome 9. The H locus is located on chromosome 19.

ABO antigens are detectable at 5 to 6 weeks in utero.[6] A newborn possesses fewer antigen copies per red cell compared with an adult. For example, adult red cells carry 610,000 to 830,000 B antigens, whereas newborn red cells carry 200,000 to 320,000 B antigens.[7] Newborns' red cells also lack the fully developed antigen structures of adults' red cells. In **cord blood** samples, ABO antigens have fewer numbers and partially developed antigen structures and may demonstrate weaker ABO phenotyping reactions. Antigen development occurs slowly until the full expression of adult levels is reached at about 2 to 4 years of age.[6]

The worldwide frequency of ABO phenotypes within the white population has been well documented. Group O and group A individuals constitute 45% and 40% of whites. These two blood groups are the most common ABO phenotypes, followed by group B with an 11% frequency and group AB with a 4% frequency.[8] ABO phenotype frequencies differ in selected populations and ethnic groups. For example, the group B phenotype has a higher frequency in blacks and Asians compared with whites (Table 5.2).

INHERITANCE AND DEVELOPMENT OF A, B, AND H ANTIGENS

A discussion of the inheritance and formation of ABO antigens requires an understanding of the H antigen, which is inherited independently of the ABO blood group system antigens. The *H* gene genetically controls the production of H antigen, which is located on a different chromosome from the ABO genetic locus. In addition to the *ABO* and *H* genes, the expression of soluble ABO antigens is influenced by inheritance of the *Se* gene (see the section "Secretor Status" later in this chapter). The *Se* gene genetically influences the formation of ABO antigens in saliva, tears, and other body fluids. Consequently, occurrence and location of the ABO antigens are influenced by three genetically independent loci: *ABO, H,* and *Se.*

ABO antigens are assembled on a common carbohydrate structure that also serves as the base for the formation of the H, Lewis, I/i, and P1 antigens. Consequently, this common carbohydrate structure is capable of antigen expression for more than one blood group system (Fig. 5.3). This common structure is analogous to an antigen building block. Because of the interrelationship between the common antigen building block and multiple

TABLE 5.2	Frequency Distributions of ABO Phenotypes (U.S. Population)		
ABO PHENOTYPE	**WHITE (%)**	**BLACK (%)**	**ASIAN (%)**
A	40	27	28
B	11	20	27
AB	4	4	5
O	45	49	40

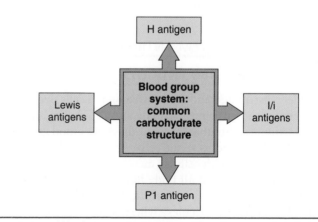

Fig. 5.3 Antigens in several blood group systems are formed from the same carbohydrate precursor structure.

blood group systems, it is important to recognize that the action of genes of one blood group system can affect the expression of antigens in another system.

Common Structure for A, B, and H Antigens

The common structure (antigen building block) for A, B, and H antigens is an **oligosaccharide chain** attached to either a protein or a lipid carrier molecule. The oligosaccharide chain comprises four sugar molecules linked in simple linear forms or complex branched structures. The two terminal sugars, D-galactose and N-acetylglucosamine, may be linked together in two different configurations. When the number 1 carbon of D-galactose is linked with the number 3 carbon of N-acetylglucosamine, the linkage is described as β1→3. Type 1 oligosaccharide chains are formed. When the number 1 carbon of D-galactose is linked with the number 4 carbon of N-acetylglucosamine, the linkage is described as β1→4. Type 2 oligosaccharide chains are formed (Fig. 5.4). Type 2 structures are associated primarily with glycolipids and glycoproteins on the red cell membrane, and type 1 structures are associated primarily with body fluids. Some type 2 glycoprotein structures are located in body fluids and secretions.[9]

Development of H Antigen

The H antigen is the only antigen in the H blood group system. This blood group system, assigned to a locus on chromosome 19, is closely linked with the *Se* locus. The *H* locus has two significant alleles: *H* and *h*. The *H* allele is a dominant allele with high frequency (>99.99%), whereas the *h* allele is classified as an amorph with rare frequency. Genes encode for the production of proteins, and the gene product of the *H* allele is a protein classified biochemically as a **transferase** enzyme. Transferase enzymes promote the transfer of a biochemical group from one molecule to another. A **glycosyltransferase** enzyme catalyzes the transfer of glycosyl groups (simple carbohydrate units) in biochemical reactions.

In the formation of H antigen, a glycosyltransferase enzyme transfers a sugar molecule, L-fucose, to either type 1 or type 2 common oligosaccharide chains. The biochemical name for this enzyme is L-fucosyltransferase (*FUT-1*). The L-fucose added to the terminal galactose of the type 1 and type 2 chain is called the **immunodominant sugar** for H antigens because the sugar confers H specificity (Fig. 5.5).[10] Formation of the H antigen is the end product of an enzymatic reaction. This formation is crucial to the expression of A and B antigens because the gene products of the *ABO* alleles require that the H antigen be the acceptor molecule. The *FUT-1* gene adds galactose to both oligosaccharide chains on red cells and in secretions. Scan the QR code for molecular information about glycosyltransferases A and B.

This section previously described the *h* allele as an amorph with no detectable gene product. The red cells from an *h* homozygote (*hh*) are classified as the **Bombay phenotype**. These rare individuals lack both H antigen and ABO antigen expression on their red cells. The Bombay phenotype is discussed in more detail at the end of this chapter.

Oligosaccharide chain: chemical compound formed by a small number of simple carbohydrate molecules

Transferase: class of enzymes that catalyzes the transfer of a chemical group from one molecule to another

Glycosyltransferase: enzyme that catalyzes the transfer of glycosyl groups (simple carbohydrate units) in biochemical reactions

Immunodominant sugar: sugar molecule responsible for specificity

Bombay phenotype: rare phenotype of an individual who genetically has inherited the *h* allele in a homozygous manner; the individual's red cells lack H and ABO antigens

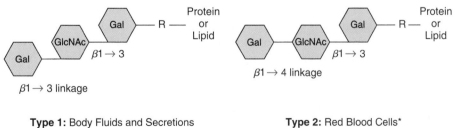
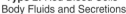

Type 1: Body Fluids and Secretions   **Type 2:** Red Blood Cells*
                                                Body Fluids and Secretions

Fig. 5.4 Type 1 and type 2 oligosaccharide chain structures. *Gal*, Galactose; *GlcNAc*, N-acetylglucosamine; ***, most type 2 chains are located on the red cells. (Modified from Brecher ME, editor: *Technical manual*, ed 15, Bethesda, MD, 2005, AABB.)

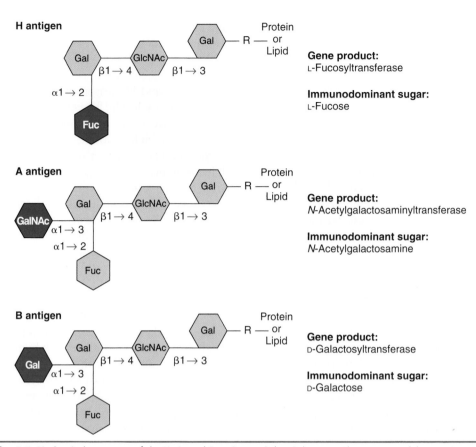

Fig. 5.5 Biochemical structures of the H, A, and B antigens. *Gal*, D-Galactose; *GlcNAc*, *N*-acetylglucosamine; *Fuc*, L-fucose; *GalNAc*, *N*-acetylgalactosamine. (Modified from Brecher ME, editor: *Technical manual*, ed 15, Bethesda, MD, 2005, AABB.)

Development of A and B Antigens

The precursor of A and B antigens is the H antigen.

Genetic control of A and B antigens has been mapped to chromosome 9. Three major alleles exist within the *ABO* locus: *A*, *B*, and *O*. The *A* and *B* alleles, similar to the *H* allele, are glycosyltransferases. The *A* allele produces *N*-acetylgalactosaminyltransferase, which transfers the sugar *N*-acetylgalactosamine to an oligosaccharide chain; the chain was previously converted to H antigen. The *B* allele produces D-galactosyltransferase, which transfers the sugar D-galactose to an oligosaccharide chain; the chain was previously converted to H antigen (see Fig. 5.5).[10] *N*-acetylgalactosamine is the immunodominant sugar for A specificity, and D-galactose is the immunodominant sugar for B specificity.

The specificity of A and B antigen is defined by immunodominant sugars: *N*-acetylgalactosamine (A antigen) and D-galactose (B antigen).

The O allele is considered nonfunctional because the resulting gene product is an enzymatically inactive protein. As a result, group O red cells carry no A or B antigens but are rich in unconverted H antigens. Adult group O red cells have about 1.7 million H antigen copies per red cell and possess the greatest concentration of H antigens per red cell.[3] Other ABO phenotypes have fewer copies of H antigens because the H antigen is the acceptor molecule for the A and B enzymes. Group A_1B phenotype possesses the lowest number of unconverted H sites. Fig. 5.6 illustrates the variation of H antigen concentration in ABO phenotypes.

Yamamoto et al[11] defined the molecular basis of the ABO phenotypes. These investigators discovered that a few mutations exist in the glycosyltransferase gene at the ABO locus. On the molecular level, the A and B glycosyltransferases differ slightly in their nucleic acid compositions. Additionally, the nucleic acid composition of the *O* allele has revealed that it does not produce an enzymatically active protein capable of acting on the H antigen precursors.

A and B antigens are not primary gene products.

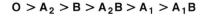

$$O > A_2 > B > A_2B > A_1 > A_1B$$

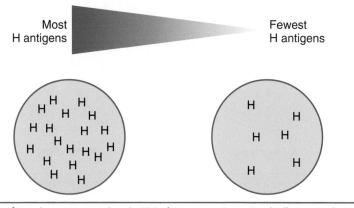

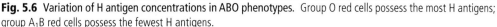

Most
H antigens

Fewest
H antigens

Fig. 5.6 Variation of H antigen concentrations in ABO phenotypes. Group O red cells possess the most H antigens; group A_1B red cells possess the fewest H antigens.

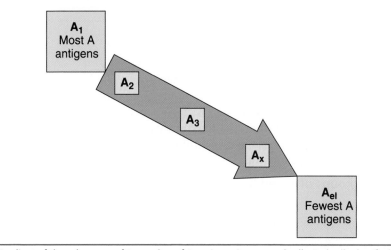

A_1
Most A
antigens

A_2

A_3

A_x

A_{el}
Fewest A
antigens

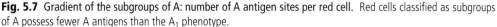

Fig. 5.7 Gradient of the subgroups of A: number of A antigen sites per red cell. Red cells classified as subgroups of A possess fewer A antigens than the A_1 phenotype.

ABO SUBGROUPS

Comparison of A_1 and A_2 Phenotypes

The ABO phenotypes can be divided into categories termed subgroups. Subgroups differ in the number of antigen copies expressed on the red cell membrane, representing a quantitative difference in antigen expression (Fig. 5.7). Some evidence also exists to support the theory of qualitative differences in antigen expression. Some subgroups possess more highly branched, complex antigenic structures, whereas others have simplified linear forms of antigen.[12]

The group A phenotype is classified into two major subgroups: A_1 and A_2. These glycosyltransferase gene products, which are genetically controlled by the A^1 and A^2 genes, differ slightly in their ability to convert H antigen to A antigen. The A_1 phenotype, encoded by the A^1 gene, exists in about 80% of group A individuals. In the A_1 phenotype, A antigens are highly concentrated on branched and linear oligosaccharide chains. The A^1 gene effectively acts on the H antigens in the production of A antigens. The A_2 phenotype, encoded by the A^2 gene, constitutes about 20% of group A individuals. In the A_2 phenotype, A antigen copies are fewer than in the A_1 phenotype. This phenotype is assembled on the simplified linear forms of the oligosaccharide chains. An alloantibody, anti-A1, can be detected in 1% to 8% of A_2 individuals and in 22% to 35% of A_2B individuals.

In routine ABO phenotyping, both A_1 and A_2 red cells agglutinate with commercially available anti-A reagents. These red cells are distinguished in serologic testing with a reagent called ***Dolichos biflorus*** lectin. This lectin is extracted from the seeds of the plant

Dolichos biflorus: plant lectin with specificity for the A1 antigen

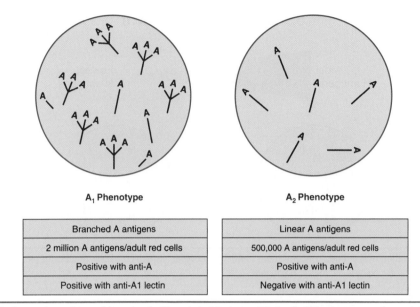

A₁ Phenotype	A₂ Phenotype
Branched A antigens	Linear A antigens
2 million A antigens/adult red cells	500,000 A antigens/adult red cells
Positive with anti-A	Positive with anti-A
Positive with anti-A1 lectin	Negative with anti-A1 lectin

Fig. 5.8 Comparison of A₁ and A₂ red cells. (From Issitt PD, Anstee DJ: *Applied blood group serology*, ed 4, Durham, NC, 1998, Montgomery Scientific Publications.)

A₁ and A₂ phenotypes demonstrate 3+ to 4+ reactions with commercial anti-A reagents.

Anti-A1 lectin is useful in resolving ABO typing problems when A₂ phenotypes develop anti-A1.

Mixed-field agglutination: agglutination pattern in which a population of the red cells has agglutinated and the remainder of the red cells is unagglutinated

Adsorption: procedure that uses red cells (known antigens) to remove red cell antibodies from a solution (plasma or antisera); group A red cells can remove anti-A from solution

Ulex europaeus: plant lectin with specificity for the H antigen

Elution: procedure that dissociates antigen–antibody complexes on red cells; freed IgG antibody is tested for specificity

Dolichos biflorus and has anti-A1 specificity. When properly diluted, the *Dolichos biflorus* lectin (anti-A1 lectin) agglutinates A₁, but not A₂, red cells. The anti-A1 lectin is not used in routine ABO testing of donors and recipients because it is unnecessary to distinguish between the A₁ and A₂ phenotypes for transfusion purposes. This reagent is useful in resolving ABO typing problems and identifying infrequent subgroups of A. Fig. 5.8 compares the A₁ and A₂ phenotypes.

Additional Subgroups of A and B

Subgroups of A

Although more infrequent than A₁ and A₂, other A subgroups have been described that involve reduced expression of A antigens. The decreased number of A antigen sites per red cell result in weak or no agglutination when tested with commercial anti-A reagents. The subgroups are genetically controlled by the inheritance of rare alleles at the *ABO* locus and collectively have a frequency of less than 1%. Because these subgroups occur so infrequently, they are mainly of academic interest. The A subgroups have been classified as A$_{int}$, A₃, A$_x$, A$_m$, A$_{end}$, A$_{el}$, and A$_{bantu}$, based on the reactivity of red cells with human anti-A and anti-A,B. Historically, human polyclonal-based anti-A,B contained an antibody with specificity toward both the A and the B antigens that could not be separated into anti-A and anti-B components. This reagent possessed an enhanced ability to detect weaker subgroups compared with anti-A. Current anti-A,B monoclonal antibody reagents blend anti-A and anti-B clones for formulations to detect the weaker subgroups.

Weak or no agglutination with commercial anti-A monoclonal antibody reagents is a key factor in recognizing a subgroup in this category. Murine monoclonal blends of commercial anti-A have been formulated to enhance the detection of these weaker subgroups in ABO phenotyping. These monoclonal antibody anti-A reagents are blended to ensure that some subgroups of A are readily detected. Some subgroups may characteristically demonstrate **mixed-field agglutination** patterns (eg, A₃ subgroup) or possess anti-A1 in the serum (eg, A₃, A$_x$, and A$_{el}$ subgroups).[13] Some subgroups of A continue to react weakly or not react with murine monoclonal blends of anti-A. In these circumstances, saliva studies for the detection of soluble forms of A and H antigens and testing with anti-H lectin (*Ulex europaeus*) may provide additional information. The amount of H antigen present on the weak subgroups of A is usually equivalent to group O red cells (3+ to 4+ reactions). Special techniques of **adsorption** and **elution** may also be necessary to demonstrate the presence of the A antigen (eg, A$_{el}$ subgroup). However, these techniques are not performed routinely.

TABLE 5.3	Serologic Characteristics of A_3, A_x, and A_{el} Subgroups						
			RED CELL AGGLUTINATION WITH				
SUBGROUP	ANTI-A	HUMAN ANTI-A,B	ANTI-H LECTIN*	ANTI-A1 LECTIN†	SOLUBLE ANTIGENS IN SALIVA‡	ANTI-A1 IN SERUM
A_3	++ mf	++ mf	+++	0	A and H	0 to ++§
A_x	weak/0	+ to ++	++++	0	H	0 to ++§
A_{el}	0	0	++++	0	H	0 to ++§

mf, Mixed field.
*Ulex europaeus.
†Dolichos biflorus.
‡If secretor.
§Variable occurrence of anti-A1.

The serologic classification of rare A subgroups is determined by the following:
- Weak or no red cell agglutination with anti-A and anti-A,B commercial reagents
- No agglutination with anti-A1 lectin
- Presence or absence of anti-A1 in the serum
- Strong agglutination reactions with anti-H
- Presence of A and H in saliva
- Adsorption and elution studies

Table 5.3 provides information regarding the serologic characteristics of A_3, A_x, and A_{el} subgroups.[10] Weak subgroups of A are difficult to classify using serologic techniques. Usually the phenotype is described as A subgroup or A subgroup B. For definitive classification, molecular techniques are available to characterize the genotype, if necessary.

Subgroups of B

B subgroups are rarer than the A subgroups. The criteria for the recognition and differentiation of these subgroups are similar to criteria of the A subgroups. Typically, these subgroups demonstrate weak or no agglutination of red cells with anti-B reagents.

Importance of Subgroup Identification in Donor Testing

Although subgroups of A and B are considered to be of academic interest, the failure to detect a weak subgroup could have serious consequences. If a weak subgroup is missed in a recipient (the individual receiving the transfusion), the recipient would be classified as group O. Classification as a group O rather than a weak subgroup would probably not harm the recipient because group O red cells would be selected for transfusion and can be transfused to any ABO phenotype. However, an error in donor phenotyping and the subsequent labeling of the donor unit as group O (rather than group A) might result in the decreased survival of the transfused cells in a group O recipient. Group O recipients would possess ABO antibodies capable of reacting with the weak subgroup antigens in vivo, resulting in the decreased survival of these transfused red cells in the recipient's circulation.

SECTION 3

GENETIC FEATURES OF ABO BLOOD GROUP SYSTEM

Inheritance of genes from the *ABO* locus on chromosome 9 follows the laws of Mendelian genetics. An individual inherits two *ABO* genes (one from each parent). The three major alleles of the ABO blood group system are *A*, *B*, and *O*. The *A* gene subsequently can be divided into the A^1 and A^2 alleles. The *A* and *B* genes express a codominant mode of inheritance, whereas the *O* allele is recessive. The A^1 allele is dominant over the A^2 allele, and both alleles are dominant over the *O* allele. The major ABO phenotypes and possible corresponding genotypes for the phenotypes are outlined in Table 5.4. Correct use of terminology regarding the ABO blood group system should be mentioned. When reference is made to the alleles A^1 and A^2, the numbers are always indicated as superscripts. In references to the A_1 and A_2 phenotypes, the numbers are always indicated in a subscript format.

TABLE 5.4	ABO Phenotypes and Possible Genotypes
PHENOTYPE	**POSSIBLE GENOTYPES**
Group A_1	A^1A^1
	A^1A^2
	A^1O
Group A_2	A^2A^2
	A^2O
Group B	BB
	BO
Group A_1B	A^1B
Group A_2B	A^2B
Group O	OO

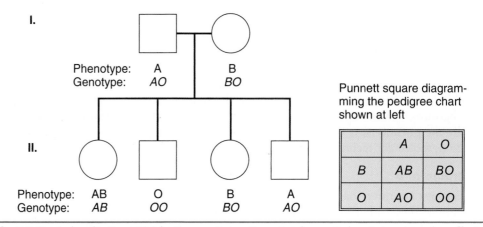

Punnett square diagramming the pedigree chart shown at left

	A	O
B	AB	BO
O	AO	OO

Fig. 5.9 Practical application: ABO inheritance patterns. Group A and group B phenotypes may produce offspring with group AB, O, B, and A phenotypes if the parents' genotypes are *AO* and *BO*.

Because the O allele is recessive, it is not always possible to determine the ABO genotype from the corresponding phenotype without family studies or molecular analysis. Red cells can be phenotyped only for the presence or absence of antigens and cannot be genotyped. Unless a family study has been performed with conclusive results, a genotype is only a probable interpretation of a phenotype. Deduction of the genotype from a family study is illustrated in Fig. 5.9. The Generation I female's phenotype is group B with possible genotypes of *BB* or *BO*, and the male's phenotype is group A with possible genotypes of *AA* or *AO*. The parental genotypes may be deduced only after phenotyping the offspring. The four offspring's phenotypes are presented in Generation II. To produce a group O offspring, both parents must have passed on the O allele. Therefore their genotypes must be *AO* and *BO*.

SECTION 4
ABO BLOOD GROUP SYSTEM ANTIBODIES

As Landsteiner recognized in his early experiments, individuals possess the ABO antibody in their serum directed against the ABO antigen absent from their red cells. Landsteiner's rule remains an important consideration in the selection of blood products, given that ABO antibodies exist in healthy individuals. These ABO antibodies, present in individuals with no known exposure to blood or blood products, were originally thought to be "naturally occurring." The current hypothesis is that biochemical structures similar to A and B antigens are present in the environment in bacteria, plants, and pollen. As a result of this environmental exposure to these similar forms of A and B antigens, individuals

TABLE 5.5	Reduction in ABO Antibody Titers
Age-Related	
Newborn	
Elderly	
Pathologic Etiology	
Chronic lymphocytic leukemia	
Congenital hypogammaglobulinemia or **acquired hypogammaglobulinemia**	
Congenital agammaglobulinemia or **acquired agammaglobulinemia**	
Immunosuppressive therapy	
Bone marrow transplant	
Multiple myeloma	

Congenital hypogamma-globulinemia: genetic disease characterized by reduced levels of gamma globulin in the blood

Acquired hypogammaglobu-linemia: lower-than-normal levels of gamma globulin in the blood associated with malignant diseases (chronic leukemias and myeloma) and immunosuppressive therapy

Congenital agammaglobulin-emia: genetic disease characterized by the absence of gamma globulin and antibodies in the blood

Acquired agammaglobulin-emia: absence of gamma globulin and antibodies associated with malignant diseases such as leukemia, myeloma, or lymphoma

Non–red blood cell stimu-lated: immunologic stimulus for antibody production is unrelated to a red cell antigen

Titers: extent to which an antibody is diluted before it loses its ability to agglutinate with antigen

respond immunologically to these antigens and produce ABO antibodies detectable in plasma and serum.[14] Consequently, the term naturally occurring is a misnomer because an immunologic stimulus is present for antibody development. The term **non–red blood cell stimulated** is more appropriate for describing the ABO antibodies.

Newborns do not produce their own ABO antibodies until they are 3 to 6 months of age.[6] ABO antibodies detected before this time are maternal in origin. Maximal ABO **titers** have been reported in children 5 to 10 years old. As a person ages, the ABO titers tend to decrease and may cause problems in ABO phenotyping. In addition to newborns and older patients, other situations exist where ABO antibody titers may be weak or not demonstrable in testing (Table 5.5).[15] Recognition of these circumstances can assist in resolving ABO phenotyping problems discussed later in this chapter.

GENERAL CHARACTERISTICS OF HUMAN ANTI-A AND ANTI-B

Immunoglobulin Class

The anti-A produced in group B individuals and the anti-B produced by group A individuals contain primarily antibodies of the IgM class along with small amounts of IgG. In contrast, anti-A and anti-B antibodies found in the serum of group O individuals are composed primarily of the IgG class. The titers of anti-A and anti-B can vary widely. In whites, the titer of anti-A is higher than anti-B; in blacks, the titers of both anti-A and anti-B are higher than those found in whites.[6]

Hemolytic Properties and Clinical Significance

IgG and IgM forms of anti-A and anti-B are capable of the activation and binding of complement and eventual hemolysis of red cells in vivo or in vitro. Because of their ability to activate the complement cascade with resultant hemolysis, the ABO antibodies are considered of **clinical significance** in transfusion medicine. An antigen–antibody reaction between a recipient's ABO antibody and the ABO phenotype of the transfused red cells can cause activation of complement and destruction of the transfused donor red cells, precipitating the clinical signs and symptoms of an acute hemolytic transfusion reaction. For example, a group A recipient has circulating anti-B antibodies in serum. If this individual were transfused with group B or AB donor red cells, the circulating anti-B would recognize the B antigen on the donor red cells and combine with the antigens. The complement system is readily activated, causing a decreased survival of transfused red cells.

Clinical significance: antibodies capable of causing decreased survival of transfused cells as in a transfusion reaction; have been associated with hemolytic disease of the fetus and newborn

In Vitro Serologic Reactions

ABO antibodies directly agglutinate a suspension of red cells in a physiologic saline environment and do not require any additional potentiators. They are optimally reactive in immediate-spin phases at room temperature (15° C to 25° C). The agglutination reactions do not require an incubation period and react immediately on centrifugation.

Anti-A and anti-B react in immediate-spin phases (direct agglutination reactions). This property is the basis of the tube test.

HUMAN ANTI-A,B FROM GROUP O INDIVIDUALS

Human anti-A,B is detected in the serum of group O individuals with unique activities beyond mixtures of anti-A and anti-B antibodies. Activity of human anti-A,B is regarded as a specificity that is cross-reactive with both A and B antigens. A cross-reactive antibody is capable of recognizing a particular molecular structure (antigenic determinant) common to several molecules. This distinguishing characteristic enables the antibody to agglutinate with red cells of group A, B, and AB phenotypes because this antibody recognizes a structure shared by both A and B antigens. Human anti-A,B also manifests the property of agglutinating red cells of infrequent subgroups of A, particularly A_x. Before the advent of monoclonal reagents, human anti-A,B was widely used to detect these infrequent subgroups in routine ABO typing. Monoclonal antibody reagents have since replaced the use of human anti-A,B in ABO phenotyping.

ANTI-A1

In accordance with Landsteiner's rule for expected ABO antibodies, sera from group O and B individuals contain anti-A antibodies. The anti-A produced by group O and B individuals can be separated by adsorption and elution techniques into two components: anti-A and anti-A1. Anti-A1 is specific for the A1 antigen and does not agglutinate A_2 red cells. The optimal reactivity of this antibody is at room temperature or lower. Anti-A1 is not considered clinically significant for transfusion purposes. Anti-A1 becomes a concern when it causes problems with ABO phenotyping results and **incompatible crossmatches** on immediate spin. Anti-A2 does not exist because the A_2 phenotype possesses the same A antigens as A_1 phenotype but in reduced quantities. Individuals with A_1 phenotype do not respond immunologically when exposed to A_2 red cells.

Incompatible crossmatches: occur when agglutination or hemolysis is observed in the crossmatch of donor red cells and patient serum, indicating a serologic incompatibility. The donor unit would not be transfused.

SECTION 5

ABO BLOOD GROUP SYSTEM AND TRANSFUSION

ROUTINE ABO PHENOTYPING

A fundamental procedure of immunohematologic testing is the determination of the ABO phenotype. The procedure is straightforward and is divided into two components: testing of the red cells for the presence of ABO antigens (or forward grouping) and testing of serum or plasma for the expected ABO antibodies (or reverse grouping). According to the *Standards for Blood Banks and Transfusion Services,* donor and recipient red cells must be tested using anti-A and anti-B reagents. Donor and recipient serum or plasma must be tested for the expected ABO antibodies using reagent A_1 and B red cells.[15] Neither human anti-A,B nor the monoclonal blend anti-A,B is required in ABO typing. Testing of cord blood and samples from infants younger than 4 months requires only red cell testing in ABO phenotyping because ABO antibody levels are not detectable.

The ABO phenotype is determined when the red cells are directly tested for the presence or absence of either A or B antigens. Serum testing provides a control for red cell testing because ABO antibodies would reflect Landsteiner's rule. Table 5.6 shows the expected reactions observed in ABO phenotyping. An **ABO discrepancy** occurs when red cell testing does not agree with the expected serum testing. Any discrepancy in ABO testing should be resolved before transfusion of recipients or labeling of donor units.

Donor blood samples are routinely typed at the time of donation. The ABO-labeled red blood cell (RBC) donor units are confirmatory typed on receipt at the hospital transfusion service.

ABO discrepancy: occurs when ABO phenotyping of red cells does not agree with expected serum testing results for the particular ABO phenotype

The procedure for ABO phenotyping is presented in the *Laboratory Manual* that accompanies this textbook.

Reverse grouping (serum or plasma testing) is not required for confirmatory testing of labeled, previously typed donor RBCs and in infants younger than 4 months of age.

SELECTION OF ABO-COMPATIBLE RED BLOOD CELLS AND PLASMA PRODUCTS FOR TRANSFUSION

In routine transfusion practices, donor products (RBCs and plasma) with identical ABO phenotypes are usually available to the recipient. This transfusion selection is referred to as providing ABO-identical (ABO group–specific) blood for the intended recipient. In

TABLE 5.6	ABO Phenotype Reactions			
	RED CELL REACTIONS WITH		SERUM OR PLASMA REACTIONS WITH	
PHENOTYPE	ANTI-A	ANTI-B	A_1 CELLS	B CELLS
Group A	+	0	0	+
Group B	0	+	+	0
Group O	0	0	+	+
Group AB	+	+	0	0

+, Agglutination; 0, no agglutination.

TABLE 5.7	Practical Application: ABO Compatibility for Whole Blood, Red Blood Cells, and Plasma Transfusions			
RECIPIENT		DONOR		
ABO PHENOTYPE	WHOLE BLOOD	RED BLOOD CELLS	PLASMA	
Group A	Group A	Groups A, O	Groups A, AB	
Group B	Group B	Groups B, O	Groups B, AB	
Group AB	Group AB	Groups AB, A, B, O	Group AB	
Group O	Group O	Group O	Groups O, A, B, AB	

situations where blood of identical ABO phenotype is unavailable, ABO-compatible (ABO group–compatible) blood may be issued to the recipient.

For RBC transfusions, ABO compatibility between the recipient and the donor is defined as the serologic compatibility between the ABO antibodies present in the recipient's serum and the ABO antigens expressed on the donor's red cells. For example, a group A recipient who concurrently demonstrates anti-B in serum would be compatible with either group A or group O donor red cells because serum anti-B would not react with either the group A or the group O red cells in vivo. However, if this individual receives a transfusion with either group B or group AB donor red cells, recipient anti-B antibodies would recognize the B antigens present on the red cells. Antigen–antibody complexes form, may activate the complement cascade, and result in the signs and symptoms of an acute hemolytic transfusion reaction. ABO compatibility applies to RBC transfusions but not to transfusions of whole blood. When whole blood is transfused, ABO-identical donor units must be provided because both plasma and red cells are present in the product. The concepts of ABO compatibility for whole blood and RBC transfusions are outlined in Table 5.7. Scan the QR code to play the Blood Typing Game.

Persons with group O red cells are called **universal donors** because the RBC product lacks both A and B antigens and could be transfused to any ABO phenotype. Group O donor RBCs can be used in times of urgency for emergency release of donor units. Conversely, group AB recipients are considered **universal recipients** because these individuals lack circulating ABO antibodies and can receive RBCs of any ABO phenotype.

When plasma products are transfused, the selection of an ABO-identical phenotype is the ideal situation. When identical ABO phenotypes are unavailable, the rationale for compatible plasma transfusions is the reverse of RBC transfusions. In this case the donor's plasma must be compatible with the recipient's red cells. Serologic compatibility exists between the ABO antibodies in the donor unit with the ABO antigens present on the recipient's red cells. Group A recipients needing plasma would be compatible with group A and AB plasma products. Because group A plasma contains anti-B and group AB has no ABO antibodies, these plasma products do not recognize the A antigen on recipient red cells. No adverse antigen–antibody reaction would ensue. For the transfusion of plasma, group AB is considered the universal donor and group O is the universal recipient (see Table 5.7).

Agglutination reactions for ABO typing are usually 3+ to 4+ in strength.

Universal donors: group O donors for RBC transfusions; these RBCs may be transfused to any ABO phenotype because the cells lack both A and B antigens

Universal recipients: group AB recipients may receive transfusions of RBCs from any ABO phenotype; these recipients lack circulating ABO antibodies in plasma

Universal donor for RBC transfusions is group O; universal donor for plasma transfusions is group AB.

Universal recipient for RBC transfusions is group AB; universal recipient for plasma transfusions is group O.

TABLE 5.8	Practical Application: Guidelines for Investigating ABO Technical Errors
Identification or Documentation Errors	
Correct sample identification on all tubes Results are properly recorded Interpretations are accurate and properly recorded	
Reagent or Equipment Errors	
Daily quality control on ABO typing reagents is satisfactory Inspect reagents for contamination and hemolysis Centrifugation time and calibration are confirmed	
Standard Operating Procedure Errors	
Procedure follows manufacturer's directions Correct reagents were used and added to testing Red blood cell suspensions are at the correct concentration Cell buttons are completely suspended before grading the reaction	

SECTION 6

RECOGNITION AND RESOLUTION OF ABO DISCREPANCIES

The recognition and resolution of ABO discrepancies are challenging aspects of problem solving in the blood bank. As defined in a previous section, an ABO discrepancy is an ABO phenotype where the results of the red cell testing do not agree with the results of expected serum testing. Discrepancies may be indicated when the following observations are noted in the results of ABO phenotyping:

- Agglutination strengths of the typing reactions are weaker than expected. Typically, the reactions in ABO red cell testing with anti-A and anti-B reagents are 3+ to 4+; the results of ABO serum testing with reagent A_1 and B cells are 2+ to 4+.
- Expected reactions in ABO red cell testing and serum testing are missing (eg, group O individual is missing one or both reactions in serum testing with reagent A_1 and B cells).
- Extra reactions are noted in either the ABO red cell or serum tests.

The source of these discrepancies can be either technical or sample-related problems. The first step in the resolution of an ABO discrepancy is to identify the source of the problem. Is the discrepancy a technical error in testing, or is the discrepancy related to the sample itself?

TECHNICAL CONSIDERATIONS IN ABO PHENOTYPING

Several types of technical errors can transpire in ABO typing and lead to erroneous results. An awareness and recognition of these technical errors can assist in the resolution of an ABO discrepancy. These technical errors can be classified into several categories, including identification and documentation errors, reagent and equipment problems, and standard operating procedure errors. By following the guidelines outlined in Table 5.8, technical sources of error can be pinpointed more readily. A new sample can be obtained to eliminate possible contamination or identification problems. In addition, red cell suspensions prepared from patient samples can be washed three times before repeated testing. When a technical error is discovered and corrected, the ABO discrepancy can be quickly resolved with repeated testing. If the discrepancy still exists after repeated testing, the possibility of a problem related to the sample itself (eg, related to the patient or donor) should be considered. Refer to Fig. 5.10 for a stepwise approach when faced with an ABO discrepancy.

SAMPLE-RELATED ABO DISCREPANCIES

Sample-related problems can be divided into two groups: ABO discrepancies that affect the ABO red cell testing and discrepancies that affect the ABO serum or plasma testing. Is the problem associated with the patient or donor red cells, or is it associated with patient

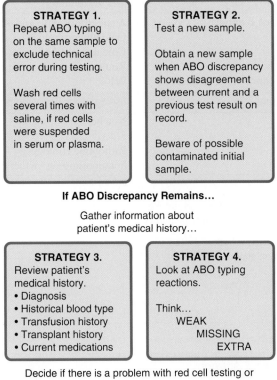

Survival Tip: First Things First...

Rule out technical errors first...
Most discrepancies are related to technical errors.

STRATEGY 1.
Repeat ABO typing on the same sample to exclude technical error during testing.

Wash red cells several times with saline, if red cells were suspended in serum or plasma.

STRATEGY 2.
Test a new sample.

Obtain a new sample when ABO discrepancy shows disagreement between current and a previous test result on record.

Beware of possible contaminated initial sample.

If ABO Discrepancy Remains...

Gather information about patient's medical history...

STRATEGY 3.
Review patient's medical history.
• Diagnosis
• Historical blood type
• Transfusion history
• Transplant history
• Current medications

STRATEGY 4.
Look at ABO typing reactions.

Think...
WEAK
MISSING
EXTRA

Decide if there is a problem with red cell testing or problem with serum/plasma testing...then investigate.

Fig. 5.10 Steps in resolution of an ABO discrepancy.

or donor antibodies? A logical approach to solving these sample-related problems is to select the side of the ABO test (red cell testing or serum or plasma testing) believed to be discrepant and to focus on the problem from this angle. The observed strengths of agglutination reactions in the testing of both the red cells and the serum or plasma are keys in determining whether to focus problem solving on a red cell or a serum/plasma problem. For success with this approach, a working knowledge of the multitude of potential problems relating to ABO red cell and serum testing is mandatory (Table 5.9). The most commonly encountered ABO discrepancies in the immunohematology laboratory are discrepancies relating to weak or missing ABO antibodies in serum/plasma testing. ABO discrepancies associated with red cell testing are reviewed first, followed by discussion of discrepancies associated with serum/plasma testing.

ABO Discrepancies Associated with Red Cell Testing

ABO discrepancies that affect the testing of red cells (forward grouping) can be classified into three categories: extra antigens present, missing or weak antigens, and mixed-field reactions. In the examples provided, either serum or plasma may be used as the sample in the ABO reverse-grouping test.

Extra Antigens Present

ABO red cell typing results may demonstrate unexpected positive agglutination reactions with commercial anti-A or anti-B reagents. Extra reactions are present in red cell testing or forward grouping. For the purposes of this textbook, the scope of the discussion on extra antigens in red cell testing is limited to the illustration of the **group A with acquired B antigen** and the **B(A) phenotype**.

Examples 1 and 2 follow to demonstrate extra antigens present with the acquired B and B(A) phenotype.

Group A with acquired B antigen: group A_1 individual with disease of the lower gastrointestinal tract, cancer of the colon and rectum, intestinal obstruction, or gram-negative septicemia who acquires reactivity with anti-B reagents in ABO red cell testing and appears as group AB

B(A) phenotype: group B individual who acquires reactivity with anti-A reagents in ABO red cell testing; in these individuals, the B gene transfers trace amounts of the immunodominant sugar for the A antigen and the immunodominant sugar for the B antigen

TABLE 5.9	Overview of ABO Discrepancies
PROBLEMS WITH RED CELL TESTING	PROBLEMS WITH SERUM/PLASMA TESTING
Extra antigens	Extra antibodies
Group A with acquired B antigen B(A) phenotype Polyagglutination Rouleaux Hematopoietic progenitor cell transplants	A subgroups with anti-A1 Cold alloantibodies Cold autoantibodies Rouleaux IVIG
Missing or weak antigens	Missing or weak antibodies
ABO subgroup Pathologic etiology Transplantation	Newborn Elderly Pathologic etiology Immunosuppressive therapy for transplantation
Mixed-field reactions	
Transfusion of group O to group A, B, or AB Hematopoietic progenitor stem cell transplants A_3 phenotype	

IVIG, Intravenous immunoglobulin.

EXAMPLE 1

Group A with Acquired B Antigen			
ABO Testing Results			
Patient Red Cells with		Patient Serum with Reagent Red Cells	
Anti-A	Anti-B	A_1	B
4+	1+	0	4+

EVALUATION OF ABO TESTING RESULTS

1. The agglutination of the patient's red cells with anti-A is strong (4+).
2. The agglutination of the patient's red cells with anti-B is weaker (1+) than usually expected (3+ to 4+).
3. These red cells react as the phenotype group AB.
4. The results of serum testing reactions are typical of a group A individual.

CONCLUSION

These reactions are typical of individuals possessing the acquired B antigen. With acquired B antigen, a group A individual possesses an extra antigen in red cell testing (notice the weaker agglutination with anti-B reagents). Anti-B is observed in the serum testing. Serum testing reactions are typical for a group A individual.

BACKGROUND INFORMATION

Deacetylating: removal of the acetyl group (CH₃CO–)

Usually only group A_1 individuals with diseases of the lower gastrointestinal tract, cancers of the colon and rectum, intestinal obstruction, or gram-negative septicemia express the acquired B antigen. The most common mechanism for this phenotype is usually associated with a bacterial **deacetylating** enzyme that alters the A immunodominant sugar, *N*-acetylgalactosamine, by removing the acetyl group. The resulting sugar, galactosamine, resembles the B immunodominant sugar, D-galactose, and cross-reacts with many anti-B reagents.[16]

In the early 1990s, an increase in the detection of acquired B antigen with certain monoclonal anti-B blood grouping reagents licensed by the U.S. Food and Drug Administration was observed.[17] The observation was linked to the use of ES-4 monoclonal anti-B clone at pH levels of 6.5 to 7.0. If the formulation of the clone was acidified to pH 6.0, the acquired B antigen was not observed.

Red cells agglutinated strongly by anti-A and weakly by anti-B in combination with a serum containing anti-B are suggestive of the acquired B antigen. These patients should receive units of group A red cells for transfusion purposes. Scan the QR code for more information about the acquired B antigen.

RESOLUTION OF ABO DISCREPANCY

1. Determine the patient's diagnosis and transfusion history. The first step in the resolution of any ABO discrepancy is to obtain more information about the patient. This information may provide additional clues about the root cause of the ABO discrepancy.
2. Test the patient's serum against autologous red cells. Anti-B in the patient's serum does not agglutinate autologous red cells with the acquired B antigen.
3. Test red cells with additional monoclonal anti-B reagents from other manufacturers that are documented not to react with the acquired B antigen or a source of human polyclonal anti-B.

EXAMPLE 2

B(A) Phenotype			
ABO Testing Results			
Patient Red Cells with		**Patient Serum with Reagent Red Cells**	
Anti-A	Anti-B	A_1	B
1+	4+	4+	0

EVALUATION OF ABO TESTING RESULTS

1. The agglutination of the patient's red cells with anti-A is weak (1+).
2. The agglutination of the patient's red cells with anti-B is strong (4+).
3. The results of serum testing are typical of a group B individual.

CONCLUSION

These reactions are characteristic of a possible B(A) phenotype. In the B(A) phenotype, a group B with an apparent extra antigen reaction is observed with anti-A in red cell testing.

BACKGROUND INFORMATION

The B(A) phenotype has been observed because of the increased sensitivity of potent monoclonal antibody reagents for ABO phenotyping.[18] These reagents can detect trace amounts of either A or B antigens that are nonspecifically transferred by the glycosyltransferase enzymes. In the B(A) phenotype, the *B* gene transfers trace amounts of the immunodominant sugar for the A antigen (*N*-acetylgalactosamine) and the immunodominant sugar for the B antigen (D-galactose) to the H antigen acceptor molecules. The trace amounts of A antigens are detected with certain clones from the monoclonal antibody reagents. A similar mechanism can cause an A(B) phenotype analogous to the acquired B antigen.

RESOLUTION OF ABO DISCREPANCY

1. Determine the patient's diagnosis and transfusion history.
2. Test red cells with additional monoclonal antibody anti-A reagents from other manufacturers or a source of human polyclonal anti-A.

Polyagglutination: property of cells that causes them to be agglutinated by naturally occurring antibodies found in most human sera; agglutination occurs regardless of blood type

Wharton's jelly: gelatinous tissue contaminant in cord blood samples that may interfere in immunohematologic tests

Other potential explanations for extra antigens in ABO red cell testing include the following:

a. **Polyagglutination** of red cells by most human sera as a result of the exposure of a hidden antigen on the red cell membrane because of a bacterial infection or genetic mutation. ABO discrepancies caused by polyagglutination are rarely detected because of the routine use of monoclonal antibody reagents, which have replaced human-derived ABO antisera.

b. Nonspecific aggregation of serum-suspended red cells because of abnormal concentrations of serum proteins or **Wharton's jelly** in cord blood samples (false-positive agglutination).

Missing or Weakly Expressed Antigens

In the category of ABO discrepancies concerning missing or weakly expressed antigens, patient or donor red cells demonstrate weaker-than-usual reactions with reagent anti-A and anti-B or may fail to demonstrate any reactivity. Phenomena associated with this category include the following:

- ABO subgroups
- Weakened A and B antigen expression in patients with leukemia or Hodgkin's disease
  Example 3 illustrates missing or weakly expressed antigens by presenting an ABO discrepancy typically observed with a subgroup of A.

EXAMPLE 3

Subgroup of A			
ABO Testing Results			
Patient Red Cells with		**Patient Serum with Reagent Red Cells**	
Anti-A	Anti-B	A_1	B
0	0	0	3+

EVALUATION OF ABO TESTING RESULTS

1. No agglutination of the patient's red cells with both anti-A and anti-B reagents is observed. The individual appears to be a group O phenotype.
2. The results of serum testing are typical of a group A individual. Agglutination of anti-B with reagent B red cells is strong (3+).

CONCLUSION

These reactions are characteristic of a missing antigen in the red cell testing. The serum testing results are those expected in a group A individual. Anti-A, found in group O individuals, is absent in the serum testing.

BACKGROUND INFORMATION

As previously discussed in this chapter, weak or missing reactions with anti-A and anti-B reagents correlate with subgroups of A and B. Subgroups of A represent less than 1% of the group A population, and the subgroups of B are even rarer. Inheritance of an alternative allele at the *ABO* locus results in a quantitative reduction of antigen sites per red cell and in weakened or missing reactions with anti-A and anti-B reagents.

RESOLUTION OF ABO DISCREPANCY

1. Determine the patient's diagnosis and transfusion history.
2. Repeat the red cell testing with extended incubation times and include human polyclonal anti-A,B or monoclonal blend anti-A,B. The extended incubation time may enhance the antigen–antibody reaction.

Additional Testing Results	
	Anti-A,B
Patient red cells	1+
Conclusion: Probable subgroup of A	

Additional Testing Results	
	Anti-A,B
Patient red cells	0
Next Step: Perform adsorption and elution studies with anti-A; these studies assist in determining the presence of A antigens on the patient's red cells	

Molecular genotyping of this patient can identify the subgroup of A and resolve the ABO discrepancy.

Mixed-Field Reactions

Mixed-field reactions can occur in red cell testing with anti-A or anti-B reagent. As noted earlier, a mixed-field reaction contains agglutinates with a mass of unagglutinated red cells. Usually a mixed-field reaction is due to the presence of two distinct cell populations. For example, testing red cells from a patient recently transfused with non–ABO-identical RBCs (group O donor RBCs to a group AB recipient) can yield mixed-field observations. In addition to the transfusion of group O RBCs to group A, B, or AB individuals, recipients of **hematopoietic progenitor transplants,** individuals with the A_3 phenotype, and patients with **Tn-polyagglutinable red cells** can demonstrate mixed-field reactions. Example 4 illustrates an ABO discrepancy showing mixed-field reactions.

The transfusion of red cell donor units or stem cell transplants can cause mixed-field reactions. They are called artificially induced chimerisms.

Hematopoietic progenitor cell transplant: replacement of hematopoietic stem cells derived from allogeneic bone marrow, peripheral stem cells, or cord blood to treat certain leukemias, immunodeficiencies, and hemoglobinopathies

Tn-polyagglutinable red cells: type of polyagglutination that occurs from a mutation in the hematopoietic tissue, characterized by mixed-field reactions in agglutination testing

EXAMPLE 4

Group B Patient Transfused with Group O RBCs			
ABO Testing Results			
Patient Red Cells with		**Patient Serum with Reagent Red Cells**	
Anti-A	Anti-B	A_1	B
0	2+mf	4+	0

mf, Mixed field.

EVALUATION OF ABO TESTING RESULTS
1. The strength of the agglutination reaction with anti-B is weaker than expected for group B individuals.
2. The anti-B mixed-field grading of reactivity is a 2+ reaction with a sufficient number of unagglutinated cells.
3. The results of serum testing are typical of a group B individual.

CONCLUSION
These results demonstrate a group B individual possibly transfused with group O RBCs.

BACKGROUND INFORMATION
In certain situations, ABO-identical RBC products might not be available for transfusion, and group O RBC products are transfused. If many group O donor RBC units are transfused with respect to the recipient's total body mass, mixed-field reactions may appear in the ABO red cell testing.

RESOLUTION OF ABO DISCREPANCY

1. Determine the patient's diagnosis and recent transfusion history.
2. Determine whether the patient is a recent hematopoietic progenitor cell recipient.
3. Investigate pretransfusion ABO phenotype history, if possible.

ABO Discrepancies Associated with Serum or Plasma Testing

ABO discrepancies that affect serum or plasma testing (reverse grouping) include the presence of additional antibodies other than anti-A and anti-B or the absence of expected ABO antibody reactions. The most commonly encountered ABO discrepancies involve the absence of expected ABO antibody reactions.

Additional Antibodies in Serum or Plasma Testing

This section of ABO discrepancies addresses the detection of anti-A1, **cold alloantibodies, cold autoantibodies,** and rouleaux in ABO typing. Example 5 is an illustration of group A_2 with anti-A1. Example 6 illustrates a cold autoantibody and cold alloantibody. Example 7 illustrates rouleaux. In all of these situations, the ABO discrepancy manifests as additional antibodies in serum or plasma testing.

Cold alloantibodies: red cell antibodies specific for other human red cell antigens that typically react at or below room temperature

Cold autoantibodies: red cell antibodies specific for autologous antigens that typically react at or below room temperature

EXAMPLE 5

Group A_2 with Anti-A1			
ABO Testing Results			
Patient Red Cells with		**Patient Serum with Reagent Red Cells**	
Anti-A	Anti-B	A_1	B
4+	0	2+	4+

EVALUATION OF ABO TESTING RESULTS

1. The agglutination pattern with anti-A and anti-B reagents is typical of a group A individual.
2. The results of serum testing with reagent A_1 and B red cells indicate a group O individual.

CONCLUSION

These results demonstrate an extra reaction in the serum testing with the reagent A_1 red cells (2+). Possible explanations for the extra reaction include an anti-A1, a cold alloantibody, a cold autoantibody, or rouleaux. This example illustrates an ABO discrepancy resulting from group A_2 with anti-A1.

RESOLUTION OF ABO DISCREPANCY

1. Determine the patient's diagnosis and transfusion history.
2. Test the patient's red cells with anti-A1 lectin to ascertain whether a subgroup of A is present.

Additional Testing Results	
Patient Red Cells Tested with Anti-A1 Lectin	Conclusion
0	Subgroup of A; suspect anti-A1 antibody

3. Test the patient's serum with three examples of A_1 and A_2 reagent red cells to confirm the presence of anti-A1 antibody.

Additional Testing Results

Patient Serum Tested with					
A$_1$ Cells	A$_1$ Cells	A$_1$ Cells	A$_2$ Cells	A$_2$ Cells	A$_2$ Cells
2+	2+	2+	0	0	0

CONCLUSION

Agglutination is observed with A$_1$ red cells providing the evidence for anti-A1. The serum does not agglutinate with A$_2$ red cells. Anti-A1 may be present in 1% to 8% of the group A$_2$ phenotype.

EXAMPLE 6

Cold Autoantibody or Cold Alloantibody in Serum/Plasma Testing

ABO Testing Results			
Patient Red Cells with		Patient Serum with Reagent Red Cells	
Anti-A	Anti-B	A$_1$	B
4+	4+	0	1+

EVALUATION OF ABO TESTING RESULTS

1. Strong agglutination reactions are observed in red cell testing and are consistent with a group AB individual.
2. The results of serum testing with reagent B red cells demonstrate a weaker extra reaction (1+). This serum testing appears to be consistent with a group A individual.

CONCLUSION

These results indicate a possible extra reaction in the serum testing with the reagent B red cells. Example 6 illustrates the presence of a cold alloantibody or a cold autoantibody.

BACKGROUND INFORMATION

Donors and patients may possess antibodies to other blood group system red cell antigens in addition to those of the ABO blood group system. These *alloantibodies* may appear as additional serum antibodies in ABO typing as one of the following specificities: anti-P1, anti-M, anti-N, anti-Le^a, and anti-Le^b. Because they react at or below room temperature, these antibodies are sometimes referred to as *cold*. Reagent A$_1$ and B red cells used in ABO serum testing may possess these antigens in addition to the A and B antigens. Screening cells, which are group O reagent red cells, are used to detect an alloantibody because they lack A and B antigens. Any serum reactivity caused by an existing ABO antibody is eliminated in the reaction with group O cells. It is logical to conclude that screening cells are valuable in distinguishing between ABO antibodies and alloantibodies.

Patients and donors may also possess serum antibodies directed toward their own red cell antigens. These antibodies are classified as autoantibodies. If autoantibodies are reactive at or below room temperature, they are also called *cold*. Cold autoantibodies usually possess the specificity of anti-I or anti-IH and react against all adult red cells, including screening cells, A$_1$ and B cells, and autologous cells. An **autocontrol** (autologous control) is tested to differentiate a cold autoantibody from a cold alloantibody. If the autocontrol is positive, the reactions observed with the A$_1$ and B cells and screening cells are probably the result of autoantibodies. See Chapter 8 for additional information on cold autoantibody test methods and techniques useful in negating their reactivity in ABO typing tests.

Autocontrol: testing a person's serum with his or her own red cells to determine whether an autoantibody is present

RESOLUTION OF ABO DISCREPANCY

1. Determine the patient's diagnosis and transfusion history.
2. Test the patient's serum with screening cells and an autocontrol at room temperature. This strategy helps distinguish whether cold alloantibody or cold autoantibody is present.

	Interpretation of Testing Results		
	Screening Cells	Autologous Red Cells	Conclusion
Patient serum	Pos*	Neg	Cold alloantibody
Patient serum	Pos	Pos	Cold autoantibody

*Positive reaction if the corresponding antigen is present on the screening cell.

3. If an alloantibody is detected, antibody identification techniques can be performed (see Chapter 8).
4. If an autoantibody is detected, special techniques to identify the antibody (a minicold panel) and remove antibody reactivity (prewarming techniques) can be used (see Chapter 8).

EXAMPLE 7

Rouleaux			
ABO Testing Results			
Patient Red Cells with		Patient Serum with Reagent Red Cells	
Anti-A	Anti-B	A_1	B
4+	4+	2+	2+

EVALUATION OF ABO TESTING RESULTS

1. Strong agglutination reactions are observed in red cell testing and are consistent with the expected results of a group AB individual.
2. Serum testing results are consistent with those of a group O individual.

CONCLUSION

Consider the possibility of extra reactions in serum testing with the reagent red cells because of an alloantibody, an autoantibody, or rouleaux. The phenomenon of rouleaux is demonstrated in this example.

BACKGROUND INFORMATION

Rouleaux can produce false-positive agglutination in testing. The red cells resemble stacked coins under microscopic examination. Increased concentrations of serum proteins can affect this spontaneous agglutination of red cells. Diseases associated with rouleaux include **multiple myeloma** and **Waldenström macroglobulinemia**. In addition to creating problems with the serum testing in ABO phenotyping, rouleaux can create extra reactions in the ABO red cell typing if unwashed red cell suspensions are used. Scan the QR code for more information.

RESOLUTION OF ABO DISCREPANCY

1. Determine the patient's diagnosis and transfusion history.
2. Wash red cell suspension and repeat the phenotyping.
3. Perform the **saline replacement technique** to help distinguish true agglutination from rouleaux (Fig. 5.11).

Missing or Weak ABO Antibodies in Serum or Plasma Testing

ABO antibodies may be missing or weakened in certain patient-related situations and may result in an ABO discrepancy. Example 8 illustrates this type of ABO discrepancy in serum/plasma testing.

Multiple myeloma: malignant neoplasm of the bone marrow characterized by abnormal proteins in the plasma and urine

Waldenström macroglobulinemia: overproduction of IgM by the clones of a plasma B cell in response to an antigenic signal; increased viscosity of blood is observed

Saline replacement technique: test to distinguish rouleaux from true agglutination

Missing or weak ABO antibodies in serum/plasma testing are the most commonly encountered ABO discrepancies.

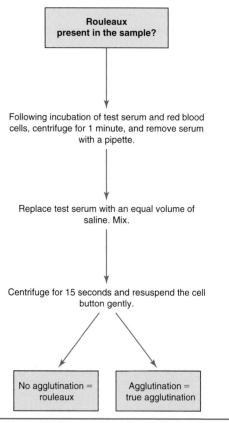

Fig. 5.11 Saline replacement technique. Rouleaux causing false-positive reactions can be distinguished from agglutination with this simple technique. (Modified from Mallory D: *Immunohematology methods and procedures,* Rockville, MD, 1993, American Red Cross.)

EXAMPLE 8

Missing or Weak ABO Antibodies in Serum or Plasma Testing			
ABO Testing Results			
Patient Red Cells with		**Patient Serum with Reagent Red Cells**	
Anti-A	Anti-B	A_1	B
0	0	0	0

EVALUATION OF ABO TESTING RESULTS
1. The agglutination pattern with anti-A and anti-B reagents is typical of a group O individual.
2. The results of serum testing with reagent A_1 and B red cells indicate a group AB individual.

CONCLUSION
Consider approaching this problem from the angle of missing serum reactions with reagent A_1 or B cells.

BACKGROUND INFORMATION
An investigation of the patient's history, including age, diagnosis, and immunoglobulin levels, provides clues to explaining the missing reactions in the serum testing. The patient's age is an important factor because the concentrations of ABO antibodies are reduced in newborns and elderly adults. Knowledge of the patient's diagnosis is essential; reduced immunoglobulin levels are also associated with several pathologic states (see Table 5.5).

In conjunction with the patient's diagnosis, the immunoglobulin levels and serum protein electrophoretic patterns are helpful data in the resolution and identification of the root cause for this ABO discrepancy.

RESOLUTION OF ABO DISCREPANCY

1. Determine the patient's diagnosis, age, and immunoglobulin levels, if available.
2. Incubate serum testing for 15 minutes at room temperature, and then centrifuge and examine for agglutination. This simple incubation step often solves the problem. If the results are still negative, place the serum testing at 4° C for 5 minutes with an autologous control. The autologous control validates the test by ensuring that positive reactions are not attributable to a cold autoantibody.

Interpretation of Additional Testing Results				
4° C	A$_1$ Red Cells	B Red Cells	Autologous Red Cells	Conclusion
Patient serum	Pos	Pos	Neg	Group O
Patient serum	Pos	Pos	Pos	Cold autoantibody

SECTION 7

SPECIAL TOPICS RELATED TO ABO AND H BLOOD GROUP SYSTEMS

CLASSIC BOMBAY PHENOTYPE

The classic Bombay phenotype is an unusual genetic occurrence associated with the ABO and H blood group systems. A 1952 report describing a family living in Bombay, India, is the source of the descriptive term for the phenotype.[1] This family's red cells were unusual because they lacked H antigens and subsequently any ABO antigen expression. Both red cells and secretions were deficient in H and ABO antigen expression. The red cell reactions were characteristic of the group O phenotype in routine ABO testing. Serum testing demonstrated reactions similar to group O individuals. Another related antibody, anti-H, was detected in the family's serum in addition to the ABO antibodies of anti-A, anti-B, and anti-A,B. The anti-H in the Bombay phenotype is of clinical significance because this antibody is capable of high thermal activity at 37° C and complement activation with resulting hemolysis.

More than 130 Bombay phenotypes have been reported with a relatively greater incidence in India.[19] Genetic family studies have identified the genotype required for this phenomenon. An individual who is homozygous for the *h* allele (*hh*) expresses the Bombay phenotype (the *H* and *h* genes of the *H* locus were previously described in this chapter). The *hh* genotype does not produce the L-fucosyltransferase necessary to transfer the immunodominant sugar, L-fucose, to the acceptor oligosaccharide chain to form the H antigen. As a result, the H antigen is not assembled on the red cells. Because H antigen is the building block for the development of the A and B antigens, A and B glycosyltransferases cannot act on their substrate to produce the corresponding antigen structures, even though the ABO alleles are inherited. The resulting phenotype lacks expression of both H and ABO antigens. Transfusion for these individuals presents an especially difficult problem because they are compatible only with the Bombay phenotype. If transfusion is necessary, stored autologous units, siblings, and rare donor files are potential options.

Bombay individuals have group O phenotype in routine ABO typing. These individuals are not compatible with group O RBC units because their serum possesses anti-H.

SECRETOR STATUS

The interrelationship of the secretor locus with the expression of ABO antigens in body fluids was noted several times throughout this chapter. There are two allelic genes at this locus: *Se* and *se*. The gene product of the *Se* allele, *FUT2,* is an L-fucosyltransferase that preferentially adds L-fucose to type 1 oligosaccharide chain structures in secretory glands. The *FUT2* gene may also act on type 2 chains in the secretory glands. The *H* gene, *FUT1,* preferentially adds fucose to type 2 chains.

Example 1

Genes inherited			Antigen expression	
			RBC	Saliva
AB	HH	SeSe ⟶	A, B, H	A, B, H
AB	HH	sese ⟶	A, B, H	None

Example 2

Genes inherited			Antigen expression	
			RBC	Saliva
OO	HH	Sese ⟶	H	H
OO	HH	sese ⟶	H	None

Fig. 5.12 Practical application: interaction of ABO, H, and secretor genes in the expression of soluble antigens in saliva. *RBC*, Red blood cell.

The *FUT2* gene is directly responsible for regulating the expression of soluble A, B, and H antigens on the glycoprotein structures located in body secretions such as saliva. An individual who inherits the *Se* allele in either a homozygous (*SeSe*) or a heterozygous (*Sese*) manner is classified as a **secretor**. About 80% of the random population inherits the *Se* allele. These individuals are classified as secretors. These individuals express soluble forms of H antigens in secretions that can be converted to A or B antigens by the A and B glycosyltransferases. These soluble antigens are found in saliva, urine, tears, bile, amniotic fluid, breast milk, exudate, and digestive fluids.[6] An individual with the genotype *sese* is classified as a **nonsecretor** with a frequency of about 20% of the random population. The allele, *se*, is an amorph. A homozygote does not convert glycoprotein antigen precursors to soluble H substance and has neither soluble H antigens nor soluble A or B antigens present in body fluids. Fig. 5.12 illustrates the genetic interaction of the *ABO, H,* and *Se* loci.

Secretor: individual who inherits *Se* allele and expresses soluble forms of H antigens in secretions

Nonsecretor: individual who inherits the genotype *sese* and does not express soluble H substance in secretions

Secretor studies may be helpful in identifying a subgroup of A or B antigens.

CHAPTER SUMMARY

- The major concepts of ABO antigens and ABO antibodies presented in this chapter are summarized in the following table.

IMPORTANT FACTS: ABO AND H BLOOD GROUP SYSTEM ANTIGENS

Widespread antigen distribution	Blood cells, tissues, body fluids, secretions
Biochemical composition	Glycolipid/glycoprotein
Common structures	Type 1 and type 2 oligosaccharide chains
Gene products	Glycosyltransferases
Immunodominant sugars	H antigen: L-fucose
	A antigen: N-acetylgalactosamine
	B antigen: D-galactose
Antigen expression	Cord blood cells: weak
Genetic loci	ABO blood group system: chromosome 9
	H system: chromosome 19
Major alleles	A^1, A^2, B, O
	H, h
Bombay phenotype	Genotype hh; no H or ABO antigens
Secretor status	Se allele; soluble H and ABO antigens

Landsteiner's rule	Serum possesses the ABO antibody directed toward the A or B antigen that is absent from red cells
Antibody production	No antibodies detectable in first few months of life; decreases in elderly adults
Antibody immunoglobulin class	IgM and IgG
In vitro reactions	At or below room temperature
Complement binding	Yes; some hemolytic
Clinical significance	Yes

CRITICAL THINKING EXERCISES

Exercise 5.1 Case Study

RT, a 37-year-old woman, is a first-time donor at your blood center. She is a healthy donor with an unremarkable medical history and no medications. Initial ABO phenotyping results indicate an ABO discrepancy.

ABO Testing Results			
Donor Red Cells with		Donor Serum with Reagent Red Cells	
Anti-A	Anti-B	A_1	B
0	4+	3+	1+

1. Evaluate the ABO phenotyping results. Is the discrepancy associated with the red cell testing or the serum testing? State the reasons for this selection.
2. How would you classify the category of ABO discrepancy shown in this problem?
3. What are the potential causes of an ABO discrepancy in this category?

Additional Testing

No technical errors were found. The donor's red cells were washed, and the ABO phenotyping was repeated. Red cell testing results were identical to the first set. In addition to A_1 and B reagent red cells, commercial screening cells and an autologous control were tested with the donor's serum. The results of the testing are depicted in the following table.

Additional Testing Results			
Donor's Serum Testing with			
A_1 Red Cells	B Red Cells	Screening Cells	Autologous Red Cells
3+	1+	1+	0

4. What conclusions can be drawn from the results of additional serum testing?
5. What additional steps are required to resolve this ABO discrepancy?

Exercise 5.2

What are the possible ABO phenotypes of offspring with parents possessing the genotypes A^1A^2 and BO?

Exercise 5.3

Group O individuals are considered universal donors for the transfusion of RBCs and universal recipients for plasma transfusions. Provide an explanation for this statement.

Exercise 5.4

Create a diagram to illustrate the genetic pathways for ABO antigen production and the Bombay phenotype.

Exercise 5.5
For a Bombay phenotype encountered in the immunohematology laboratory:
1. Predict the agglutination reactions of the patient's red cells with the following reagents: anti-A, anti-B, anti-A,B, and *Ulex europaeus*.
2. Predict the agglutination reactions of the patient's serum sample with the following reagent red cells: A_1, B, and O.

Exercise 5.6
Why does an individual with the genotype *AB, HH,* and *sese* possess A, B, and H antigens on red cells but does not have any soluble forms of these antigens in the saliva?

STUDY QUESTIONS

1. Given the following ABO typing results, what is a potential conclusion for these results?

ABO Testing Results			
Patient Red Cells with		Patient Serum with Reagent Red Cells	
Anti-A	Anti-B	A_1	B
4+	4+	1+	0

   a. expected results for a group O individual
   b. expected results for a group AB individual
   c. discrepant results; patient has A antigen on red cells with anti-A in serum
   d. discrepant results; patient has B antigen on red cells with no anti-B in serum

2. What are the gene products of the *A* and *B* genes?

   a. glycolipids
   b. glycoproteins
   c. oligosaccharides
   d. transferase enzymes

For questions 3 through 5, use the following ABO typing results:

ABO Testing Results			
Patient Red Cells with		Patient Serum with Reagent Red Cells	
Anti-A	Anti-B	A_1	B
0	0	4+	4+

3. What is the ABO interpretation?

   a. group O
   b. group A
   c. group B
   d. group AB

4. What ABO phenotypes would be compatible if the patient required a transfusion of RBCs?

   a. group AB, O, A, or B
   b. group O or B
   c. group AB or O
   d. only group O

5. What ABO phenotypes would be compatible if the patient required a transfusion of fresh frozen plasma?

    a. group AB, O, A, or B
    b. group O or B
    c. group AB or O
    d. only group O

6. What term describes using known sources of reagent antisera (known antibodies) to detect ABO antigens on a patient's red cells?

    a. Rh typing
    b. reverse grouping
    c. direct antiglobulin test
    d. forward grouping

7. Which result is discrepant if the red cell typing shown in the following chart is correct?

ABO Testing Results			
Patient Red Cells with		Patient Serum with Reagent Red Cells	
Anti-A	Anti-B	A_1	B
0	4+	0	0

    a. negative reaction with group B cells
    b. positive reaction with anti-B
    c. negative reaction with group A_1 cells
    d. no discrepancies in these results

8. What ABO antibody is expected in this patient serum based on the following information?

Patient Red Cells with	
Anti-A	Anti-B
0	0

    a. anti-B
    b. anti-A
    c. anti-A and anti-B
    d. none

9. According to Landsteiner's rule, if a patient has no ABO antibodies after serum testing, what ABO antigens are present on the patient's red cells?

    a. A
    b. B
    c. both A and B
    d. none

10. Select the ABO phenotypes, in order from most frequent to least frequent, that occur in whites:

    a. A, B, O, AB
    b. O, A, B, AB
    c. B, A, AB, O
    d. AB, O, B, A

11. Which of the following statements is true about ABO antibody production?

    a. ABO antibodies are present in newborns
    b. ABO titers remain at constant levels throughout life
    c. ABO antibodies are stimulated by bacteria and other environmental factors
    d. All of these statements are true

12. What immunoglobulin class is primarily associated with ABO antibodies?

    a. IgA
    b. IgG
    c. IgE
    d. IgM

13. What immunodominant sugar confers B blood group specificity?

    a. D-galactose
    b. L-fucose
    c. N-acetylgalactosamine
    d. L-glucose

14. An individual has the genotype of *AO, hh*. What antigens would be present on the red cells of this individual?

    a. A only
    b. A and H
    c. A and O
    d. none of the above

15. What gene controls the presence of soluble H substance in saliva?

    a. *H*
    b. *A*
    c. *Se*
    d. *B*

16. Which lectin agglutinates A_1 red cells?

    a. *Dolichos biflorus*
    b. *Ulex europaeus*
    c. *Dolichos europaeus*
    d. *Ulex biflorus*

17. What immunodominant sugar determines the specificity of H antigens?

    a. D-galactose
    b. L-fucose
    c. N-acetylgalactosamine
    d. L-glucose

18. Which of the following situations may produce ABO discrepancies in the serum testing?

    a. newborn
    b. patient with hypogammaglobulinemia
    c. cold alloantibody
    d. all of the above

19. What soluble antigen forms are detectable in saliva based on the following genotype: *AB, HH, SeSe?*
    a. none (nonsecretor)
    b. only H
    c. A, B, and H
    d. A and B

20. Which ABO discrepancy is the best explanation for the results shown in the following chart?

ABO Testing Results			
Patient Red Cells with		Patient Serum with Reagent Red Cells	
Anti-A	Anti-B	A_1	B
4+	0	2+	4+

    a. an elderly patient
    b. subgroup of A
    c. deterioration of reagents
    d. hypogammaglobulinemia

Answers to Study Questions can be found on page 387.

ⓔ Additional student resources, including review questions, a laboratory manual, and case studies, can be found on the Evolve website.

REFERENCES

1. Issitt PD, Anstee DJ: *Applied blood group serology*, ed 4, Durham, NC, 1998, Montgomery Scientific Publications.
2. Table of blood group antigens v4.0 141124: International Society of Blood Transfusion. http://www.isbtweb.org/working-parties/red-cell-immunogenetics-and-blood-group-terminology. Accessed May 2015.
3. Reid ME, Lomas-Francis C, Olsson ML: *The blood group antigen facts book*, ed 3, San Diego, CA, 2012, Elsevier Academic Press.
4. Landsteiner K: Zur Kenntnis der antifermentativen, lytischen und agglutinierenden Wirkungen des Blutserums und der Lymphe, *Zbl Bakt* 27:357, 1900.
5. von Decastello A, Sturli A: Über die Isoagglutinine im Serum gesunder und kranker Menschen, *Munchen Med Wochenschr* 95:1090, 1902.
6. Klein HG, Anstee DJ: *Mollison's blood transfusion in clinical medicine*, ed 12, West Sussex, England, 2014, Wiley Blackwell.
7. Economidou J, Hughes-Jones N, Gardner B: Quantitative measurements concerning A and B antigen sites, *Vox Sang* 12:321, 1967.
8. Mourant AE, Kopeâc AC, Domaniewska-Sobczak K: *The distribution of the human blood groups and other biochemical polymorphisms*, ed 2, London, England, 1976, Oxford University Press.
9. Fung MK: *Technical manual*, ed 18, Bethesda, MD, 2014, AABB.
10. Pittiglio DH: Genetics and biochemistry of A, B, H and Lewis antigens. In Wallace ME, Gibbs FL, editors: *Blood group systems: ABH and Lewis*, Arlington, VA, 1986, AABB.
11. Yamamoto F, Clausen H, White T, et al.: Molecular genetic basis of the histo-blood group ABO blood group system, *Nature* 345:229, 1990.
12. Fukuda MN, Hakamori S: Structures of branched blood group A-active glycosphingolipids in human erythrocytes and polymorphism of A- and H-glycolipids in A_1 and A_2 subgroups, *J Biol Chem* 257:446, 1982.
13. Lopez M, Benali J, Bony V, et al.: Activity of IgG and IgM ABO antibodies against some weak A (A_3, A_x, A_{end}) and weak B (B_3, B_x) red cells, *Vox Sang* 37:281, 1979.
14. Nance ST: Serology of the ABH and Lewis blood group systems. In Wallace ME, Gibbs FL, editors: *Blood group systems: ABH and Lewis*, Arlington, VA, 1986, AABB.
15. Levitt J: *Standards for blood banks and transfusion services*, ed 29, Bethesda, MD, 2014, AABB.
16. Gerbal A, Maslet C, Salmon C: Immunological aspects of the acquired B antigen, *Vox Sang* 28:398, 1975.
17. Beck ML, Kowalski MA, Kirkegaard JR, et al.: Unexpected activity with monoclonal anti-B reagents, *Immunohematology* 8:22, 1992.
18. Beck ML, Yates AD, Hardman J, et al.: Identification of a subset of group B donors reactive with monoclonal anti-A reagent, *Am J Clin Pathol* 92:625, 1989.
19. Bhatia HM: Serologic reactions of ABO and Oh (Bombay) phenotypes due to variations in H antigens. In Mohn JF, Plunkett RW, Cunningham RK, et al.: *Human blood groups: Proceedings of the Fifth International Convocation on Immunology*, Basel, Switzerland, 1977, Karger.

Rh BLOOD GROUP SYSTEM

CHAPTER OUTLINE

LEARNING OBJECTIVES

On completion of this chapter, the reader should be able to:

1. Explain how the D antigen received the terminology of Rh.
2. Compare and contrast the current genetic theory of the inheritance of Rh blood group system antigens with theories proposed by Fisher-Race and Wiener.
3. Discuss the biochemistry of the Rh blood group system, including the gene products and antigen structures.
4. Translate between the Fisher-Race and Wiener terminology.
5. Express phenotyping results for the Rh blood group system antigens in the terminology currently accepted by the International Society of Blood Transfusion.
6. Predict the most probable Rh genotype given the Rh antigen typing results (phenotype).
7. Define weak D and list the genetic circumstances that can cause this phenotype.
8. Describe the appropriate application and test procedure for the weak D antigen.
9. Interpret results of the weak D test when the control is positive, and explain why this would occur.
10. Define compound antigens, and give two examples of this phenotype.
11. Distinguish the G antigen from other antigens in the Rh blood group system, and explain the significance of anti-G.
12. Explain the relationship of the RHAG blood group system to the Rh$_{null}$ and Rh$_{mod}$ phenotypes.
13. Describe the characteristics of the Rh blood group system antibodies and their clinical significance with regard to transfusion and hemolytic disease of the fetus and newborn (HDFN).
14. Compare and contrast the antibody and antigen characteristics of the LW blood group system to the Rh blood group system.
15. Solve case studies with data from Rh phenotyping.

The Rh blood group system is highly complex, polymorphic, and the second most important blood group system after the ABO blood group system. Since the initial discovery of the D antigen in 1939, the Rh blood group system has grown to include more than 50 related antigens. This chapter focuses on the five principal antigens—D, C, E, c, and e—and their corresponding antibodies, which account for most clinical transfusion issues.

SECTION 1
HISTORICAL OVERVIEW OF THE DISCOVERY OF THE D ANTIGEN

The terms "Rh-positive" and "Rh-negative" refer to the presence or absence of the D red cell antigen; these terms are also known as "D-positive" and "D-negative." In contrast to the ABO blood group system, the absence of the D antigen or other Rh blood group system antigens on the red cell does not typically correspond with the presence of the antibody in the plasma. In other words, individuals who phenotype as "group A, D–negative" would have anti-B in their serum but not anti-D. The production of anti-D and other Rh blood group system antibodies requires immune red cell stimulation from red cells positive for the antigen. This exposure may occur during transfusion or pregnancy.

The discovery of the Rh blood group system, as with many other blood group systems, followed the investigation of an adverse transfusion reaction or hemolytic disease of the fetus and newborn (HDFN). In 1940, Levine and Stetson linked the cause of HDFN to an antibody in the Rh blood group system.[1] They named the system Rh, based on the characteristics of the maternal antibody with one reported by Landsteiner and Weiner. Landsteiner and Weiner reported an antibody made from stimulating guinea pigs and rabbits with Rhesus macaque monkey red cells.[2] The Rh antibody agglutinated 85% of human red cells tested and was nonreactive with 15%. From this discovery, the population was characterized as Rh positive or Rh negative. Later experiments demonstrated that the Rh antibody made in the guinea pigs and rabbits was similar, but not identical, to the anti-Rh produced by humans. The two antibodies were different. The rhesus antibody specificity was directed toward another red cell antigen, named LW in honor of Landsteiner and Wiener. The name of the Rh blood group system had been established by then and was not changed.

SECTION 2
GENETICS, BIOCHEMISTRY, AND TERMINOLOGY

GENETICS AND BIOCHEMISTRY OF THE Rh BLOOD GROUP SYSTEM

The current theory of genetic control of Rh antigen expression was enhanced with the ability to characterize the amino acid sequences produced by genes that code for proteins on the red cell membrane. Originally postulated by Tippett,[3] the Rh blood group system antigens were encoded by two closely linked genes—*RHD* and *RHCE*—on chromosome 1. *RHD* determines the D antigen expression on the surface of red cells. D-negative individuals have no genetic material at the site.[4] An antithetical "d" antigen does not exist. Adjacent to the *RHD* locus, the gene *RHCE* determines the C, c, E, and e antigen specificities. Alleles present at this locus include *RHCE*, *RHCe*, *RHcE*, and *RHce*. The antigens CE, Ce, cE, and ce are expressed (Fig. 6.1).[5] The *RHCE* gene codes for similar polypeptides, distinguished by two amino acid sequences as illustrated in Fig. 6.2.[6] The assortment

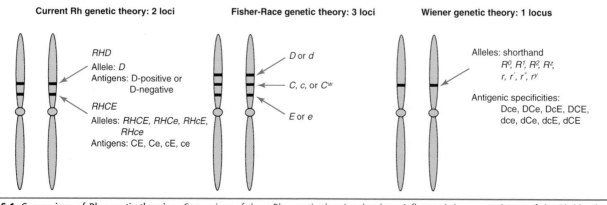

Fig. 6.1 Comparison of Rh genetic theories. Comparison of three Rh genetic theories that have influenced the nomenclature of the Rh blood group system. Modern molecular techniques have established that the Rh blood group system antigens are determined by two genetic loci.

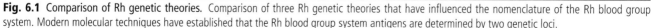

of other antigens in the Rh blood group system occurs as a result of variations of these polypeptides embedded in the cell membrane bilayer in unique configurations. The *RHD* gene, which codes for the D antigen, can vary by many more amino acids, creating more variability among individuals. These differences between individuals help explain why exposure to D antigen can result in a likely immune response.[7] A list of commonly encountered Rh antigens is provided in Table 6.1.

The products of both the *RHD* and the *RHCE* genes are proteins of 416 amino acids that traverse the membrane 12 times and display short loops of amino acids on the exterior (see Fig. 6.2).[7] The Rh blood group system polypeptides, in contrast to most blood group–associated proteins, carry no carbohydrate residues. Rh antigens have been detected only on red cell membranes. Specific antibodies also do not recognize Rh proteins when the proteins are separated from the membrane.[8] The functions of the Rh antigens on the red cells might be related to **cation** transport and membrane integrity.[9] The lack of Rh blood group system antigens, called Rh$_{null}$, causes a membrane abnormality that shortens red cell survival. Rh$_{null}$ is discussed in further detail later in this chapter.

> The *RH* genes have many mutations. Investigators have noted more than 150 alleles in the *RHD* gene and more than 60 alleles in the *RHCE* gene. These mutations rarely change the serology of the red cell reactions in phenotyping.[10]

Cation: An ion or group of ions having a positive charge

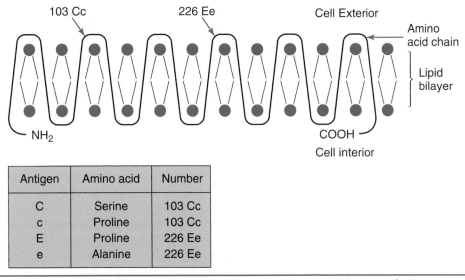

Antigen	Amino acid	Number
C	Serine	103 Cc
c	Proline	103 Cc
E	Proline	226 Ee
e	Alanine	226 Ee

Fig. 6.2 Model of the Rh polypeptide. Model of the differences in the amino acid sequence for the antigens produced by the *RHCE* gene. The basic structure is similar. Differences in the amino acid at the residue number indicated determine the serologic typing to be C or c, E or e.

TABLE 6.1 Common Antigens in the Rh Blood Group System: Equivalent Notations

NUMERIC	FISHER-RACE	OTHER NAMES	ISBT NO.
Rh1	D	Rh +	004001
Rh2	C		004002
Rh3	E		004003
Rh4	c		004004
Rh5	e		004005
Rh6	ce	*cis*-ce or f	004006
Rh7	Ce	*cis*-Ce	004007
Rh8	C^w		004008
Rh9	C^x		004009
Rh10	ce^s	V	004010
Rh12	G		004012

ISBT, International Society of Blood Transfusion.

Another gene, Rh-associated glycoprotein (*RHAG*), resides on chromosome 6.[11] This gene is important to the expression of the Rh antigens. *RHAG* encodes a glycosylated polypeptide (protein with attached carbohydrates) with a structure very similar to the Rh proteins. The RHAG forms complexes with the Rh proteins and must be present for Rh antigen expression. By itself, the RHAG does not express any Rh antigens. The International Society of Blood Transfusion (ISBT) has assigned a blood group system to the RHAG.

Rh TERMINOLOGIES

This section describes four different terminologies used in the Rh blood group system. Two terminologies, Fisher-Race and Weiner, were derived from genetic theories of Rh inheritance. These systems reflect serologic observations and inheritance theories based on family studies. Because these systems are used interchangeably in the transfusion setting, it is necessary to understand these theories well enough to "translate" from one to another. Fisher-Race terminology is used to name the antibody found in a patient specimen. Weiner terminology is used to identify red cell phenotypes on the antibody identification panel cells, etc. Two additional systems were developed because of a need for a universal language compatible with computers. The third terminology, Rosenfield, describes the presence or absence of an Rh antigen. The ISBT created the fourth terminology. Blood bank professionals must be familiar with all of these terminologies when discussing the Rh blood group system. Table 6.1 lists the equivalent notations for the more common Rh antigens.

Fisher-Race: CDE Terminology

Fisher and Race[12] postulated that the Rh blood group system antigens were inherited as a gene complex or haplotype that codes for three closely linked sets of alleles. The *D* gene is inherited at one locus, *C* or *c* genes are inherited at the second locus, and *E* or *e* genes are inherited at the third locus. Each parent contributes one haplotype or set of Rh genes. Fig. 6.1 illustrates this concept. Each gene expresses an antigen that is given the same letter as the gene. When referring to the gene, the letter is italicized. For example, the gene that produces the C antigen is *C*. Each red cell antigen can be recognized by testing with a specific antibody. The original theory assumed the *d* allele was present when the *D* allele was absent. According to the Fisher-Race theory, the order of the genes on the chromosome is *DCE*; however, it is often written alphabetically as *CDE*.

Wiener: Rh-Hr Terminology

In contrast to the Fisher-Race theory, Wiener[13] postulated that alleles at *one* gene locus were responsible for expression of the Rh blood group system antigens on red cells. Each parent contributes one *RH* gene. The inherited form of the gene may be identical (homozygous) to or different (heterozygous) from each parent. According to Wiener, eight alleles exist at the *RH* gene locus: R^0, R^1, R^2, R^z, r, r', r'', and r^y. The gene encodes a structure on the red cell called an **agglutinogen,** identified by its parts or factors. These factors are identified with the same antisera that agglutinate the D, C, c, E, and e antigens mentioned earlier in the Fisher-Race nomenclature. The difference between the Wiener and Fisher-Race theories is the inheritance of the Rh blood group system on a *single* gene locus rather than *three* separate genes. The antigen complex or agglutinogen comprises factors that are identifiable as separate antigens (Table 6.2). For example, in Wiener terminology, the R^1 gene codes for the Rh_1 agglutinogen, which is made up of factors Rh_0, rh', and hr'' that correspond to D, C, and e antigens, respectively. The *r* gene codes for the rh agglutinogen, made up of factors hr' and hr'' that correspond to c and e antigens, respectively. The longhand factor notations of Rh_0, rh', hr', rh'', and hr'' that correspond to D, C, c, E, and e antigens, respectively, are outdated and rarely used.

Wiener terminology can be easily translated to Fisher-Race terminology when the following points are kept in mind: R is the same as D; r indicates no D antigen; the number 1 and the character ' denote C; and the number 2 and the character '' denote E (Table 6.3). For example, in Wiener nomenclature, c, D, and E factors or antigens would be written as

Agglutinogen: term referring to a group of antigens or factors that are agglutinated by antisera

TABLE 6.2	Wiener Theory: Genes and Antigens
GENE (WIENER)	**ANTIGENS (FISHER-RACE)**
R^0	cDe
R^1	CDe
R^2	cDE
R^z	CDE
r	ce
r'	Ce
r''	cE
r^y	CE

Note: Factors in the Wiener terminology are easily translated to the Fisher-Race terminology, which defines the antigens more clearly.

TABLE 6.3	Converting Fisher-Race Terminology to Wiener Terminology		
FISHER-RACE ANTIGEN	**WIENER TERMINOLOGY**		**EXAMPLES**
D	R (D+)	r (D−)	$DCe = R_1$
C	1	'	$Ce = r'$, $DCe = R_1$
E	2	''	$cE = r''$, $DcE = R_2$
CE	z	y	$DCE = R_z$, $CE = r_y$
ce	0		$ce = r$

Uppercase R indicates that the D antigen is present; lowercase r indicates that the D antigen is absent; 1 and ' indicate C; 2 and '' indicate E; 0 indicates ce; z indicates CE (with R); y indicates CE (with r).

R_2. Although most workers prefer the Fisher-Race terminology to Wiener terminology, it is often easier to describe a phenotype as R_2R_2 than as D+, C−, c+, E+, e−. Subscripts refer to antigens, whereas italics and superscripts indicate genes.

Rosenfield: Numeric Terminology

Both the Wiener and the Fisher-Race terminologies are based on genetic concepts. The Rosenfield system was developed to communicate phenotypic information more suited for computerized data entry; it does not address genetic information.[14] In this system, each antigen is given a number that corresponds to the order of its assignment in the Rh blood group system. A red cell's phenotype is expressed with Rh followed by a colon and the numbers corresponding to the tested antigens. If a red cell sample is negative for the antigen tested, a minus sign is written before the number. For example, red cells that tested D+, C+, E−, c+, e+ would be written as Rh:1,2,−3,4,5. Table 6.1 compares Fisher-Race and numeric terminology.

INTERNATIONAL SOCIETY OF BLOOD TRANSFUSION: STANDARDIZED NUMERIC TERMINOLOGY

The ISBT, in an effort to standardize blood group system nomenclature, assigned a six-digit number to each blood group specificity.[15] The first three numbers represent the system, and the remaining three represent the antigen specificity. The assigned number of the Rh blood group system is 004, and the remaining three numbers correspond to the Rosenfield system. For example, the ISBT number for the C antigen is 004002. An ISBT "symbol," or alphanumeric designation similar to the Rosenfield terminology, is used to refer to a specific antigen. The term Rh is written in uppercase letters, and the antigen number immediately follows the system designation. The ISBT symbol for C is RH2. A partial list of Rh antigens that includes the ISBT numeric designation is given in Table 6.1.

R_1 is an antigen expression for DCe, which uses the subscript 1. R^1 is the allele for the antigen expression, which uses italics and the superscript 1.

DETERMINING THE GENOTYPE FROM THE PHENOTYPE

The term phenotype refers to the test results obtained with specific antisera, and the term genotype refers to the genetic makeup of an individual. The genotype cannot be determined without family studies or molecular testing but can be inferred from the phenotype based on the frequency of genes in a population. Five antisera, used to determine the Rh blood group system phenotypes, include anti-D, anti-C, anti-c, anti-E, and anti-e. Agglutination with the antisera indicates that the antigen is present on the red cell; no agglutination indicates the absence of the antigen.

TABLE 6.4 Order of Frequency of the Common Rh Blood Group System Haplotypes

WHITE		BLACK	RARE (BOTH RACES)
CDe (R_1)	Highest	cDe (R_0)	Ce (r′)
ce (r)		ce (r)	cE (r″)
cDE (R_2)	↓	CDe (R_1)	CE (r_y)
cDe (R_0)	Lowest	cDE (R_2)	CDE (R_Z)

Note: The information in this table is useful when predicting the most probable genotype after the phenotype or antigen typing determination. Knowing that a *cDe/cDe* or R^0/R^0 genotype is more common in blacks would be important if D-positive, C-negative units were requested.

TABLE 6.5 Rh Phenotypes and Genotypes

	RESULTS WITH ANTISERA					GENOTYPE		GENOTYPE FREQUENCY (%)	
ANTI-D	ANTI-C	ANTI-E	ANTI-C	ANTI-E	PHENOTYPE	CDE	RH-HR	WHITE	BLACK
+	+	−	+	+	CcDe	*CDe/ce*	R^1r	**31**	9
						CDe/cDe	R^1R^0	3	**15**
						Ce/cDe	r′R⁰	<1	2
+	+	−	−	+	CDe	*CDe/CDe*	R^1R^1	**18**	3
						CDe/Ce	R¹r′	2	<1
+	−	+	+	+	cDEe	*cDE/ce*	R^2r	**10**	6
						cDE/cDe	R^2R^0	1	**10**
+	−	+	+	−	cDE	cDE/cDE	R²R²	2	1
						cDE/cE	R²r″	<1	<1
+	+	+	+	+	CcDEe	*CDe/cDE*	R^1R^2	**12**	4
						CDe/cE	R¹r″	1	<1
						Ce/cDE	r′R²	1	<1
+	−	−	+	+	cDe	*cDe/ce*	R^0r	3	**23**
						cDe/cDe	R⁰R⁰	<1	**19**
−	−	−	+	+	ce	*ce/ce*	rr	15	7
−	+	−	+	+	Cce	Ce/ce	r′r	<1	<1
−	−	+	+	+	cEe	cE/ce	r″r	<1	<1
−	+	+	+	+	CcEe	Ce/cE	r′r″	<1	<1

Note: The more common genotypes and genotype frequencies are shown in bold. This information shows the more probable genotypes given Rh antigen phenotype determinations. Depending on the race of the individual, a different genotype of the red cells might be predicted.

When the phenotype is known, the most probable genotype can be determined by knowing the most common Rh blood group system genes for the race of the person being tested (Table 6.4). In the white population, the four most common genes encountered, in order of frequency from highest to lowest, are *CDe (R¹)*, *ce (r)*, *cDE (R²)*, and *cDe (R⁰)*. In the black population, the order of gene frequency from highest to lowest is *cDe (R⁰)*, *ce (r)*, *CDe (R¹)*, and *cDE (R²)*. The genes *Ce (rʹ)*, *cE (rʺ)*, *CDE (Rᶻ)*, and *CE (rʸ)* are not commonly found in either race. If a red cell specimen were phenotyped as D+, C+, E−, c+, e+, the phenotype would be CcDe. When inferring the genotype from the white population, the combination *CDe/ce* or *R¹r* would be the most probable genotype. In the black population, the most probable genotype would be *CDe/cDe* or *R¹R⁰* because the *R⁰* allele is more common than the *r* allele. Table 6.5 lists phenotypes determined by reactions with specific antisera and the most probable genotype based on gene frequency in the population.

Pedigree diagrams illustrate inheritance patterns. In Fig. 6.3, the inheritance of the Rh blood group system is diagrammed to illustrate the concept that the Rh blood group system is inherited as a haplotype. Because the *RHD* and *RHCE* loci are close on chromosome 1, it is easy to follow the inheritance of the gene complex using Wiener terminology. A Punnett square, which can predict phenotypes and genotypes, can also be used to illustrate the probability of being D-positive or D-negative (Fig. 6.4).

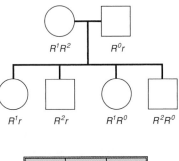

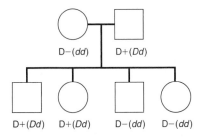

Fig. 6.3 Inheritance of Rh haplotypes. Because the genes coding for the Rh blood group system are very close on the chromosome, Rh antigens are inherited as haplotypes. This inheritance is illustrated in a pedigree chart and in a Punnett square.

Fig. 6.4 Inheritance of the D antigen. Predicting the probability of D-positive offspring from a D-negative mother (*dd*) and a heterozygous (*Dd*) father. The *d* gene does not exist and is used only for illustrative purposes. From this mating, 50% of the children could be D-positive.

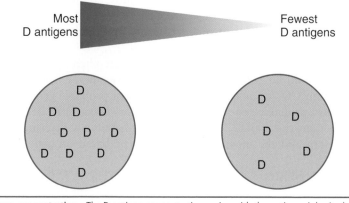

$$-D- > R^2R^2 > R^1R^1 > R^1r \text{ or } R^0r > R^1r' \text{ or } R^0r'$$

Fig. 6.5 **D antigen concentration.** The D antigen concentration varies with the antigens inherited at the *RHCE* gene. The D-deletion phenotype has the most D antigen sites. The *C* gene weakens the D antigen expression if inherited on the opposite chromosome. R^2R^2 cells show a higher D expression than R^1R^1 cells. When anti-D reacts with R^2R^2 cells, the red cells would typically demonstrate a stronger pattern of agglutination.

Immunogenicity: ability of an antigen to stimulate an immune response

Because of the high immunogenicity of the D antigen, testing for the presence or absence of the D antigen is included in routine blood typing along with the ABO antigens.

Weak D: weak form of the D antigen that requires the indirect antiglobulin test for its detection

The weak D test requires a control because the test uses an antiglobulin phase. Red cells with a positive direct antiglobulin test (DAT) will agglutinate in the IAT. A control for the routine D phenotype is present if negative reactions with anti-A and anti-B are observed. These reagents all have similar diluents.

SECTION 3

ANTIGENS OF THE Rh BLOOD GROUP SYSTEM

D ANTIGEN

The D antigen is the most immunogenic antigen in the Rh blood group system. **Immunogenicity** refers to the ability of an antigen to elicit an immune response. As high as 70% to 85% of D-negative people receiving a D-positive red blood cell (RBC) transfusion have been reported to produce an antibody with anti-D specificity.[16,17] Other reports have placed a 50% to 70% probability of immunization.[18] For that reason, a D-negative patient should receive D-negative RBC units. Fig. 6.5 illustrates the variation of the D antigen concentration in different phenotypes. Scan the QR codes for more information.

Weak D

Most red cells can be phenotyped for the D antigen directly with anti-D commercial reagents. Although the antibody to D antigen is typically of the IgG class, reagent manufacturers have developed monoclonal anti-D antibodies for concurrent use with anti-A and anti-B testing. When the D antigen is weakly expressed on the red cell, its detection may require the indirect antiglobulin test (IAT) (Fig. 6.6). Red cells that are positive for D only by the IAT are referred to as **weak D**. Recently the serologic weak D definition has been modified to reactivity of RBCs with anti-D reagent giving no or weak (≤2+) reactivity in initial testing with moderate or strong reactivity with antihuman globulin (AHG). Table 6.6 shows the interpretation of this test, which must always include a control. The Rh or D control is a reagent made by manufacturers that consists of all additives except the D antibody. It is used to determine whether agglutination by anti-D at immediate-spin is false positive, which could be due to the reagent additives, such as albumin. The Rh or D control tested at the antiglobulin phase determines whether patient cells are already coated with IgG antibodies before testing. Reagent manufacturers specify the use of controls in their package inserts, and it is important to become familiar with these guidelines. Chapter 3 discusses Rh reagents in detail. If the control is positive, additional serologic techniques may be required.

Older terminology classified weak D antigens as D^u. The IAT used to determine whether a weak form of D is present is still sometimes referred to as the D^u test, although this is incorrect terminology.[19] Newer monoclonal antibody reagents for Rh blood group system antigens have enhanced the ability to detect the weaker D antigens without additional IAT testing.

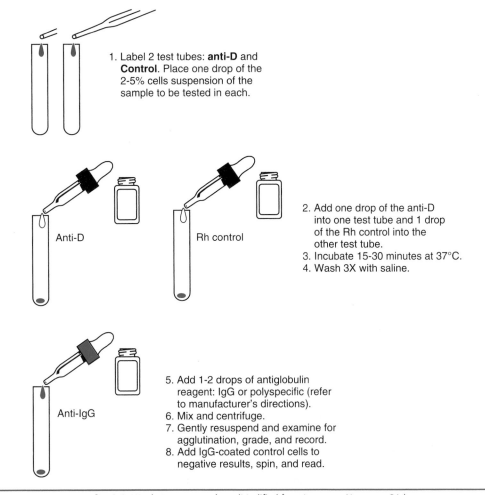

Fig. 6.6 Weak D test procedure. (Modified from Immucor, Norcross, GA.)

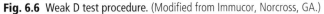

| TABLE 6.6 | Weak D Test: Interpretation with Control Results | | |

| | REACTION WITH | | |
SAMPLE NO.	ANTI-D	CONTROL	INTERPRETATION
1	+	0	D-positive
2	0	0	D-negative
3	+	+	Unable to interpret

Note: The weak D test is an antiglobulin test used to detect the D antigen on the cell. Because the test uses anti-IgG to demonstrate the presence of the D antigen, preexisting IgG on the cell would cause a "false-positive" result, as in sample no. 3. The control must be negative for the presence of IgG for the weak D test to be valid as in samples 1 and 2.

Weaker D expression can result from several different genetic circumstances outlined briefly in the following section. They are weak D due to genetics, position effect, and partial D. Only the weak D due to genetics requires detection of the D antigen by the IAT.

Weak D: Genetic

Some *RHD* genes code for a weaker expression of the D antigen. This quantitative variation in the *RHD* gene is more common in blacks and is often part of the *cDe (R_0)* haplotype. An IAT using anti-D is usually required to detect this form of D antigen.

Weak D: Position Effect

Weaker expression of the D antigen can be found when the *Ce (r')* gene is inherited in *trans* to the *RHD* gene (Fig. 6.7). Genes inherited in *trans* are inherited on opposite chromosomes. The *Ce (r')* gene paired with a *CDe (R^1)* or a *cDe (R^0)* gene weakens the

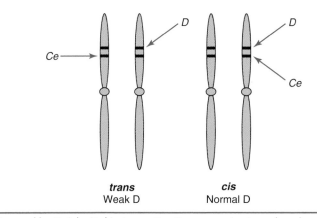

trans
Weak D

cis
Normal D

Fig. 6.7 Weak D caused by *Ce* inherited in *trans*. D antigen expression is weaker when the *D* and *Ce* genes are inherited on the opposite chromosome.

expression of the D antigen. Weak D antigen due to position effect is usually detected with monoclonal anti-D reagents because of the increased sensitivity of monoclonal reagents. The occurrence of the *Ce (r′)* gene is less than 2%.

Weak D: Partial D

Although rare, some individuals who are positive for the D antigen can make an alloantibody that appears to be anti-D after exposure to D-positive red cells. Investigation of this phenomenon revealed that some D-positive cells could be missing parts of the D antigen complex. When these individuals are exposed to the "whole D" antigen, they can make an antibody to the part they are missing. In the past, the **partial D** phenotype was termed *D variant* or *D mosaic*. Lomas et al.[20] established nine partial D phenotypes, which are classified by their parts or epitopes. The nine-epitope model was later expanded to accommodate new reaction patterns with different monoclonal anti-D reagents.[21] Red cells of most partial D phenotypes react as strongly with monoclonal antibody anti-D reagents as red cells composed of the complete D antigen. For this reason, partial D phenotypes are infrequently detected. A partial D phenotype should be suspected if a D-positive individual makes an antibody that reacts with D-positive cells but is nonreactive with his or her own cells.[19] In addition, the partial D phenotype should be suspected if two different manufacturers' monoclonal anti-D reagents are used and the interpretation as D-positive or D-negative does not agree. In this circumstance, the clone used to manufacture the reagent may vary in its ability to detect all the epitopes or parts of the D antigen. The types of weak D are summarized in Table 6.7.

Significance of Testing for Weak D

The AABB *Standards* requires testing for weak D on donor red cells that do not directly agglutinate with anti-D reagents using a method designed to detect weak expression of D.[22] There is no requirement for a test that uses an IAT.[19] Weak D–positive units are labeled D-positive and should be transfused only to D-positive recipients. A D control or an autocontrol is an important part of the weak D test because it verifies that a positive result is not due to red cells already coated with antibodies. If red cells are coated with IgG antibodies before testing with anti-D at the antiglobulin phase, the test is invalid and additional procedures are required to determine the D antigen status of the donor. Scan the QR code for more information.

Testing for weak D on potential transfusion recipient samples is not required. Many facilities perform only the direct test for the D antigen and do not complete the antiglobulin procedure if the reaction is negative. This policy may be most cost effective in terms of time and reagents because most D-negative individuals do not test positive for the weak D antigen. Patients are classified as D-negative and transfused with D-negative blood.

Some facilities test for weak D on recipient samples. If a weak D phenotype is detected, D-positive blood is provided. Although unlikely, a patient with a weak D antigen because of the partial D phenotype can theoretically make anti-D. The partial D phenotype is uncommon and with current monoclonal antibody reagents usually does not require the antiglobulin test for detection.

Partial D: D antigen that is missing part of its typical antigenic structure

DVI is a partial D antigen that is common in people of European ancestry. Anti-D produced by women with partial DVI has caused fatal hemolytic disease. Currently licensed commercial reagents are nonreactive with partial DVI red cells. Therefore these individuals would be classified as D-negative for transfusion and RhIG prophlaxis.[19]

The weak D test should not be performed on red cells with a positive direct antiglobulin test because false-positive results would occur.

TABLE 6.7	Weak D Summary	
TYPES OF WEAK D EXPRESSION	**DETECTED BY**	**CAN MAKE ANTI-D**
Genetic, reduced D antigen	Weak D test	No
Ce in *trans* to *RHD* (example: R^0r')	Monoclonal reagents	No
Partial D	Most monoclonal reagents and/or weak D test	Yes, antibody to the missing epitope

TABLE 6.8	Summary of Less Common Rh Blood Group System Antigens and Antibodies	
ANTIGEN	**ANTIGEN CHARACTERISTICS**	**ANTIBODY CHARACTERISTICS**
ce or f	*cis*-product antigen; present when c and e are inherited as a haplotype	Rare antibody; can cause HTR and HDFN; c– or e– blood is f–
Ce or Rh7	*cis*-product antigen; present when C and e are inherited as a haplotype	Anti-Ce is often made by D+ patients who make anti-C
C^w	Low-frequency antigen, found in 2% of whites and rarely in blacks; most C^w+ are also C+	Can be naturally occurring; immune examples can cause HDFN and HTR
C^x	Low (<0.01%) occurrence; C^x+ is C+	Rare, can cause mild HTR and HDFN
V or Ce^s	Found in 30% of blacks and <1% of whites	Often found with other antibodies; can cause HTR but not HDFN
G	Present on most D+ and all C+ cells	Antibody appears to be anti-D and anti-C; can cause HDFN and HTR
Rh29 or total Rh	Present on all red cells except Rh_{null} cells	Anti-Rh29 is made by Rh_{null} individuals (amorph and regulator)
RH:17	Present on all red cells except -D- cells (D deletion)	Antibody made by individuals who are -D-
hr^s	e-like antigens (e variants) produced by all Rh genes that make e; antigen hr^s is associated with weak e antigen typing	Antibodies found when an e+ person makes an apparent anti-e

HDFN, Hemolytic disease of the fetus and newborn; *HTR*, hemolytic transfusion reaction.

RhIG: Rh immune globulin (RhIG) is purified anti-D prepared from immunized donors and is given to D-negative mothers to prevent the formation of anti-D

Weak D testing is required for donors who initially phenotype as D-negative. Policies regarding typing for weak D in potential transfusion recipients vary among institutions.

Weak D testing is also performed on prenatal evaluations and Rh immune globulin (**RhIG**) workups. The decision to give RhIG to weak D–positive women during prenatal evaluations varies among institutions. It is unknown if prophylaxis would be successful in the case of a mother with a partial D phenotype with a D-positive infant. This clinical situation is discussed further in the chapter on HDFN (Chapter 12). Some debate about these policies exists; however, the important element in weak D testing by the IAT is that the interpretation is correct and uses proper controls to detect cells already sensitized with IgG antibodies.

OTHER Rh BLOOD GROUP SYSTEM ANTIGENS

Antigens in the Rh blood group system other than D, C, E, c, and e are alternative forms or variations produced by the *RHD* and *RHCE* genes. These antigens, corresponding antibodies, and clinical relevance are outlined in the following section. Table 6.8 provides a summary of less common antigens and antibody characteristics. Scan the QR code for a quiz on the blood group system.

Compound Antigens

Examples of **compound antigens** in the Rh blood group system include the following:
- Rh6 (ce or f)
- Rh7 (Ce)
- Rh27 (cE)
- Rh22 (CE)

A compound antigen is the additional antigen product formed when certain genes code for an additional protein. For example, when c and e are inherited as *RHce*, another epitope called "f" is expressed in addition to the c and e antigens. This epitope can also elicit its own immune response. The f antigen would not be present on the red cell if the person's genotype was *DCe/DcE* even though the red cells would type positive for both the c and the e antigens. In this case the *c* and *e* alleles were inherited from the *RHCe* and *RHcE* genes, and f would not be formed. Compound antigens, previously referred to as *cis* products, indicate that the antigens were coded from a haplotype rather than a single gene coding for a single protein.[19] Table 6.9 summarizes the compound antigen combinations.

Antibodies to compound antigens are infrequently encountered. If they were identified, locating antigen-negative units would require the use of common Rh antisera, such as anti-E, anti-C, anti-c, and anti-e. For example, if anti-f were identified, RBC units that are c-negative or e-negative would also be negative for the f antigen. When RBCs are required, units that are negative for one of the antigens creating the compound antigen can be safely transfused.

G Antigen

The G antigen is located on red cells that possess C or D antigens. Red cells that are negative for both the D and the C antigen are negative for the G antigen. Because an antibody to G reacts with red cells that are either D-positive or C-positive, the specificity appears to be anti-D and anti-C. Antibodies to G appear as an anti-D plus an anti-C; however, the specificities cannot be separated. In other words, anti-G antibodies mimic the reactions observed with anti-D and anti-C antibodies. In some cases, a D-negative person may receive D−, C+ red cells and appear to produce anti-C as well as anti-D. The antibody produced in this case was most likely anti-G. Distinguishing anti-G, anti-D, and anti-C antibodies requires adsorption and elution procedures.[18] Extensive testing to identify anti-G is not usually necessary. Individuals making anti-G or what appears to be anti-D or anti-C should receive red cells that are negative for *both* D and C antigens. Rare cells exist that are negative for D and positive for G (r^G). G is not a compound antigen; G is present when D *or* C is inherited. Scan the QR code for more information on G antigen.

UNUSUAL PHENOTYPES

Unusual phenotypes in the Rh blood group system are rarely encountered in routine blood bank testing. Unusual phenotypes include cells that have diminished or undetectable Rh blood group system antigen expression. Understanding the inheritance patterns and cell characteristics of unusual phenotypes provides insight into the genetics and biochemistry of the system. **Null phenotypes,** found in many blood group systems, have led to an understanding of the role of the antigen on the red cell. Serologically, null phenotypes have provided the mechanism to categorize blood group systems.

TABLE 6.9	Compound Antigens on Rh Proteins	
COMPOUND ANTIGEN	**RH PROTEIN**	**FISHER-RACE/WIENER NOTATION**
ce or f	Rhce	Dce (R_0) or ce (r)
Ce or Rh7	RhCe	DCe (R_1) or Ce (r′)
cE or Rh27	RhcE	DcE (R_2) or cE (r″)
CE or Rh22	RhCE	DCE (R_z) or CE (r_y)

D-Deletion Phenotype

Rare Rh phenotypes demonstrate no reactions when the red cells are tested with anti-E, anti-e, anti-C, or anti-c. Genetic material was deleted or rendered nonfunctional at the *RHCE* site. Red cells that lack C/c or E/e antigens may demonstrate stronger D antigen activity (see Fig. 6.5). Individuals who have the "D-deletion" phenotype may produce an antibody that reacts as a single specificity (anti-Rh17) or separable specificities such as anti-e and anti-C. An individual who produces anti-Rh17 would require D-deleted RBC units if transfusions are necessary. The D-deletion phenotype is written as -D- or D—.

Rh$_{null}$ Phenotype

The Rh$_{null}$ phenotype appears to have no Rh antigens and can be produced from two distinct genetic mechanisms. Cells that type as Rh$_{null}$ have membrane abnormalities that shorten their survival and cause hemolytic anemia of varying severity.[23] Antibodies produced by immunized individuals who lack all Rh antigens may be directed to "total-Rh" (Rh29) or to an individual Rh-antigen specificity. If an anti-Rh29 is detected, Rh$_{null}$ cells are needed for transfusion. Donations from siblings, autologous donations, and donations from the rare donor registry could be potential sources of compatible RBC units.

The inheritance of the Rh$_{null}$ phenotype can result from a **regulator gene** or an amorph gene. A regulator gene, *RHAG* (Rh associated glycoprotein), is inherited on chromosome 6 and codes for the thirtieth-named blood group system. Although the RHAG blood group system does not carry any Rh system antigens, its presence is essential for the expression of the Rh system antigens. *RHAG* mutations are associated with the absence of expression of Rh antigens.[7] In the regulator type Rh$_{null}$, the Rh genes are inherited but are not expressed. The amorph Rh$_{null}$ phenotype is less well understood. The *RHD* gene is absent, and there is a lack of expression of the *RHCE* gene, causing neither protein to be produced.[24]

Regulator gene: gene inherited at another locus or chromosome that affects the expression of another gene

Rh$_{mod}$ Phenotype

The Rh$_{mod}$ phenotype is similar to the regulator Rh$_{null}$. In this phenotype, red cells lack most of their Rh antigen expression because of the inheritance of a modified *RHAG* gene. Hemolytic anemia is also a characteristic of this phenotype.

The absence or altered conformation of the RHAG protein is primarily responsible for the Rh$_{null}$ and Rh$_{mod}$ phenotypes.[25]

SECTION 4
Rh ANTIBODIES

GENERAL CHARACTERISTICS

Rh blood group system antibodies are usually made by exposure to Rh antigens through transfusion or pregnancy. Antibodies to Rh blood group system antigens show similar serologic characteristics. Most antibodies are IgG (IgG$_1$) and bind at 37° C; agglutination is observed by the IAT. Enhancement with high-protein, low-ionic-strength saline (LISS), proteolytic enzymes, and polyethylene glycol (PEG) potentiators is useful in identification procedures. Some Rh antibodies may also be IgM (anti-E) or found in individuals who never underwent transfusion or were never pregnant (anti-C^W). Stronger reactivity with homozygous antigen expression (dosage) is characteristic of antibodies to C, c, E, and e, although this is not typical of anti-D. Anti-D is typically stronger with R$_2$R$_2$ red cells because these cells have more D antigen sites. Rh antibodies are not associated with complement activation detectable by hemolysis in tube testing or the use of polyspecific AHG reagent.

When an R$_1$R$_1$ individual makes an anti-E, anti-c often may be present, although possibly weak or undetectable. Because of this association, some clinical laboratories provide both c-negative and E-negative blood when anti-E is identified. It is recommended that more sensitive methods to detect anti-c be used when anti-E is present.

CLINICAL CONSIDERATIONS

Transfusion Reactions

Antibodies to Rh blood group system antigens can cause hemolytic transfusion reactions. Although antibodies often remain detectable for many years, their reactivity in agglutination procedures can decrease to undetectable levels. Exposure to the antigen when the antibody has formed produces a rapid secondary immune response. Antigen-negative RBCs should be transfused if antibodies to Rh blood group system antigens are identified or have been previously noted in the patient's history. It is important to check previous records of patients who may be transfused for a history of red cell antibodies that may have developed from previous transfusions or pregnancies.

Hemolytic Disease of the Fetus and Newborn

HDFN was initially observed in infants of D-negative women with D-positive mates. First pregnancies were usually unaffected. Infants from subsequent pregnancies were often stillborn or severely anemic and jaundiced. The initial pregnancy stimulated the mother to produce anti-D from the exposure to D-positive cells that occurred during birth when the infant's and mother's circulations mixed. Because maternal anti-D antibodies can cross the placenta, fetal red cells in subsequent pregnancies were destroyed by the mother's antibody. RhIG protects D-negative mothers against the production of anti-D after delivery. Anti-C, anti-c, anti-E, and anti-e are not protected by RhIG and can cause HDFN. An important aspect of prevention of HDFN is antibody screening early in pregnancy and the determination of the D antigen status of mothers to ascertain RhIG candidacy.

SECTION 5
LW BLOOD GROUP SYSTEM

RELATIONSHIP TO THE Rh BLOOD GROUP SYSTEM

The LW blood group system is presented here because of its phenotypic relationship to the Rh blood group system. The antigens and antibodies are similar in serologic properties but are not genetically related. As discussed earlier, the LW antibody, made by guinea pigs and rabbits that were immunized with red cells from rhesus macaque monkeys in early experiments, is similar to the anti-D antibody. Anti-LW reacts strongly with D-positive cells and weakly with D-negative cells. Rh_{null} cells are negative for LW antigens as well. The theory suggesting a precursor relationship between the Rh blood group system and LW antigens has been discounted, although the membrane biochemistry is still being studied.[26] A summary of LW system antigens and antibodies appears in Table 6.10.

The *LW* locus is mapped to chromosome 19. The LW system alleles are *LW^a*, *LW^b*, and *LW*. LW(a+b−) is the most common phenotype in the population because the *LW^a* gene is of high frequency. The *LW* gene is an amorph, and inheriting two *LW* genes produces the rare LW(a−b−) phenotype. Antibodies to the LW system are clinically significant and rare.

TABLE 6.10	LW Blood Group System	
GENOTYPE	**PHENOTYPE**	**CHARACTERISTICS**
LW^aLW^a or *LW^aLW*	LW(a+b−)	Most common (97%) LW phenotype
LW^aLW^b	LW(a+b+)	3%
LW^bLW^b or *LW^bLW*	LW(a−b+)	Rare
LWLW	LW(a−b−)	Rare; can make anti-LW, which reacts more strongly with D+ cells

CHAPTER SUMMARY

The major concepts of the Rh blood group system regarding inheritance theories, nomenclature, antigens, and antibodies are summarized in the following table.

SUMMARY OF Rh BLOOD GROUP SYSTEM ANTIGENS

Biochemical Composition	Polypeptides with no carbohydrate residues
Gene Products	416 amino acids that traverse the membrane 12 times
Current Genetic Theory	Two genes, *RHD* and *RHCE;* alleles include *RHCE, RHCe, RHcE,* and *RHce*
Fisher-Race Theory	Three genes; alleles include *D/d, C/c,* and *E/e*
Wiener Theory	One gene; alleles include R^0, R^1, R^2, R^z, r, r', r'', and r^y
Rosenfield/Numeric Terminology	Numeric D = Rh1, C = Rh2, E = Rh3, c = Rh4, e = Rh5
ISBT: Standard Numeric	Rh blood group system is 004; each antigen has a number as shown in Rosenfield system
Genetic Loci	Chromosome 1
Weak D	D antigen negative or agglutinated with some anti-D on immediate-spin and detected by IAT
Compound Antigens	ce or f, Ce or Rh7, CE or Rh22, and cE or Rh27
G Antigen	Present whenever the D or C antigen is on the red blood cell
Rh_{null} Phenotype	Results from an amorph gene or *RHAG* regulator gene; no Rh antigens, abnormal red blood cell membrane

SUMMARY OF Rh BLOOD GROUP SYSTEM ANTIBODIES

Antibody Production	Red blood cell stimulation through transfusion or pregnancy
Immunoglobulin Class	IgG; usually IgG1 and IgG3
In vitro Reactions	Binds at 37° C; agglutination observed using IAT
Enhancement	LISS, proteolytic enzymes, albumin, and PEG
Complement Binding	No
Clinical Significance	Yes; can cause delayed transfusion reactions and HDFN
Dosage	Yes; stronger reactions with homozygous expression

CRITICAL THINKING EXERCISES

Exercise 6.1
A transfusion recipient from an outside facility needs four units of R_2R_2 RBCs for transfusion. From this request, determine the following:
1. What Rh blood group system antigens are present on R_2R_2 RBCs?
2. What Rh blood group system antigens are not present on R_2R_2 RBCs?
3. What is the frequency of finding compatible R_2R_2 RBC units?
4. Write R_2R_2 donor units in Fisher-Race and Rosenfield terminology.

Exercise 6.2
The following reactions were obtained by testing red cells from a male donor with Rh blood group system antisera:

Rh Antisera	Donor RBC Reaction
Anti-D	+
Anti-C	+
Anti-E	0

Rh Antisera	Donor RBC Reaction
Anti-c	0
Anti-e	+
Rh control	0

+, Agglutination; 0, no agglutination.

1. What is the Rh phenotype?
2. Determine the most probable Rh genotype if the donor is white.
3. If the donor were black, would the most probable Rh genotype be different in this case?
4. What Rh antibodies could this donor make after transfusion?
5. Is this Rh phenotype rare or common?

Exercise 6.3

A 65-year-old patient with cancer was tested. The following table shows the results.

Anti-A	Anti-B	Anti-D	D Control	A_1 Cells	B Cells	Interpretation
4+	4+	1+	1+	0	0	AB, D-positive

1. Is the interpretation of the patient's blood type correct?
2. What test is recommended to solve the Rh typing discrepancy?
3. Should a weak D test be performed if the patient has a positive direct antiglobulin test?
4. If the patient needs a transfusion before the resolution of the discrepancy, what blood type should this patient receive?

Exercise 6.4

The following results were obtained from a first-time blood donor:

Anti-A	Anti-B	Anti-D	Weak D	D Control	A_1 Cells	B Cells	Interpretation
4+	0	0	2+	0 ✓	0	4+	

✓ = IgG sensitized red cells agglutinated.

1. Interpret the blood donor's ABO and D phenotyping.
2. Discuss the validity of the testing.
3. Why is it unnecessary to perform an Rh control with the immediate-spin anti-D test?
4. If the transfusion service did not perform weak D testing on recipients, what type of blood would this patient receive for an RBC transfusion?

Exercise 6.5

A 25-year-old man received five units of group O, D-negative RBCs in the emergency room after a serious car accident. His blood type, which was determined from a sample collected before transfusion, was group O, D-negative. A sample was resubmitted 2 weeks after the accident for pretransfusion testing before orthopedic surgery. The antibody screen was positive, and the antibodies identified were anti-D and anti-C.

1. What are possible explanations for the antibodies identified?
2. What additional testing should be performed to explain the problem?
3. If the blood type of the units he received was correct, what is the probable Rh phenotype of the units that he received?
4. What antigen or antigens should be negative if he needs RBC transfusions in the future?
5. Based on your knowledge of Rh antigen frequency, will it be difficult to obtain these units?

Exercise 6.6
Based on your knowledge about factors relating to immunogenicity, why are the Rh antigens (especially D antigen) considered highly immunogenic?

STUDY QUESTIONS

1. How is the Rh genotype *CDE/cDE* written in Wiener notation?
   a. R^0R^1
   b. R^yR^2
   c. R^2R^1
   d. R^zR^2

2. In Rosenfield notation, the phenotype of a donor may be written as Rh:1,−2,−3,4,5. What is the correct phenotype in Fisher-Race (CDE) notation?
   a. cDe
   b. CcDe
   c. CcDE
   d. CDEe

3. Anti-f was identified in a patient. Because commercial antisera are not available, what is the best course of action to locate compatible RBC units?
   a. crossmatch E-negative units
   b. contact the rare donor registry
   c. release O, D-negative units
   d. crossmatch c-negative units

4. A patient's Rh phenotype was D+, c+, e+, C−, E−. What is the most likely race of this donor?
   a. black
   b. white
   c. Asian
   d. Native American

5. What test is needed to determine weak D antigen status?
   a. the IAT
   b. the DAT
   c. anti-D^u typing sera
   d. anti-D antisera with a LISS potentiator

6. Which of the following red cell genotypes would react negatively with anti-G?
   a. R^0r
   b. *rr*
   c. R^2r
   d. *r′r*

7. What statement is true relative to the results of a weak D test performed on a patient with a positive direct antiglobulin test?
   a. accurate as long as the check cells were positive
   b. unreliable because of immunoglobulins already on the cell
   c. reliable if a high-albumin anti-D was used
   d. false-negative because of antibody neutralization

8. Which of the following is associated with the Rh$_{null}$ phenotype?
   a. elevated D antigen expression
   b. increased LW antigen expression
   c. the Bombay phenotype
   d. red cell membrane abnormalities

9. What is the name of the blood group system that was originally identified as the Rh blood group system?
   a. Kell
   b. Lutheran
   c. Lewis
   d. LW

10. A donor tested D-negative using commercial anti-D reagent. The weak D test was positive. How should the RBC unit be labeled?
    a. D-positive
    b. D-negative
    c. D variant
    d. varies with blood bank policy

11. Which offspring is *not* possible from a mother who is R$_2$r and a father who is R$_1$r?
    a. *DcE/DcE*
    b. *DCe/DcE*
    c. *DcE/ce*
    d. *ce/ce*

12. What is the common form of antibodies produced upon exposure to Rh blood group system antigens?
    a. naturally occurring IgM
    b. immune IgG
    c. immune IgM
    d. naturally occurring IgG and IgM

13. Which of the following genotypes is heterozygous for the C antigen?
    a. R^1r
    b. R^2R^2
    c. R^1R^1
    d. *r′r′*

14. What is the likelihood that two heterozygous D-positive parents will have a D-negative child?
    a. less than 1%
    b. not possible
    c. 25%
    d. 75%

15. Which of the following genotypes could make anti-Ce (Rh7)?
    a. R^2R^2
    b. R^1R^0
    c. R^1R^2
    d. *r′r*

16. Which of the following phenotypes would react with anti-f?
    a. rr
    b. R$_1$R$_1$
    c. R$_2$R$_2$
    d. R$_1$R$_2$

17. A donor is tested with Rh antisera; given the following results, what is the most probable Rh genotype?

Rh Antisera	Donor RBC Reaction
Anti-D	+
Anti-C	+
Anti-E	0
Anti-c	+
Anti-e	+
Rh control	0

+, Agglutination; *0*, no agglutination.

    a. R^1R^1
    b. R^1r
    c. R^0r
    d. R^2r

18. Anti-D was detected in the serum of a D-positive person. What is a possible explanation?
    a. the antibody is really anti-G
    b. compound antibody was formed
    c. regulator gene failure
    d. missing antigen epitope

19. An antibody to the E antigen was identified in a patient who received multiple transfusions. What is the *most likely* phenotype of the patient's red cells?
    a. R_1R_1
    b. R_2R_2
    c. R_1r
    d. r'r'

20. The regulator gene *RHAG:*
    a. is inherited on chromosome 1
    b. is responsible for the Rh_{mod} phenotype
    c. must be inherited to express LW antigens
    d. is responsible for the D-deletion phenotype

Answers to Study Questions can be found on page 387.

Additional student resources, including review questions, a laboratory manual, and case studies, can be found on the Evolve website.

REFERENCES

1. Levine P, Stetson RE: An unusual case of intragroup agglutination, *JAMA* 113:126, 1939.
2. Landsteiner K, Wiener AS: An agglutinable factor in human blood recognized by immune sera for rhesus blood, *Proc Soc Exp Biol N Y* 43:223, 1940.
3. Tippett P: A speculative model for the Rh blood groups, *Ann Hum Genet* 50:241, 1986.
4. Colin Y, Cherif-Zahar B, Le Van Kim C, et al.: Genetic basis of the RhD-positive and RhD-negative blood group polymorphism as determined by Southern analysis, *Blood* 78:2747, 1991.
5. Mouro I, Colin Y, Cherif-Zahar B, et al.: Molecular genetic basis of the human Rhesus blood group system, *Nat Genet* 5:62, 1993.
6. Arge P, Cartron JP: Molecular biology of the Rh antigens, *Blood* 78:551, 1991.
7. Westhoff CM: The Rh blood group system in review: a new face for the next decade, *Transfusion* 44:1663, 2004.
8. Cherif-Zahar B, Bloy C, Le Van Kim C, et al.: Molecular cloning and protein structure of a human blood group Rh polypeptide, *Proc Natl Acad Sci USA* 87:6243, 1990.
9. Daniels G, Lomas-Francis C, Wallace M, et al.: Epitopes of Rh D: serology and molecular genetics. In Silberstein LE, editor: *Molecular and functional aspects of blood group antigens*, Bethesda, MD, 1995, AABB.

10. Blumenfeld CO, Patnaik SK: Allelic genes of blood group antigens: a source of human mutations and cSNPs documented in Blood Group Antigen Gene Mutation Database, *Hum Mutat* 23:8–16, 2004.

11. Ridgewell K, Spurr NK, Laguda B, et al.: Isolation of cDNA clones for a 50 kDa glycoprotein associated with Rh (rhesus) blood group antigen expression, *Biochem J* 287:223–228, 1992.

12. Race RR: The Rh genotypes and Fisher's theory, *Blood* 2:27, 1948.

13. Wiener AS: Genetic theory of the Rh blood types, *Proc Soc Exp Biol Med* 54:316, 1943.

14. Rosenfield RE, Allen Jr FH, Swisher SN, et al.: A review of Rh serology and presentation of a new terminology, *Transfusion* 2:287, 1962.

15. Lewis M, Anstee DJ, Bird GWG, et al.: Blood group terminology 1990: the ISBT working party on terminology for red cell surface antigens, *Vox Sang* 58:152, 1990.

16. Pollack W, Ascari WQ, Kochesry RJ, et al.: Studies on Rh prophylaxis: relationship between doses of anti-Rh and size of antigenic stimulus, *Transfusion* 11:355, 1971.

17. Urbaniak SJ, Robertson AE: A successful program of immunizing Rh-negative male volunteers for anti-D production using frozen/thawed blood, *Transfusion* 21:64, 1981.

18. Issitt PD: *Applied blood group serology*, ed 3, Miami, FL, 1985, Montgomery Scientific.

19. Fung MK: *Technical manual*, ed 18, Bethesda, MD, 2014, AABB.

20. Lomas C, McColl K, Tippett P: Further complexities of the Rh antigen D disclosed by testing category D^{II} cells with monoclonal anti-D, *Transfus Med* 3:67, 1993.

21. Reid ME, Lomas-Francis C, Olsson ML: *The blood group antigen facts book*, ed 3, San Diego, CA, 2012, Academic Press.

22. Levitt J, editor: *Standards for blood banks and transfusion services*, ed 29, Bethesda, MD, 2014, AABB.

23. Schmidt PJ: Hereditary hemolytic anemias and the null blood types, *Arch Intern Med* 139:570, 1979.

24. Cherif-Zahar B, Raynal V, Le Van Kim C, et al.: Structure and expression of the RH locus in the Rh-deficiency syndrome, *Blood* 82:656, 1993.

25. Daniels G: *Rh and RHAG blood group systems, in human blood groups*, ed 3, Oxford, UK, 2013, Wiley-Blackwell http://dx.doi.org/10.1002/9781118493595.ch5.

26. Bloy C, Hermand P, Cherif-Zahar B, et al.: Comparative analysis by two-dimensional iodopeptide mapping of the RhD protein and LW glycoprotein, *Blood* 75:2245, 1990.

OTHER RED CELL BLOOD GROUP SYSTEMS, HUMAN LEUKOCYTE ANTIGENS, AND PLATELET ANTIGENS

7

CHAPTER OUTLINE

LEARNING OBJECTIVES

On completion of this chapter, the reader should be able to:

1. Identify the major antigens classified within the other blood group systems.
2. Predict the frequencies of the observed phenotypes and the association of phenotypes with ethnic group diversity.
3. Describe the biochemical characteristics of antigens within each blood group system.
4. Discuss the genetic mechanisms for antigen inheritance in each blood group system. Predict the null phenotypes associated with genetic variations.

5. Compare and contrast the serologic characteristics and clinical relevance of the antibodies associated with each blood group system.
6. Identify unique characteristics of selected blood group systems, their associations with disease, and their biological functions.
7. Solve complex antibody problems using serologic characteristics of blood group system antibodies.
8. Select donor units that are compatible for transfusion to patients with multiple and rare antibodies.
9. Differentiate high-frequency and low-frequency antigens in antibody identification problems.
10. Using the principles of tissue matching, select the best potential graft given the HLA typing and antibody specificities.
11. Predict the probable HLA typing results in a family study performed for graft selection.
12. Compare and contrast the class I and II MHC complexes with regard to antigens, their associated immune cells, and their role in immunity.
13. Explain the role of HLA testing in platelet transfusion support.
14. Outline the serologic test methods used in HLA typing and antibody identification.
15. Discuss the role of platelet antigens in transfusion medicine.

SECTION 1

WHY STUDY OTHER BLOOD GROUP SYSTEMS?

In addition to the antigens of the ABO and Rh blood group systems, more than 300 unique antigens have been documented on red cells. At the time of publication, the International Society of Blood Transfusion (ISBT) has defined 36 blood group systems. As previously discussed, the antigens of the ABO and Rh blood group systems are of primary importance in transfusion. The antibodies to ABO and Rh blood group system antigens are capable of effecting a decreased survival of transfused red cells and playing a role in the pathogenesis of hemolytic disease of the fetus and newborn (HDFN). Antigens assigned to other blood group systems can also elicit immune responses in transfusion or pregnancy. Some of these antibodies produced are considered clinically relevant in transfusion medicine. Knowledge of the blood group systems provides the foundation for solving complex antibody problems in a logical and efficient manner.

In traditional terms, the blood group antigen has been considered the target of a red cell alloantibody or autoantibody. The antigen–antibody complex may trigger a process leading to the immune-mediated destruction of red cells. Primary efforts in the blood bank have revolved around resolving problems relating to this pathophysiologic role.

In addition to these pathophysiologic roles, the molecular cloning of blood group genes has provided insight into the primary functional roles of these blood group antigens. Studies have linked blood group systems with unique roles in the following physiologic functions related to red cell membranes[1]:

- Molecules that function in transporting water-soluble molecules across the lipid bilayer for intake of nutrients and excretion of waste products
- Molecules that function in the complement pathway
- Molecules that play a role in the ability of cells to adhere to other cells
- Molecules that function as structural proteins to maintain red cell shape and mechanical deformability
- Molecules with suggested enzymatic activities

In addition to serving these physiologic functions, red cell antigens can function as microbial receptors for infection by microorganisms (bacteria, viruses, or protozoan parasites). For example, the Duffy antigens, Fy^a and Fy^b, serve as the attachment sites for certain malarial parasites. An overview of the relationships of the blood group systems and their unique functional roles is presented in Table 7.1.[1]

This chapter also includes the facts relative to antigens not present on red cells. These antigens include the human leukocyte (HLA) and platelet antigens. In addition to red cell antigens, these antigens are important in transfusion and transplantation medicine.

TABLE 7-1	Functional Roles of Some Blood Group Systems
Glycosyltransferases	
ABO, P1PK, Lewis, and H blood group systems	
Structural Relationship to Red Cell	
MNS, Diego, and Gerbich blood group systems	
Transport Proteins	
Rh, Kidd, Diego, Colton, and Kx blood group systems	
Complement Pathway Molecules	
Chido/Rodgers, Cromer, and Knops blood group systems	
Adhesion Molecules	
Lutheran, Xg, Landsteiner–Wiener, and Indian blood group systems	
Microbial Receptors	
MNS, Duffy, P, Lewis, and Cromer blood group systems	
Biologic Receptors	
Duffy, Knops, and Indian blood group systems	

Note: Many of these functional relationships were predicted based on molecular cloning studies and remain under investigation.

HLA antigens elicit HLA antibodies, similar to red cell antibodies, because of exposure to foreign antigens during transfusions of blood products and from pregnancy. Platelets also possess inherited membrane proteins that can elicit an immune response. Platelet antibodies are not commonly formed because there is less platelet antigen variability in the population.

ORGANIZATION OF CHAPTER

This chapter highlights the major facts relating to the antigens and antibodies of the other blood group systems. Each blood group system section begins with a box that outlines the major features of each system. The following information is featured:

- ISBT blood group system symbol
- ISBT blood group system number
- Clinical significance of the blood group system antibodies

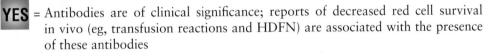 **YES** = Antibodies are of clinical significance; reports of decreased red cell survival in vivo (eg, transfusion reactions and HDFN) are associated with the presence of these antibodies

NO = Antibodies are not of clinical significance; there is no association of decreased red cell survival in vivo (eg, transfusion reactions and HDFN) with the presence of the antibodies

- Immunoglobulin class of most antibodies produced: IgM or IgG immunoglobulin class
- Optimal in vitro antibody-binding temperature

 = Antibodies bind at 37° C

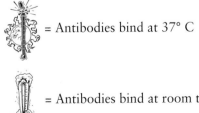 = Antibodies bind at room temperature or lower

- Optimal in vitro reaction method

RT = Agglutination reactions are observed at room temperature or lower or with a buffered gel card if using gel technology

AHG = Agglutination reactions are enhanced in indirect antiglobulin tests (IATs) or using the antiglobulin methods of gel technology or solid phase red cell adherence assays (SPRCAs)

- Antibody reactivity with enzyme-treated reagent red cells (ficin or papain)

 = No significant changes in the strength of agglutination reactions are observed with papain and ficin enzyme-treated reagent red cells

E↑ = Agglutination reactions with papain or ficin enzyme-treated reagent red cells are increased in strength (eg, enhanced)

Ⓔ = No agglutination is observed with papain or ficin enzyme-treated reagent red cells; the agglutination reactions disappear with enzyme-treated reagent red cells

VAR = Variable agglutination reactions are observed with papain or ficin enzyme-treated reagent red cells

- Dosage

YES = Antibodies can exhibit dosage in antibody identification panels

NO = Antibodies characteristically do not exhibit dosage in antibody identification panels

OCC = Some antibodies may demonstrate dosage

VAR = Individual variation in dosage expression

SECTION 2
KELL BLOOD GROUP SYSTEM

ISBT System Symbol	ISBT System Number	Clinical Significance	Antibody Class	Optimal Temperature	Reaction Phase	Effect of Enzymes	Dosage
KEL	006	**YES**	IgG		AHG	E → NO EFFECT	OCC

CHARACTERISTICS AND BIOCHEMISTRY OF KELL ANTIGENS

Kell Antigens Facts

In 1946 Coombs et al[2] reported the detection of a new blood group antibody in a patient named Kelleher after using their antiglobulin test. This antibody was associated with a case of HDFN, a disease characterized by the decreased survival of fetal red cells because of their sensitization with maternal immunoglobulin G (IgG) antibodies. This antibody, anti-Kell, defined a red cell antigen that was designated the Kell antigen; the Kell blood group system was established. Since its discovery 60 years ago, the Kell blood group system has grown into a complex polymorphism of 35 red cell antigens.[3] Numeric and alphabetic terminologies similar to those of the Rh blood group system have evolved for the Kell blood group system. Any references to the blood group system as an entity are called Kell, whereas appropriate references to the antigens within the system are made through the numeric or alphabetic notations. The original names of the Kell antigens are appropriately used only in an historical context. The correct terminology for the original antigen is K or KEL1 rather than Kell.

TABLE 7.2	Summary of Antigens: Kell Blood Group System[3]

Antithetical Antigens: High Frequency and Low Frequency

K (KEL1) and k (KEL2)
Kp^a (KEL3), Kp^b (KEL4), and Kp^c (KEL21)
Js^a (KEL6) and Js^b (KEL7)
K11 (KEL11) and K17 (KEL17)
K14 (KEL14) and K24 (KEL24)

Antithetical Antigens: Low Frequency

VLAN (KEL25) and VONG (KEL28)

High-Frequency Antigens

Ku (KEL5)
K12 (KEL12)
K13 (KEL13)
K16 (KEL16)
K18 (KEL18)
K19 (KEL19)
Km (KEL20)
K22 (KEL22)
TOU (KEL26)
RAZ (KEL27)
KALT (KEL29)
KTIM (KEL30)
KUCI (KEL32)
KANT (KEL33)
KASH (KEL34)
KELP (KEL35)
KETI (KEL36)
KHUL (KEL37)
KYOR (KEL38)

Low-Frequency Antigens

Ul^a (KEL10)
K23 (KEL23)
KYO (KEL31)

Note: K8 and K9 are obsolete; K15 (Kx) is no longer included in the Kell system.

Population studies determined that the K (KEL1) antigen has about a 9% frequency in the white population. Its antithetical antigen, k or KEL2 (originally designated as Cellano), possesses a 99.8% frequency in whites and was first reported in 1949.[4] Additional pairs of high-frequency and low-frequency antithetical antigens intrinsic to the Kell blood group system were discovered over the next several years. These antigens were designated Kp^a or KEL3 (originally designated as Penny) and Kp^b or KEL4 (originally designated as Rautenberg).[5,6] The Kp^b (KEL4) antigen possesses a high frequency (99.9%), whereas the Kp^a (KEL3) antigen is rarely expressed in the white population (2%). The Js^a or KEL6 antigen (originally designated as Sutter) and the Js^b or KEL7 antigen (originally designated as Matthews) were added to the Kell blood group system as a pair of high-frequency and low-frequency antithetical antigens.[7,8] The Js^a antigen has a 20% frequency in the black population and a <0.01% frequency in whites. At the present time, 35 red cell antigens are assigned to the Kell blood group system, which are summarized in Table 7.2. Similarities to the Rh blood group system include the confinement of Kell antigens to red cells and the presence of detectable antigens on fetal red cells. Because of this early antigen development, Kell antibodies have been implicated in HDFN cases.

Red cell antigens classified as high frequency are present in greater than 99% of the population. Red cell antigens classified as low frequency are present in less than 10% of the population.

High-frequency and low-frequency red cell antigens may be inherited together in an antithetical manner, which means on opposite alleles.

K, Kp^a, and Js^a red cell antigens are extremely rare in Asian populations.[9]

Biochemistry of Kell Antigens

In biochemical terms, the Kell blood group system antigens are located on a glycoprotein that is integral to the red cell membrane.[10] The Kell glycoprotein is covalently linked to

Sulfhydryl reagents: reagents that disrupt the disulfide bonds between cysteine amino acid residues in proteins; DTT, 2-ME, and AET function as sulfhydryl reagents

Kell blood group system red cell antigens are not destroyed when treated with papain or ficin enzymes.

"Kell" should not be used when referring to K antigen or anti-K. The term refers to whole glycoprotein as described in the biochemistry section.

another protein, Kx, which defines the Kx blood group system. Special studies of the Kell glycoprotein have revealed that 4000 to 18,000 Kell antigen sites exist per red cell.[11] The biological role of the Kell glycoprotein has been characterized as a zinc endopeptidase, which is central to zinc binding and catalytic activity.[3]

The Kell antigens are characteristically sensitive to treatment with **sulfhydryl reagents,** such as 2-mercaptoethanol (2-ME), dithiothreitol (DTT), or 2-aminoethylisothiouronium bromide (AET). These reagents reduce the disulfide bonds, which results in a disruption of multiple disulfide bonds in the protein. An antigen with a three-dimensional highly folded protein structure is susceptible to any agent that interferes with its tertiary structure. Molecular cloning studies have demonstrated that the Kell glycoprotein possesses an extensively folded disulfide-bonded region. This factor explains Kell antigen sensitivity to disulfide-reducing agents.[12] Treatment of red cells with these sulfhydryl reagents creates red cells that lack Kell antigens. Ethylenediaminetetraacetic acid (EDTA)-glycine acid (EGA, Immucor, Norcross, GA), a reagent that dissociates IgG from red cells, also destroys Kell antigens.[9]

Immunogenicity of Kell Antigens

The K (KEL1) antigen is strongly immunogenic. The immunogenicity of the K antigen ranks second to the D antigen in terms of eliciting an immune response in transfusions. Studies reported that 1 in 10 K-negative individuals who are transfused with K-positive donor red cells develop anti-K in response to transfusion. Other antigens within the Kell blood group system are less immunogenic. Antibodies to these antigens are not commonly observed because of a combination of two factors: antigen frequency and immunogenicity of structure.

K_0 or Kell$_{null}$ Phenotype

A red cell phenotype lacking expression of the Kell glycoprotein, and consequently the Kell antigens, was identified by Chown et al[13] in 1957. This null phenotype is designated K_0 or Kell$_{null}$. The inheritance of two recessive K_0 genes in a homozygote (K_0K_0) results in the null phenotype. These individuals lack all Kell system antigens but express another related antigen, Kx antigen. This antigen is discussed later in this chapter.

The alloantibody stimulated immunologically in K_0 individuals who have received transfusions has been called anti-Ku or anti-KEL5 and is clinically significant for transfusion purposes. Anti-Ku is produced because the Ku antigen is present on all red cells except K_0 cells. Immunized K_0 individuals require transfusion with rare K_0 donor units. Rare donor units can be obtained by contacting the American Rare Donor Program sponsored by the AABB and the American Red Cross.

GENETICS OF THE KELL BLOOD GROUP SYSTEM

The Kell blood group system gene, *KEL*, is located on chromosome 7. The Kell locus is the site of the different Kell genes that produce the antigens of the Kell blood group system. Five sets of alleles that produce the Kell system's antithetical antigens exist within the Kell locus. These alleles include the following:

- *K* and *k*
- *Kp^a* and *Kp^b*
- *Js^a* and *Js^b*
- *K11* and *K17*
- *K14* and *K24*
- *VLAN* and *VONG* (both low-frequency antigens)

The high-incidence genes include *k*, *Kp^b*, *Js^b*, and *K11*. This haplotype is common in all populations. Low-incidence genes include *K*, *Kp^a*, *Js^a*, and *K17*. The incidence of low-frequency alleles varies among different ethnic groups. The *K*, *Kp^a*, and *K17* alleles are more common in the white population, whereas the *Js^a* allele is more common in the black population.[14] Table 7.3 summarizes the common phenotypes and their frequency distribution of the Kell blood group system.

TABLE 7.3 Common Phenotypes and Frequencies in the Kell Blood Group System

PHENOTYPE	FREQUENCY (%)	
	WHITE	BLACK
K–k+	91	98
K+k–	0.2	Rare
K+k+	8.8	2
Kp(a+b–)	Rare	0
Kp(a–b+)	97.7	100
Kp(a+b+)	2.3	Rare
Js(a+b–)	0	1
Js(a–b+)	100	80
Js(a+b+)	Rare	19

From Reid ME, Lomas-Francis C, Olsson ML: *The blood group antigen facts book,* ed 3, San Diego, CA, 2012, Academic Press.

Other unrelated genetic loci may affect the expression of Kell antigens on red cells. The Kell antigens may be modified by regulator genes on the X chromosome in relation to the Kx blood group system as discussed later in this chapter.

CHARACTERISTICS OF KELL ANTIBODIES

Most Kell system antibodies possess the following characteristics:

- Immunoglobulin class is IgG.
- Antibodies are produced in response to antigen exposure through transfusion or pregnancy.
- Antibodies agglutinate optimally in the IAT.
- Antibodies usually do not bind complement.
- Antibodies have been associated with hemolytic transfusion reactions and HDFN.
- Enzyme treatment of red cells shows no enhancement or depression of antibody reactivity.
- Depressed reactivity of anti-K is observed in some low-ionic-strength solution (LISS) reagents.

Anti-K is the most commonly observed antibody of the Kell blood group system in the transfusion service. Most examples of anti-K are IgG and react well in IATs and sometimes at room temperature. Despite its low frequency (9%), the K antigen's high degree of immunogenicity is responsible for the occurrence of the antibody in a patient population. Examples of IgM anti-K elicited from exposure to some bacteria may also be present in a patient population.[3]

Antibodies to k, Kp[b], and Js[b] are not commonly detected because individuals who lack these high-incidence antigens are scarce. An antibody to one of these antigens should be considered when a patient's serum reacts with most or all panel cells in antibody identification studies. Anti-k and anti-Kp[b] production are associated with the white population, whereas anti-Js[b] is associated with the black population. Sources of compatible donor red cell units are difficult to obtain when dealing with an antibody to a high-frequency antigen. Suitable donors often may be obtained from the patient's siblings or the American Rare Donor Program.

Antibody production to the Kp[a] and Js[a] antigens is also infrequent in a patient population because both antigens possess low frequencies. Donor units possessing these antigens are uncommon; exposure to these antigens by transfusion recipients is minimal.

Anti-K will react well with K+k+ and K+k– red cells in antibody panels.

The association of certain antibodies and race can assist in the resolution of antibody identification. For example, anti-Js[b] is associated with the black population.

Few examples of non–red cell–stimulated anti-K were reported in healthy male donors with no transfusion history. In other examples, a microbial infection was implicated as the immunizing agent.[9]

SECTION 3
Kx BLOOD GROUP SYSTEM

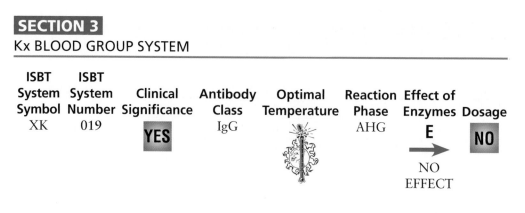

ISBT System Symbol	ISBT System Number	Clinical Significance	Antibody Class	Optimal Temperature	Reaction Phase	Effect of Enzymes	Dosage
XK	019	YES	IgG		AHG	E → NO EFFECT	NO

Kx ANTIGEN AND ITS RELATIONSHIP TO THE KELL BLOOD GROUP SYSTEM

As previously discussed in the genetics section, the autosomal gene responsible for the production of the Kell glycoprotein is located on chromosome 7. Another gene, assigned to the X chromosome and designated as *XK*, encodes a protein called Xk that carries the Kx antigen. Kx antigen has been assigned to the Kx blood group system. A discussion of this blood group system is included here because the absence of Kx antigen in the McLeod phenotype (discussed in the next section) weakens the expression of Kell antigens.

Although the Kx antigen is genetically independent of the Kell antigens, it possesses a phenotypic relationship to the Kell blood group system. Red cells with normal Kell phenotypes carry trace amounts of Kx antigen. Red cells from K_0 individuals possess elevated levels of Kx antigen.

MCLEOD PHENOTYPE

When the *XK* gene is not inherited, Kx antigen is not expressed on the red cells. The absence of Kx antigen from red cells and a concurrent reduced expression of the Kell blood group system antigens are characteristically associated with a red cell abnormality known as the McLeod phenotype. Individuals with the McLeod phenotype have red cell morphologic and functional abnormalities characterized by decreased red cell survival (Fig. 7.1). The McLeod phenotype is very rare and is seen almost exclusively in males

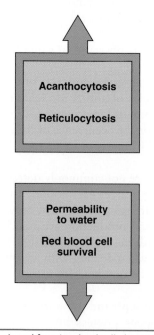

Acanthocytosis: presence of abnormal red cells with spurlike projections in the circulating blood

Reticulocytosis: increase in the number of reticulocytes in the circulating blood

Fig. 7.1 McLeod phenotype: morphologic and functional red cell abnormalities. Individuals expressing the McLeod phenotype have decreased red cell survival with increased hematologic **acanthocytosis** and **reticulocytosis**.

TABLE 7.4	Summary of Kell Blood Group System Phenotypes and Kx Antigen			
	ANTIGEN EXPRESSION		POSSIBLE SERUM	NORMAL RED CELL
PHENOTYPE	KELL	Kx	ANTIBODIES?	MORPHOLOGY?
Common	Normal	Weak	Kell alloantibodies	Yes
K_0	None	↑↑↑	Anti-Ku	Yes
McLeod	↓↓↓	None	Anti-KL (anti-Kx and anti-Km)	Acanthocytes
DTT-treated	None	↑	Not applicable	Not applicable

↓↓↓, Marked reduction; ↑↑↑, marked increase; ↑, slight increase.
Modified from Reid ME, Lomas-Francis C, Olsson ML: *The blood group antigen facts book*, ed 3, San Diego, CA, 2012, Academic Press.

because of the X chromosome–borne gene. The Kx antigen, the McLeod phenotype, and the K_0 phenotype are summarized in Table 7.4.

MCLEOD SYNDROME

The McLeod phenotype is just one phenomenon attributed to the McLeod syndrome. Individuals with McLeod syndrome, in addition to having red cell abnormalities, may possess associated defects of muscular and neurologic origins. Elevated levels of creatine kinase accompany the syndrome. The correlation of depressed Kell antigens and these defects currently is undetermined. The X-linked disorder of **chronic granulomatous disease** is occasionally associated with McLeod syndrome. In this disorder, the normal functional properties of phagocytic white blood cells are impaired. The phagocytes are able to engulf but not kill microorganisms. Because of this functional defect, patients possess an increased susceptibility to infections. A genetic deletion of chromosomal material encompassing both genetic loci on the X chromosome accounts for the association of the McLeod phenotype and chronic granulomatous disease.

Chronic granulomatous disease: inherited disorder in which the phagocytic white blood cells are able to engulf, but not kill, certain microorganisms

SECTION 4
DUFFY BLOOD GROUP SYSTEM

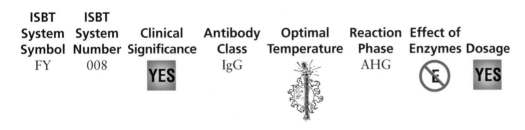

ISBT System Symbol	ISBT System Number	Clinical Significance	Antibody Class	Optimal Temperature	Reaction Phase	Effect of Enzymes	Dosage
FY	008	YES	IgG		AHG	(E with no symbol)	YES

CHARACTERISTICS AND BIOCHEMISTRY OF DUFFY ANTIGENS

Duffy Antigens Facts

The Duffy blood group system was first described in 1950 when a previously unrecognized antibody was discovered in the serum of a hemophiliac who received multiple transfusions, Mr. Duffy.[15] The antigen that defined this antibody was called Fy^a (FY1). Its antithetical antigen, Fy^b (FY2), was described the following year.[16] When phenotypic studies of the Fy^a and Fy^b antigens were performed, investigators observed that whites commonly had phenotypes Fy(a+b+), Fy(a–b+), or Fy(a+b–). Sanger et al[17] reported in 1955 that most blacks lacked both Fy^a and Fy^b antigens and had the phenotype Fy(a–b–). The Fy(a–b–) phenotype is rare among whites.

TABLE 7.5 Common Phenotypes and Frequencies in the Duffy Blood Group System

PHENOTYPE			FREQUENCY (%)	
REACTIONS WITH ANTI-Fy^a	REACTIONS WITH ANTI-Fy^b	INTERPRETATION	WHITE	BLACK
+	0	Fy(a+b−)	17	9
0	+	Fy(a−b+)	34	22
+	+	Fy(a+b+)	49*	1
0	0	Fy(a−b−)	Rare	68†

*Most common phenotype in the white population.
†Most common phenotype in the black population.
From Reid ME, Lomas-Francis C, Olsson ML: *The blood group antigen facts book*, ed3, San Diego, CA, 2012, Academic Press.

TABLE 7.6 Summary of Antigens and Their Characteristics in the Duffy Blood Group System

Fy^a and Fy^b	Antithetical antigens Expressed on cord blood cells Sensitive to ficin or papain treatment Receptors for *Plasmodium vivax* and *Plasmodium knowlesi*
Fy3	Expressed on cord blood cells Resistant to ficin or papain treatment Red cells that are Fy(a−b−) are also Fy:-3
Fy5	Expressed on cord blood cells Resistant to ficin or papain treatment Common in whites Altered expression in Rh$_{null}$ phenotype Possible antigen interaction between Duffy and Rh proteins
Fy6	Expressed on cord blood cells Red cells that are Fy(a−b−) are also Fy:-6 Sensitive to ficin or papain treatment Antigen has been defined by murine monoclonal antibodies; no human anti-Fy6 has been described

Note: Fy4 is obsolete in this system.

Common phenotypes and frequencies of the Duffy antigens are presented in Table 7.5, which shows that phenotype frequencies differ significantly between whites and blacks. A white Australian woman with the rare Fy(a−b−) phenotype was the first to produce anti-Fy3, which reacted with all Fy(a+) and Fy(b+) red cells.[18] This Duffy antigen was called Fy3. Additional antigens (Fy5 and Fy6) have been assigned to the system, which now includes five antigens. Duffy antigens are well developed at birth and detectable on fetal red cells. As with the Kell blood group system antigens, the Duffy antigens have not been identified on granulocytes, lymphocytes, monocytes, or platelets. The Fy^a and Fy^b antigens are considered of greatest importance for transfusion purposes. The antigens in this blood group system are summarized in Table 7.6.

Biochemistry of Duffy Antigens

The Duffy antigens have been mapped to a glycoprotein of the red cell membrane.[19] Molecular studies of the Duffy glycoprotein determined that the glycoprotein spans the lipid bilayer of the membrane multiple times. The Fy^a, Fy^b, and Fy6 antigens are susceptible to proteolytic degradation by the enzymes papain and ficin. When red cells are treated with papain or ficin, these antigens are destroyed.

In 1993 Horuk et al[20] identified the Duffy glycoprotein as an erythrocyte receptor for numerous proinflammatory **chemokines**. These chemokines are involved in the activation

The Fy^x phenotype expresses weak Fy^b antigen not detected by anti-Fy^b.

Chemokines: group of cytokines involved in the activation of white blood cells during migration across the endothelium of white blood cells. In this functional role, the Duffy glycoprotein is capable of binding molecules responsible for cell-to-cell communication. Research suggests that the Duffy glycoprotein functions as a biological sponge for these excess chemokines.

GENETICS OF DUFFY BLOOD GROUP SYSTEM

In 1968, Donahue et al[21] showed that the Duffy gene, *FY (DARC),* was located on chromosome 1. Their report marked the first assignment of a human gene to a specific chromosome. The Duffy blood group system locus is **syntenic** with the Rh blood group system locus and consists of the following alleles:
- *FYA* allele, which encodes Fy^a antigen
- *FYB* allele, which encodes Fy^b, FY3, FY5, and FY6 antigens
- *FYA* and *FYB* are codominant alleles
- *FY* allele, which encodes no identifiable Duffy antigen

CHARACTERISTICS OF DUFFY ANTIBODIES

Discussion of Duffy antibodies is limited to anti-Fy^a and anti-Fy^b. Common characteristics of anti-Fy^a and anti-Fy^b include the following:
- The antibodies are stimulated by antigen exposure through transfusion or pregnancy.
- Agglutination reactions are best observed in IATs.
- Immunoglobulin class is IgG.
- The antibodies usually do not bind complement.
- The antibodies possess clinical significance in transfusion and are an uncommon cause of HDFN.
- Anti-Fy^a and anti-Fy^b are nonreactive with enzyme-treated cells because these enzymes degrade the antigens.
- Weaker examples of Duffy antibodies demonstrate stronger agglutination reactions with the homozygous expression of antigen [Fy(a–b+) or Fy(a+b–)] versus the heterozygous expression of antigen [Fy(a+b+)]; antibodies are detecting dosage of antigen expression.
- Anti-Fy^a is more commonly observed than anti-Fy^b, indicating that Fy^b is a poor immunogen.

DUFFY SYSTEM AND MALARIA

Most African and African American blacks are resistant to infection from certain forms of malarial parasites. Miller et al[22] first made the connection between malaria and the Duffy blood group system in 1975. These investigators showed that Fy(a–b–) red cells were not invaded by *Plasmodium knowlesi* parasites. Later observations confirmed that *P. knowlesi* and *Plasmodium vivax* invaded Fy(a+) or Fy(b+) red cells, but Fy(a–b–) red cells were resistant to infection. The Duffy antigens serve as biological receptor molecules to assist the attachment of the merozoite to the red cell. The high incidence of the Fy(a–b–) phenotype in the West African population supports the hypothesis that this phenotype offered a selective evolutionary advantage for resistance to *P. vivax* infection. However, resistance to *Plasmodium falciparum* is not a characteristic of the Fy(a–b–) phenotype.

SECTION 5
KIDD BLOOD GROUP SYSTEM

Fy^a and Fy^b antigens are destroyed with enzymes. Their corresponding antibodies do not react with enzyme-treated red cells.

Syntenic: genetic term referring to genes closely situated on the same chromosome without being linked

FY allele produces no Duffy glycoprotein on the red cell. *FYFY* homozygotes have the phenotype Fy(a–b–). This phenotype is found in 70% of African Americans and 100% of Gambians.[9]

FY allele provides a genetic selective advantage in geographic areas where *P. vivax* is endemic.

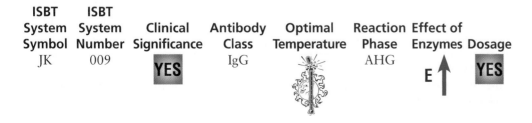

ISBT System Symbol	ISBT System Number	Clinical Significance	Antibody Class	Optimal Temperature	Reaction Phase	Effect of Enzymes	Dosage
JK	009	YES	IgG		AHG	E ↑	YES

TABLE 7.7 Common Phenotypes and Frequencies in the Kidd Blood Group System

PHENOTYPE			FREQUENCY (%)	
REACTIONS WITH ANTI-Jk^a	REACTIONS WITH ANTI-Jk^b	INTERPRETATION	WHITES	BLACKS
+	0	Jk(a+b−)	26.3	51.1*
0	+	Jk(a−b+)	23.4	8.1
+	+	Jk(a+b+)	50.3†	40.8
0	0	Jk(a−b−)	Rare	Rare

*Most common phenotype in the black population.
†Most common phenotype in the white population.
From Reid ME, Lomas-Francis C, Olsson ML: *The blood group antigen facts book,* ed 3, San Diego, CA, 2012, Academic Press.

CHARACTERISTICS AND BIOCHEMISTRY OF KIDD ANTIGENS

Kidd Antigens Facts

In contrast to the polymorphism of the Rh and Kell blood group systems, the Kidd blood group system is relatively uncomplicated at both the serologic and the genetic levels. The unique characteristic of the Kidd blood group system arises from the challenge for the transfusion service personnel to detect Kidd alloantibodies in vitro. The Kidd antibodies are often linked to extravascular hemolysis in delayed hemolytic transfusion reactions, where removal of antibody-sensitized red cells is facilitated by the reticuloendothelial system.

Three antigens—Jk^a, Jk^b, and Jk3—define the Kidd blood group system. The original reports of the antibodies to Jk^a and Jk^b appeared in the early 1950s.[23,24] The discovery of the Jk(a−b−) phenotype, or the Kidd null phenotype, followed.[25] Individuals with this null phenotype are usually from the Far East and Pacific Island areas and may produce an antibody, anti-Jk3. Anti-Jk3 reacts serologically as an inseparable combination of anti-Jk^a and anti-Jk^b. This unique antibody defined an antigen specified as Jk3. The Jk3 antigen is present whenever Jk^a or Jk^b antigens are also produced. This antigen is analogous to the Fy3 antigen in that Fy3 antigen is present on Fy(a+) and Fy(b+) red cells. Kidd antigens develop early in fetal life and are detectable on fetal red cells. In general, the Kidd antigens do not rank high in terms of red cell immunogenicity. The Kidd antigens are not denatured after exposure to routine proteolytic enzyme reagents. The common phenotypes and frequencies of the Kidd antigens are presented in Table 7.7.

Biochemistry of Kidd Antigens

Heaton and McLoughlin[26] reported the first evidence clarifying the biochemical structure of the Kidd antigens in 1982. These investigators showed that Jk(a−b−) red cells were more resistant to lysis in the presence of 2 M urea than red cells possessing either the Jk^a or Jk^b antigens. Red cells of normal Kidd phenotypes swell and lyse rapidly on exposure to 2 M urea. From these observations, they suggested that the molecule expressing the Kidd antigens was a urea transporter because the absence of the Kidd antigens resulted in a defect in urea transport. More recently, it was reported that the Kidd blood group and urea transport function of human erythrocytes were carried by the same multipass glycoprotein.[27] From a practical perspective, screening methods based on the property of resistance to 2 M urea can be used to identify rare Jk(a−b−) donor units.

GENETICS OF THE KIDD BLOOD GROUP SYSTEM

The Kidd blood group system has been assigned to a genetic locus, *JK*, located on chromosome 18. Characteristics of the alleles within the locus include the following:
• *JKA* allele encodes the Jk^a and Jk3 antigens and is codominant with the *JKB* allele.

TABLE 7.8 Characteristics of Antibodies in the Kell, Duffy, and Kidd Blood Group Systems

CHARACTERISTIC	KELL SYSTEM	DUFFY SYSTEM	KIDD SYSTEM
Red cell stimulated	Yes	Yes	Yes; weak antibody
IgG	Yes	Yes	Yes
Reactive with AHG	Yes	Yes	Yes
Effect of enzymes	No effect	No reactivity	Enhanced
Clinical significance	Yes	Yes	Yes
Unique features	Anti-K most common		Bind complement
	Anti-Js^b more common in blacks		Common cause of delayed hemolytic transfusion reactions
	Anti-Kp^b more common in whites		

- *JKB* allele encodes the Jk^b and Jk3 antigens and is codominant with the *JKA* allele.
- *JK* allele is a silent allele that produces neither Jk^a nor Jk^b antigens; it is a common allele in Polynesians, Filipinos, and Chinese; the *JKJK* genotype results in a Jk(a–b–) phenotype.
- Jk(a–b–) phenotype can also be derived by the action of a dominant suppressor gene, *In(Jk)*.

CHARACTERISTICS OF KIDD ANTIBODIES

As previously mentioned, the alloantibodies produced in response to Kidd antigen exposure are of clinical significance for transfusion recipients. Their importance lies in their characteristic weak reactivity in vitro combined with the capacity to effect severe red cell destruction in vivo. After immune stimulation, antibody titers increase and may quickly decrease to undetectable levels. Delayed hemolytic transfusion reactions and extravascular hemolysis are commonly associated with the antibodies of this blood group system. In addition, rare examples of Kidd antibodies capable of the activation and binding of complement proteins may cause intravascular red cell destruction in a transfusion reaction. A patient's previous records should be consulted before selecting donor units to reduce the incidence of these transfusion reactions.

Common characteristics of anti-Jk^a and anti-Jk^b include the following:
- The immunoglobulin class is IgG.
- Agglutination reactions are best observed by the IAT.
- The antibodies show dosage of Kidd antigens on red cells; weak examples of antibodies demonstrate stronger agglutination reactions with the homozygous expression of antigen [Jk(a–b+) or Jk(a+b–)] versus the heterozygous expression of antigen [Jk(a+b+)].
- Some antibodies may bind complement.
- The antibodies are produced in response to antigen exposure through transfusion or pregnancy.
- The antibodies usually appear in combination with multiple antibodies in the sera of individuals who have formed other red cell antibodies.
- Antibody detection is aided with enzyme reagents, LISS, and polyethylene glycol (PEG).
- The antibodies do not store well; antibody reactivity quickly declines in vitro.

Because antibodies to the Kell, Duffy, and Kidd blood group antigens are of great clinical significance, their recognition in antibody identification testing is vital to ensure that patients receive antigen-negative donor red cell units when necessary. Each of these blood group systems shares similar antibody characteristics. Table 7.8 compares the important characteristics of these system antibodies.

SECTION 6

LUTHERAN BLOOD GROUP SYSTEM

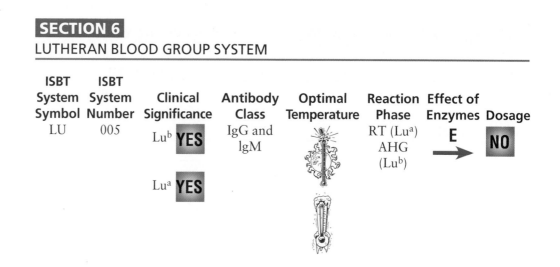

ISBT System Symbol	ISBT System Number	Clinical Significance	Antibody Class	Optimal Temperature	Reaction Phase	Effect of Enzymes	Dosage
LU	005	Lu^b **YES** Lu^a **YES**	IgG and IgM		RT (Lu^a) AHG (Lu^b)	E →	**NO**

CHARACTERISTICS AND BIOCHEMISTRY OF LUTHERAN ANTIGENS

Lutheran Antigens Facts

The Lutheran blood group system comprises 20 antigens. The Auberger antigens, Au^a and Au^b, first reported in 1961 and 1989, respectively, were added to the Lutheran system and assigned to LU18 and LU19.[28] Lutheran antigens have not been found on lymphocytes, granulocytes, monocytes, or platelets. In addition, Lutheran antigens are weakly expressed on cord blood cells. Most Lutheran antigens are of high incidence; corresponding red cell alloantibodies are infrequently encountered in the transfusion service.

The two primary antigens of this system include the antithetical antigens, Lu^a (LU1) and Lu^b (LU2). Antibodies to these antigens are occasionally observed in patient samples. Lu^a (LU1) and Lu^b (LU2) antigens are resistant to ficin and papain treatment of red cells. Individuals in most populations have the Lu(a–b+) phenotype (Table 7.9).

The Lu$_{null}$ phenotype, Lu(a–b–), rarely occurs and may manifest itself in any of the following three unique genetic mechanisms:

- Recessive: only true Lu$_{null}$ phenotype; homozygosity for a rare recessive amorph, *LU*, at the *LU* locus
- Dominant inhibitor or In(Lu) phenotype: heterozygosity for a rare dominant inhibitor gene, *In(Lu)*, that is not located at the *LU* locus
- X-linked suppressor gene: inherited in a recessive manner as Lu$_{mod}$ phenotype

Biochemistry of Lutheran Antigens

In biochemical studies using monoclonal antibodies, the Lutheran antigens were located on a membrane glycoprotein.[29] The biological importance of the Lutheran glycoproteins may be linked to adhesion properties and the mediation of intracellular signaling.[3]

GENETICS OF THE LUTHERAN BLOOD GROUP SYSTEM

The *LU* locus has been assigned to chromosome 19 and is linked to the *Se* (secretor) locus. The *H*, *Le*, and *LW* genetic loci are also located on chromosome 19. The *LUA* and *LUB* codominant alleles genetically encode the production of the low-frequency antigen Lu^a and the high-frequency antigen Lu^b.

CHARACTERISTICS OF LUTHERAN ANTIBODIES

Important serologic characteristics of the Lutheran antibodies are outlined as follows.

Anti-Lu^a

- Anti-Lu^a may be present without immune red cell stimulation.
- Immunoglobulin classes are IgM and IgG.

TABLE 7.9 Common Phenotypes and Frequencies in the Lutheran Blood Group System			
PHENOTYPE			
REACTIONS WITH ANTI-Lu^a	REACTIONS WITH ANTI-Lu^b	INTERPRETATION	FREQUENCY (%): MOST POPULATIONS
+	0	Lu(a+b–)	0.2
0	+	Lu(a–b+)	92.4
+	+	Lu(a+b+)	7.4
0	0	Lu(a–b–)	Rare

From Reid ME, Lomas-Francis C, Olsson ML: *The blood group antigen facts book*, ed 3, San Diego, CA, 2012, Academic Press.

- Optimal in vitro agglutination reactions are observed at room temperature.
- Anti-Lu^a has a characteristic mixed-field pattern of agglutination; small loose agglutinates are surrounded by unagglutinated free red cells.
- It has no clinical significance in transfusion; mild cases of HDFN have been reported.

Anti-Lu^b

- Anti-Lu^b is a rare antibody because of the antigen's high incidence.
- Immunoglobulin class is IgG.
- Most examples of anti-Lu^b agglutinate at the antiglobulin phase.
- Some examples of anti-Lu^b show a mixed-field agglutination pattern.
- Anti-Lu^b has been associated with transfusion reactions and mild cases of HDFN.

SECTION 7
LEWIS BLOOD GROUP SYSTEM

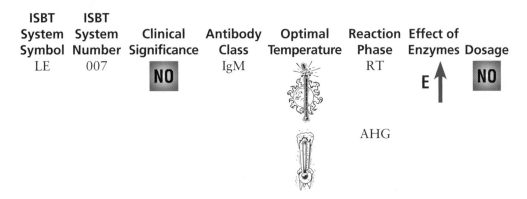

ISBT System Symbol	ISBT System Number	Clinical Significance	Antibody Class	Optimal Temperature	Reaction Phase	Effect of Enzymes	Dosage
LE	007	NO	IgM		RT / AHG	E ↑	NO

CHARACTERISTICS AND BIOCHEMISTRY OF LEWIS ANTIGENS

Lewis Antigens Facts

The Lewis antigens, in contrast to other blood group antigens, are manufactured by tissue cells and secreted into body fluids.[30] Lewis antigens are found primarily in secretions and plasma and are adsorbed onto the red cell membrane. In contrast to the antigens of the Kell, Duffy, and Kidd blood group systems, the Lewis antigens are not integral to the red cell membrane. The development of the Lewis antigen structure begins in the first week after birth and may continue for 6 years. The Lewis system is similar to the ABO system in that the antigen development depends on three sets of independently inherited genes. Lewis genes encode a glycosyltransferase that adds a sugar to an antigen precursor structure. The Lewis antigen system is not particularly relevant from a clinical standpoint because Lewis antibodies do not usually cause in vivo red cell destruction. The antibodies

TABLE 7.10   Lewis System Phenotypes and Frequencies

REACTIONS WITH ANTI-Le^a	REACTIONS WITH ANTI-Le^b	INTERPRETATION	FREQUENCY (%) WHITES	BLACKS
+	0	Le(a+b−)	22	23
0	+	Le(a−b+)	72	55
0	0	Le(a−b−)	6	22
+	+	Le(a+b+)	Rare	Rare

From Fung MK: *Technical manual,* ed 18, Bethesda, MD, 2014, AABB.

are common, however, and an understanding of antigen genetics and biochemistry is helpful in the discernment of the serologic characteristics. Frequency distributions of the Lewis antigens appear in Table 7.10.

Biochemistry of Lewis Antigens

Lewis determinants are carbohydrates on glycolipids and glycoproteins. The product of the Lewis gene (*LE/FUT3*) is L-fucosyltransferase, which adds L-fucose to the number 4 carbon of N-acetylglucosamine of type 1 precursor structures. The type of precursor *FUT3* uses determines the Lewis antigen gene product. In individuals without the *SE* (secretor) gene, the structure acquires Le^a antigen specificity and is adsorbed onto the red cell membrane, which creates the Le(a+) phenotype. If type 1 H structures are also present in the secretions, the *FUT3* Lewis transferase adds L-fucose to this structure. This resulting product, Le^b, is adsorbed preferentially over the Le^a glycoprotein onto the red cell membrane. As discussed in Chapter 5, the difference between type 1 and type 2 structures is the linkage between the carbons of D-galactose and N-acetylglucosamine on the H precursor chain. In type 2 H chains, the number 4 carbon is unavailable for fucose attachment; type 2 chains never express Lewis antigen activity.

Newborn red cells possess the Le(a−b−) phenotype. As the Lewis antigens begin to develop, the cells may type as Le(a+b+) until the transition to Le(a−b+) is complete. Reliable Lewis phenotyping may be impossible until about 6 years of age. During pregnancy, Lewis antigens are greatly reduced on red cells.[3]

The Le^b antigen is the receptor for *Helicobacter pylori*, a gram-negative bacterium associated with gastritis, peptic ulcer disease, gastric carcinoma, and the Norwalk virus.[9]

Le^a antigen cannot be converted into Le^b antigen. Le(b+) individuals will always have some undetectable Le^a antigen and phenotype as Le(a−b+).

Lewis antigens can be lost from the red cells in infectious mononucleosis, alcoholic cirrhosis and pancreatitis, and pregnancy.

INHERITANCE OF LEWIS SYSTEM ANTIGENS

The Lewis system depends on three genes to produce the Lewis antigen structures: *H*, *Se* (secretor), and *Le* (Lewis). The *H*, *Se*, and *Le* gene products are glycosyltransferases called *FUT1*, *FUT2*, and *FUT3*, respectively. The *Se* gene enables the *H* gene transferase to act in the secretions. The *le*, *h*, and *se* genes are amorphs and produce no detectable products. If an *Le* gene is inherited, Le^a antigens are found in the secretions and are adsorbed onto the red cells, regardless of the secretor status. If the *Se* gene is inherited in addition to the *Le* gene, the Lewis transferase converts the available H-soluble structure to a Le^b antigen, and the red cells adsorb Le^b instead of Le^a. This concept is illustrated in Fig. 7.2. If the gene inherited from both parents is *le*, no antigen structure is present on the red cells.

A summary of Lewis inheritance and biochemistry concepts is provided in Table 7.11. Table 7.12 summarizes the genes, plasma products, and red cell phenotypes that arise from the *Le*, *Se*, and *H* genes.

CHARACTERISTICS OF LEWIS ANTIBODIES

Lewis antibodies occur almost exclusively in the serum of Le(a−b−) individuals, usually without known red cell stimulus.[30] Le(a−b+) individuals do not produce anti-Le^a, and it is rare to find anti-Le^b in an Le(a+b−) individual. Anti-Le^a or anti-Le^b can be found in an Le(a−b−) individual. Lewis antibodies are IgM and have no clinical significance. If a donor unit of Lewis antigen–positive blood was transfused to a patient with a Lewis antibody,

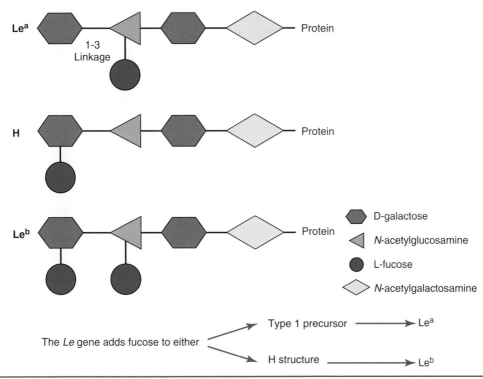

Fig. 7.2 Formation of the Lewis antigens.

TABLE 7.11	Summary of Lewis Inheritance and Biochemistry Concepts

- Le^a and Le^b are *not* alleles.
- Le(a–b+) red cell phenotype arises from the inheritance of an *Le*, *Se*, and *H* gene.
- Individuals who have a phenotype of Le(a+b–) are not secretors, with the exception of the Bombay phenotype.
- Bombay phenotype (*hh*) cannot express the Le^b antigen.
- A person can be a nonsecretor (*sese*) and still secrete Le^a into body fluids.
- Lewis antigens found in the secretions are glycoproteins.
- Lewis antigens found in plasma are glycolipids.
- Red cells adsorb only glycolipids, not glycoproteins, onto the membrane.
- Adult red cells with a phenotype of Le(a+b+) are very rare.

TABLE 7.12	Lewis Genes and Red Cell Phenotypes	
GENES PRESENT	**ANTIGENS IN SECRETIONS**	**RED CELL PHENOTYPE**
Le sese H	Le^a	Le(a+b–)
Le Se H	Le^a Le^b H	Le(a–b+)
lele sese H	None	Le(a–b–)
lele Se H	H	Le(a–b–)
Le sese hh	Le^a	Le(a+b–)
Le Se hh	Le^a	Le(a+b–)
lele sese hh	None	Le(a–b–)
lele Se hh	None	Le(a–b–)

the Le^a or Le^b antigens in the donor plasma would readily neutralize Lewis antibodies. For this reason, it is exceedingly rare for Lewis antibodies to cause decreased survival of transfused Le(a+) or Le(b+) cells. Phenotyping donor blood for the presence of Lewis antigens when a recipient has an anti-Lewis antibody is unnecessary. Crossmatching for compatibility using anti-IgG antihuman globulin, with or without prewarming, provides a good indication of transfusion safety.[31] If room temperature reactions are not used in the antibody screen or antibody identification panel, anti–Lewis antibody reactivity will be avoided. Lewis antibodies have not been implicated in HDFN because the antibodies do not cross the placenta and the antigens are not well developed at birth. Anti-Le^a and anti-Le^b are found during and immediately after pregnancy more often than would be expected.

Serologic Characteristics

Lewis system antibodies can be challenging to identify because the reactions can have a wide temperature range. The challenges include the following:
- Agglutination is observed at immediate-spin, 37° C, and the antiglobulin phase.
- Agglutination is often fragile and easily dispersed.
- Enzymes enhance anti-Le^b antibody reactivity.
- Hemolysis is sometimes seen in vitro, especially if fresh serum is used, because anti-Le^a efficiently binds complement.
- Neutralization techniques using commercially prepared Lewis substance may be helpful to confirm the presence of a Lewis antibody or eliminate the reactions to identify other antibodies mixed in the serum.

> Neutralization is an antibody identification technique that combines a soluble antigen with antibody in vitro. If the patient's serum contains the antibody, the soluble antigen makes the antibody inactive.

> Patients with Lewis antibodies do not require antigen-negative RBC blood products. RBC units that are crossmatch compatible by IAT at 37° C are safe to transfuse.

SECTION 8
I BLOOD GROUP SYSTEM AND i ANTIGEN

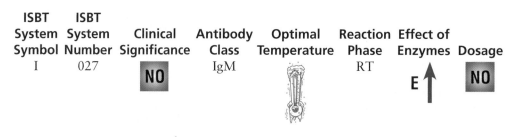

ISBT System Symbol	ISBT System Number	Clinical Significance	Antibody Class	Optimal Temperature	Reaction Phase	Effect of Enzymes	Dosage
I	027	NO	IgM		RT	E ↑	NO

I AND i ANTIGENS FACTS

> Red cell antigens that have not been assigned to a blood group system are classified in blood group collections. The blood group collections contain two or more antigens that are related serologically, biochemically, or genetically. However, these antigens do not fit the criteria for a blood group system.

The I blood group system is composed of one antigen named I, which was assigned to a blood group system in 2002. The product of the *I* gene is *N*-acetylglucosaminyltransferase and is the branching transferase. The i antigen remains in Ii Blood Group Collection 207. The gene for the production of the i antigen has not been identified and is formed from the sequential action of multiple gene products encoding glycosyltransferases. I and i are not antithetical antigens.[3] The i antigen is expressed on newborn and cord blood cells, whereas the I antigen is expressed on adult cells. Anti-I is a commonly encountered autoantibody with optimal reactivity at colder temperatures. The antibody has no clinical significance because it does not elicit red cell destruction during transfusion or pregnancy. However, this antibody often causes a great deal of confusion in serologic testing.

BIOCHEMISTRY OF I AND i ANTIGENS

The I and i antigens exist on the precursor A, B, and H oligosaccharide chains at a position closer to the red cell membrane. The I antigen is associated with branched chains, and the i antigen is associated with linear chains (Fig. 7.3). The I and i antigens are present on both glycolipid and glycoprotein structures on the red cell membrane. They also can be found as soluble glycoprotein antigens in plasma and in body secretions such as human milk and amniotic fluid.

The I antigen is not well developed at birth; linear chains of the oligosaccharide precursor chain are found predominantly in newborns. As the straight chains develop into

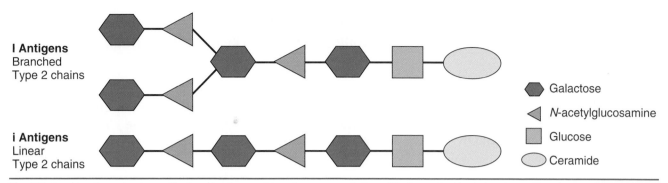

I Antigens
Branched
Type 2 chains

i Antigens
Linear
Type 2 chains

- ⬡ Galactose
- ◁ *N*-acetylglucosamine
- ▢ Glucose
- ⬭ Ceramide

Fig. 7.3 I and i antigen structures. The I and i antigens exist on the precursor A, B, and H oligosaccharide chains at a position closer to the red cell membrane. The I antigen is associated with branched chains, and the i antigen is associated with linear chains.

branched chains through the action of the branching transferase, the i antigen converts into the I antigen structure over a 2-year period. Adult red cells possess a strong expression of I antigen and trace amounts of i antigen. Conversely, cord cells possess a strong expression of i antigen and a weak expression of I antigen.

SEROLOGIC CHARACTERISTICS OF AUTOANTI-I

Anti-I is usually found as a cold-reacting, **clinically insignificant** IgM autoantibody. Most individuals possess an autoanti-I detectable at 4° C. Anti-I is often detected when samples are tested at room temperature. Anti-I varies in its reactivity with different adult red cells because the branching oligosaccharide chain structures vary.[30] Because anti-I binds complement, polyspecific antiglobulin reagents may detect the C3d component attached to the red cell. When anti-I is detected, efforts to avoid its reactivity are often accomplished with **prewarming techniques.** This procedure is discussed further in the chapter on antibody identification (Chapter 8). The use of enzyme reagents in antibody detection enhances anti-I reactivity.

Anti-I also reacts as a compound antibody. It is often found as an anti-IH and exhibits stronger agglutination with red cells having greater numbers of H antigens, such as group O and group A_2 cells. This antibody is also clinically insignificant. When crossmatching a group A individual, this specificity is noted if agglutination reactions are stronger with panel and screening reagent red cells than with group A donor units.

DISEASE ASSOCIATION

Strong autoanti-I is associated with *Mycoplasma pneumoniae* infections and **cold hemagglutinin disease.** Anti-i is associated with infectious mononucleosis, lymphoproliferative disease, and occasionally cold hemagglutinin disease. In these situations, if transfusion becomes necessary, finding serologically compatible blood may be more difficult. I-negative or i-negative donor units are not required. Serologic techniques to evaluate these antibodies are discussed in Chapter 8.

> Autoanti-I can interfere with ABO serum testing and compatibility testing. The frequency of alloanti-I is rare.

> Autoanti-i is an uncommon cold agglutinin that reacts strongly with cord blood cells or i_{adult} red cells.

Clinically insignificant: antibody that does not shorten the survival of transfused red cells or has been associated with HDFN

Prewarming technique: patient serum and test cells are prewarmed separately before combining to prevent reactions of cold antibodies binding at room temperature and activating complement

Cold hemagglutinin disease: autoimmune hemolytic anemia produced by an autoantibody that reacts best in colder temperatures (<37° C)

SECTION 9

P1PK BLOOD GROUP SYSTEM, GLOBOSIDE BLOOD GROUP SYSTEM, AND GLOBOSIDE BLOOD GROUP COLLECTION

P1PK BLOOD GROUP SYSTEM: P1, P^k, AND NOR ANTIGENS

ISBT System Symbol	ISBT System Number	Clinical Significance	Antibody Class	Optimal Temperature	Reaction Phase	Effect of Enzymes	Dosage
P1PK	003	NO	IgM		RT	E↑	VAR

GLOBOSIDE BLOOD GROUP SYSTEM: P ANTIGEN

GLOBOSIDE BLOOD GROUP COLLECTION: LKE AND PX2 ANTIGENS

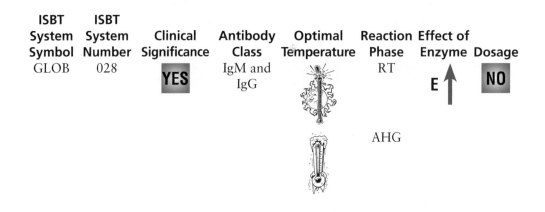

ISBT System Symbol	ISBT System Number	Clinical Significance	Antibody Class	Optimal Temperature	Reaction Phase	Effect of Enzyme	Dosage
GLOB	028	YES	IgM and IgG		RT / AHG	E ↑	NO

FACTS: P1PK AND GLOB BLOOD GROUP SYSTEM ANTIGENS, LKE, AND PX2 ANTIGENS

The P1PK blood group system includes three antigens, P1, P^k, and NOR, and three phenotypes, P_1, P_2, and the null phenotype p. The P antigen in the GLOB (globoside) blood group system is also involved in these phenotypes because P^k is the precursor of the P antigen. Structurally related to the ABH antigens, these blood group antigens also exist as glycoproteins and glycolipids. The antigens are formed by the action of glycosyltransferases, and the P1 antigen is present in soluble form in some secretions. Three antigens (P1, P, and P^k) produce five distinct phenotypes: P_1, P_2, p, P_1^k, and P_2^k. These phenotypes and their corresponding antigens are shown in Table 7.13.

The most common phenotypes in the P1PK blood group system are P_1 and P_2, analogous to the A_1 and A_2 phenotypes in the ABO system. Individuals with the P_1 phenotype have both P and P1 antigens on their red cells. Individuals with the P_2 phenotype express only P antigen on their red cells and may produce an anti-P1. The P1 antigen is poorly developed at birth and is variably expressed on adult cells. The P1 antigen expression decreases on storage of the red cells and exists in a soluble form detected in plasma and **hydatid cyst fluid.**

P and P^k antigens are high-frequency antigens. Their relevance in routine testing is uncommon because antibodies to these antigens are very rare. The P^k antigen expression is found on most red cells in varying amounts except those red cells with the p phenotype.[3] Table 7.14 summarizes the antigen and antibody characteristics of the P1PK and GLOB blood group systems.

The LKE and PX2 antigens are assigned to the Globoside Blood Group Collection and are associated with the P1, P^k, and P antigens. LKE and PX2 antigens occur with high frequency in the population. PX2 is expressed more strongly on red cells of the p phenotype.[3] Anti-PX2 appears to be naturally occurring.[3]

ANTIGEN BIOCHEMISTRY

Expression of the P^k, P, and P1 antigens proceeds through the stepwise addition of sugars to lactosylceramide. The P^k antigen is first synthesized through the addition of the carbohydrate galactose by galactosyltransferase 1. The P^k antigen serves as the substrate for N-acetylgalactosaminyltransferase 1, which adds N-acetylgalactosamine to the terminal galactose to make the P antigen.

The P1 antigen is formed by the addition of a carbohydrate to the paragloboside precursor chain. Paragloboside is a type 2 precursor, which serves as the substrate for both the P1 and H antigens. The addition of galactose to the paragloboside produces the P1 antigen. The addition of fucose to the paragloboside produces the H antigen. The structural difference between these two antigens is one carbohydrate molecule. The formation of the P1PK and GLOB blood group antigens is shown in Fig. 7.4.

The P_1 and P_2 phenotypes account for more than 99% of donors.[9]

Hydatid cyst fluid: fluid obtained from a cyst of the dog tapeworm

NOR antigen was assigned to the P1PK system in 2012. The antigen occurs in the population at a low frequency. It has been found in two families to date (American and Polish).[3]

TABLE 7.13   P1PK and GLOB Blood Group Systems Phenotypes, Antigens, and Frequencies

| PHENOTYPE | ANTIGENS | FREQUENCIES (%) | |
		BLACKS	WHITES
P_1	P1 P P^k	94	79
P_2	P P^k	6	21
P_1^k	P1 P^k	Very rare	Very rare
P_2^k	P^k	Very rare	Very rare
p	—	Very rare	Very rare

TABLE 7.14   P1PK and GLOB Blood Group Systems Antigen and Antibody Characteristics

PHENOTYPE	ANTIGEN CHARACTERISTICS	POSSIBLE ANTIBODIES	ALLOANTIBODY CHARACTERISTICS
P_1	Red cells express P, P1, and P^k antigens P1 antigen is not well developed at birth Most common phenotype	None	Not applicable
P_2	Lacks P1 antigen but expresses P and P^k antigens Second most common phenotype	Anti-P1	IgM; room temperature; not clinically significant Variable reactions with adult cells
P_1^k	Red cells express P1 and P^k antigens Very rare phenotype	Anti-P	Clinically significant; associated with spontaneous abortions (rare)
P_2^k	Red cells express only P^k antigens Very rare phenotype	Anti-P and anti-P1	Anti-P and anti-P1 characteristics
p	Null phenotype of system Negative for P, P1, and P^k antigens Very rare phenotype	Anti-PP1P^k (Tj^a)	Hemolytic; clinically significant; can be separated into three specificities

P1PK AND GLOB BLOOD GROUP SYSTEM ANTIBODIES

Anti-P1

Anti-P1 is a frequently encountered alloantibody in the serum of P_2 individuals and does not require red cell immune stimulation. This antibody is an IgM cold-reactive agglutinin enhanced with enzymes. Commercially available P1 substance can be used to neutralize the antibody to confirm the antibody presence or eliminate the reactions.

Anti-P1 rarely decreases red cell survival. Providing P1-positive RBC units is acceptable for transfusion, if compatible at the antiglobulin phase.[32] If reactions are interfering with the crossmatch, avoiding the immediate-spin reading usually eliminates the antibody reactions.

Other alloantibodies in these systems are rarely encountered and are summarized in Table 7.14.

Autoanti-P

Autoanti-P is associated with an immune hemolytic anemia called **paroxysmal cold hemoglobinuria** (PCH). Autoanti-P is an IgG antibody known as the Donath–Landsteiner

Paroxysmal cold hemoglobinuria: rare autoimmune disorder characterized by hemolysis and hematuria associated with exposure to cold

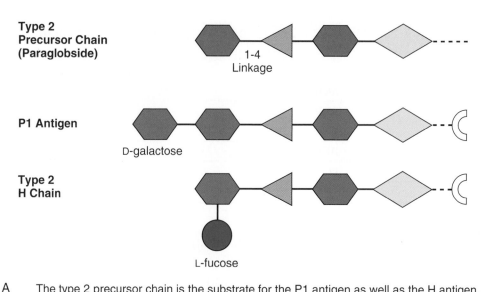

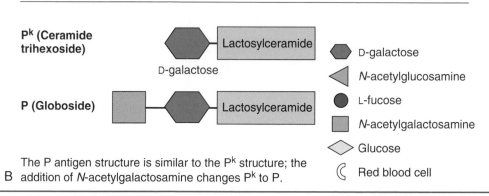

A   The type 2 precursor chain is the substrate for the P1 antigen as well as the H antigen.

The P antigen structure is similar to the Pk structure; the
B   addition of N-acetylgalactosamine changes Pk to P.

Fig. 7.4 P1PK and GLOB system antigen structures. **A,** P1 antigen. **B,** Pk and P antigen structure.

Biphasic hemolysin: antibody, such as the Donath–Landsteiner antibody, that requires a period of cold and warm incubations to bind complement with resulting hemolysis

antibody. This **biphasic hemolysin** binds to P-positive (P_1 or P_2) red cells at lower temperatures in the extremities. Complement is attached, which produces hemolysis when the red cells are subsequently warmed to 37° C. This rare autoantibody may appear transiently in children after viral infections and in adults with tertiary syphilis. The autoantibody reacts weakly or not at all in routine in vitro test methods and requires the Donath–Landsteiner test for confirmation. A summary of this test appears in Fig. 7.5.

Patients with autoanti-P may have a weakly positive direct antiglobulin test because of complement coating. If transfusion becomes necessary, P-negative blood is not required. However, the RBC unit may be administered through a **blood warmer.**[33] Patients should be kept warm at all times. Scan the QR code for more information.

Blood warmer: medical device that prewarms donor blood to 37° C before transfusion

Anti-PP1Pk

Individuals with the null phenotype (p phenotype) can make an antibody with anti-PP1Pk specificity. This antibody was originally called anti-Tjª and can be separated into three antibody specificities. Anti-PP1Pk often exhibits hemolysis in vitro and is clinically significant. Patients with anti-PP1Pk require RBC transfusions from donors with the p phenotype.[34]

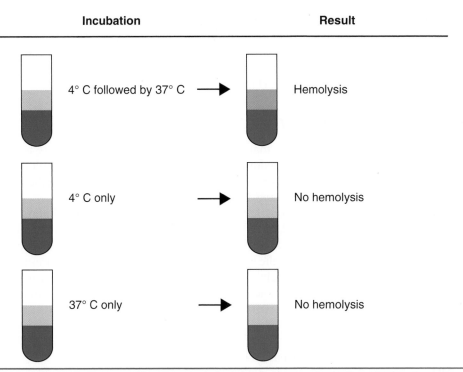

Fig. 7.5 Donath–Landsteiner test. After the patient's freshly drawn serum and red cells are incubated, complement binds only at lower temperatures and causes hemolysis when the tube is warmed to 37° C.

SECTION 10
MNS BLOOD GROUP SYSTEM

M AND N ANTIGENS

ISBT System Symbol	ISBT System Number	Clinical Significance	Antibody Class	Optimal Temperature	Reaction Phase	Effect of Enzymes	Dosage
MNS	002	NO	IgM		RT AHG	Ɇ	YES

S AND s ANTIGENS

ISBT System Symbol	ISBT System Number	Clinical Significance	Antibody Class	Optimal Temperature	Reaction Phase	Effect of Enzymes	Dosage
MNS	002	YES	IgG		AHG	VAR	YES

The MNS system includes 46 antigens that are expressed primarily on red cells.[3] Molecular genetics have provided insight into the genetic nature of the various MNS system antigens, many of which result from crossing over, gene recombination, and substitutions. This section limits the discussion of the MNS antigens and antibodies to M (MNS1), N (MNS2), S (MNS3), s (MNS4), and U (MNS5).

GENETICS AND BIOCHEMISTRY

The two genes (*GYPA* and *GYPB*) that encode the MNS system antigens are located on chromosome 4. Because of their proximity, they are usually inherited as a haplotype. One gene codes for M or N, and the other codes for S or s. The most frequently inherited haplotype is Ns, followed by Ms, MS, and NS.

The genes *GYPA* and *GYPB* code for **glycophorin** A (GPA) and glycophorin B (GPB), respectively. *GYPA* codes for the M and N antigens, and *GYPB* codes for the S and s antigens.

The structures that carry the MNS blood group system antigens are glycoproteins; because most of the sugars carry **sialic acid** structures, the membrane structures are called sialoglycoproteins.[35] The MN sialoglycoprotein (GPA) and the Ss sialoglycoprotein (GPB) structures are similar but distinct. The amino acid sequence makes each a unique structure; Fig. 7.6 compares the antigen structures.

GPA: M and N Antigens

Characteristics of M and N antigens include the following:

- GPA consists of 131 amino acids, with 72 outside the cell membrane.

Glycophorin: glycoprotein that projects through the red cell membrane and carries many blood group antigens

Sialic acid: constituents of the sugars attached to proteins on red cells that lend a negative charge to the red cell membrane

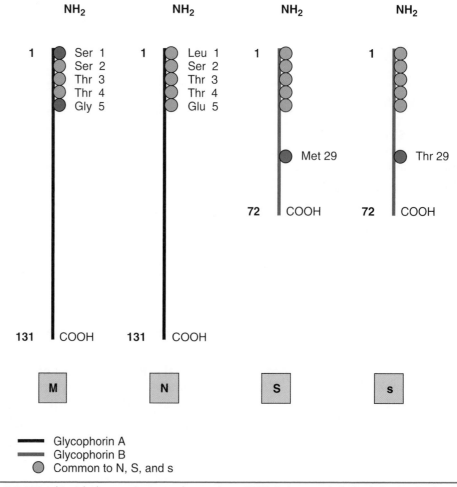

Fig. 7.6 MN and Ss sialoglycoprotein structural comparison. *COOH,* Carboxy terminal; *Gly,* glycine; *Leu,* leucine; *Glu,* glutamic acid; *Met,* methionine; *NH₂,* Amino terminal; *1,* amino acid 1; *131,* amino acid 131; *Ser,* serine; *Thr,* threonine.

TABLE 7.15 Antibody Characteristics in the MNS System

ANTIBODY	IMMUNOGLOBULIN CLASS	CLINICALLY SIGNIFICANT	EFFECT OF FICIN	CHARACTERISTICS
M	IgM*	No	Removed	Rarely reported to cause HDFN or HTR; stronger reactions with cells from homozygote
N	IgM	No	Removed	Weak, cold reactive
S	IgG	Yes	Variable	
s	IgG	Yes	Variable	
U	IgG	Yes	Resistant	Reacts with all S+ or s+ red cells; U-negative cells are found only in blacks

HDFN, Hemolytic disease of the fetus and newborn; HTR, hemolytic transfusion reaction.
*Sometimes can be whole or partially IgG.[30]

- M and N antigens differ at positions 1 and 5; the first and fifth amino acid residues for the M antigen structure are serine and glycine, respectively, whereas the N antigen structure has leucine and glutamic acid at positions 1 and 5, respectively.
- Inheriting M or N in the homozygous state [(M+N−) or (M−N+)] greatly enhances the strength of the antigen expression.

GPB: S, s, and U Antigens

Characteristics of S, s, and U antigens include the following:
- GPB consists of 72 amino acids, with 43 outside the cell membrane.
- S and s antigens differ at amino acid position 29; S antigen has methionine at that position, whereas s antigen has threonine.
- The U antigen is located near the membrane and is always present when S or s is inherited.
- Absence of or altered GPB expression would result in red cells phenotyping as S−s−U−.

GPB carries the same first 26–amino acid sequence as the N antigen of the GPA structure. Inheriting S or s provides antigenic activity similar to N called the "N" antigen. This N-like structure may prevent N-negative individuals from forming an anti-N antibody.[34] However, anti-N formed by N-negative individuals and reagent anti-N do not react with "N" because there are too few antigen copies to support agglutination.[36]

ANTIBODIES OF THE MNS BLOOD GROUP SYSTEM

Antibodies to the antigens included in the MNS system vary in their clinical significance and serologic properties. They are summarized in Table 7.15.

Anti-M

Examples of IgM and IgG forms of anti-M have been reported. Anti-M occurs naturally and is considered a clinically insignificant antibody.[30] Examples of anti-M that react at the antiglobulin phase after a prewarming procedure should be considered clinically significant. Anti-M is rarely implicated in HDFN.

Anti-M may demonstrate variable reactions with different manufacturers' panel or screening cells because of the pH of the preservative.[37] Some examples of anti-M react better at a pH of 6.5. Anti-M demonstrates marked dosage because agglutination reactions are stronger with homozygous expressions of the antigen (eg, M+N− reagent red cells have a stronger reaction than M+N+ reagent red cells).

Anti-N

Anti-N is a rarely encountered IgM cold-reacting antibody that is not usually clinically significant. Examples of an N-like antibody have been found more frequently in dialysis

TABLE 7.16	Phenotype Frequencies in MNS System	
	PHENOTYPE FREQUENCIES (%)	
ANTIGEN	WHITES	BLACKS
M+	78	74
N+	72	75
S+	55	31
s+	89	93
U+	99.9	99

From Reid ME, Lomas-Francis C, Olsson ML: *The blood group antigen facts book*, ed 3, San Diego, CA, 2012, Academic Press.

Anti-M is commonly observed. Anti-N is rare. Most anti-M and anti-N are not clinically significant. When M or N antibodies reactive at 37° C are detected, antigen-negative or compatible RBC units should be provided.[12]

patients exposed to formaldehyde-sterilized dialyzer membranes. This anti-N–like antibody is also not clinically significant and may be a result of an altered N antigen structure on the red cells.[37]

Anti-S, Anti-s, and Anti-U

Anti-S, anti-s, and anti-U are clinically significant IgG antibodies that can cause decreased red cell survival and HDFN. It is not difficult to find compatible blood for patients who have made anti-S or anti-s. Table 7.16 shows the frequency of S and s antigens in the population. The U antigen is a high-incidence antigen, occurring in more than 99% of the population. Anti-U is rare but should be considered when serum from a previously transfused or pregnant black person contains an antibody to a high-incidence antigen. The probability of anti-U existence can be established by showing that the person is S– and s–. U-negative blood is found in less than 1% of the black population and is not found in white donors. The Rare Donor Registry may need to be contacted if a patient with an anti-U needs a transfusion.

SECTION 11
MISCELLANEOUS BLOOD GROUP SYSTEMS

This section addresses the blood groups that are less commonly encountered in routine transfusion medicine. In many of these systems, the clinical significance of the antibodies associated with the system is unknown or not well documented because of the scarcity of examples. Antibodies to the antigens in these systems are infrequent because most are of either high frequency or low frequency, and others are of low immunogenicity. Table 7.17 summarizes these systems or collections. Low-frequency antigens that do not belong to a collection or system are not included. The use of molecular techniques has added to the knowledge of genetics and antigen products and in some instances has altered their classification.

TABLE 7.17	Miscellaneous Blood Groups and Antigens			
NAME	ANTIGEN SYMBOL	ISBT NO.	ANTIGENS	CHARACTERISTICS
Diego	Di, Wr	010	Di^a Di^b Wr^a Wr^b	Di^a is more common in South American Indians anti-Wr^a is commonly found with other antibodies
Cartwright	Yt	011	Yt^a Yt^b	Variably sensitive to enzymes; sensitive to DTT
Xg	Xg	012	Xg^a	Inherited on X chromosome; frequency varies with sex
Scianna	SC	013	SC:1 SC:2 SC:3	
Dombrock	Do	014	Do^a Do^b Gy^a Hy Jo^a	Hy phenotype is found only in blacks; anti-Do^a and anti-Do^b antibodies are rarely found as a single specificity
Colton	Co	015	Co^a Co^b Co3	Anti-Co^b is rarely found as a single specificity
Chido/Rodgers	Ch/Rg	017	Ch Rg	Antigens are sensitive to enzymes and found in plasma; antibodies have HTLA characteristics

Continued

TABLE 7.17	Miscellaneous Blood Groups and Antigens–cont'd			
NAME	ANTIGEN SYMBOL	ISBT NO.	ANTIGENS	CHARACTERISTICS
Gerbich	Ge	020	**Ge2 Ge3 Ge4** Wb Ls^a An^a Dah	All antigens except for Ge4 are sensitive to enzymes
Cromer	Cr	021	**Cr^a Tc^a** Tc^b Tc^c **Dr^a Es^a IFC WES^a** WES^b **UMC**	Antigen is also found in plasma; located on decay-accelerating factor
Knops	Kn	022	**Kn^a** Kn^b **McC^a Sl^a Yk^a**	Antigen depression in SLE, PNH, and AIDS; antigens are weakened by ficin treatment; antibodies have HTLA characteristics
Cost	Cs	205	**Cs^a** Cs^b	Part of a blood group collection rather than a system
VEL	Vel	034	**Vel**	Variable antigen expression on red cells; both IgG and IgM antibodies are associated with hemolytic reactions; antibodies react best with enzyme-treated red cells
JMH	JMH	026	**JMH**	Autoanti-JMH is often found in elderly patients with absent or weak antigen expression; antibodies have HTLA characteristics; antigens are sensitive to enzymes and DTT
Sd^a	Sd^a	901.012	**Sd^a**	Antigen found in guinea pig and human urine; antibodies are typically weak and agglutination is mixed field; reduction of Sd^a expression during pregnancy

Note: Items in **boldface** indicate antigens of high incidence.

AIDS, Acquired immunodeficiency syndrome; *DTT,* dithiothreitol; *HTLA,* high-titer, low-avidity; *PNH,* paroxysmal nocturnal hemoglobinuria; *SLE,* systemic lupus erythematosus.

SECTION 12

HUMAN LEUKOCYTE ANTIGEN (HLA) SYSTEM AND PLATELET ANTIGENS

HUMAN LEUKOCYTE ANTIGENS

Testing Applications in the Clinical Laboratory

Most nucleated cells such as leukocytes and tissue cells possess inherited antigens on the cell surface called human leukocyte antigens. HLA antigens and the antibodies they elicit are involved in transfusion and transplantation medicine. HLA antibodies, similar to red cell antibodies, result from exposure to foreign antigens during transfusions of blood products and from pregnancy.

These antibodies can cause poor platelet response, or **refractoriness,** in patients requiring platelet transfusions. To improve platelet response, donor platelets that are HLA matched with the recipient may be necessary. HLA antibodies are also responsible for reactions that cause chills and fever in some patients receiving red cell transfusions. In this situation, blood products that are "leukocyte reduced" to avoid HLA antigens and residual cytokines usually prevent further reactions. HLA testing is not routine in the transfusion service or blood bank setting; however, an understanding of its inheritance, nomenclature, and application is important for optimal patient support. Table 7.18 lists applications of HLA testing.

Organ and hematopoietic progenitor cell transplants rely on HLA matching for the best outcome. In addition, HLA testing is used to assess risk factors for disease susceptibility. These tests are not diagnostic for the associated diseases but are used to assess relative risk. A growing application of HLA typing has been in pharmacogenomic applications. Certain HLA antigens are associated with optimal drug therapy regimens for certain diseases.[38]

Inheritance and Nomenclature of HLA

The genes encoding the expression of the HLA antigens are part of the major histocompatibility complex (MHC) gene system located on chromosome 6. Although the MHC system

Refractoriness: unresponsiveness to platelet transfusions due to HLA-specific or platelet-specific antibodies or platelet destruction from fever or sepsis; responsiveness is measured by posttransfusion platelet counts

was first recognized and named from experiments in tissue transplantation, the role of the MHC is essential in the recognition of self and nonself, the coordination of cellular and humoral immunity, and the immune response to antigens.

The MHC genes contain an estimated 33 to 40 genes grouped into three regions. The regions are known as class I, class II, and class III (Fig. 7.7). The class I region encodes genes from the classic transplantation molecules: HLA-A, HLA-B, and HLA-C; the class II region encodes molecules HLA-DR, HLA-DP, and HLA-DQ; and the class III region includes genes coding some complement proteins (C2 and C4) and cytokines. Linkage disequilibrium in the HLA system occurs because these genetic loci are very close. The MHC genes that encode HLA antigens are inherited as haplotypes. Each sibling could potentially share at least one haplotype with the other and has a 25% chance of having the same HLA typing. For this reason, siblings are likely matches when organ or bone marrow transplants are required.

Each person inherits one haplotype from each parent, and both haplotypes are expressed. This inheritance pattern is illustrated in the example in Fig. 7.8. There are

TABLE 7.18	HLA Testing Applications

- Hematopoietic progenitor cell transplants
- Solid-organ transplants
- Platelet selection for refractory patients
- Disease association
  - Ankylosing spondylitis—B27
  - Celiac disease—DQ2
- Optimize certain drug therapy regimens
  - Abacavir sensitivity (for HIV treatment) and B*57:01 allele[43]

HIV, Human immunodeficiency virus.

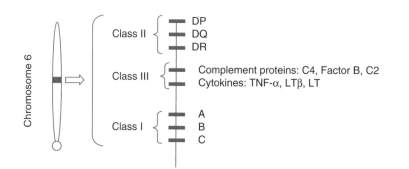

Fig. 7.7 Major histocompatibility complex (MHC).

MOTHER

A2	A11
B7	B44
Cw7	Cw12
DR17	DR13
DQ2	DQ8

FATHER

A1	A3
B8	B35
Cw3	Cw5
DR4	DR8
DQ5	DQ7

Potential offspring:

Child 1

A2	A1
B7	B8
Cw7	Cw3
DR17	DR4
DQ2	DQ5

Child 2

A2	A3
B7	B35
Cw7	Cw5
DR17	DR8
DQ2	DQ7

Child 3

A11	A1
B44	B8
Cw12	Cw3
DR13	DR4
DQ8	DQ5

Child 4

A11	A3
B44	B35
Cw12	Cw5
DR13	DR8
DQ8	DQ7

Fig. 7.8 Example of the inheritance pattern of class I and class II HLA antigens. Each child inherits a complete set of HLA alleles as a unit from each parent's chromosome. There is a 25% chance that two children in a family will inherit the same sets and have identical HLA typing.

TABLE 7.19 HLA Nomenclature

GENETIC LOCUS	ANTIGEN	NUMBER OF ANTIGENS	ALLELE EXAMPLE
A	A1 to A80	26	A*01:01
B	B5 to Bw6	62	B*07:02
C	Cw1 to Cw10	10	C*01:02
DR	DR1 to DR18	24	DRB1*01:01
DQ	DQ1 to DQ9	9	DQB1*05:01
DP	DP1 to DP6	6	DPB1*01:01

http://hla.alleles.org/nomenclature/stats.html. Accessed August 2015.

hundreds of possible alleles at each locus (Table 7.19). Each antigen expression is identified with a unique number that is determined by either serologic (antigen–antibody reactions) or molecular methods. The MHC region is the most polymorphic system of genes in humans because of the many possible alleles at each location. The probability that any two individuals will express the same HLA antigens is extremely low.

The naming of the HLA antigens consists of a letter designating the locus, including A, B, C, DR, DQ, and DP, and a number indicating the antigen, for example, A2, B27, Cw7, DR1, DQ5. For the C locus, the "w" is included in the nomenclature to distinguish HLA C-locus antigens from complement components. The HLA nomenclature began when the only test method was the serologic lymphocytotoxicity assay. Today, more accurate and specific molecular typing assays are used. Because of the increased sensitivity of the typing methods and knowledge of the glycoprotein structure of the HLA antigens, the number of alleles that can be determined continues to increase, whereas the total number of antigens has remained the same. In 2015, 13,412 HLA and related alleles were described by the HLA nomenclature.[39] The World Health Organization is responsible for standardizing the HLA nomenclature. For example, using the correct nomenclature, A2 is expressed as A2 for antigen-level resolution determined by serologic testing, HLA-A*02 for low-resolution typing, and HLA-A*02:01 if high-resolution testing is performed. Allele-level, high-resolution typing is particularly important for hematopoietic graft survival. Scan the QR code for more information about HLA nomenclature, alleles, and antigens.

> The HLA genes are highly polymorphic. Several alleles exist at each locus.

Testing and Identification of HLA and Antibodies

Testing to Identify HLA

As described earlier in this chapter, red cell antigens and antibodies are primarily identified by agglutination reactions or hemagglutination test methods. Because of the nature of leukocyte antigens and antibodies, agglutination techniques are not effective. Serologic identification of HLA antigens requires the lymphocytotoxicity test method. In addition, HLA typing is also performed using molecular technology as described in Chapter 4.

Class I antigens are found on the surface of platelets, leukocytes, and most nucleated cells in the body. Mature red cells lack HLA antigens, although reticulocytes express HLA class I antigens. HLA class II antigens are found on the antigen-presenting cells—macrophages, dendritic cells, and B cells. In the circulation, the number of cells expressing class I antigens is greater than the number of cells with class II antigens. Because class II antigens are not found on platelets, it is not necessary to match class II antigens when HLA-compatible platelets are requested.

In serologic typing methods, a suspension of T or B lymphocytes is added to microtiter plates containing known antibody specificities. After incubation, rabbit complement is added. If the antibody on the plate matches the antigen on the cell, complement is activated, causing cell injury or a positive reaction. Cell damage is detected by the addition of a dye. This injury allows the dye to enter the cell, providing a visual means to distinguish the positive cells from nonreactive cells. Each well is scored while viewing under the microscope, and a pattern of reactivity determines the class I or class II typing (Fig. 7.9).

Serologic typing of the HLA antigens is not always clear because antibodies can often react to more than one epitope (cross-reactive). In many cases, specific antibodies are not developed to recognize the many different HLA antigens that can be expressed. For these reasons, sensitive and specific molecular methods are replacing and supplementing this with the lymphocytotoxicity test.

Antibody Detection and Identification

ABO compatibility is essential for the success of all solid-organ transplants. Second to ABO compatibility, careful matching of HLA antigens in patients with existing antibodies is important for long-term graft survival for kidney, heart, and lung transplants. Fig. 7.10 shows that the degree of HLA matching for kidney transplants corresponds to the survival of the graft.[40] The soluble nature of HLA antigens in the liver allows for a greater flexibility in the selection of donor tissue for liver transplants, even when preformed antibodies exist. Organ transplant candidates are periodically screened for developing HLA antibodies so that a suitable match can be determined when an organ becomes available.

Patients can become sensitized to HLA antigens by the following types of exposures to alloantigens[41]:

Pregnancies. About 30% to 50% of women with three or more pregnancies develop HLA antibodies. In some women, the antibodies are present for just a short time (weeks to months), whereas they may persist for many years in other women.

Blood transfusions. About 50% of patients who receive multiple transfusions develop antibodies. Today, most patients who require blood transfusions receive leukocyte-reduced blood, which decreases the chances for a patient to become sensitized.

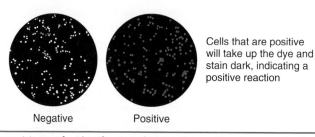

Cells that are positive will take up the dye and stain dark, indicating a positive reaction

Negative   Positive

Fig. 7.9 Lymphocytotoxicity test for identification of HLA antigens. Complement and a dye combine to determine whether there is antigen–antibody recognition. Complement-mediated cell membrane damage occurs if the antigen and antibody form a complex. The damaged membrane becomes permeable to the dye, which enters the cell, creating a positive reaction. Dye exclusion is a negative reaction.

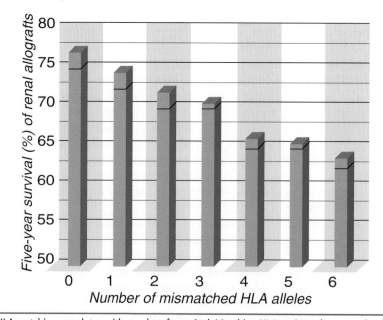

Fig. 7.10 HLA matching correlates with renal graft survival. Matching HLA antigens between the donor and recipient significantly improves renal allograft survival. The data represent deceased (cadaver) grafts. (From Abbas AK, Lichtman AH, Pillai S: *Cellular and molecular immunology*, ed 7, Philadelphia, PA, 2011, Saunders.)

Previous transplant. About 90% of patients develop HLA antibodies within 2 weeks of a failed graft.

The term panel-reactive antibody (PRA) was developed from serologic tests performed on microtiter trays composed of a panel of common antigens. A higher PRA meant that the recipient had many reactions and was less likely to be compatible with available organs.

With the increase in sensitivity and specificity of newer solid-phase methods, PRA determined by serologic methods has been replaced with a **calculated panel-reactive antibody (CPRA)**.[41] This number is based on the antigens that the organ candidate is reactive against, called **unacceptable antigens,** and provides a statistical guide for determining reactivity within the population. The calculation uses a formula and HLA frequencies derived from HLA types found in more than 12,000 donors. This number is used as one assessment in determining a candidate's placement on the waitlist for available organs.

Crossmatching the recipient serum with the T cells and B cells from the potential donor is another important procedure to avoid rejection caused by antibodies to the donor tissue. Crossmatching is possible for kidney and pancreas transplants when there is sufficient time; however, it is not always possible with heart, lung, and heart/lung transplants. The **mixed lymphocyte culture (MLC)**, historically used for crossmatching, has been replaced with immunofluorescent flow cytometric techniques.[42]

PLATELET ANTIGENS

Platelets possess inherited membrane proteins that can also elicit an immune response. Platelet antibodies are less frequently found because there is less antigen variability in the population. Antibodies to platelet antigens are the major cause of **neonatal alloimmune thrombocytopenia (NAIT)**, in which maternal alloantibodies against antigen inherited from the father can cause fetal platelet destruction. Platelet antibodies cause **posttransfusion purpura (PTP)**. These antibodies destroy the transfusion recipient's platelets after transfusion. Platelet antibodies can also decrease the expected increment of platelets after a platelet transfusion.

The most common platelet antibody is directed against HPA-1a antigen, also known as Pl^{A1}. HPA-1a is present on the platelets of about 98% of the population.[12] In cases of NAIT, in which the mother's antibody is directed against the infant's platelet antigen, therapy involves either washed maternal platelets or antigen-negative platelets from a donor who is negative for HPA-1a antigen. Platelet recipients who have become refractory, in addition to HLA matching, can be crossmatched with a test method designed to detect platelet antigen incompatibility.

Calculated panel-reactive antibody (CPRA): estimates the percentage of donors that would be incompatible with a transplant candidate, based on the candidate's antibodies to HLA antigens

Unacceptable antigens: antigens that the potential graft recipient is reacting against; antibodies to these antigens could reduce the graft survival

Mixed lymphocyte culture (MLC): in vitro reaction of T cells from one individual against MHC antigens on leukocytes from another individual; the technique measures the response of HLA class II differences between donor and recipient cells, usually through radioactive measurements of DNA synthesis. This test was historically used for compatibility and D (class II) antigen typing.

Neonatal alloimmune thrombocytopenia: antibody destruction of a newborn's platelets caused by antibodies formed from prior pregnancies and directed to paternal antigens

Posttransfusion purpura: antibody destruction of platelets after transfusion

CHAPTER SUMMARY

Appreciating the unique characteristics of each blood group system is helpful in understanding the serologic and clinical features of the associated antibodies. A summary of the clinical significance of the blood group systems is found in the following table. With the exception of the ABO system, IgM antibodies are usually not clinically significant and react at room temperature. IgG antibodies require the antiglobulin test and are clinically significant.

SUMMARY OF CLINICAL SIGNIFICANCE OF BLOOD GROUP SYSTEMS[3]

Clinical Significance	Blood Group System Alloantibodies
Clinically significant	ABO, Rh, Kell, Kidd; Duffy; S, s, and U, Lutheran (Lu^b)
Usually clinically insignificant	I, Lewis, M, N, P1, Lutheran (Lu^a)

Modified from Reid ME, Lomas-Francis C, Olsson ML: *The blood group antigen facts book*, ed 3. San Diego, CA, 2012, Academic Press.

Being familiar with the antigen and antibody characteristics of each blood group system is essential in performing pretransfusion testing. The following table serves as a quick reference for the important concepts described in this chapter.

Continued

CHAPTER SUMMARY—cont'd

SYSTEM	ANTIGENS	FREQUENCY (%) WHITE	FREQUENCY (%) BLACK	IN VITRO REACTIONS PHASE	IN VITRO REACTIONS ENZYME	IG CLASS	COMMENTS
Kell	K	9	2	AHG	→	IgG	Antigens in the Kell system are destroyed by DTT.
	k	99.9	99.8	AHG	→	IgG	
	Kp^a	2	<1	AHG	→	IgG	
	Kp^b	99.9	>99.9	AHG	→	IgG	
	Js^a	<1	20	AHG	→	IgG	
	Js^b	>99.9	99	AHG	→	IgG	
Duffy	Fy^a	66	10	AHG	⊘	IgG	Fy(a–b–) is protective against malaria.
	Fy^b	83	23	AHG	⊘	IgG	
Kidd	Jk^a	77	91	AHG	↑	IgG	Kidd antibodies are associated with delayed transfusion reactions.
	Jk^b	73	49	AHG	↑	IgG	
Lutheran	Lu^a	7.6	5.3	RT	→	IgM	Antibodies may exhibit mixed-field reactions.
	Lu^b	99.8	99.9	AHG	→	IgG	
Lewis	Le^a	22	23	RT	↑	IgM	Lewis antigens are found in plasma and red cells.
	Le^b	72	55	RT	↑	IgM	Le^b arises from *H*, *Le*, and *Se* genes
I	I	>99.9	>99.9	RT	↑	IgM	Anti-I is frequently found as a cold autoantibody.
	i	<1	<1	RT	↑	IgM	I is negative on cord cells.
P1PK	P1	79	94	RT	↑	IgM	
MNS	M	78	74	RT	⊘	IgM	The M and N antigens show dosage in antibody panels.
	N	72	75	RT	⊘	IgM	
	S	55	31	AHG	var	IgG	S–s– are also U-negative.
	s	89	93	AHG	var	IgG	

DDT, Dithiothreitol.

The HLA System and Platelet Immunology

- Genes encoding the expression of the HLAs are part of the MHC found on chromosome 6 and code for class I (A, B, C), class II (DR, DQ, DP), and class III complement proteins.
- HLA antigens are inherited as a haplotype and are important in recognition of self and nonself, coordination of cellular and humoral immunity, and the immune response to antigens.
- Antibodies directed against HLA or platelet antigens can cause a refractory or poor platelet response to transfused platelets. HLA-matched or HLA-compatible platelets may be considered.

CRITICAL THINKING EXERCISES

Exercise 7.1
The blood bank received a call requesting two units of "Kell-negative" RBCs for a patient with anti-K.
1. Discuss why this request is incorrect.
2. What should the request have stated?

Exercise 7.2
List the red cell antibodies with serologic reactivity usually enhanced with enzyme-treated panel cells.

Exercise 7.3
A patient has a history of the following alloantibodies: anti-S, anti-Le^b, and anti-Jk^a.
1. Which of these antibodies are clinically significant?
2. How would you test for compatible RBC units?
3. How would enzyme-treated panel cells react with this mixture of antibodies?

Exercise 7.4
A patient has a history of a previously identified autoanti-I. The current sample is nonreactive with screening cells when tested at room temperature. What are the implications of this result in a current request for the transfusion of two units of RBCs?

Exercise 7.5
Explain how you would differentiate a Donath–Landsteiner antibody from a cold autoantibody.

Exercise 7.6
A prenatal sample contains the alloantibody, anti-Js^b.
1. Is this antibody clinically significant?
2. What is the most probable race of this patient?
3. What reagents would be helpful in the workup of this antibody?

Exercise 7.7
A physician requests phenotypically matched donor RBC units for a very young sickle cell patient. The patient's phenotype is D+, C–, E–, c+, e+, K+, S–, s+, M–, N+; Le(a–b–); Fy(a–b–); Jk(a+b–).
1. Which donor population (race) would you test to find a close match?
2. Which antigens are not important to match because of the corresponding antibody's clinical significance?

Exercise 7.8
A patient has a phenotype of Le(a–b+).
1. Is this patient a secretor or a nonsecretor?
2. What genes are responsible for conferring Le^a and Le^b antigens on the red cells?

Exercise 7.9
A patient was admitted for surgery with a history of a previous anti-U. You are directed to test this patient's siblings because U-negative donor units are rare. No commercial antiserum is available for testing. What other antisera could you use to determine the phenotype of the patient's siblings?

Exercise 7.10
1. Does a patient with an anti-Vel present a problem for provision of compatible donor units?
2. How would Vel-negative units be located?

Exercise 7.11
What are the Xg blood group system phenotypes of the male and female offspring from the mating of an Xg(a+) male and an Xg(a–) female?

Exercise 7.12
A patient who is not responding to platelet transfusions requires an HLA-matched platelet transfusion. The patient's HLA type is performed and is reported as A2, A11, B8, B35. A donor is called with a compatible type to donate for this patient. Why were the class II antigens not considered for matching?

Exercise 7.13
Parents of a kidney transplant candidate were tested for a potential compatible kidney because the candidate demonstrated HLA antibodies. The patient's HLA antigens were typed as A1, A2, B27, B50, DR17, and DR11. Antibodies identified were specific for A3, B18, and DR7 antigens.
1. If the mother's HLA typing is A1, A3, B35, B27, DR4, and DR11 and the father's typing is A2, A24, B50, B44, DR11, and DR17, what antigens did the father contribute?
2. List the probable HLA types of the candidate's three siblings. Select the kidney or kidneys with the best match.

STUDY QUESTIONS

1. Which blood group system possesses the Js^b and Kp^a antigens?
   a. Duffy
   b. Lutheran
   c. Kell
   d. Kidd

2. Which of the following antibodies is commonly associated with delayed transfusion reactions?
   a. anti-Lu^a
   b. anti-S
   c. anti-Jk^b
   d. anti-M

3. Which phenotype is associated with a resistance to *Plasmodium vivax?*
   a. Fy(a–b–)
   b. Jk(a–b–)
   c. Le(a–b–)
   d. Lu(a–b–)

4. Enzyme-treated reagent red cells used in antibody identification can enhance antibody reactions. Which of the following antibodies is not enhanced with the use of enzyme-treated red cells?
   a. anti-M
   b. anti-Le^a
   c. anti-Jk^b
   d. anti-I

5. Which of these antibodies are typically IgM? You may select more than one answer.
   a. anti-K
   b. anti-S
   c. anti-U
   d. anti-N
   e. anti-Le^b
   f. anti-Jk^b
   g. anti-P1

6. Which of the following reagents destroys the Kell system antigens?
   a. ficin
   b. albumin
   c. PEG
   d. DTT

7. Which blood group system's antigens are associated with glycophorin A and glycophorin B?
   a. Duffy
   b. Kidd
   c. Lewis
   d. MNS

8. Which of the following antibodies is characteristically clinically insignificant?
   a. anti-Kp^b
   b. anti-S
   c. anti-Le^b
   d. anti-Fy^a

9. Which of the following red cell phenotypes is associated with the McLeod phenotype?
   a. Rh$_{null}$ phenotype
   b. K$_0$ phenotype
   c. U-negative phenotype
   d. absence of Kx antigens

10. What statement is true regarding a phenotype of Lu(a–b–)?
    a. rare in whites but not blacks
    b. rare in blacks but not whites
    c. rare in all populations
    d. common in all populations

11. What is the common specificity of cold autoantibodies?
    a. I
    b. M
    c. P1
    d. S

12. What alloantibody is associated with individuals possessing the p phenotype?
    a. anti-P2
    b. anti-p
    c. anti-P
    d. anti-Tj^a

13. Select the alleles within the Lewis system.
    a. *Le, le*
    b. *Le^a, Le^b*
    c. *Le, Se, H*
    d. *Le, Le*

14. Which of the following antibodies requires the antiglobulin test for in vitro detection?
    a. anti-M
    b. anti-P1
    c. anti-U
    d. anti-I

15. What procedure helps distinguish between an anti-Fy^a and anti-Jk^a in an antibody mixture?
    a. lowering the pH of the patient's serum
    b. using a thiol reagent
    c. testing at colder temperatures
    d. testing ficin-treated panel cells

16. What statement is true relative to anti-K?
    a. agglutinates in IAT phases of the antibody screen
    b. is usually of the IgM antibody class
    c. does not agglutinate with K+k+ panel cells
    d. loses reactivity in enzyme phases

17. Which of the following antigens is poorly expressed on cord blood cells?
    a. K
    b. M
    c. Le^b
    d. D

18. Reagent antibody screening cells may not detect antibodies directed against low-incidence antigens. Which antibody is most likely to go undetected?
    a. Vel
    b. S
    c. Kp^a
    d. K

19. Select the disease commonly associated with the McLeod phenotype.
    a. infectious mononucleosis
    b. chronic granulomatous disease
    c. Hodgkin disease
    d. PCH

20. Which set of antibodies could you possibly find in a patient with no history of transfusion or pregnancy?
    a. anti-I, anti-S, and anti-P1
    b. anti-M, anti-c, and anti-B
    c. anti-A, anti-I, and anti-D
    d. anti-B, anti-I, and anti-Le^a

21. What is the most likely Lewis phenotype of a nonsecretor?
    a. Le(a–b–)
    b. Le(a+b+)
    c. Le(a+b–)
    d. Le(a–b+)

22. Anti-N is identified in a white patient who requires a blood transfusion. If 10 donor RBCs were tested, how many of these units would most likely be negative for the N antigen?
    a. 0
    b. 3
    c. 7
    d. 10

23. Which of the following antibodies is neutralized by pooled human urine?
    a. anti-Cs^a
    b. anti-Sd^a
    c. anti-Ch
    d. anti-Vel

24. The red cells of a donor have a U-negative phenotype. What red cell antibody would not react with these red cells?
    a. anti-M
    b. anti-S
    c. anti-P1
    d. anti-K

25. Which of the following blood group systems is associated with a depression of the antigens in chronic granulomatous disease?
    a. Duffy
    b. Kidd
    c. P
    d. Kell

26. Which of the following cells expresses HLA class II antigens?
    a. B cells
    b. platelets
    c. erythrocytes
    d. T cells

27. The mixed lymphocyte culture (MLC) is an older technique in the HLA laboratory used to determine:
    a. HLA-A antigens
    b. HLA-C antigens
    c. HLA antibody identification
    d. HLA-D antigens and compatibility

28. What term describes a poor platelet response to transfused platelets due to the presence of HLA or platelet antibodies?
    a. haplotype
    b. refractory
    c. vasoactive
    d. thrombocytopenia

29. How do patients become sensitized to HLA antigens?
    a. pregnancies
    b. blood transfusions
    c. previous transplants
    d. all of the above

30. Which of the following HLA antigens is not characterized as class I?
    a. C
    b. A
    c. DR
    d. B

Answers to Study Questions can be found on page 387.

 Additional student resources, including review questions, a laboratory manual, and case studies, can be found on the Evolve website.

REFERENCES

1. Lublin DM: Functional roles of blood group antigens. In Silberstein LE, editor: *Molecular and functional aspects of blood group antigens*, Bethesda, MD, 1995, AABB.
2. Coombs RR, Mourant AE, Race RR: In vivo isosensitization of red cells in babies with hemolytic disease, *Lancet* 1:264, 1946.
3. Reid ME, Lomas-Francis C, Olsson ML: *The blood group antigen facts book*, ed3, San Diego, CA, 2012, Academic Press.

4. Levine P, Backer M, Wigod M, et al.: A new human hereditary blood property (Cellano) present in 99.8% of all bloods, *Science* 109:464, 1949.
5. Allen FH, Lewis SJ: Kp^a (Penney), a new antigen in the Kell blood group system, *Vox Sang* 2:81, 1957.
6. Allen FH, Lewis SJ, Fudenberg HH: Studies of anti-Kp^b, a new alloantibody in the Kell blood group system, *Vox Sang* 3:1, 1958.
7. Gibett ER: Js, a "new" blood group system antigen found in Negroes, *Nature* 181:1221, 1958.
8. Walker RH, Argall CI, Steane EA, et al.: Anti-Js^b, the expected antithetical antibody of the Sutter blood group system, *Nature* 197:295, 1963.
9. Fung MK: *Technical manual*, ed 18, Bethesda, MD, 2014, AABB.
10. Marsh WL, Redman CM: The Kell blood group system: a review, *Transfusion* 30:158, 1990.
11. Parsons SF, Judson PA, Anstee DJ: Monoclonal antibodies against Kell glycoprotein: serology, immunochemistry, and quantitation of antigen sites, *Transfus Med* 3:137, 1993.
12. Lee S, Zambas ED, Marsh WL, et al.: Molecular cloning and primary structure of Kell blood group protein, *Proc Natl Acad Sci USA* 88:6353, 1991.
13. Chown F, Lewis M, Kaita H: A new Kell blood group phenotype, *Nature* 180:711, 1957.
14. Issitt PD, Antsee DJ: *Applied blood group serology*, ed 4, Durham, NC, 1998, Montgomery Scientific.
15. Cutbush M, Mollison PL, Parker DM: A new human blood group, *Nature* 165:188, 1950.
16. Ikin EW, Mourant AE, Pettenkoffer JH, et al.: Discovery of the expected haemagglutinin, anti-Fy^b, *Nature* 168:1077, 1951.
17. Sanger R, Race RR, Jack J: The Duffy blood groups of New York Negroes: the phenotype Fy(a–b–), *Br J Haematol* 1:370, 1955.
18. Albrey JA, Vincent EE, Hutchinson J, et al.: A new antibody, anti-Fy3, in the Duffy blood group system, *Vox Sang* 20:29, 1971.
19. Moore S, Woodrow CF, McClelland DB: Isolation of membrane components associated with human red cell antigens Rh(D), (c), (E) and Fy, *Nature* 295:529, 1982.
20. Horuk R, Chitnis CE, Darbonne WC, et al.: A receptor for the malarial parasite *Plasmodium vivax*: the erythrocyte chemokine receptor, *Science* 261:1182, 1993.
21. Donahue RP, Bias WB, Renwick JH, et al.: Probable assignment of the Duffy blood group locus to chromosome 1 in man, *Proc Natl Acad Sci USA* 61:949, 1968.
22. Miller LH, Mason SJ, Dvorak JA, et al.: Erythrocyte receptors for (*Plasmodium knowlesi*) malaria: Duffy blood group determinants, *Science* 189:561, 1975.
23. Allen FH, Diamond LK, Niedziela B: A new blood group antigen, *Nature* 167:482, 1951.
24. Plaut G, Ikin EW, Mourant AE, et al.: A new blood group antibody. anti-Jk^b, *Nature* 171:431, 1953.
25. Pinkerton FJ, Mermod LE, Liles BA, et al.: The phenotype Jk(a–b–) in the Kidd blood group system, *Vox Sang* 4:155, 1959.
26. Heaton DC, McLoughlin K: Jk(a–b–) RBCs resist urea lysis, *Transfusion* 28:197, 1982.
27. Olivès B, Mattei MG, Huet M, et al.: Kidd blood group and urea transport function of human erythrocytes are carried by the same protein, *J Biol Chem* 270:15607, 1995.
28. Zelinski T, Kaita H, Coghlan G, et al.: Assignment of the Auberger red cell antigen polymorphism to the Lutheran blood group system: genetic justification, *Vox Sang* 61:275, 1991.
29. Parsons SF, Mallinson G, Holmes CH, et al.: The Lutheran blood group glycoprotein, another member of the immunoglobulin superfamily, is widely expressed in human tissues and is developmentally regulated in human liver, *Proc Natl Acad Sci USA* 92:5496, 1995.
30. Rosse WF, Sherwood JB: Cold-reacting antibodies: differences in the reaction of anti-I antibodies with adult and cord red blood cells, *Blood* 36:28–42, 1970.
31. Waheed A, Kennedy MS, Gerhan S: Transfusion significance of Lewis system antibodies: report on a nationwide survey, *Transfusion* 21:542, 1981.
32. Anstall HB, Blaylock RC: The P blood group system: biochemistry, genetics and clinical significance. In Moulds JM, Woods LL, editors: *Blood groups: P, I, Sd^a and Pr*, Arlington, VA, 1991, AABB.
33. Mollison PL, Engelfriet CP, Contreras M: *Blood transfusion in clinical medicine*, ed 9, Oxford, UK, 1993, Blackwell Scientific.
34. Anstall HB, Urie PM: Transfusion therapy in special clinical situations. In Anstall HB, Urie PM, editors: *A manual of hemotherapy*, New York, NY, 1986, John Wiley & Sons.
35. Stroup M, Treacy M: *Blood group antigens and antibodies*, Raritan, NJ, 1982, Ortho Diagnostics.
36. Issitt P: *Applied blood group serology*, ed 3, Miami, FL, 1985, Montgomery Scientific.
37. Holliman SM: The MN blood group system: distribution, serology and genetics. In Unger PJ, Laird-Fryer B, editors: *Blood group systems: MN and Gerbich*, Arlington, VA, 1989, AABB.
38. Brecher ME: *Technical manual*, ed 17, Bethesda, MD, 2011, AABB.
39. Robinson J, Halliwell JA, Hayhurst JH, et al.: The IPD and IMGT/HLA database: allele variant databases, *Nucleic Acids Research* 43:D423, 2015.
40. Abbas AK, Lichtman AH, Pillai S: *Cellular and molecular immunology*, ed 7, Philadelphia, PA, 2011, Saunders.
41. Organ Procurement and transplant network: http://optn.transplant.hrsa.gov/. Accessed December 2011.
42. Rodey GE: *HLA beyond tears*, ed 2, Durango, CO, 2000, Denovo.
43. Mallal S, Phillips E, Carosi G, et al.: HLA-B*5701 screening for hypersensitivity to abacavir, *N Engl J Med* 358:568, 2008.

ANTIBODY DETECTION AND IDENTIFICATION

8

CHAPTER OUTLINE

LEARNING OBJECTIVES

On completion of this chapter, the reader should be able to:

1. Define atypical or unexpected antibodies.
2. Explain the production of alloantibodies as related to exposure to blood group systems.
3. Evaluate antibody screen and direct antiglobulin test (DAT) reactions to predict the most likely category of antibody problem.
4. Compare and contrast autocontrol and DAT.
5. Explain why patient information helps in the process of antibody identification.
6. Describe the reagent red cell panel and antigram with regard to antigen configuration and ABO type.
7. Analyze the phase of reactions to determine the potential clinical significance of an antibody.
8. Correlate an antibody's reaction strength to the dosage of an antigen, and identify how dosage can assist in antibody resolution.
9. Interpret panel reactions using the process of "ruling out."
10. Explain the "rule of three" with regard to antibody identification.
11. Identify different methods for working with multiple antibodies in a serum sample.
12. Differentiate warm autoantibody reactions from an antibody to a high-frequency antigen.
13. Explain the importance of a control when performing antibody neutralization.
14. Discuss the use of and the potential problems with the prewarm procedure.
15. Apply methods to enhance the serologic reactions of weak IgG antibodies.
16. Explain the process of identifying the specificity of a cold autoantibody and techniques to avoid cold autoantibody reactivity.
17. Describe the process and limitations of adsorption techniques as they apply to warm and cold autoantibodies.
18. Illustrate the elution procedure, and list the methods and application of this test.
19. Analyze antibody panels, and perform antibody identifications,
20. Perform antibody screens and antibody identification panel testing.

One of the most important tests in pretransfusion and prenatal testing is the antibody screen. The detection of antibodies directed against red cell antigens is an important tool for the blood bank technologist. The AABB's *Standards for Blood Banks and Transfusion Services* requires the use of antibody screen to detect clinically significant antibodies in both the blood donor and transfusion recipient.[1] The detection of unexpected antibody in the screen of a patient or donor initiates the identification process, which can seem like detective work. The term unexpected refers to antibodies other than ABO blood group system antibodies. These unexpected antibodies can be made in response to a transfusion of red cells or exposure to fetal cells during pregnancy or delivery. Because these antibodies are directed to a non–self-antigen, they are called alloantibodies. Autoantibodies are antibodies, usually formed by a disease process or medication, made to a person's own red cells.

Determining the specificity of antibodies, or antibody identification, necessitates the knowledge of blood group system antigen and antibody characteristics outlined in previous chapters and an understanding of the reagents used to enhance or eliminate reactions. Clues are often subtle and elusive, and the process must be methodical and accurate. Except for a simple antibody with one specificity, each sample is often unique and may necessitate several different approaches to reach a conclusive identification. Proficiency and confidence in antibody resolution come from experience and an understanding of basic theoretical concepts involved in the process. It is also important to review the unique blood group antigen and antibody characteristics discussed in previous chapters. This chapter outlines the theory behind problem-solving techniques.

> The only expected blood group antibodies in a patient's sample are ABO antibodies, which follow Landsteiner's law.

SECTION 1
ANTIBODY DETECTION

ANTIBODY SCREEN

The purpose of an antibody screen is to detect any potentially clinically significant antibody in a donor's or recipient's sample. Studies have demonstrated that only a small percentage of the healthy population (from 0.02% to 2%) has detectable red cell antibodies.[2,3] In contrast, 14% to 50% of individuals in chronically transfused populations, such as sickle cell anemia patients, may demonstrate red cell alloantibodies.[4]

Antibody screens are performed to detect antibodies in the following people:
- Patients requiring transfusion
- Women who are pregnant or after delivery
- Patients with suspected transfusion reactions
- Blood and plasma donors

The antibody screen involves incubating the patient's serum or plasma with screening cells at 37° C and performing an indirect antiglobulin test (IAT) for the detection of IgG antibodies. Antibody screening cells are group O reagent red cells. These cells are tested with the patient's serum to determine whether an unexpected antibody exists. Fig. 8.1 is an example of an antigram for a two-cell screen. An antigram lists the antigens present in the reagent red cell suspension. A reaction to one or both of the screen cells demonstrates the presence of an atypical antibody. Some workers prefer the three-cell screen because it provides a D-negative cell and homozygous cells for the Duffy and Kidd blood groups. The most common clinically significant antibodies react with a two-cell or three-cell screen. Initial conclusions regarding the type of antibody can often be

Cell	Rh							MNSs				P1	Lewis		Lutheran		Kell		Duffy		Kidd					
	D	C	E	c	e	f	Cw	M	N	S	s	P1	Lea	Leb	Lua	Lub	K	k	Fya	Fyb	Jka	Jkb				
I R1R1 (56)	+	+	0	0	+	0	0	+	+	0	+	0	+	0	0	+	+	+	+	0	+	+				
II R2R2 (89)	+	0	+	+	0	0	0	0	+	+	0	+	0	+	0	+	0	+	0	+	+	0				

Fig. 8.1 Antibody screen red cell antigram.

made when the antibody screen is complete. A summary of typical screen results with the tentative interpretations is listed in Fig. 8.2. Careful attention to the antibody screen results can save time when proceeding to the panel. The screen provides the initial clues that begin the antibody identification process. Scan the QR code for the antibody screen procedure.

Equally important as the detection of clinically significant antibodies is the recognition of false-positive reactions and the potential causes. Reactions that appear to be agglutination but are not can cause unnecessary testing and delay if transfusions are needed. False-positive reactions can be caused by rouleaux, antibodies to preservatives, fibrin, contamination of the sample, and presence of cryoprecipitate from frozen samples. Polyethylene glycol (PEG) can cause false-positive reactions if the reactions are read at 37° C. Before extensive workups are initiated, investigating the patient's diagnosis, reviewing methodologies, and obtaining a new sample are recommended.

> The procedure for the antibody screen and other procedures discussed in this chapter are included in the *Laboratory Manual* that accompanies this textbook.

> A positive antibody screen occurs because of prior exposure to red cell antigens from pregnancy or transfusions.

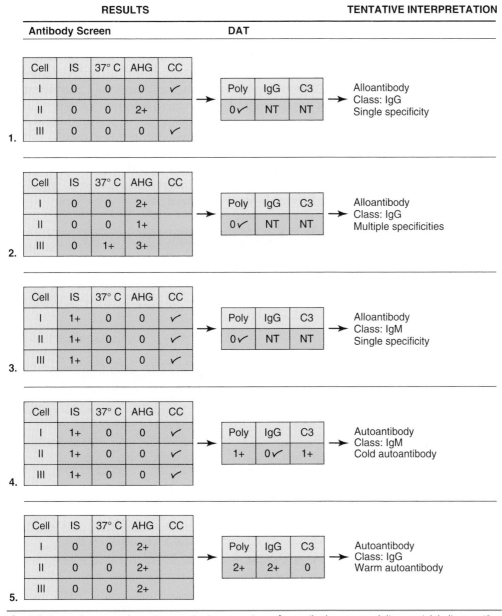

Fig. 8.2 Screen interpretations. Presumptive interpretations after antibody screen and direct antiglobulin test. *IS,* Immediate-spin; *37° C,* 37° C incubation; *AHG,* antihuman globulin; *CC,* check cells; ✓, check cells agglutinate; *NT,* not tested; *Poly,* polyspecific antiglobulin reagent; *C3,* anticomplement reagent; *IgG,* anti-IgG reagent.

AUTOCONTROL AND DIRECT ANTIGLOBULIN TEST

In antibody identification, the autocontrol and the direct antiglobulin test (DAT) can provide important information regarding antibody specificity. An autocontrol tests the patient's serum with his or her red cells and includes the potentiator used in the antibody screen or panel. The control is usually incubated with the antibody identification panel. For proper interpretation, the control is read in the reaction phases appropriate for the potentiator. The DAT is performed on the patient's cells without serum and potentiator or an incubation step. Testing an autocontrol routinely with the screen is optional; most workers prefer to perform a DAT only if the screen is positive.[5] The autocontrol and DAT provide useful information in determining whether the patient's antibody is directed against his or her red cells or against transfused cells, in the case of a recent transfusion.

POTENTIATORS AND ALTERNATIVE METHODS IN ANTIBODY SCREEN AND IDENTIFICATION PROCEDURES

Potentiators are commonly used in both antibody screening and identification procedures to increase the speed and sensitivity of the antibody attachment to the red cell antigen. The chapter on reagents explained the theory of each type of enhancement medium—low-ionic-strength saline (LISS), bovine serum albumin (BSA), polyethylene glycol (PEG), and proteolytic enzymes. Alternative methods such as solid-phase and gel technology are incorporated into routine screening and antibody identification procedures. Each method has limitations and advantages. Selection of potentiators and laboratory methods for antibody detection and identification is usually based on the patient population, workload, and degree of expertise in the laboratory.

The uses and limitations of LISS, BSA, PEG, and enzyme potentiators, along with gel technology and solid-phase techniques, are outlined in Table 8.1. Appreciating the differences and limitations of the potentiators and methods helps the technologist select the most appropriate one for the antibody involved.

TABLE 8.1	Comparison of Potentiators and Methods	
POTENTIATOR	**USE**	**LIMITATIONS**
Low-ionic-strength saline (LISS)	Sensitive, economical, and allows for shorter incubation time	Enhances cold autoantibodies Some weak anti-K antibodies may be missed Equal parts of plasma/serum and LISS are important If the ionic strength of a LISS procedure is altered, there is a decreasing sensitivity of the test system.
Bovine serum albumin (BSA)	Affects second stage of agglutination Reduces the repulsion between red cells but does not shorten the incubation time Does not enhance warm autoantibodies	Needs longer incubation time Not sensitive for most antibodies except in Rh blood group system
Polyethylene glycol (PEG)	Shows increased sensitivity Often detects the presence of antibodies not found with BSA or LISS	Enhances warm autoantibodies IgM antibodies do not react well or at all with this potentiator Recommend using anti-IgG AHG, not anti-IgG, -C3d AHG No 37° C readings May require extra wash

TABLE 8.1	Comparison of Potentiators and Methods—cont'd	
POTENTIATOR	**USE**	**LIMITATIONS**
Enzymes: ficin, papain	Eliminates presence of Fy^a, Fy^b, M, and N antigens; S and s antigens are variably affected	Enhance cold and warm autoantibodies
	Loss of reactivity in the panel for any antibodies present to the antigens stated earlier	Can be used as additional tools for investigating complex antibody problems but should not be used as the only method
	Enhances Rh, JK, LE, P1 antibodies	
Gel technology	Avoids cold reactive antibodies	Enhances warm autoantibodies
	Shows increased sensitivity Can be automated	Weak anti-K and some anti-E may be missed due to LISS-suspended red cells
Solid phase (SPRCA)	Avoids cold reactive antibodies	Enhances warm autoantibodies
	Shows increased sensitivity Can be automated	Weak anti-K may be missed due to LISS potentiators
		Manual method may be difficult to read

AHG, Antihuman globulin.

PATIENT HISTORY

Before beginning antibody identification procedures, it is essential to obtain a complete transfusion, medical, and pregnancy history. Transfusions within the last 3 months present the possibility of a mixed red cell population and recent antibody stimulation. The patient may not be aware of any red cell antibodies. If the patient moved to a different hospital, this information might not have transferred. Communication with previous medical facilities where the patient may have undergone transfusion is often helpful.

Patient information such as diagnosis, race, and age offers additional clues to the nature of the antibody problem. Some diseases are associated with the development of certain antibodies. For example, a patient with systemic lupus erythematosus or carcinoma is frequently associated with a warm autoantibody, whereas pneumonia may result in a cold autoimmune process. Patients with sickle cell disease can have both multiple alloantibodies and autoantibodies. Generally, patients younger than 50 years old or healthy blood donors do not possess autoantibodies. Some antibodies are associated only with certain races because of the frequency of antigens in certain populations. For example, anti-Js^b antibody is associated with the black population.

> A patient's transfusion and pregnancy history can provide important clues to the antibodies made to red cell antigens.

SECTION 2
ANTIBODY IDENTIFICATION

INITIAL PANEL

Testing the serum or plasma against a panel of reagent red cells usually follows the detection of the antibody in the screen. A panel, similar to the screening cells, consists of group O reagent red cells with phenotypes for most common antigen specificities. Manufacturers prepare panels with various antigen configurations, which may include 10, 11, 15, 16, or 20 cells and be considered extended antibody screens. Initial testing of the panel cells uses the same potentiators as those in the antibody screen. An autocontrol is included with the panel, especially if not routinely tested with the antibody screen. Some procedural variation exists among transfusion services and reference laboratories regarding antibody identification procedures. This chapter follows the most widely accepted procedures and provides brief discussions regarding alternative methods.

The panel "map," or antigram, is unique to each panel lot number where reactions are recorded for interpretation of the results. It is important to grade reactions consistently

TABLE 8.2	Key to Reactions and Abbreviations
Key to Reactions	
0	No agglutination or hemolysis
+w	Very tiny agglutinates; cloudy background
1+	Small agglutinates; cloudy background
2+	Medium agglutinates; clear background
3+	Several large agglutinates; clear background
4+	One solid agglutinate
H	Hemolysis
✓	IgG sensitized red cells agglutinate
NT	Not tested
Key to Abbreviations	
IS	Immediate-spin
RT	Room temperature
IAT	Indirect antiglobulin test
AHG	Antihuman globulin
DAT	Direct antiglobulin test
Poly	Polyspecific antiglobulin reagent
CC	IgG sensitized red cells
LISS	Low-ionic-strength saline
PEG	Polyethylene glycol
37	37° C incubation

while following specific laboratory guidelines; procedure manuals often represent this as the "key." This key to reactions provides a higher degree of accuracy in interpretations and the ability of another technologist to review or perform additional testing. The key used for the antibody problems presented in this chapter is shown in Table 8.2.

After results are recorded for each phase and negative reactions are confirmed with check cells (IgG-sensitized reagent red cells), the panel can be interpreted. The interpretation guidelines in Table 8.3 outline important concepts in evaluating antibody screen results. These guidelines should be used in the examples of antibody problems that follow. Scan the QR code for the antibody identification procedure.

PANEL INTERPRETATION: SINGLE ANTIBODY SPECIFICITY

Refer to Panels 8.1 and 8.2 for the following discussion of interpreting a single antibody.

Autocontrol

The autocontrol determines whether alloantibody or autoantibody specificity exists. The autocontrol is a suspension of the patient's red cells with the patient's serum. Incubated with the panel cells, the autocontrol is read at the same phases as the panel. The autocontrol is typically included at the end of the panel, indicated on the panel as "patient cells." If the autocontrol is positive and the DAT is negative, the potentiator may be causing false-positive results. In that case, the panel should be repeated using a different type of potentiator or no enhancement solution. Usually a positive autocontrol or positive DAT indicates an autoantibody or an antibody produced against recently transfused red cells. Autoantibodies are of the cold or warm type, depending on the optimal reaction temperature; they are discussed in later in this chapter. Panel 8.1 has a negative autocontrol, which indicates an alloantibody exists in the patient's serum.

The autocontrol and DAT help determine whether an autoantibody or alloantibody is present. A positive autocontrol and negative DAT indicates a false-positive result.

TABLE 8.3	Guidelines for Interpretation of a Panel	
LOOK AT	**RESULT**	**INTERPRETATION**
Autocontrol	Negative	Alloantibody
	Positive	Autoantibody or drug interaction
		Delayed transfusion reaction; transfused cells are sensitized with antibody
Reaction phases	Room temperature or immediate-spin	Cold or IgM antibody
	37° C reactions	May be cold (IgM) if reactions started at room temperature
		May be warm (IgG) if reactions are not seen at room temperature but noticed at AHG
	AHG	Warm or IgG antibody; clinically significant
Reaction strength	Single strength	Probably one antibody specificity
	Varying strengths	More than one antibody or one antibody showing dosage
Ruling out	Negative reactions	If no reaction was observed, the antibody to the antigen on the panel was probably not present
		If the antigen on the panel is heterozygous, the antibody may be showing dosage; rule out carefully
	Positive reactions	*Never* rule out using positive reactions
Matching the pattern	Single antibody	If the specificity is a single antibody, the pattern of positive reactions matches one of the antigen columns
	Multiple antibodies	When more than one antibody is present, it is difficult to match a pattern unless the phases or reaction strengths are unique
Rule of three	Three positives	Is the suspected antibody reactive with at least three panel cells that are antigen-positive?
	Three negatives	Is the suspected antibody negative with at least three panel cells that do not possess the antigen?
Patient's phenotype	Negative	If the patient does not possess the antigen, it is possible to make the antibody
	Positive	Transfused red cells are present if patient received a unit of RBCs within last 3 months
		Suspected antibody is incorrect

AHG, Antihuman globulin; *RBCs,* red blood cells.

Panel 8.1   Single Antibody Specificity

Cell	Rh							MNSs				P1	Lewis		Lutheran		Kell		Duffy		Kidd		*LISS*			
	D	C	E	c	e	f	C^w	M	N	S	s	P1	Le^a	Le^b	Lu^a	Lu^b	K	k	Fy^a	Fy^b	Jk^a	Jk^b	*IS*	*37*	*AHG*	*CC*
1 R1R1 (51)	+	+	0	0	+	0	0	+	+	+	0	+	0	+	0	+	+	+	0	+	+	0	*0*	*0*	*2+*	
2 R1R1* (32)	+	+	0	0	+	0	+	+	0	0	+	+	0	+	0	+	0	+	0	+	+	+	*0*	*0*	*0*	✓
3 R2R2* (64)	+	0	+	+	0	0	0	0	+	0	+	+	+	0	0	+	+	+	0	0	+	+	*0*	*0*	*2+*	
4 r'r* (75)	0	+	0	+	+	+	0	+	0	+	+	+	0	+	0	+	0	+	+	0	+	+	*0*	*0*	*0*	✓
5 r"r* (87)	0	0	+	+	+	+	0	+	+	+	+	+	0	+	0	+	0	+	+	0	+	0	*0*	*0*	*0*	✓
6 rr* (98)	0	0	0	+	+	+	0	+	+	+	+	+	+	0	0	+	0	+	+	0	+	+	*0*	*0*	*0*	✓
7 rr* (76)	0	0	0	+	+	+	0	+	0	+	0	0	0	+	0	+	+	0	+	+	0	+	*0*	*0*	*3+*	
8 rr* (53)	0	0	0	+	+	+	0	+	0	+	+	+	0	0	0	+	0	+	0	+	0	+	*0*	*0*	*0*	✓
9 rr* (23)	0	0	0	+	+	+	0	+	+	+	+	0	+	0	0	+	0	+	+	+	+	0	*0*	*0*	*0*	✓
10 R1R1* (34)	+	+	0	0	+	0	+	0	+	+	0	+	0	+	0	+	0	+	0	+	+	+	*0*	*0*	*0*	✓
Autocontrol: patient's red cells and patient serum																							*0*	*0*	*0*	✓

*Use negative reactions to rule out.
+, Antigen present; *0*, antigen absent.

Phases

> The phase of the reaction helps determine whether an IgG or IgM antibody is present.

The phase or reaction temperature at which agglutination appears is an indication that the antibody is IgG or IgM. Typically, IgM antibodies react at room temperature or on immediate-spin. IgM antibodies such as anti-Le^a, anti-Le^b, anti-M, anti-N, anti-I, and anti-P1 should be suspected if immediate-spin reactions are detected. IgG antibodies react at the antiglobulin phase. Reactions at different phases may indicate more than one antibody and a combination of IgG and IgM antibodies. The example in Panel 8.1 illustrates an IgG antibody.

Reaction Strength

> Dosage example: red cells M+N– plus anti-M = 3+ and red cells M+N+ plus anti-M = 1+.

The strength of the antibody reaction is a clue to the number of antibodies present. Reactions of varying strengths suggest more than one antibody. In Panel 8.1, all reactions are fairly strong and of similar strength (2+ and 3+). Antibodies such as anti-K, anti-D, anti-E, anti-e, anti-c, and anti-C are commonly stronger than anti-Fy^a, anti-Fy^b, anti-Jk^a, anti-Jk^b, anti-S, and anti-s. The strength of the reaction also varies with the antigen dosage. If a panel cell is homozygous, a stronger reaction may be noticed. In some cases, weak antibodies may not even react with heterozygous antigen expression.

Ruling Out

> **Rule out:** to eliminate the possibility that an antibody exists in the serum based on its nonreactivity with a particular antigen

Panel cells that give negative reactions (0) with all tested phases are used to **rule out** antibodies. This process is illustrated in Panel 8.2. Begin with the first negative panel cell reaction, which is cell 2. Looking across the panel, place a line through the antigen specificity that is positive (+) on the panel. If an antigen–antibody reaction did not occur, the antibody did not react with the antigen on the panel cell and it can be eliminated as a possible antibody. Panel cells that are heterozygous, particularly in the Duffy, Kidd, and MNS system, should *not* be crossed out because the antibody might have been too weak to react or is exhibiting dosage. Continue ruling out using the panel cells that gave a negative reaction. The process of ruling out has narrowed the antibody possibilities down to anti-K and anti-Lu^a.

Panel 8.2	Ruling Out and Determining a Specificity																										
	Rh							MNSs				P1	Lewis		Lutheran		Kell		Duffy		Kidd		LISS			
Cell	D	C	E	c	e	f	Cw	M	N	S	s	P1	Lea	Leb	Lua	Lub	K	k	Fya	Fyb	Jka	Jkb	IS	37	AHG	CC
1 R1R1 (51)	+	+	0	0	+	0	0	+	+	+	0	+	0	+	0	+	+	+	0	+	+	0	0	0	2+	
2 R1R1 (32)	+	+	0	0	+	0	+	+	0	0	+	+	0	+	0	+	0	+	0	+	+	+	0	0	0	✓
3 R2R2 (64)	+	0	+	+	0	0	0	0	+	0	+	+	+	0	0	+	+	+	0	0	+	+	0	0	2+	
4 r'r (75)	0	+	0	+	+	+	0	+	0	+	+	+	0	+	0	+	0	+	+	0	+	+	0	0	0	✓
5 r"r (87)	0	0	+	+	+	+	0	+	+	+	+	+	0	+	0	+	0	+	+	0	+	0	0	0	0	✓
6 rr (98)	0	0	0	+	+	+	0	+	+	+	+	+	+	0	0	+	0	+	+	0	+	+	0	0	0	✓
7 rr (76)	0	0	0	+	+	+	0	+	0	+	0	0	0	+	0	+	+	0	+	+	0	+	0	0	3+	
8 rr (53)	0	0	0	+	+	+	0	+	0	+	+	+	0	0	0	+	0	+	0	+	0	+	0	0	0	✓
9 rr (23)	0	0	0	+	+	+	0	+	+	+	+	0	+	0	0	+	0	+	+	+	+	0	0	0	0	✓
10 R1R1 (34)	+	+	0	0	+	0	+	0	+	+	0	+	0	+	0	+	0	+	0	+	+	0	0	0	0	✓
Patient cells																							0	0	0	✓

Interpretation: Anti-K and anti-Lu^a are not crossed out. Anti-K matches the reaction pattern. Three positive cells and three negative cells are demonstrating, "satisfying the rule of 3." Note that cell 7 is homozygous for the *K* gene. The reaction is stronger (showing dosage) with this panel cell as compared with cells 1 and 3.
+, Antigen present; *0*, antigen absent.

Matching the Pattern

The next step in panel interpretation is to look at the reactions that are positive and match the pattern. When a single antibody is present, the pattern of reactions observed matches one of the antigen columns. In this example, agglutination was observed with panel cells 1, 3, and 7, and the K antigen is present on these cells. Therefore the antibody identity is anti-K. The other potential antibody specificity is not ruled out; Lu^a is a low-frequency antigen (<2% of the population). Because the antigens are rare in the population, the probability of producing an antibody to them is low. For this reason, they can be ruled out without further testing. Additional antigens that are of low frequency in the population that are sometimes listed on panels are V, C^W, Kp^a, and Js^a. Antibodies to these antigens are also typically ruled out but may be considered if the patient has been multiply transfused or has an incompatible **crossmatch**. (The crossmatch is discussed in the next chapter.) A "special antigen typing" column is often found on a panel antigram that may also provide clues if reactions do not fall within the patterns of the more commonly found antibodies.

Low-Incidence (Frequency) Antigens			
Lu^a	Kp^a	V	VS
C^w	Wr^a	Js^a	Co^b

Rule of Three

Identifying antibodies involves performing tests and making a conclusion based on antibody reaction patterns. To make a scientific conclusion, these reactions must be statistically greater than the reactions in a random event. The **p value**, or probability value, must be 0.05 or less for identification to be considered valid.[6] To obtain this probability, at least three antigen-positive red cells that react and three antigen-negative red cells that do not react should be observed. In the example in Panel 8.1, three antigen-positive cells (panel cells 1, 3, and 7) and seven antigen-negative cells (panel cells 2, 4, 5, 6, 8, 9, and 10) were observed. Therefore the **"rule of three"** was met. If there were not enough cells in this panel to determine sufficient probability, additional cells from another panel would be selected for testing. This panel is known as a selected cell panel.

NOTE: The *Technical Manual* allows either a rule of 3 or rule of 2 for proving antibody identity. This discussion illustrated the rule of 3.

Patient's Phenotype

Individuals do not make alloantibodies to antigens they possess (self-antigens). Another way to confirm antibody identification is to test the patient's red cells to ensure they are negative for the antigen corresponding to the identified antibody. Testing red cells should be performed only if no recent transfusions have occurred. Red cells from transfused donor units may remain in the circulation for 3 months and may cause misleading and incorrect results if different cell populations are present. The accurate phenotype of a recently transfused patient would necessitate **cell separation** techniques to separate transfused and autologous red cells. Cell separation techniques can be found in the methods section of the *AABB Technical Manual*. In laboratories with access to molecular methods, it is possible to determine the genotype of the recipient who has been multiply transfused.[7]

MULTIPLE ANTIBODIES

When patients have more than one antibody, additional techniques are needed to resolve the problem. Panels 8.3, 8.4, and 8.5 illustrate an approach to multiple antibody identification.

Following the guidelines outlined in Table 8.3, several conclusions can be made in Panel 8.3:
- The autocontrol is negative; an alloantibody should be suspected.
- Reactions only at the antihuman globulin (AHG) phase suggest an IgG antibody.
- The reaction strength is variable (1+ to 3+), which suggests more than one antibody and/or an antibody that exhibits dosage.

- Anti-E and anti-Fy^a cannot be ruled out after crossing out antigens that did not react with the antibody.
- Matching the pattern is more difficult when more than one antibody specificity exists.
- Under the rule of three, two E-positive panel cells were reactive (panel cells 3 and 5) with the patient's sample. However, panel cell 5 is positive for *both* E and Fy^a antigens and cannot be included. Four E-negative panel cells were nonreactive (panel cells 1, 2, 8, and 10). The rule of three was not met for confirmation of anti-E. Two more E-positive panel cells that are Fy(a–) need to be tested.
- Five Fy(a+) panel cells reacted (panel cells 4, 5, 6, 7, and 9) with the patient's sample. However, panel cell 5 is positive for *both* E and Fy^a antigens and cannot be included. Four Fy(a–) panel cells (panel cells 1, 2, 8, and 10) were nonreactive. The rule of three was met for confirmation of anti-Fy^a. Anti-Fy^a is also showing dosage in the panel. Panel cells 4 and 6 are Fy(a+b–) and have a 2+ reactivity; panel cells 7 and 9 are Fy(a+b+) and have a 1+ reactivity.
- The patient's red cell phenotype is E-negative and Fy(a–), providing additional support that these antibodies could be present.

Panel 8.3   Multiple Antibodies

Cell	D	C	E	c	e	f	C^w	M	N	S	s	P1	Le^a	Le^b	Lu^a	Lu^b	K	k	Fy^a	Fy^b	Jk^a	Jk^b	IS	37	AHG	CC
			Rh						MNSs			P1	Lewis		Lutheran		Kell		Duffy		Kidd			LISS		
1 R1R1 (51)	+	+	0	0	+	0	0	+	+	+	0	+	0	+	0	+	+	+	0	+	+	0	0	0	0	✓
2 R1R1 (32)	+	+	0	0	+	0	+	+	0	0	+	+	0	+	0	+	0	+	0	+	+	+	0	0	0	✓
3 R2R2 (64)	+	0	+	+	0	0	0	0	+	0	+	+	+	0	0	+	+	+	0	0	+	+	0	0	3+	
4 r'r (75)	0	+	0	+	+	+	0	+	0	+	+	+	0	+	0	+	0	+	+	0	+	+	0	0	2+	
5 r"r (87)	0	0	+	+	+	+	0	+	+	+	+	+	0	+	0	+	0	+	+	0	+	0	0	0	3+	
6 rr (98)	0	0	0	+	+	+	0	+	+	+	+	+	+	0	0	+	0	+	+	0	+	+	0	0	2+	
7 rr (76)	0	0	0	+	+	+	0	+	0	+	0	0	0	+	0	+	+	0	+	+	0	+	0	0	1+	
8 rr (53)	0	0	0	+	+	+	0	+	0	+	+	+	0	0	0	+	0	+	0	+	0	+	0	0	0	✓
9 rr (23)	0	0	0	+	+	+	0	+	+	+	+	0	+	0	0	+	0	+	+	+	+	0	0	0	1+	
10 R1R1 (34)	+	+	0	0	+	0	+	0	+	+	0	+	0	+	0	+	0	+	0	+	+	0	0	0	0	✓
Patient cells			0																0				0	0	0	✓

Interpretation: Anti-Fy^a and anti-E.
+, Antigen present; 0, antigen absent.

Multiple Antibody Resolution

Selected cells are often used to complete the requirements for the "rule of three" to confirm the antibody specificities that are initially suspected. Cells may be "selected" from other panels without running the entire panel. In this example, Panel 8.4 shows another panel that can be used to select additional E-positive, Fy(a–) cells. Panel cells 3 and 10 are E-positive and Fy(a–). When tested with the patient's serum, 3+ reactivity is observed in the AHG phase of the panel. Anti-E specificity has now been confirmed by the rule of three.

If the same panel manufacturer is used to select more cells, it is important to check that the donor number or code is not the same as the panel cell used in the original panel. This number is usually indicated in the first column of the panel. The donor codes for the selected cells used in Panel 8.4 are 45 and 92, which are not the same as the original cells in Panel 8.3. If the number were the same, it would mean that the same panel cell is being repeated. It is also important to remember that negative-reacting screening cells in initial testing may provide additional information for confirmation.

Panel 8.4   Selected Cell Panel

Cell	D	C	E	c	e	f	Cw	M	N	S	s	P1	Lea	Leb	Lua	Lub	K	k	Fya	Fyb	Jka	Jkb	IS	37	AHG
			Rh						MNSs			P1	Lewis		Lutheran		Kell		Duffy		Kidd		LISS		
1 r"r (22)	0	+	0	+	+	0	0	+	+	+	0	+	0	+	0	+	+	+	0	+	+	0			
2 R1R1 (72)	+	+	0	0	+	0	+	+	0	0	+	+	0	+	0	+	0	+	0	+	+	+			
3 R2R2 (45)	+	0	(+)	+	0	0	0	0	+	0	+	+	+	0	0	+	+	+	(0)	0	+	+	0	0	3+
4 r"r (28)	0	0	+	+	+	+	0	+	0	+	+	+	0	+	0	+	0	+	+	0	+	+			
5 rr (88)	0	0	0	+	+	+	0	+	+	+	+	+	0	+	0	+	0	+	0	0	+	0			
6 rr (38)	0	0	0	+	+	+	0	+	+	+	+	+	+	0	0	+	0	+	+	0	+	+			
7 rr (74)	0	0	0	+	+	+	0	+	0	+	0	0	0	+	0	+	+	0	+	+	0	+			
8 rr (21)	0	0	0	+	+	+	0	+	0	+	+	+	0	0	0	+	0	+	0	+	0	+			
9 rr (67)	0	0	0	+	+	+	0	+	+	+	+	0	+	0	0	+	0	+	+	+	+	0			
10 R2R2 (92)	+	0	(+)	+	0	0	0	0	+	+	0	+	0	+	0	+	0	+	(0)	+	+	0	0	0	3+

Interpretation: Selected cells for determining that an anti-E was present in the serum along with the anti-Fy^a.
+, Antigen present; 0, antigen absent.

TABLE 8.4   Enzyme Treatment Summary

BLOOD GROUP	REACTIVITY WITH ENZYMES
Rh, P1, I, Kidd, Lewis	Antibody reactions in panels are enhanced
M, N, S, Duffy	Antigens are destroyed (S and s variable) by enzyme treatment
Kell	Unaffected

Additional Techniques

Proteolytic enzymes can be used to eliminate or enhance antibody activity. The Fy^a, Fy^b, S, M, and N antigenic activity is eliminated using enzyme methods. However, the antibodies to antigens of the Rh, Kidd, and Lewis systems are greatly enhanced using enzymes in the test system (Table 8.4). Enzymes act by removing the sialic acid residues from the red cell membrane, eliminating some red cell antigens while exposing others. Two procedures can be used for enzyme treatment, as follows:

* One-stage enzyme technique

  In a one-stage procedure, patient serum, enzyme (papain), and red cells are incubated together.

* Two-stage enzyme technique

  Panel or screening cells are pretreated with enzymes (ficin or papain) and washed. The pretreated cells are used without other enhancement media in the antiglobulin test. Enzyme-treated red cells can be prepared before use or purchased commercially.

After enzyme treatment, red cells are retested with the serum to determine whether the antibody (or mixture of antibodies) is still reacting. In the example shown in Panel 8.5, the following conclusions can be made:

* If no agglutination is present after enzyme treatment, the loss of panel cell reactions indicates that an antibody present in the patient's sample was specific for an antigen denatured by enzymes. Panel cells 4, 6, 7, and 9 were not reactive after ficin treatment because the Fy^a antigen was denatured, and the anti-Fy^a in the patient's sample had no antigen for antibody binding.

One-stage enzyme technique: antibody identification technique that requires the addition of the enzyme to the cell and serum mixture

Two-stage enzyme technique: treatment of the red cells with an enzyme before the addition of the serum

- Panel cell 5 could be used to confirm the anti-E specificity. The Fy^a antigen was eliminated with ficin, and the anti-E reaction remained.

When using an enzyme-treated cell, observing agglutination only at the AHG phase is recommended to avoid false-positive reactions. Because enzymes denature some antigens, it should not be used as the only antibody detection or identification method.

Panel 8.5	Ficin-Treated Panel																											
		Rh						MNSs				P1	Lewis		Lutheran		Kell		Duffy		Kidd		LISS			Ficin		
Cell	D	C	E	c	e	f	C^w	M	N	S	s	P1	Le^a	Le^b	Lu^a	Lu^b	K	k	Fy^a	Fy^b	Jk^a	Jk^b	37	AHG	CC	AHG	CC	
1 R1R1 (51)	+	+	0	0	+	0	0	+	+	+	0	+	0	+	0	+	+	+	0	+	+	0	0	0	✔	0	✔	
2 R1R1 (32)	+	+	0	0	+	0	+	+	0	0	+	+	0	+	0	+	0	+	0	+	+	+	0	0	✔	0	✔	
3 R2R2 (64)	+	0	(+)	+	0	0	0	0	+	0	+	+	+	0	0	+	+	+	0	0	+	+	0	3+		(3+)		
4 r'r (75)	0	+	0	+	+	+	0	+	0	+	+	+	0	+	0	+	0	+	+	0	+	+	0	2+		0	✔	←
5 r''r (87)	0	0	(+)	+	+	+	0	+	+	+	+	+	0	+	0	+	0	+	+	0	+	0	0	2+		(3+)		
6 rr (98)	0	0	0	+	+	+	0	+	+	+	+	+	+	0	0	+	0	+	+	0	+	+	0	2+		0	✔	←
7 rr (76)	0	0	0	+	+	+	0	+	0	+	0	0	+	0	+	+	+	0	+	+	0	+	0	1+		0	✔	←
8 rr (53)	0	0	0	+	+	+	0	+	0	+	+	+	0	0	0	+	0	+	0	+	0	+	0	0	✔	0	✔	
9 rr (23)	0	0	0	+	+	+	0	+	+	+	+	0	+	0	0	+	0	+	+	+	+	0	0	1+		0	✔	←
10 R1R1 (34)	+	+	0	0	+	0	+	0	+	+	0	+	0	+	0	+	0	+	0	+	+	0	0	0	✔	0	✔	
Patient cells																	.						0	0	✔	0	✔	

Interpretation: ← arrow shows where ficin treatment of panel cells removed the Fy^a antigen, causing the antibody to no longer react with the panel cells. The treated panel more clearly shows the anti-E antibody.
+, Antigen present; 0, antigen absent.

ANTIBODIES TO HIGH-FREQUENCY ANTIGENS

Antibodies to high-frequency antigens (ie, antigens with a high incidence) present another type of identification challenge. If an antigen occurs in the population at a 98% or greater frequency, it is considered high frequency or high incidence. Typical reaction patterns are illustrated in Panel 8.6. By using the panel interpretation guidelines (see Table 8.3), the following conclusions can be made to give direction for additional testing:

- The autocontrol is negative; therefore an alloantibody should be suspected.
- The phases show that the reactions are occurring only at the AHG phase, which suggests an IgG antibody.
- The reaction strengths are similar in reaction strength (2+ to 3+), which suggests a single specificity.
- Because only one negative cell exists on the panel, panel cell 7 eliminates the possibility of anti-c anti-e, anti-f, anti-M, anti-S, anti-Le^b, anti-Lu^b, anti-K, and anti-Jk^b. Antibodies that are not ruled out are anti-D, anti-C, anti-E, anti-C^w, anti-N, anti-s, anti-P1, anti-Le^a, anti-Lu^a, anti-k, and anti-Jk^a. These specificities remain as possible antibodies in the sample. Because the antigens Fy^a and Fy^b are heterozygous on panel cell 7, they should not be used to rule out potential antibodies to these antigens.
- In matching the pattern, anti-k fits the pattern under the k antigen column when looking across at the potential specificities. Because it was not ruled out, the tentative antibody identification is an anti-k.
- Under the rule of three, two additional k-negative cells need to be "selected" from other panels and tested to conclude that an anti-k exists.
- The frequency of being negative for the k antigen is less than 1 in 500; therefore if the patient is k-negative, the specificity is probably anti-k.

Panel 8.6 Antibody to a High-Frequency Antigen

Cell	D	C	E	c	e	f	Cw	M	N	S	s	P1	Lea	Leb	Lua	Lub	K	k	Fya	Fyb	Jka	Jkb	IS	37	AHG	CC
			Rh						MN	Ss		P1	Lew	is	Luth	eran	Ke	ll	Du	ffy	Ki	dd		LIS	S	
1 R1R1 (51)	+	+	0	0	+	0	0	+	+	+	0	+	0	+	0	+	+	+	0	+	+	0	0	0	3+	
2 R1R1 (32)	+	+	0	0	+	0	+	+	0	0	+	+	0	+	0	+	0	+	0	+	+	+	0	0	3+	
3 R2R2 (64)	+	0	+	+	0	0	0	0	+	0	+	+	+	0	0	+	+	+	0	0	+	+	0	0	3+	
4 r'r (75)	0	+	0	+	+	+	0	+	0	+	+	+	0	+	0	+	0	+	+	0	+	+	0	0	2+	
5 r''r (87)	0	0	+	+	+	+	0	+	+	+	+	+	0	+	0	+	0	+	+	0	+	0	0	0	2+	
6 rr (98)	0	0	0	+	+	+	0	+	+	+	+	+	+	0	0	+	0	+	+	0	+	+	0	0	2+	
7 rr (76)	0	0	0	+	+	+	0	+	0	+	0	0	0	+	0	+	+	(0)	+	+	0	+	0	0	0	✓
8 rr (53)	0	0	0	+	+	+	0	+	0	+	+	+	0	0	0	+	0	+	0	0	0	+	0	0	2+	
9 rr (23)	0	0	0	+	+	+	0	+	+	+	+	0	+	0	0	+	0	+	+	+	+	0	0	0	2+	
10 R1R1 (34)	+	+	0	0	+	0	+	0	+	+	0	+	0	+	0	+	0	+	0	+	+	0	0	0	3+	
Patient cells																		0					0	0	0	✓

Interpretation: Anti-k.
+, Antigen present; 0, antigen absent.

Additional Testing

Although the antibody specificity determined in Panel 8.6 is probably an anti-k after testing the two additional k-negative selected cells, the antibodies that were not ruled out still need to be investigated. Additional k-negative selected cells should be tested; however, this strategy is difficult because k-negative panel cells are not common. Instead, the patient's red cells can be phenotyped for the antigens corresponding to the antibodies not ruled out (ie, D, C, E, Cw, N, s, etc.) If the patient is positive for any of these antigens, the corresponding antibody can be ruled out. Remember, the autocontrol was negative; the antibody is an alloantibody.

Eliminating the antigen reactivity by dithiothreitol (DTT) treatment is another approach to working with anti-k.[7] DTT is a reagent used to denature the Kell system antigens on red cells. It works by disrupting the tertiary structure of proteins, which makes them unable to bind with the specific antibody. Treating k-positive cells with DTT, followed by retesting, would eliminate the anti-k agglutination. Potential antibodies "underlying" the anti-k could then be investigated. The use of DTT is not a routine procedure in most transfusion services. It is most useful when antibodies to the high-frequency Kell system antigens are suspected: k, Kp^b, and Js^b. DTT treatment of panel cells is not necessary when identifying anti-K, -Kp^a, and -Js^a.

Additional clues when working with antibodies to high-frequency antigens are summarized in Table 8.5. The potential of multiple antibodies underlying the high-frequency antibody adds to the challenge. Rare reagent red cells used to identify an antibody to a high-incidence antigen and rule out underlying antibodies are not common on panels. Samples may be referred to an immunohematology reference laboratory, where an inventory of frozen rare blood cells and rare antisera is available for further testing.

High-Titer, Low-Avidity Antibodies

Some antibodies to high-incidence antigens may have the characteristic high-titer, low-avidity (HTLA) reaction pattern. These antibodies are typically weak (low avidity) and can often be diluted out to relatively high titer despite the weak reaction strengths. HTLA antibodies react at the AHG phase; are inconsistent; and are not usually enhanced with other potentiators such as PEG, increased incubation time, or the addition of more serum. They have not been implicated in causing transfusion reactions or hemolytic disease of the

TABLE 8.5	Clues for Identifying High-Frequency Antibodies
CLUE	**ANTIBODIES AFFECTED**
Room temperature reactions	I, H, P, P1, PP1P^k
Negative with ficin-treated cells	Ch, Rg, JMH
Negative with DTT-treated cells	JMH, Yt^a, Js^b, Kp^b, k, LW
Weakened with DTT-treated cells	Lu^b, Do^b, Kn^a
Weak reactions at AHG	Lu^b, Ch, Rg, Cs^a, Kn^a, McC^a, Sl^a, JMH, Sd^a
Negative or weak on cord blood cells	Sd^a, Ch, Rg, Lu^b, I, Vel, Le^a, Le^b
Stronger on cord blood cells	i, LW
Variable expression on RBCs	Lu^b, Kn^a, Sl^a, I, P1, Sd^a, Ch, Rg, McC^a, JMH, Vel
Race association: black	U, Js^b, Sl^a, At^a, Hy, Tc^a, Cr^a
Race association: white	Kp^b, Lan
Mixed field and refractile microscopically	Sd^a
High-titer, low-avidity antibodies	Ch, Rg, Yk^a, Cs^a, JMH,* Kn^a, McC^a

DTT, Dithiothreitol; *AHG*, antihuman globulin; *RBCs*, red blood cells.
*JMH can be an autoantibody; occurs in older patients.

TABLE 8.6	Characteristics of High-Titer, Low-Avidity Antibodies

Inconsistent reactions that are sometimes not reproducible
Usually not clinically significant
Often found with other antibodies
Variable reactions among panel cells
Not usually enhanced with polyethylene glycol, low-ionic-strength saline, or enzymes
Nonreactive with autologous cells
Weak reactions at antiglobulin phase often only microscopic
Reactions may be weaker on older red cells
Titration and inhibition may be useful techniques in classification and identification of these
   antibodies

fetus and newborn (HDFN). It is not important to identify the specificity of the HTLA antibody. Clinically significant antibodies may be masked by the HTLA reactions. Table 8.6 summarizes some characteristics of the different HTLA antibodies and provides clues for investigation and identification.[8]

ANTIBODIES TO LOW-FREQUENCY ANTIGENS

Patients who make antibodies to multiple antigen specificities often make antibodies to antigens of low incidence. Antibodies to low-incidence antigens can also sometimes occur alone and may be suspected when the screen is negative and the crossmatch is positive. A panel with only one reactive panel cell suggests this type of antibody. Identification of the antibody is limited to the available panel cells and should never be a reason to delay transfusion. The "special type" column found on panels can be used to find additional selected cells for identification. An extended cell profile is often available from most reagent manufacturers; it lists the less common specificities found on panel cells in detail.

Antibodies to low-incidence antigens include anti-C^w, anti-Wr^a, anti-V, anti-VS, anti-Co^b, anti-Kp^a, anti-Js^a, and anti-Lu^a. When blood is needed, crossmatching for compatibility through the AHG phase is acceptable. Using reagent antisera to screen RBC units for transfusion is not necessary, and in most labs antisera is not available. If an antibody to a low-frequency antigen is identified in a pregnant woman, testing the serum against the father's red cells can predict the possibility of incompatibility with the fetus (assuming the parents are ABO compatible). Titration studies to determine an increase in titer during pregnancy can be performed using the father's red cells.

ENHANCING WEAK IgG ANTIBODIES

Weak IgG antibodies are sometimes difficult to identify because the reaction patterns may not fit probable specificities. Repeating the panel with a different enhancement medium, increasing the serum-to-cell ratio, or increasing the incubation time may be necessary. Panel 8.7 illustrates this concept. The antibody (anti-c) reacted only with homozygous cells in the panel tested with LISS. Repeating the panel using PEG enhanced the anti-c reactions significantly. If the serum-to-cell ratio or incubation time is altered to enhance reaction strength, the package inserts for the enhancement media should be reviewed for specific limitations. Reagent red cells from different manufacturers may also give variable results because of preservatives and slight differences in the pH of the red cell suspension. If suspected, washing the panel cells once before use may eliminate the problem. Using panel cells before the expiration date is very important because some antigens deteriorate with storage. Obtaining a fresher sample from the patient may also enhance the antibody activity. Determining the identity of weak reacting antibodies is especially important if the patient recently received a transfusion. A new antibody may be developing and can be initially very weak. Fig. 8.3 summarizes approaches for resolving a weak antibody.

Panel 8.7	Polyethylene Glycol (PEG) Enhancement																										
	Rh							MNSs				P1	Lewis		Lutheran		Kell		Duffy		Kidd		LISS			PEG	
Cell	D	C	E	c	e	f	Cʷ	M	N	S	s	P1	Leᵃ	Leᵇ	Luᵃ	Luᵇ	K	k	Fyᵃ	Fyᵇ	Jkᵃ	Jkᵇ	*37*	AHG	*CC*	AHG	*CC*
1 R1R1 (51)	+	+	0	0	+	0	0	+	+	+	0	+	0	+	0	+	+	+	0	+	+	0	*0*	0	✓	0	✓
2 R1R1 (32)	+	+	0	0	+	0	+	+	0	0	+	+	0	+	0	+	0	+	0	+	+	+	*0*	0	✓	0	✓
3 R2R2 (64)	+	0	+	+	0	0	0	0	+	0	+	+	+	0	0	+	+	+	0	0	+	+	*0*	1+		2+	
4 r'r (75)	0	+	0	+	+	+	0	+	0	+	+	+	0	+	0	+	0	+	+	0	+	+	*0*	0	✓	(2+)	
5 r"r (87)	0	0	+	+	+	+	0	+	+	+	+	+	0	+	0	+	0	+	+	0	+	0	*0*	+w		2+	
6 rr (98)	0	0	0	+	+	+	0	+	+	+	+	+	+	0	0	+	0	+	+	0	+	+	*0*	+w		2+	
7 rr (76)	0	0	0	+	+	+	0	+	0	+	0	0	0	+	0	+	+	0	+	+	0	+	*0*	1+		2+	
8 rr (53)	0	0	0	+	+	+	0	+	0	+	+	+	0	0	0	+	0	+	0	+	0	+	*0*	1+		2+	
9 rr (23)	0	0	0	+	+	+	0	+	+	+	+	0	+	0	0	+	0	+	+	+	+	0	*0*	1+		2+	
10 R1R1 (34)	+	+	0	0	+	0	+	0	+	+	0	+	0	+	0	+	0	+	0	+	+	0	*0*	0	✓	0	✓
Patient cells																							*0*	0	✓	0	✓

Interpretation: Anti-c, which may have been misidentified without PEG enhancement.
+, Antigen present; *0*, antigen absent.

COLD ALLOANTIBODIES

"Cold" or IgM antibodies typically react at immediate-spin, room-temperature, and sometimes 37° C phases. These antibodies are usually clinically insignificant because they do not cause red cell destruction if antigen-positive RBC donor units are transfused. When the crossmatch is performed, the antibody activity often has to be avoided to find serologically compatible blood.

The specificities of the cold-reacting alloantibodies are anti-P1, anti-M, anti-N, anti-Leᵃ, and anti-Leᵇ. The antibody is usually identified by noting reactions at immediate-spin that may not carry through to the AHG phase, although 37° C reactions are sometimes seen. Panel 8.8 is an example of a "typical" anti-Le[b] identification panel. Antibodies to P1, M, and N sometimes do not react with all antigen-positive cells because variability often exists in antigen strength. Anti-M and anti-N demonstrate dosage. Anti-P1 reactions vary greatly with the age of the cells used and may not always react with all P1-positive panel cells. To enhance weak reactions or reactions not fitting the expected pattern, incubation at or below room temperature is recommended. After antibody identification, techniques to avoid the reactivity are used to identify underlying clinically significant antibodies and perform a crossmatch.

Neutralization techniques are useful procedures for working with certain antibodies to determine whether clinically significant antibodies are masked by their reactions. In a neutralization procedure, soluble forms of Lewis, P1, Sd[a], Ch, and Rg antigens are added to the patient's serum to inhibit the reactivity of the antibody in a red cell panel. Lewis and P1 substances are available commercially. Sd[a] substance is found in urine from antigen-positive individuals. Chido and Rodgers antigens are found in plasma from individuals positive for these antigens or a pool of several plasma sources. When performing a neutralization procedure, controls must be tested along with the neutralized serum. The control is untreated diluted patient's serum. It indicates that the negative reactions after neutralization are due to the elimination of antibody reactivity and not simply dilution of the antibody in question. An example of potential outcomes of the neutralization technique, along with the control, is illustrated in Table 8.7.

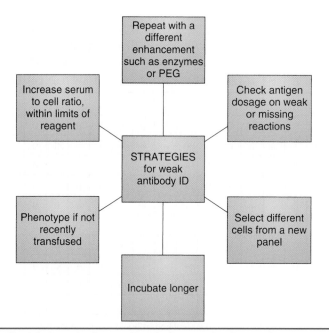

Fig. 8.3 Strategies for a weak antibody or one that does not fit a pattern.

TABLE 8.7	Neutralization of Anti-Leb		
SELECTED CELLS USED FOR TESTING	CONTROL: SERUM + SALINE	NEUTRALIZATION: SERUM + LEWIS SUBSTANCE	INTERPRETATION
1. Le(a–b+)	1+	0	Lewis antibody was neutralized
2. Le(a–b+)	1+	1+	Lewis antibody was not neutralized or diluted
3. Le(a–b+)	0	0	Antibody was probably diluted

Note. This table illustrates the importance of the control when performing neutralization.
1+, Small agglutinates, clear background; *0*, no agglutination or hemolysis.

Panel 8.8 Cold-Reacting Alloantibody

Cell	D	C	E	c	e	f	Cʷ	M	N	S	s	P1	Leᵃ	Leᵇ	Luᵃ	Luᵇ	K	k	Fyᵃ	Fyᵇ	Jkᵃ	Jkᵇ	IS	37	AHG	CC
1 R1R1 (51)	+	+	0	0	+	0	0	+	+	+	0	+	0	+	0	+	+	+	0	+	+	0	2+	1+	+w	
2 R1R1 (32)	+	+	0	0	+	0	+	+	0	0	+	+	0	+	0	+	0	+	0	+	+	+	2+	1+	+w	
3 R2R2 (64)	+	0	+	+	0	0	0	0	+	0	+	+	+	0	0	+	+	+	0	0	+	+	0	0	0	✓
4 r'r (75)	0	+	0	+	+	+	0	+	0	+	+	+	0	+	0	+	0	+	+	0	+	+	2+	1+	+w	
5 r"r (87)	0	0	+	+	+	+	0	+	+	0	+	+	0	+	0	+	0	+	+	0	+	0	1+	1+	+w	
6 rr (98)	0	0	0	+	+	+	0	+	+	+	+	+	+	0	0	+	0	+	0	+	+	+	0	0	0	✓
7 rr (76)	0	0	0	+	+	+	0	+	0	+	0	0	0	+	0	+	+	0	+	+	0	+	2+	1+	+w	
8 rr (53)	0	0	0	+	+	+	0	+	0	0	+	0	0	+	0	+	0	+	0	+	0	+	0	0	0	✓
9 rr (23)	0	0	0	+	+	+	0	+	+	+	+	0	+	0	0	+	0	+	+	+	+	0	0	0	0	✓
10 R1R1 (34)	+	+	0	0	+	0	+	0	+	0	+	+	0	+	0	+	0	+	0	+	+	0	1+	1+	+w	
Patient cells																							0	0	0	✓

Reactions are the strongest at IS; therefore a cold-reacting IgM antibody should be suspected, and ruling out should be done at this phase. Interpretation: anti-Leᵇ.
+, Antigen present; 0, antigen absent.

SECTION 3

AUTOANTIBODIES AND AUTOIMMUNE HEMOLYTIC ANEMIA

The first section of this chapter explained the detection and identification process involving alloantibodies. As previously discussed, the initial investigation of an antibody includes a DAT or autocontrol that, if positive, could be caused by a cold autoantibody, warm autoantibody, drug mechanism, HDFN, or a delayed transfusion reaction. (Refer to the summary in Table 8.8.)

This section describes the techniques used in the investigation of the DAT and serum reactions caused by cold and warm autoantibodies. These autoantibodies are developed in a condition known as **autoimmune hemolytic anemia** (AIHA). The autoantibodies lead to a transient or chronic anemia through the destruction of the individual's red cells in vivo. AIHA can be classified by the characteristics of the type of autoantibody produced: cold AIHA (IgM antibody) or warm AIHA (IgG antibody). Certain drugs can also induce AIHA. AIHA patients present in the transfusion service with a low hemoglobin and a positive DAT. In addition, these patients may have free autoantibody in their samples.

The principal investigation focuses on the recognition of the presence of an autoantibody and determination of any underlying clinically significant alloantibodies. The specificity of cold and warm autoantibodies is usually not relevant because autoantibodies are reactive with all reagent red cells, donor red cells, and autologous cells, regardless of the

Autoimmune hemolytic anemia: immune destruction of autologous red cells

TABLE 8.8   Interpreting a Positive Direct Antiglobulin Test

ASSOCIATED WITH	SPECIFICITY	SERUM ANTIBODY
Transfusion reaction	IgG	Specific alloantibody
Warm autoimmune disease	IgG (C3)	Reacts with all cells at antihuman globulin phase
Cold autoimmune disease; pneumonia	C3	Reacts with all cells at colder temperatures
Drug interaction	IgG (C3)	Serum may be nonreactive
Clot tube stored at 4° C	C3	None
HDFN; maternal antibodies on infant's RBCs	IgG	Alloantibody or ABO antibody from mother on blood cells

HDFN, Hemolytic disease of the fetus and newborn; RBCs, red blood cells.

Detecting and identifying underlying alloantibodies masked by an autoantibody is the primary concern when performing a workup of an autoantibody.

Adsorption: procedure that uses red cells (known antigens) to remove red cell antibodies from a solution (plasma or antisera); group A red cells can remove anti-A from solution

antigens present. Detecting and identifying underlying alloantibodies masked by the auto-antibody is the chief focus of the investigation. To detect and identify underlying antibod-ies, serologic techniques have two strategies:

- Avoid interference of the autoantibody
- Remove the autoantibody from the serum by **adsorption**

The first clue to an autoantibody is a positive DAT and/or autocontrol, along with serum antibodies that are reactive with most or all reagent red cells tested. The patient's diagnosis, age, transfusion history, and medication history are important to determine the classification and direction of an autoantibody investigation. In addition, the performance of the DAT on a clotted specimen may result in false-positive complement reaction with anti-C3d and polyspecific AHG reagents. Samples collected in ethylenediamine tetraacetic acid (EDTA) anticoagulant are preferred for performing a DAT to avoid unnecessary test-ing due to false-positive reactions.

COLD AUTOANTIBODIES AND COLD AIHA

Cold AIHA is caused by IgM autoantibodies, which optimally react at temperatures below 37° C. Cold AIHA disease is called cold agglutinin disease (CAD). A brief description of auto-immune disorders caused by cold autoantibodies will enhance the reader's understanding of the techniques needed to identify the cold autoantibodies.

Cold Agglutinin Disease

In CAD, patients may have a history of mild anemia, *Mycoplasma pneumoniae* infection, or infectious mononucleosis. A chronic form of CAD is often seen in elderly patients with associated lymphoma, chronic lymphocytic leukemia, or Waldenström macroglobulin-emia.[6] CAD can be observed in an EDTA sample where the red cells are agglutinated at room temperature and may even appear to be clotted. In vivo, the cold autoantibody binds to the red cells circulating in the body's colder extremities such as fingers, toes, nose, and ears, initiating the complement cascade. As blood returns to the warmer core tem-peratures, the cold autoantibodies dissociate from the patient's red cells. The complement cascade initiated by the antigen–antibody binding continues. The autoantibody specificity in CAD is most often autoanti-I and less commonly autoanti-i. Hemolytic cold autoanti-bodies found in CAD may necessitate transfusion support in extreme cases.

Paroxysmal Nocturnal Hemoglobinuria

Paroxysmal cold hemoglobinuria (PCH) is a rare autoimmune disorder characterized by hemolysis and hematuria associated with exposure to cold. As discussed in the previous chapter, autoanti-P is associated with this immune hemolytic anemia. This rare autoanti-body may appear transiently in children after viral infections and in adults with tertiary syphilis. Auto-anti-P is an IgG antibody reacting weakly or not at all in routine in vitro test methods. The Donath-Landsteiner test is required for confirmation of PCH. Another autoantibody implicated in PCH is anti-Pr.[9] Patients with autoanti-P may have a weak positive direct antiglobulin test because of complement coating. If transfusion becomes necessary, P-negative blood is not required. However, administration of the RBC unit should be through a blood warmer. Patients should be kept warm at all times.

Dealing with Cold Autoantibodies

Recognizing the presence of a cold autoantibody is the first step in beginning the investiga-tion. Cold autoantibodies can have reactions at several phases, and each example may be different in the reaction strength and phase noted. As illustrated in Example 4 in Fig. 8.2, the "typical" cold autoantibody is initially observed demonstrating reactions at room tem-perature, and the DAT is often positive due to the presence of complement component C3d.

Panel 8.9 further illustrates the nonspecificity of the antibody reactions, phases, and consistent reaction strengths. Complement-coated patient red cells and panel cells that react at room temperature are the most significant clues in recognizing a cold autoanti-body. Although the use of gel technology, solid phase, and PEG do not routinely test at the room-temperature phase, cold autoantibodies can attach at room temperature and still demonstrate reactions at AHG. Sometimes the cold antibody may not be detected in the screen but may become apparent because of an ABO discrepancy in non–group O patients. Serologic manifestations of cold autoantibodies can be quite variable, which contributes to the difficulty in problem resolution.

Determining the specificity of the cold autoantibody is helpful to ascertain that additional techniques are reliable. Locating RBC donor units that are negative for the antigen corresponding to the cold autoantibody is not necessary.

Panel 8.9 Cold Autoantibody

Cell	D	C	E	c	e	f	C^w	M	N	S	s	P1	Le^a	Le^b	Lu^a	Lu^b	K	k	Fy^a	Fy^b	Jk^a	Jk^b	IS	37	AHG	CC
1 R1R1 (51)	+	+	0	0	+	0	0	+	+	+	0	+	0	+	0	+	+	+	0	+	+	0	2+	1+	+w	
2 R1R1 (32)	+	+	0	0	+	0	+	+	0	0	+	+	0	+	0	+	0	+	0	+	+	+	2+	1+	1+	
3 R2R2 (64)	+	0	+	+	0	0	0	0	+	0	+	+	+	0	0	+	+	+	0	0	+	+	2+	1+	+w	
4 r'r (75)	0	+	0	+	+	+	0	+	0	+	+	+	0	+	0	+	0	+	+	0	+	+	2+	1+	+w	
5 r"r (87)	0	0	+	+	+	+	0	+	+	+	+	+	0	+	0	0	0	+	+	0	+	0	1+	1+	+w	
6 rr (98)	0	0	0	+	+	+	0	+	+	+	+	+	+	0	0	+	0	+	+	0	+	+	1+	1+	+w	
7 rr (76)	0	0	0	+	+	+	0	+	0	+	0	0	0	+	0	+	+	0	+	+	0	+	1+	1+	+w	
8 rr (53)	0	0	0	+	+	+	0	+	0	+	+	+	0	0	0	+	0	+	0	+	0	+	2+	1+	+w	
9 rr (23)	0	0	0	+	+	+	0	+	+	+	+	0	+	0	0	+	0	+	+	+	+	0	2+	1+	1+	
10 R1R1 (34)	+	+	0	0	+	0	+	0	+	+	0	+	0	+	0	+	0	+	0	+	+	0	1+	1+	+w	
Patient cells																							2+	1+	1+	

+, Antigen present; 0, antigen absent.

Cold Autoantibody Specificity

Sometimes antibody reactivity that does not fit a particular pattern is attributed to a cold autoantibody. Proceeding with techniques to avoid a suspected cold antibody that was not there can cause misleading interpretations. Some practitioners advocate establishing the presence of a cold autoantibody before continuing.[10] The tool first used is called a cold panel, which is a set of selected reagent red cells that aids in determining the presence of a suspected cold autoantibody (Fig. 8.4). The most common cold autoantibody specificities are anti-I, anti-H, and anti-IH. Because the I antigen is not well developed at birth, cord blood cells (I-negative) can be useful in determining the specificity. Hospitals with neonatal units usually have access to group O cord samples, which can be used for this purpose. Some manufacturers also have these I-negative reagent cells available on panels. Autoanti-IH and anti-H are more commonly found in the serum of group A_1 and A_1B individuals because their red cells have the least amount of H antigen. Differentiating between anti-I, anti-H, and anti-IH is not necessary but can be accomplished by adding A_1 and A_2 cells to the panel.

		SC I	SC II	AC	Cord	Cord	A₁	A₂	Group O
A	4° C	3+	3+	3+	0	0	NT	NT	individual with anti-I

		SC I	SC II	AC	Cord	Cord	A₁	A₂	Group A
B	4° C	3+	3+	3+	1+	1+	1+	2+	individual with cold anti-IH

Fig. 8.4 Minicold panel.

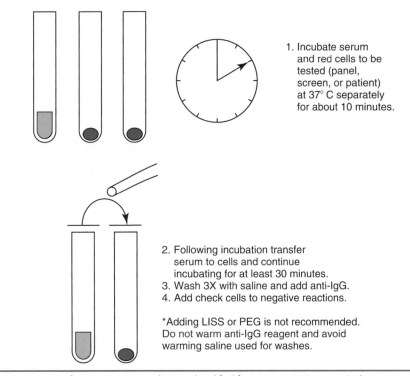

1. Incubate serum and red cells to be tested (panel, screen, or patient) at 37° C separately for about 10 minutes.

2. Following incubation transfer serum to cells and continue incubating for at least 30 minutes.
3. Wash 3X with saline and add anti-IgG.
4. Add check cells to negative reactions.

*Adding LISS or PEG is not recommended. Do not warm anti-IgG reagent and avoid warming saline used for washes.

Fig. 8.5 Prewarm technique. (Modified from Immucor, Norcross, GA.)

Avoiding Cold Autoantibody Reactivity

After the cold autoantibody's presence is confirmed as the cause of the reactivity, serologic techniques are used that *avoid* the cold autoantibody's reactivity. This technique will determine whether the presence of an underlying alloantibody is also present in the patient's sample. This section outlines the reasons for this approach, as follows:

- *Avoid anticomplement in the AHG test:* The use of anti-IgG antiglobulin reagent rather than polyspecific reagent may help eliminate the cold autoantibody reactions at the AHG phase. This reagent does not detect the attachment of complement. Many laboratories routinely use this reagent for this reason.[10]
- *Eliminate the IS and 37° C reading:* By not reading at immediate-spin and the 37° C reaction phase, the attachment of cold autoantibodies can be avoided. Some laboratories do this routinely to avoid detection of cold autoantibodies in testing.
- *Avoid LISS enhancement:* Using 22% BSA as an enhancement instead of LISS avoids some cold autoantibodies enhanced by LISS. If albumin is used, an extended incubation is suggested.
- *Perform prewarm technique:* If the procedures listed in the preceding section still do not eliminate a cold autoantibody that is carrying through to the AHG phase, the prewarm technique may be necessary. Fig. 8.5 outlines this technique. Warming the serum and cell suspension to 37° C in separate tubes avoids the antibody attachments that occur at or below room temperature. **Caution:** Use this technique carefully because it can reduce the strength of clinically significant alloantibodies masked by the cold autoantibody.[11] Washing with warm saline after the 37° C incubation and before anti-IgG addition is not recommended because clinically significant antibodies can be removed from the cells, causing antibodies to be missed.[12] In addition, anti-IgG should not be warmed. Because enhancement media are not used, sensitivity is decreased in the prewarmed procedure.[13]

Adsorption Techniques

If the cold autoantibody persists after implementing the aforementioned techniques, the cold antibody requires removal from the serum in an adsorption technique. If the patient has not been transfused in the last 3 months, an **autoadsorption** can be performed. If

Autoadsorption: attachment of the patient's antibodies to the patient's own red cells and subsequent removal from the serum

Allogeneic adsorption: use of blood from a genetically different individual, such as reagent or donor cells that have been phenotyped for common red cell antigens, to remove alloantibodies and autoantibodies

TABLE 8.9	Adsorption Techniques	
ADSORPTION TECHNIQUE	**DESCRIPTION**	**LIMITATIONS**
Rabbit erythrocyte stroma (RESt)	Removes cold (IgM) antibodies, particularly anti-I specificities	May adsorb anti-B and other IgM antibodies[15]
Cold autoadsorption	Patient red cells are used to remove cold autoantibodies to determine whether alloantibodies are present	Do not use if recently transfused
Warm autoadsorption	Patient red cells are used to remove warm autoantibodies to determine whether alloantibodies are present	Do not use if recently transfused
Differential (allogeneic) adsorption	Uses known phenotyped red cells to separate specificities: • Warm autoantibodies from alloantibodies • Alloantibodies with several specificities	May adsorb alloantibody to a high-frequency antigen

the patient has been transfused, the use of **allogeneic** red cells or **rabbit erythrocyte stroma** (RESt, Immucor, Norcross, GA) adsorption is necessary.[6] Table 8.9 compares the adsorption techniques. After the cold autoantibody is adsorbed, the adsorbed serum is retested with a panel to determine whether underlying alloantibodies exist in the serum.

Rabbit erythrocyte stroma: red cell membranes from rabbits used for adsorption of IgM antibodies such as anti-I

WARM AUTOANTIBODIES AND WARM AUTOIMMUNE HEMOLYTIC ANEMIA

Warm autoantibodies are more common than cold autoantibodies. Similar to cold autoantibodies, the clinical significance and serologic manifestations can vary greatly. Warm autoimmune hemolytic anemia (WAIHA) can be **idiopathic** with no underlying disease process, or it may be a result of a pathologic disorder or medications used to treat various diseases. This AIHA results from IgG-class autoantibodies, which react best at 37° C. In vivo, the warm autoantibody coats the patient's red cells. If autoantibody level is high, the red cells become saturated with autoantibody, leaving excess autoantibody to circulate in the plasma. **Panagglutination** of red cells is observed in the antibody screen, identification, and crossmatch procedures at the IAT phase. Patients with WAIHA may have a positive DAT with IgG autoantibodies only, or with a combination of IgG autoantibodies and C3d. The patient's diagnosis, medication history, and transfusion history are important in determining whether a warm autoantibody has been detected and the best approach to problem resolution.

Idiopathic: pertains to a condition without disease or recognizable cause; spontaneous origin

Panagglutination: antibody that agglutinates all red cells tested, including autologous red cells

Serologic Results in WAIHA

The initial antibody screen and DAT results commonly found in a patient with a warm autoantibody are found in example 5 of Fig. 8.2. A typical panel may react as shown in Panel 8.10. Antibody reactions are usually seen with most panel cells, autocontrol, and screening cells. The DAT result is positive and demonstrates that the patient's cells are usually coated with IgG antibodies and sometimes complement. The typical initial serologic and clinical description of a warm autoantibody is outlined in Table 8.10. Because warm autoantibodies react best with LISS, PEG, and enzymes, retesting with 22% albumin as an enhancement may eliminate some or all of the autoantibody reactivity.

The goal in testing a sample with a suspected warm autoantibody is to determine whether an underlying alloantibody exists. Although laboratories may have limited resources to perform autoantibody workups, understanding the theory of the procedures is important. This section describes some of the procedures used when working with a warm autoantibody.

Panel 8.10   Warm Autoantibody

Cell	D	C	E	c	e	f	Cw	M	N	S	s	P1	Lea	Leb	Lua	Lub	K	k	Fya	Fyb	Jka	Jkb	IS	37	AHG	CC
			Rh						MNSs			P1	Lewis		Lutheran		Kell		Duffy		Kidd			LISS		
1 R1R1 (51)	+	+	0	0	+	0	0	+	+	+	0	+	0	+	0	+	+	+	0	+	+	0	0	0	3+	
2 R1R1 (32)	+	+	0	0	+	0	+	+	0	0	+	+	0	+	0	+	0	+	0	+	+	+	0	0	3+	
3 R2R2 (64)	+	0	+	+	0	0	0	0	+	0	+	+	+	0	0	+	+	+	0	0	+	+	0	0	3+	
4 r'r (75)	0	+	0	+	+	+	0	+	0	+	+	+	0	+	0	+	0	+	+	0	+	+	0	0	3+	
5 r"r (87)	0	0	+	+	+	+	0	+	+	+	+	+	0	+	0	+	0	+	+	0	+	0	0	0	3+	
6 rr (98)	0	0	0	+	+	+	0	+	+	+	+	+	+	0	0	+	0	+	+	0	+	+	0	0	3+	
7 rr (76)	0	0	0	+	+	+	0	+	0	+	0	0	0	+	0	+	+	0	0	+	0	+	0	0	3+	
8 rr (53)	0	0	0	+	+	+	0	+	0	+	+	0	0	+	0	+	0	+	0	+	0	+	0	0	3+	
9 rr (23)	0	0	0	+	+	+	0	+	+	+	+	0	+	0	0	+	0	+	+	0	+	0	0	0	3+	
10 R1R1 (34)	+	+	0	0	+	0	+	0	+	+	0	+	0	+	0	+	0	+	0	+	+	0	0	0	3+	
Patient cells																							0	0	3+	

Interpretation: an autoantibody is typically reactive at the AHG phase with all panel cells and the autocontrol. A similar reaction strength is usually observed with panel cells, screen cells, and crossmatches.

+, Antigen present; 0, antigen absent.

TABLE 8.10   Typical Warm Autoantibody Characteristics

TESTS	RESULTS
Screen and panel	All screen cells, panel cells, and crossmatch testing reactive at antihuman globulin phase
Direct antiglobulin test	Positive because of IgG on red cells; C3 may also be on red cells
Eluate	Usually reactive with all reagent red cells tested
Hb/Hct	Low Hb/Hct, usually requiring transfusion support, may be chronic or acute
Compatibility test	Determine whether there is an underlying alloantibody before transfusion

Hb/Hct, Hemoglobin/hematocrit.

Warm Autoantibody Specificity

The specificity of a warm autoantibody is sometimes directed to the Rh blood group system, especially to the "e" antigen. In this case the patient's serum appears to have an anti-e specificity, although the patient's red cells are e-positive and have a positive DAT. In the case of an autoantibody with anti-e specificity, testing e-negative panel cells can be performed to determine whether an underlying specificity exists. Crossmatching e-negative units provides serologically compatible blood. If chronic hemolysis exists, providing e-negative blood might increase the red cell survival.[6] More frequently in WAIHA, the antibody reactivity is directed toward all red cells of the normal Rh phenotype.

Elution

Use of Elution in WAIHA

In cases of WAIHA, it is often helpful to identify the specificity of the IgG attached to patient's red cells when the DAT is positive. To identify the antibody, the IgG attached to the red cells must be removed from the red cells. To achieve this goal, the IgG antibody is dissociated from the red cells into a solution for specificity testing. This procedure is called an elution, and the recovered antibody in the solution is an **eluate** (Fig. 8.6). Elution methods work by disturbing the antigen and antibody bond, allowing for antibody removal from the red cell membrane. Various elution methods are listed in Table 8.11. Acid elution is the most commonly used method due to commercially prepared elution kits with reliability in antibody recovery. The acid elution reduces the pH, which results in antibody disassociation from the red cell

Eluate: antibody removed from red cells to be used for antibody identification

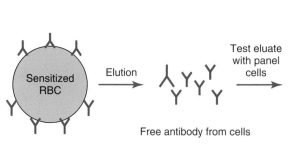

Cell number	D	C	E	c	e	f	M	N	S	s	P1	Le^a	Le^b	K	k	Fy^a	Fy^b	Jk^a	Jk^b	IS	37	AHG
1	0	+	0	+	+	+	+	+	+	+	+	+	0	+	+	+	+	+	0			
2	+	+	0	0	+	0	+	+	0	+	+	0	+	0	+	0	+	+	0			
3	+	+	0	0	+	0	+	0	+	+	+	0	+	+	+	+	+	0	+			
4	+	0	+	+	0	+	+	+	0	+	+	+	0	0	+	0	+	+	+			
5	0	0	+	+	+	+	0	+	+	0	+	0	+	0	+	0	+	+	+			
6	0	0	0	+	+	+	+	0	0	+	+	0	+	0	+	+	0	+	+			
7	0	0	0	+	+	+	+	+	+	+	+	0	0	+	0	+	0	+	+			
8	0	0	0	+	+	+	+	+	0	+	+	0	0	+	+	0	0	+	0			
9	0	0	0	+	+	+	+	0	+	0	0	+	0	0	+	0	+	+	+			
10	0	0	0	+	+	+	+	0	0	+	0	0	+	0	+	+	0	+	0			
11	0	0	0	+	+	+	0	+	0	+	0	0	+	0	+	+	+	+	+			
Patient typing																						
Interpretation:																						

Fig. 8.6 Principle of the elution technique.

TABLE 8.11	Elution Methods			
METHOD	**ANTIBODY REMOVAL**	**BENEFITS**		**LIMITATIONS**
Glycine acid	Lower pH	Rapid and sensitive; commercially available		
Heat Freeze-thaw	Physical	Rapid; effective for ABO antibodies; inexpensive		Not sensitive for antibodies other than ABO
Ether Methylene chloride Chloroform	Organic solvent	Sensitive; inexpensive		Hazardous, carcinogenic, or flammable

membrane. Organic solvents can be used for elutions because the chemicals denature antigens by dissolving the red cell lipid bilayer.[6] Heat elution methods produce conformational changes to red cells and antibody molecules. The freeze-thaw elution method lyses red cells to disrupt antigen–antibody bonds. Freeze-thaw and heat elution should be used only when testing for ABO antibodies on red cells because their sensitivity is limited.

In preparing an eluate, the red cells are initially washed several times to remove antibody that may be in the serum from the test system. Antibodies present in the serum should not be confused with the antibody attached to the red cells. To ensure this adequate washing, the "last wash" saline is tested with screening cells. If washing is sufficient, results of this test should be negative. When the eluate is prepared, it is tested against panel cells or other reagent red cells in a method similar to serum testing to determine the specificity. The eluate is usually reactive with all panel cells tested when working with a warm autoantibody. This observation helps confirm the presence of a warm autoantibody.

Nonreactive eluates may also be associated with warm autoantibodies. Antibodies to medications and nonspecific binding of proteins to red cell membranes can cause a positive DAT and a negative eluate. Evaluation of patients' medications and clinical symptoms should be considered in determining whether a warm autoantibody exists when the eluate is nonreactive. In addition, patients who show serologic evidence of warm autoimmune disease might not always demonstrate the same reactions in the serum and eluate with each transfusion request. Eluates are not useful if only complement is attached to the red cell.

Other Uses of Elution: Investigation of Transfusion Reactions and HDFN

Eluates prepared from recently transfused patients who are experiencing a possible delayed serologic or hemolytic reaction usually demonstrate the alloantibody causing the reaction. An eluate prepared from a newborn's red cells with a positive DAT demonstrates an antibody that was passed to the infant by the mother during pregnancy. Identification of this antibody is important if HDFN is suspected. Testing the eluate against a panel of red cells helps determine the antibody specificity causing a positive DAT.

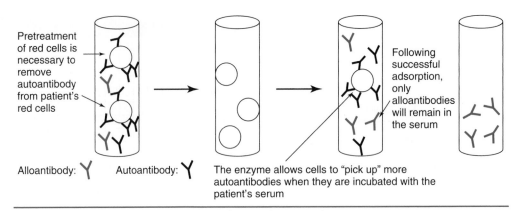

Fig. 8.7 Autologous adsorption technique.

Adsorption in WAIHA

Autologous Adsorption Procedure

As discussed in the section describing cold autoantibodies, adsorption procedures may be necessary to remove the autoantibody from the serum to determine whether an underlying alloantibody exists; an autologous adsorption may be performed. Before autologous adsorption procedures, the patient's transfusion history should be reviewed. If the patient has been transfused within the last 3 months, transfused red cells may exist in the patient's circulation. An autoadsorption is not appropriate in this circumstance because the transfused cells may adsorb the alloantibody necessary to identify.

In a warm autoadsorption procedure, initial pretreatment of the patient's red cells with DTT is necessary to remove as many of the in vivo attached autoantibodies as possible. In addition, treating the red cells with enzymes such as papain and ficin increases the capacity of cells to attach more autoantibodies. The combination of DTT and enzymes is sometimes referred to as "ZZAP" and is commercially available as W.A.R.M. reagent (Immucor, Norcross, GA). After treatment of the red cells, the patient's serum is combined with his or her red cells. An incubation period of 30 to 60 minutes is required to remove the nonspecific warm antibody (Fig. 8.7). After removal of the serum from the red cells, the adsorbed serum is retested with reagent red cells to detect and identify any underlying alloantibody.

Differential or Allogeneic Adsorption Procedure

Differential adsorption: adsorption or attachment of antibodies in the serum to specific known antigens, usually to different aliquots of red cells

For patients transfused within the preceding 3 months, a **differential,** or allogeneic, **adsorption** technique should be performed to investigate underlying alloantibodies. An allogeneic adsorption uses known red cell types that either match the patient's phenotype or represent a combination of antigens that selectively remove certain known antibody specificities. Often a set of three separate adsorptions is performed, which includes an R_1R_1 cell, R_2R_2 cell, and rr cell. Each tube adsorbs the autoantibody and leaves underlying alloantibodies in the serum. As in the autoadsorption procedure, enzyme pretreatment of red cells enhances autoantibody uptake. After incubation of the patient's serum with the allogeneic red cells, the adsorbed serum is removed. It is retested against screening or panel cells to determine whether underlying alloantibodies exist. Fig. 8.8 outlines autologous adsorption and differential adsorption procedures.

Methods to Phenotype Red Cells in WAIHA

Another challenge in working with warm autoantibody samples is phenotyping red cells that are coated with IgG. If a typing reagent requiring the antiglobulin phase, such as anti-Fy[a], is used to test IgG-coated red cells, a false-positive result occurs. To phenotype the red cells, treatment with chloroquine diphosphate or an EDTA-glycine-HCl solution such as EGA (Immucor, Norcross GA) may be necessary before antigen typing. Chloroquine diphosphate and EDTA-glycine-HCl disassociate the IgG from the red cell without damaging the antigen characteristics.[6] Follow the manufacturers' directions and test controls to avoid erroneous results. It is also important to check the patient's transfusion history.

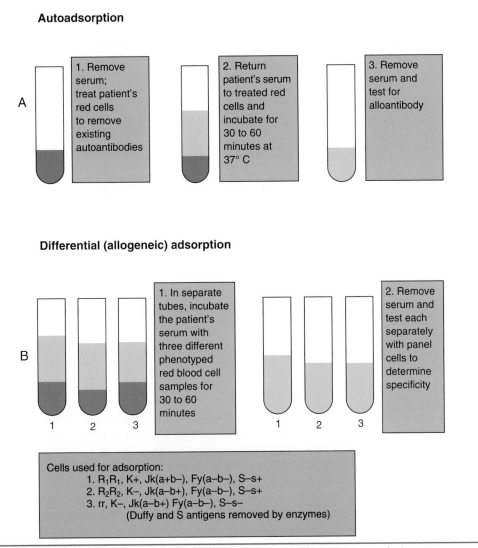

Autoadsorption

A

1. Remove serum; treat patient's red cells to remove existing autoantibodies

2. Return patient's serum to treated red cells and incubate for 30 to 60 minutes at 37° C

3. Remove serum and test for alloantibody

Differential (allogeneic) adsorption

B

1. In separate tubes, incubate the patient's serum with three different phenotyped red blood cell samples for 30 to 60 minutes

2. Remove serum and test each separately with panel cells to determine specificity

Cells used for adsorption:
1. R₁R₁, K+, Jk(a+b–), Fy(a–b–), S–s+
2. R₂R₂, K–, Jk(a–b+), Fy(a–b–), S–s+
3. rr, K–, Jk(a–b+) Fy(a–b–), S–s–
(Duffy and S antigens removed by enzymes)

Fig. 8.8 Adsorption procedure outline. **A,** Autoadsorption. **B,** Differential (allogeneic) adsorption.

If transfused cells are still circulating, the antigen typing may be misleading. Molecular methods are alternative techniques that can provide an accurate phenotype when the DAT and/or transfused cells are a problem.[7]

In summary, warm autoantibodies represent more complicated antibody identification procedures. Patients with WAIHA may require frequent transfusions, which further complicates the serologic results. Good communication with the physician caring for the patient must be initiated early to assess alternatives to transfusion and monitor the clinical symptoms associated with immune red cell destruction.

Drug-Induced Autoantibodies

Medications sometimes induce the formation of autoantibodies and may cause serologic manifestations similar to autoimmune disease. Drug mechanisms are classified as drug dependent and drug independent, depending on whether interference is detected serologically. In a drug-dependent mechanism, the DAT is positive but the serum is nonreactive with screen and panel cells. Reactions occur in vitro only by adding the drug to the test.[6] In a drug-independent mechanism, the DAT and screen and panel cells are positive and resemble a warm autoantibody in vitro. Classification of drug interactions by serologic techniques is typically beyond the scope of most laboratories.[14] Understanding the mechanisms and recognizing the drugs associated with a positive DAT and serum antibodies are helpful in testing and reporting results. This knowledge often is helpful to physicians,

TABLE 8.12   Drug Mechanisms Associated with a Positive Direct Antiglobulin Test

CATEGORY	MECHANISM	DESCRIPTION	ASSOCIATED DRUGS
Drug-independent	Unknown	Drug causes autoimmune process that resolves itself when the drug is discontinued	Fludarabine, methyldopa
		Appears serologically like a warm autoantibody	
Drug-dependent	Nonimmune protein adsorption	Drug causes modification of red cell membrane, causing proteins to attach	Cephalosporin, cefotetan, ceftriaxone, nonsteroidal antiinflammatory drugs
		Demonstrated by antibodies that react in the presence of the drug	
	Covalently binds to RBC membrane proteins	Drug attaches to red cell membrane; antibody to the drug causes red cell clearance by macrophages	Penicillin, cefotetan
		Demonstrated by treating cells with drug in vitro	

RBC, Red blood cell.

who may want to reconsider certain medications that may be causing cell destruction and serologic problems. Drug mechanisms are summarized in Table 8.12, and a more comprehensive list of drugs associated with a positive DAT and warm autoantibodies can be found in the *AABB Technical Manual.*[6]

CHAPTER SUMMARY

The process of alloantibody identification and resolving complex autoantibody problems becomes easier and more interesting with experience. Fig. 8.9, which incorporates an acronym for the words "BLOOD BANK," outlines some of the clues in antibody identification that are helpful in resolving the problems. The use of case studies is a good way to develop and enhance the problem-solving process necessary in becoming proficient in antibody identification. Antibody problems generally fall into the following categories:

- *Single antibody specificity* has a pattern that is easily identifiable, with a panel following the rules of interpretation. Confirmation that the patient or donor is negative for the corresponding antigen helps confirm the specificity.
- *Multiple antibodies* necessitate the use of carefully selected cells and additional techniques such as enzymes. Distinguishing multiple specificities necessitates attention to detail and a good understanding of antibody characteristics. The determination of the patient's red cell phenotype is also useful.

B	Blood typing problem?
L	Last transfusion or pregnancy?
O	Observe reactions at each phase
O	0.05 probability (use rule of 3)
D	Dosage
B	Black or white race?
A	Autocontrol results?
N	Negatives for ruling out
K	Know your reagents

Fig. 8.9 Clues for antibody identification.

- *Antibodies to high-frequency antigens* should be suspected if all panel cells are positive. Identification depends on locating cells that are negative for high-frequency antigens and determining whether underlying antibodies exist.
- *Antibodies to low-frequency antigens* are usually found with other antibodies. Identification depends on the availability of additional cells for testing. Transfusions should not be delayed to determine specificity.
- *Weak IgG antibodies* often can be enhanced by using a different potentiator, increasing the serum-to-cell ratio, or increasing incubation time. The detection of newly formed alloantibodies in recently transfused patients is especially important.
- *Cold alloantibodies* are usually clinically insignificant. Avoiding the reactions or using neutralization or prewarm techniques to eliminate agglutination is sometimes necessary.
- *Autoantibodies* are of either the cold or the warm type, and they should be suspected if the autocontrol or DAT is positive. Determining the existence of underlying alloantibodies is important to avoid additional hemolysis. Techniques such as adsorption and elution are usually performed to identify the antibody on the red cell and the alloantibody in the serum.

In each type of antibody problem, a methodical process is necessary to take into account important clues and reach an accurate conclusion. Being comfortable with many types of antibody situations is an appreciable goal for the immunohematologist.

CRITICAL THINKING EXERCISES

Exercise 8.1

A sample from a 55-year-old white male donor demonstrated a positive antibody screen during routine processing testing. The antibody identification panel's results are shown. Refer to the panel to answer the following questions:

			Rh						MNSs			P1	Lewis		Lutheran		Kell		Duffy		Kidd		LISS			
Cell	D	C	E	c	e	f	Cʷ	M	N	S	s	P1	Leᵃ	Leᵇ	Luᵃ	Luᵇ	K	k	Fyᵃ	Fyᵇ	Jkᵃ	Jkᵇ	IS	37	IgG	CC
1 R1R1	+	+	0	0	+	0	0	+	+	+	+	+	0	+	0	+	+	+	0	+	+	0	0	0	1+	
2 R1R1	+	+	0	0	+	0	+	+	0	0	+	+	0	+	0	+	0	+	0	+	+	+	0	0	0	✔
3 R2R2	+	0	+	+	0	0	0	0	+	0	+	+	+	0	0	+	+	+	+	0	+	+	0	0	0	✔
4 r″r	0	0	+	+	+	+	0	+	0	+	0	+	0	+	0	+	0	+	+	0	+	+	0	0	2+	
5 rr	0	0	0	+	+	+	0	+	+	+	+	+	0	+	0	+	0	+	+	0	+	0	0	0	1+	
6 rr	0	0	0	+	+	+	0	+	+	+	+	+	+	0	0	+	0	+	0	0	+	+	0	0	1+	
7 R0R0	+	0	0	+	+	+	0	+	0	0	0	0	0	+	0	+	+	+	+	+	0	+	0	0	0	✔
8 rr	0	0	0	+	+	+	0	+	0	+	+	+	0	0	0	+	0	+	0	+	0	+	0	0	1+	
9 rr	0	0	0	+	+	+	0	+	+	+	0	0	+	0	0	+	0	+	+	+	+	0	0	0	2+	
10 R1R1	+	+	0	0	+	0	+	0	+	0	+	+	0	+	0	+	0	+	0	+	+	0	0	0	0	✔
Patient cells																							0	0	0	✔

1. What phase in the panel is showing antibody reactivity?
2. What does this reaction phase suggest regarding the immunoglobulin class of antibody?
3. Is this antibody an alloantibody or an autoantibody? Defend your answer.
4. What is the antibody's most likely specificity?
5. Are there antibodies that cannot be ruled out on this panel?
6. What additional testing should be performed to verify the specificity?
7. What caused the antibody production in this donor?
8. Referring to the antigram, which panel cell or cells are homozygous for the S antigen?
9. Which panel cell is probably U-negative? Defend your answer.

Exercise 8.2

A sample from a 25-year-old obstetric patient was referred to the hospital for antibody identification. One of the antibody screening cells was weakly positive using LISS enhancement. A panel was tested with the following results listed.

Cell	D	C	E	c	e	f	Cw	M	N	S	s	P1	Lea	Leb	Lua	Lub	K	k	Fya	Fyb	Jka	Jkb	IS	37	AHG	CC
1 R1R1	+	+	0	0	+	0	0	+	+	+	0	+	0	+	0	+	+	+	0	+	+	0	1+	0	0	✓
2 R1R1	+	+	0	0	+	0	+	+	0	0	+	+	0	+	0	+	0	+	0	+	+	+	2+	1+	1+	
3 R2R2	+	0	+	+	0	0	0	0	+	0	+	+	+	0	0	+	+	+	0	0	+	+	0	0	0	✓
4 r'r	0	+	+	+	+	+	0	+	0	+	+	+	0	+	0	+	0	+	+	0	+	+	3+	2+	1+	
5 rr	0	0	0	+	+	+	0	+	+	0	+	+	0	+	0	+	0	+	0	0	+	0	1+	0	0	✓
6 rr	0	0	0	+	+	+	0	+	+	+	+	+	+	0	0	+	0	+	+	0	+	+	1+	0	0	✓
7 rr	0	0	0	+	+	+	0	0	+	+	0	0	0	+	0	+	+	0	+	+	0	+	0	0	0	✓
8 rr	0	0	0	+	+	+	0	+	0	+	+	+	0	0	0	+	0	+	0	+	0	+	3+	2+	1+	
9 rr	0	0	0	+	+	+	0	+	+	+	+	0	+	0	0	+	0	+	+	+	+	0	1+	0	0	✓
10 R1R1	+	+	0	0	+	0	+	0	+	+	0	+	0	+	0	+	0	+	0	+	+	0	0	0	0	✓
Patient cells																							0	0	0	✓

1. What phase in the panel is showing the strongest antibody reactivity?
2. What does this reaction phase suggest regarding the immunoglobulin class of antibody?
3. Is this antibody an alloantibody or an autoantibody? Defend your answer.
4. Could this antibody cross the placenta?
5. What is the antibody's most likely specificity?
6. If the panel cells were enzyme treated and retested, what would be the expected reactions?
7. Is this antibody usually clinically significant? Define clinically significant.

Exercise 8.3

A sample from a 65-year-old white male was submitted for a two-unit crossmatch. He is scheduled for an outpatient transfusion at the cancer clinic. A transfusion history indicated that he received two units of RBCs 4 months ago. Results of the ABO and D phenotypes and antibody screen follow:

Anti-A	Anti-B	Anti-D	A₁ cells	B cells	ABO/D interpretation
4+	0	3+	0	3+	A, D–positive

		LISS		
	IS	37° C		AHG
SC I	0	0		2+
SC II	0	0		2+

1. Is it possible to make an initial interpretation regarding the immunoglobulin class of the antibody?
2. What additional testing should be performed?
3. What additional medical history should be obtained for this patient?

Exercise 8.3 Additional Testing

The laboratory's policy is to perform a DAT only on samples with a positive screen unless specifically ordered. This patient's DAT results are shown in the table.

Polyspecific AHG	Anti-IgG	Anti-C3
3+	3+	0

1. Based on the DAT results, what type of antibody problem should be suspected?
2. When a DAT is positive, what procedure can be performed to identify the antibody attached to the red cells?

Exercise 8.3 Antibody Identification Panel Results

An antibody panel was performed using LISS in all phases of the antibody screen. All panel cells were positive (2+) by the IAT performed with anti-IgG. The autocontrol was 3+. An elution was performed, and the eluate reacted 3+ with all panel cells (the last wash was negative).

1. What is the specificity of the antibody?
2. What additional procedures are necessary before releasing units?
3. Would different procedures be necessary if the patient had been transfused within the last 3 months?

Exercise 8.4

A sample from a 70-year-old white female was submitted for pretransfusion workup for hip surgery in 1 week. Two units of autologous RBCs were reserved for this patient. Because the physician anticipated the need for additional units, routine compatibility testing procedures were performed. The patient had no history of recent transfusions. Results of the ABO and D phenotypes and antibody screen follow:

Anti-A	Anti-B	Anti-D	A₁ cells	B cells	ABO/D interpretation
0	0	3+	4+	4+	O, D–positive

	LISS		
	IS	37° C	IAT (Anti-IgG)
SC I	2+	1+	+w
SC II	2+	1+	+w

1. Based on the antibody screen results, what antibody class is demonstrating?
2. What is the specificity of this antibody: alloantibody or autoantibody?
3. What additional testing should be performed to determine the answer to question 2?

Exercise 8.4 Additional Testing

The patient's DAT results are shown in the table.

Polyspecific AHG	Anti-IgG	Anti-C3
1+	0 (check cells 2+)	1+

1. Do the results of the DAT confirm your suspicions? Defend your answer.
2. What additional testing should be performed to confirm the antibody specificity?

Exercise 8.4 Additional Testing

A "minicold panel" was tested and yielded the following results:

	SC I	SC II	Cord 1	Cord 2	Auto
4° C	3+	3+	0	0	3+

1. What is the probable specificity of the antibody?
2. What procedures could be performed to avoid the antibody's serologic reactivity?

Exercise 8.5

A patient's sample is demonstrating weak reactions in the IAT phase of an antibody identification panel. You are suspecting the presence of a Kidd antibody but cannot confirm it. What is the next test that you could do to confirm the antibody's specificity?

STUDY QUESTIONS

1. What is the purpose of the antibody screen?
   a. detects most clinically significant antibodies
   b. detects all low-frequency antibodies
   c. helps to distinguish between an alloantibody and autoantibody
   d. can be omitted if the patient has no history of antibodies

2. Select a characteristic of HTLA antibodies.
   a. typically react at room temperature
   b. can be enhanced with PEG

c. are usually clinically insignificant

d. are associated with HDFN

3. Which statement is a characteristic associated with anti-I?
   a. It has weaker reactions with stored blood.
   b. It can be neutralized with commercially prepared substance.
   c. It reacts best at 37° C.
   d. It does not react with cord blood cells.

4. A multiple antibody problem was resolved using enzymes. Panel cell reactions were eliminated for one antibody specificity after testing with enzyme-treated red cells. Which of the following antibodies was probably present?
   a. anti-c
   b. anti-I
   c. anti-Jk^a
   d. anti-Fy^a

5. What is the definition of an antibody demonstrating dosage?
   a. homozygous red cells were stronger
   b. heterozygous red cells were stronger
   c. red cells reacted best with PEG
   d. red cells reacted best at 4° C

6. The neutralization technique was performed on a sample containing an anti-Le^b. The control and the Lewis-neutralized sera were both negative when retested with panel cells. How would you interpret the results of this test?
   a. the anti-Le^b was successfully neutralized and no underlying antibodies were found
   b. the panel cells were not washed sufficiently
   c. the sample was probably diluted
   d. the antibody originally identified was probably not anti-Le^b

7. Which p-value is achieved in antibody identification with the rule of three?
   a. 0.09
   b. 0.02
   c. 0.05
   d. 0.15

8. What would the DAT results demonstrate if the test was performed on a clotted sample stored at 4° C?
   a. in vivo complement attachment
   b. in vivo IgG attachment
   c. in vitro complement attachment
   d. in vitro IgM attachment

9. Which of the following antibodies may not be detected in the antibody screen?
   a. anti-Js^b
   b. anti-V
   c. anti-k
   d. anti-s

10. What is the name of the procedure that removes intact antibodies from the red cell membranes?
    a. autoadsorption
    b. neutralization
    c. enzyme pretreatment
    d. elution

11. What is the name of the procedure that removes antibody from serum or plasma using the individual's own red cells?
    a. autoadsorption
    b. differential adsorption
    c. neutralization
    d. elution

12. An antibody reacted in the screen at 37° C and did not react at the AHG phase. Which of the following antibodies would you suspect?
    a. anti-s
    b. anti-e
    c. anti-N
    d. anti-Jk^a

13. What is the period when no antigen typing should be performed on a patient's red cells after transfusion?
    a. up to 30 days
    b. up to 2 months
    c. up to 3 months
    d. up to 6 months

14. DTT is useful in evaluating a sample when which antibody is suspected?
    a. anti-Js^b
    b. anti-Kp^b
    c. anti-k
    d. all of the above

15. Why are additional procedures required when working up a warm autoantibody?
    a. identify the warm autoantibody specificity in the serum
    b. locate RBC units that are compatible with the autoantibody
    c. identify potential underlying alloantibodies
    d. identify the antibodies coating the red cells

Answers to Study Questions can be found on page 387.

Additional student resources, including review questions, a laboratory manual, and case studies, can be found on the Evolve website.

REFERENCES

1. Levitt J, editor: *Standards for blood banks and transfusion services*, ed 29, Bethesda, MD, 2014, AABB.
2. Giblett ER: Blood group alloantibodies: An assessment of some laboratory practices, *Transfusion* 17:299, 1977.
3. Boral L, Henry JB: The type and screen: A safe alternative and supplement in selected surgical procedures, *Transfusion* 17:163, 1977.
4. Tremi A, King K: Red blood cell alloimmunization. Lessons from sickle cell disease, *Transfusion* 53:692–695, 2013.
5. Judd WJ, Barnes BA, Steiner EA, et al.: The evaluation of a positive direct antiglobulin test (autocontrol) in pretransfusion testing revisited, *Transfusion* 26:220, 1986.
6. Fung MK: *Technical manual*, ed 18, Bethesda, MD, 2014, AABB.
7. Alexander L: Personalized therapy reaches transfusion medicine, *AABB News*, Nov 2011.
8. Moulds MK: Selection of procedures for problem solving weak reactions in the antiglobulin phase. In Wallace ME, Green TS, editors: *Selection of procedures for problem solving*, Arlington, VA, 1996, AABB.
9. Judd WJ, Wilkinson SL, Issitt PD, et al.: Donath-Landsteiner hemolytic anemia due to an anti-Pr-like biphasic hemolysin, *Transfusion* 26:423–4225, 1986.
10. Pierce SR: Anomalous blood bank results. In Dawson RB, editor: *Troubleshooting the crossmatch*, Washington, DC, 1997, AABB.
11. Judd WJ: Controversies in transfusion medicine. Prewarmed tests: con, *Transfusion* 35:271, 1995.
12. Mallory D: Controversies in transfusion medicine. Prewarmed tests: pro—why, when, and how—not if, *Transfusion* 35:268, 1995.

13. Leger RM, Garratty G: Weakening or loss of antibody reactivity after prewarm technique, *Transfusion* 43:1611, 2003.
14. Johnson SJ, Fueger JT, Gottschall JL: One center's experience: the serology and drugs associated with drug-induced immune hemolytic anemia—a new paradigm, *Transfusion* 47:697, 2007.
15. Shan Y, et al.: Immunoglobulin M red blood cell alloantibodies are frequently adsorbed by rabbit erythrocyte stroma, *Transfusion* 50, 2010.

SUGGESTED READING

Judd WJ, Johnson S, Storry J: *Judd's methods in immunohematology*, ed 3, Bethesda, MD, 2008, AABB Press.

COMPATIBILITY TESTING

CHAPTER OUTLINE

LEARNING OBJECTIVES

On completion of this chapter, the reader should be able to:

1. Define compatibility testing and the crossmatch.
2. List the procedures included in the routine compatibility test, and explain their purpose.
3. Explain the AABB's *Standards for Blood Banks and Transfusion Services* as related to compatibility testing.
4. Select the appropriate plasma, platelets, and cryoprecipitated products for recipients with all possible ABO and D types.
5. Propose strategies for transfusion when compatible blood cannot be located.
6. Select alternative phenotypes of ABO and D donor units if ABO-identical red blood cells (RBCs) are not available in the blood bank inventory.
7. Outline the limitations of the crossmatch with regard to prevention of transfusion reactions.

8. Summarize the advantages and disadvantages related to the computer crossmatch.
9. Compare and contrast the purpose and application of the immediate-spin crossmatch and antiglobulin crossmatch.
10. Explain the elements of patient identification and their importance in compatibility testing.
11. Explain the use of a type and screen protocol and a Maximum Surgical Blood Order Schedule.
12. Evaluate laboratory results in compatibility testing.
13. Provide compatible donor RBCs for patients with multiple antibodies.
14. Explain the benefits of patient blood management.
15. Identify strategic elements in the urgent release of blood and blood components.

Compatibility testing is a term often considered synonymous with crossmatching.[1] However, in the transfusion service, a broader view of this term is taken. Compatibility testing includes recipient identification, sample collection and handling, and required pretransfusion testing. This approach ensures the greatest compatibility (no adverse reactions from transfused blood) technically possible between the donor unit and the proposed recipient. Compatibility testing encompasses all the steps highlighted in Fig. 9.1. The process begins with the transfusion request and ends with the transfusion of blood product to the patient. Because the antibody screen, ABO and D phenotyping, and donor testing are discussed elsewhere in this book, this chapter concentrates on the issues related to crossmatching—a component of compatibility testing—and provides an overview of important steps in the process of compatibility testing.

Compatibility testing: all steps in the identification and testing of a potential transfusion recipient and donor blood before transfusion in an attempt to provide a blood product that survives in vivo and provides its therapeutic effect in the recipient

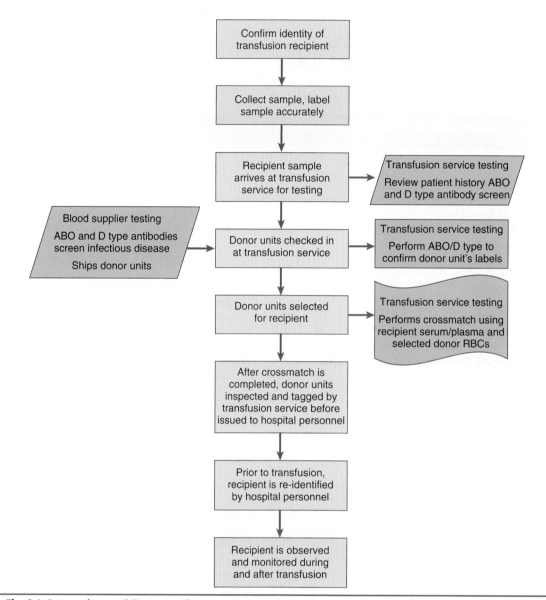

Fig. 9.1 Process of compatibility testing. The process begins at the recipient and ends with a safe transfusion into the recipient.

HISTORY OF BLOOD TRANSFUSION

The history of compatibility testing and transfusion practices is an interesting progression of events that begins with the discovery of the circulation of blood in 1628 by William Harvey,[2] an event that made the first human venous transfusions possible. The first in vivo transfusion was attempted with animal blood, and later human blood, using a quill or a metal apparatus introduced into a recipient's vein. Early recipients often died because no understanding existed of ABO blood group system antibodies (elucidated by Landsteiner in 1900) or of other blood group system alloantibodies.

Direct transfusions were performed again in the first decade of the twentieth century with some success, despite the lack of compatibility testing (Fig. 9.2). A crossmatch procedure was first attempted in 1907 in New York by Weil and Ottenberg. Sera of recipient and donor were separately subjected to lengthy room-temperature incubation with red cells from the opposite sources to detect hemolysins. Major and minor crossmatches were part of routine testing. Antibody screening did not become routine until the late 1950s to mid-1960s. Progress from the era of no testing to a century of rapid discoveries led to a proliferation of testing protocols that peaked in the 1960s. A movement existed for the

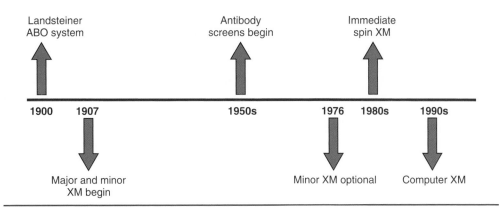

Fig. 9.2 Important events in compatibility testing. *XM,* Crossmatch.

discovery and characterization of every possible blood group antigen and the detection of every corresponding antibody. Over the past several decades, however, the forces of cost containment, practicality, and safety abbreviated, and ultimately eliminated, many of the previous testing protocols from routine practice. The AABB made the minor crossmatch unnecessary in 1976. In the 1980s the abbreviated, or immediate-spin, crossmatch was implemented in the absence of antibodies in the current antibody screen or the patient's past record. In the 1990s the blood banking community proposed the elimination of the in vitro crossmatch under certain defined circumstances and the adoption of the computer crossmatch. Scan the QR code for a more detailed review of the history of blood transfusion from the American Red Cross.

SECTION 1
PRINCIPLES OF THE CROSSMATCH

WHAT IS A CROSSMATCH?

Crossmatching is routinely performed only with donor products containing red cells. A crossmatch must be performed for red cell transfusions; the exception is situations requiring an urgent need for blood. The term crossmatch implies a crossway mixing of donor and recipient blood components.[3]

The crossmatch procedure involves the mixing of serum or plasma from the recipient with red cells from the donor (Fig. 9.3). Hemolysis or agglutination at any phase or step of the process indicates the presence of recipient antibodies interacting with donor red cell antigens and a mismatch between donor and recipient (Table 9.1). A crossmatch is interpreted as compatible when no agglutination and no hemolysis are present in testing. The donor unit is acceptable for transfusion purposes. A crossmatch is interpreted as incompatible when agglutination or hemolysis is present in testing. The donor unit is unacceptable for transfusion purposes.

PRINCIPLES OF CROSSMATCH TESTING

The rationale for the performance of the crossmatch is twofold. The crossmatch was added to compatibility testing to prevent life-threatening or uncomfortable transfusion reactions and maximize in vivo survival of transfused red cells.

The crossmatch procedure attempts to fulfill these goals in the following ways:
- The crossmatch serves as a double-check of ABO errors caused by patient misidentification or donor unit mislabeling.
- If the recipient possesses a clinically significant antibody or a history of one, the crossmatch provides a second means of antibody detection and checks the results of the antibody screen.

The crossmatch is designed to detect donor units unlikely to survive normally once transfused. The test must be rapid and simple enough to be practical. Actual

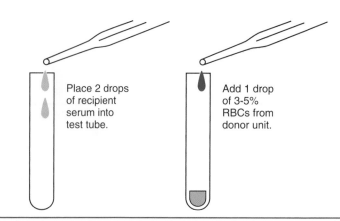

Fig. 9.3 Crossmatch. Patient serum is crossmatched with donor red cells. The minor crossmatch used donor serum crossmatched with patient red cells. Antibody screen testing on donor samples has replaced the minor crossmatch. (Modified from Immucor, Norcross, GA.)

TABLE 9.1	Compatible Versus Incompatible Crossmatch
CROSSMATCH INTERPRETATION	**APPEARANCE**
Compatible	No agglutination and no hemolysis
Incompatible	Agglutination or hemolysis

measurement of the survival rates of transfused red cells in vivo may be the best crossmatch. This technique can be performed directly through the use of radioisotope labeling, but is impractical for regular use. Instead posttransfusion hematocrit or hemoglobin values are often determined to provide a working measure of a successful transfusion. One unit of transfused RBCs should increase the hematocrit by 3% and the hemoglobin by 1 g/dL.

STANDARDS AND REGULATIONS GOVERNING THE CROSSMATCH

The AABB *Standards* provides the most inclusive summary of crossmatch standards. The crossmatch procedure must be performed using the recipient's serum or plasma and donor red cells taken from a **segment** originally attached to the blood product bag. The exception is an emergency situation in which blood may be released for transfusion before crossmatch.

The crossmatch defined by the AABB *Standards*[4] is a technique that "shall use methods that demonstrate ABO incompatibility and clinically significant antibodies to red cell antigens and shall include an antiglobulin test." Again, an exception is provided. If no clinically significant antibodies were detected in the current sample or in the patient's past records, an immediate-spin crossmatch is permitted to fulfill the requirement of detecting ABO incompatibility. The AABB provision for a computer crossmatch as an alternative to these requirements is presented later in this chapter.

CROSSMATCH PROCEDURES

There are two classifications of the crossmatch procedure: serologic crossmatch and computer crossmatch (Fig. 9.4).

Serologic Crossmatch

The serologic crossmatch procedure tests the recipient's serum or plasma with the red cells from the donor unit in either an immediate-spin crossmatch or an antiglobulin crossmatch. A crossmatch can be performed using two main methods: hemagglutination (tube and gel testing) and solid-phase red cell adherence.

Segment: sealed piece of integral tubing from the donor unit bag that contains a small aliquot of donor blood; used in the preparation of red cell suspensions for crossmatching

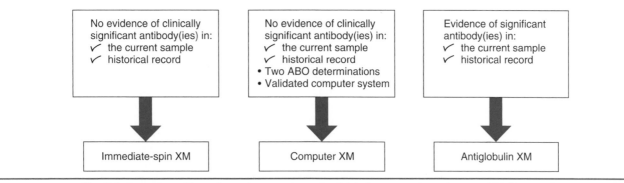

Fig. 9.4 Comparison of immediate-spin, computer, and antiglobulin crossmatch requirements. *XM,* Crossmatch.

Immediate-Spin Crossmatch

The immediate-spin crossmatch may be used for recipients with no evidence of clinically significant antibody or antibodies in the current sample and in the historical record. In this procedure, recipient serum or plasma and donor red cell suspensions are mixed and observed for agglutination. This procedure meets the AABB standard for detecting ABO incompatibility and can only be done using the tube method.

Antiglobulin Crossmatch

If the patient demonstrates a clinically significant antibody in the current antibody screen or has a history of such antibodies, antigen-negative units should be crossmatched using the antiglobulin crossmatch procedure. Commercial high-titered antiserum is required when selecting these antigen-negative donor units. For the antiglobulin crossmatch, a reading is required only at the antiglobulin phase; crossmatches performed using gel or solid-phase red cell adherence have only antiglobulin-phase results. In the tube method, the antiglobulin crossmatch procedure usually includes an immediate-spin phase, a 37° C incubation period, and an antiglobulin phase. Enhancement media used in the antibody screen are usually added to the crossmatch tubes to mirror the conditions in which the antibody was detected.

When a crossmatch is performed on a patient with a warm autoantibody, some laboratories use patient's serum or plasma that is not adsorbed. The crossmatch is reported as incompatible. Other laboratories use the adsorbed serum to screen and select nonreactive units for transfusion for patients with underlying clinically significant alloantibodies. These units would be issued as "serologically compatible with adsorbed serum." However, this practice can also be misinterpreted as a false sense of security for transfusion.[5]

Computer (Electronic) Crossmatch

A computer or electronic crossmatch uses a computer to make the final check of ABO compatibility in the selection of appropriate units for transfusion. The same prerequisite pertains to the computer crossmatch and the immediate-spin method: the recipient does not possess clinically significant antibody or antibodies in the current or any previous sample. The computer program should provide a flag indicating the recipient's eligibility or ineligibility for computer crossmatch. The AABB *Standards*[4] contains the required provisions for an acceptable computer crossmatch. Table 9.2 summarizes criteria for the computer crossmatch.

Keystroke errors are easy to make when using a computer. The system must alert the user to nonsense entries or mismatches with hard-coded ABO logic tables and require confirmation points along the way, which forces the user to verify or accept crucial conclusions with an additional entry. The bar coding of blood components and recipient specimens adds another measure of safety.

The first large-scale implementation of a computer crossmatch protocol occurred in 1992 at the University of Michigan Hospital, under an AABB exemption that met the Food and Drug Administration (FDA) requirements for alternative compatibility procedures.[6] The FDA *Code of Federal Regulations* (640.120) requires that transfusion services seek approval in writing for its use.

There should be no delays in the centrifugation step of the immediate-spin crossmatch or reading the reaction. If the immediate-spin crossmatch is not properly performed, false-negative results may occur with failure to detect ABO incompatibility.

Refer to the *Laboratory Manual* that accompanies this textbook for details of the immediate-spin and antiglobulin crossmatch procedures.

TABLE 9.2	Computer Crossmatch Requirements

- Computer-system validation on site and assurance that ABO-compatible Whole Blood or Red Blood Cell components were selected for transfusion
- Two determinations of recipient's ABO group are made
  ABO phenotype determination has been performed on a current sample.
  Second ABO phenotyping interpretation may be a retype of the same current sample, a second current sample, or a comparison with previous records.
  Note: Performing tests on two separately drawn specimens is preferred. In situations where only one sample is available for testing, repeat testing may be performed on the same specimen. FDA recommends the repeat test should be performed either by a different technologist or by the same technologist using different reagents.[13]
- Computer system includes donor unit information: product name, ABO and D phenotype, unique number, and interpretation of ABO confirmation test
- Computer system includes two unique recipient identifiers, recipient ABO and D phenotyping, antibody screen results, and interpretation of compatibility
- Logic to alert user to ABO incompatibility between donor unit and recipient and between donor unit label and ABO confirmation test
- Method to verify correct entry of all data before release of blood or blood components

From Levitt J, editor: *Standards for blood banks and transfusion services*, ed 29, Bethesda, MD, 2014, AABB.

The computer crossmatch has numerous advantages, including the following:
- Increased time efficiency
- Reduced volume of sample needed on large crossmatch orders
- Greater flexibility in staffing
- Better management of blood bank inventory
- Potential for a centralized transfusion service

LIMITATIONS OF CROSSMATCH TESTING

The performance of acceptable crossmatch testing does not guarantee a successful transfusion outcome. Adverse transfusion reactions may still occur. The risks of viral transmission, allergic reactions, and white blood cell reactions are complications that can be consequences of transfusions. These adverse complications of transfusions are discussed in a subsequent chapter.

The antibody screen and the crossmatch have inherent limitations as separate tests and should be used together. A recipient could have a negative antibody screen result and an incompatible crossmatch. A negative antibody screen does not guarantee that the recipient's serum does not have clinically significant red cell antibodies.[7] The negative antibody screen means that the recipient's serum contains no antibodies that react with the screening cells by the method used. In this example, a recipient might possess an antibody directed against a low-incidence antigen not contained in the commercial screening cells, and a crossmatch might detect this situation. An antibody detected with screening cells might not react with a weak expression of the antigen on donor cells in a crossmatch, leading to the situation of a positive antibody screen with compatible crossmatch.

A compatible crossmatch also does not guarantee the optimal survival of red cells. Aspects of the patient's clinical course (eg, bleeding, red cell sequestration) may limit the benefit of the transfusion. A delayed transfusion reaction could occur if a preexisting, undetectable recipient antibody is boosted in strength by the infusion of the corresponding antigen in the donor unit and rapidly destroys the donor red cells.

Even if red cell destruction does not occur, a recipient may become alloimmunized to the donor antigens, rendering subsequent compatibility workups more time consuming and complicated. Non–life-threatening transfusion reactions may also occur, making the transfusion uncomfortable for the recipient (eg, hives, low-grade fever, chills, itching).

Antibodies can be missed in compatibility testing if:
- The corresponding antigen is absent from screening cells
- The antibody is so weak that it detects only homozygous expressions of the antigen (dosage effect)
- The antibody is detectable only by a method not routinely employed (eg, in the presence of a particular enhancement medium)
- Antibody history is unknown

TABLE 9.3	Unexpected Incompatibilities in Immediate-Spin Crossmatch	
PROBLEM	**CAUSES**	**RESOLUTIONS**
ABO phenotyping errors	Patient identification error Sample labeling error	Repeat ABO testing Redraw patient
Unexpected antibodies	Cold alloantibody (M, P1) Anti-A1 in A_2 patient Cold autoantibody (I, IH)	Test panel cells Test A_2 cells Determine clinical significance

PROBLEM SOLVING INCOMPATIBLE CROSSMATCHES

Because pretransfusion testing encompasses antibody screening and identification and crossmatching, interpreting incompatibilities in conjunction with the results of these tests is important. Table 9.3 summarizes the causes of incompatible crossmatches in the immediate-spin crossmatch and presents suggestions for resolutions.[7] Scan the QR code for a complete list of causes of positive pretransfusion test results.

The antiglobulin crossmatch is more commonly performed in the presence of a clinically significant antibody or previous history of one. Problem solving has revolved around identification of the antibody's specificity and the location of antigen-negative donor units. An incompatible antiglobulin crossmatch occasionally may be detected. Often the primary reason for this incompatibility is the presence of a preexisting positive direct antiglobulin test (DAT) in the donor unit. Scan the QR code to have fun with the Crazy Crossmatch exercise.

SECTION 2
PRINCIPLES OF COMPATIBILITY TESTING

OVERVIEW OF STEPS IN COMPATIBILITY TESTING

As discussed in the introduction of this chapter, compatibility testing is a process that begins and ends with the recipient. The process involves many steps and requirements designed to ensure the recipient's safety for the transfusion. The steps are outlined in Table 9.4 and are discussed individually.

Recipient Blood Sample

Safe and accurate pretransfusion testing begins with the recipient's blood sample, properly collected and labeled with accurate patient identification procedures.

Patient Identification and Sample Labeling Requirements

Minimum labeling requirements are defined in the AABB *Standards*[4]: "Patient samples shall be identified with an affixed label bearing sufficient information for unique identification of the patient, including two independent identifiers." The two independent identifiers should include the patient's first and last name and a unique identification number such as birth date, driver's license, or photographic ID.

The patient must be positively identified by comparing the requisition and sample label to the identification band attached to the patient (not to the wall or the bed). The patient should also state his or her name without prompting from the phlebotomist. A caregiver may identify the patient if the patient is incoherent or a language barrier exists. Commercial identification band systems are available whereby a number on the patient's band is also attached to the specimen, request form, and eventual blood product to be transfused. Bar-coding technology has been applied to patient identification systems and has been implemented in many laboratories.

The sample must be labeled at the bedside. To prevent a possible sample mix-up, prelabeled tubes should never be used. The label must include first and last name of recipient; unique identification number; date of collection; and signature, initials, or a method to identify the phlebotomist. The label must also be legible and indelible (Fig. 9.5).

Accurate patient identification is a fundamental practice for patient safety. The majority of hemolytic transfusion reactions occur due to misidentification of patients or sample labeling errors.[7]

Good laboratory practice recommends labeling blood sample tubes in the presence of the patient.

TABLE 9.4	Steps in Compatibility Testing

- Accurate patient (recipient) identification
- Proper sample collection, labeling, and handling
- Review of recipient's past blood bank records
- ABO and D phenotyping, antibody screening, and infectious disease testing on donor units
- ABO and D phenotyping and antibody screening of recipient; crossmatch of recipient's sample with donor units
- If the recipient possesses a clinically significant antibody, donor units are screened for the corresponding antigen and crossmatched using antigen-negative units
- Tagging, inspecting, and issuing blood products
- Re-identification of recipient before transfusion
- Careful observation of recipient's vital signs after transfusion and monitoring of posttransfusion hematocrit and hemoglobin levels for efficacy of transfusion

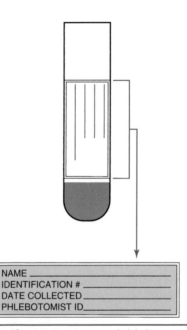

NAME _____
IDENTIFICATION # _____
DATE COLLECTED_____
PHLEBOTOMIST ID_____

Fig. 9.5 Recipient sample labeling.

Information on the label must match the request form. This request form must also include the types of blood products being ordered and the requesting physician's name. The request form is in effect a prescription. Other useful information on the request form includes the location of the patient, sex, diagnosis, date of the proposed transfusion, and priority indicator (eg, routine, stat, transfuse on date, preoperative, standby).

Sample Collection Tubes

Patient samples for compatibility testing may be serum or plasma.[7] Plasma samples are preferred. Plain tubes with a red top (no anticoagulant) and purple or pink top (ethylenediaminetetraacetic acid [EDTA]) tubes are most commonly used. Many laboratories have adopted the pink-stoppered blood collection tubes for blood bank samples. The collection tubes are spray-coated with K_2EDTA and provide anticoagulated blood with plasma and red cells for testing. Historically, any form of anticoagulated blood sample was discouraged for compatibility testing. Anticoagulants inhibit complement protein activation. In addition, there is the possible presence of fibrin in plasma. Most clinically significant antibodies are now recognized not to depend solely on the presence of complement for their detection. Considerable time can be saved in emergencies in not waiting for a blood specimen to clot, especially when most crossmatches are performed at immediate-spin, where fibrin is less likely to interfere.

Age of Sample

Samples should be collected no more than 3 days (date of draw is day 0) of the scheduled transfusion if the patient has been transfused or was pregnant in the previous 3 months or the history is unclear or unknown.[4] This practice ensures that the sample used in testing reflects the recipient's current immunologic status. Many laboratories prefer to standardize their operations by setting a 3-day limit for all pretransfusion testing samples.

If a reliable history exists of no recent pregnancy or transfusion and no current or past unexpected antibodies, the sample may be kept and reused. This practice allows preoperative testing before a patient's surgical procedure and crossmatching at the time of need. In some settings where patients are being repeatedly transfused, new samples may be required for these patients (eg, every other day). This decision must be made after considering the volume of extra work and expense entailed compared with the number of new transfusion-induced antibodies detected.

Considerations in Sample Collection and Appearance

Serum or plasma hemolyzed during the collection process is an unacceptable specimen, and the sample should be collected again. Mechanical hemolysis may be caused by the use of small-gauge needles, trauma to a vein, the forcing of blood into the tube, or the further addition of blood to a partially clotted sample. Mechanical hemolysis can mask the detection of antibody-induced hemolysis (a positive reaction in some examples of ABO, P1, Lewis, Kidd, or Vel system antibodies).

Samples potentially diluted with intravenous fluids (eg, Ringer's lactate) are also unacceptable because of the chance of missing a weak antibody or the inducement of false-positive reactions caused by the molecules in the intravenous fluid. Blood samples for the blood bank and all other laboratory testing should always be collected from below an intravenous site, preferably from a different vein and ideally from the other arm. If the intravenous site is the only site for drawing blood, the intravenous catheter should be turned off and flushed with saline, and the first 5 to 10 mL of blood should be discarded.

Comparison with Previous Records

Before beginning any testing, technologists need to perform a record check for the patient. The record check searches and reviews historical information relative to the patient. This information includes previous ABO/Rh results, presence of clinically significant antibodies, difficulties in blood typing, any adverse reaction to transfusion, any special transfusion requirements, and any special unit availability (autologous or directed). The AABB *Standards*[4] requires comparison of results of current blood typing with the historical record of ABO and D phenotyping. It also mandates that all previous records be consulted for typing anomalies, presence of clinically significant antibodies, significant transfusion reactions, and special transfusion requirements. Inconsistencies or problems must be investigated and resolved before proceeding with transfusion.

Repeat Testing of Donor Blood

The transfusing facility is responsible for confirming the correct ABO labeling of all donor blood (whole blood or RBCs) received from the donor center if the units were not previously confirmed. The AABB *Standards*[4] dictates that the ABO phenotype must be retested on all units and that the D typing must be retested on all units labeled "negative." For instance, if a D-negative unit was mislabeled D-positive, the unit would be transfused to a D-positive person, and no clinical harm would result. However, if a D-positive unit was mislabeled D-negative, the unit would be selected for a D-negative recipient and could produce an immunization to the D antigen in this individual. Testing for the weak D antigen is not required in repeat testing of donor blood. Retyping is performed by making a red cell suspension of the donor blood from a segment attached to the donor bag. Records of these repeat tests must be kept for 5 years. Any discrepancy with the typing on the label must result in rejection of the unit and notification to the collecting facility. Plasma and platelet products do not require retyping. Fig. 9.6 shows RBC donor units with attached segments.

Patient samples and a segment from the donor unit used for crossmatching must be stored for at least 7 days after transfusion in the event that a transfusion reaction investigation is necessary.[4]

Hemolyzed or lipemic samples create difficulty in the interpretation of crossmatch results.

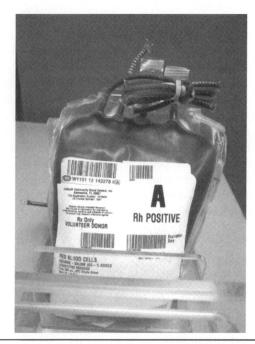

Fig. 9.6 Labeled donor RBC units with attached segments. The segments are attached to each donor unit and are used as a sample of the donor unit RBCs for crossmatch and retyping.

ABO phenotype, ABO type, and ABO group are terms used to describe the detectable ABO red cell antigens. These terms are used interchangeably in the blood bank literature.

Pretransfusion Testing on Recipient Sample

Pretransfusion testing on the recipient's sample includes the determination of the patient's ABO and D phenotype, an antibody screen, and a crossmatch.

ABO and D Phenotype of Recipient

The recipient's ABO and D phenotype is established to transfuse ABO-compatible and D-compatible blood components. For ABO group determination, the recipient's red cells are tested with commercial anti-A and anti-B reagents. The recipient's serum or plasma is also tested with reagent red cells, group A_1 and group B. Any ABO discrepancy should be resolved before any blood is transfused. If transfusion is required before resolution of the ABO discrepancy, group O RBCs should be administered.

For D antigen typing, the recipient's red cells must be tested with commercial anti-D reagent with appropriate observations or controls to avoid a false-positive interpretation. In D phenotyping discrepancies, the recipient should be transfused with D-negative RBCs until the D phenotype has been established. Weak D testing on a recipient is not necessary.[4] The transfusion of D-negative RBCs to recipients of the weak D phenotype causes no deleterious effects. Some transfusion services perform weak D testing on recipient samples to identify patients who can be transfused with D-positive blood components and to conserve the D-negative blood components. Routine testing for other Rh antigens is not necessary.

Antibody Detection Test

The recipient is also tested for expected and unexpected antibodies before components containing red cells are issued for transfusion. Antibody screening methods should detect as many clinically significant antibodies as possible and as few clinically insignificant antibodies as possible. The antibody screening procedure should be completed in a timely manner to prevent delays of transfusion. The AABB *Standards*[4] requires the use of unpooled reagent red cells in antibody screen methods used for the detection of clinically significant antibodies in recipients' samples.

Crossmatch Test

As stated earlier, a crossmatch must be performed for RBC transfusions, with the exception of circumstances requiring an urgent need for blood. The crossmatch uses

TABLE 9.5	ABO Compatibility for Whole Blood, Red Blood Cells, and Plasma Transfusions		
RECIPIENT	DONOR		
ABO PHENOTYPE	WHOLE BLOOD	RED BLOOD CELLS	PLASMA
A	A	A, O	A, AB
B	B	B, O	B, AB
AB	AB	AB, A, B, O	AB
O	O	O	O, A, B, AB

procedures to demonstrate ABO incompatibility and clinically significant antibodies to red cell antigens.

Selection of ABO Donor Units

Whenever possible, recipients should receive ABO-identical blood. If the component for transfusion contains 2 mL or more of red cells, the donor's red cells must be ABO compatible with the recipient's plasma.[7] In the transfusion of plasma products, the ABO antibodies in the transfused plasma should be compatible with the recipient's red cells. Table 9.5 reviews compatibility of ABO grouping for whole blood, RBCs, and plasma.

Selection of D Antigen Donor Units

D-positive blood components should be selected for D-positive recipients. D-negative recipients should receive RBCs that are D-negative to avoid immunization to the D antigen, especially women of childbearing age. If the recipient has a clinically unexpected antibody, the recipient should receive antigen-negative blood. If there is difficulty obtaining crossmatch-compatible donor units, the medical director should be involved in the decision to pursue transfusion.

Selection of Antigen-Negative Donor Units for Recipients with Antibodies

The provision of antigen-negative donor units for transfusion to recipients with blood group antibodies may be difficult, expensive, and unnecessary. Poole and Daniels[8] proposed a policy for the selection of suitable donor units for recipients with blood group antibodies using information about the antibody's history of clinical significance and availability of compatible blood. Antigen-negative RBC donor units were recommended for ABO, Rh, Kell, Duffy, and Kidd blood group system antibodies, anti-Co[a] and anti-Vel. Donor units that are crossmatch compatible in the antiglobulin phase were recommended for recipients with anti-A1, anti-P1, anti-Lu[a], anti-Do[a], anti-Do[b], and anti-Co[b]. The transfusion of donor units that are crossmatch compatible with anti-M and anti-N is a generally accepted practice, provided the antibodies are not reactive at 37° C. Antigen-negative donor units are not required.

> See Chapter 4 for the calculations of the number of donors required to find antigen-negative–compatible units for a patient with multiple antibodies.

Tagging, Inspecting, Issuing, and Transfusing Blood Products

When the appropriate compatibility testing has been completed and the unit or units are suitable for transfusion, a tag is produced and attached to each donor unit. The donor unit tag must clearly state the patient's full name and identification number, name of the product, donor number, expiration date, ABO and D phenotype of the unit, interpretation of the crossmatching test (if performed), and identity of the person doing the testing or selection of the unit (Table 9.6). If compatibility testing is incomplete or shows incompatibility, this information must be indicated in bold on the tag.

A physician's order for blood or a blood product must be on file for the transfusion to occur. Ideally, the person requesting the donor unit presents a transfusion request form to the blood bank staff indicating the desired product and the intended recipient. This form is checked carefully and independently by both persons against the unit tag. The unit tag information is also checked against the unit label. The expiration date is carefully checked to ensure that outdated units are not issued. The unit is visually checked for discoloration,

TABLE 9.6	Requirements for the Tag on the Crossmatched Donor Unit

- Intended recipient's two independent identifiers
- Unique donor unit number or pool number
- Interpretation of compatibility tests, if performed

From Levitt J, editor: *Standards for blood banks and transfusion services,* ed 29, Bethesda, MD, 2014, AABB.

TABLE 9.7	Requirements for the Issue of Blood and Blood Components

- Physician's order
- Intended recipient's two independent identifiers, ABO group, and D phenotype
- Donation identification number, donor ABO group, and, if required, the Rh type
- Interpretation of crossmatch tests, if performed
- Blood product expiration date and, if applicable, time
- Special transfusion requirements, if applicable
- Date and time of issue

From Levitt J, editor: *Standards for blood banks and transfusion services,* ed 29, Bethesda, MD, 2014, AABB.

> The visual check of the donor unit before issue is an important step. Bacterial contamination of units or traumatized donor units can be detected.

clots, or other abnormal appearance. These checks are documented with the name of the person issuing the unit and the person picking it up. The date and time of issue and the unit's ultimate destination are also documented (Table 9.7). After the transfusion is complete, a copy of the tag is attached to the patient's chart.

Patient identification is crucial for safe transfusion and is the ultimate responsibility of the nursing or medical personnel who hang the unit. A wristband with the patient's full name and identification number must be on the patient and must exactly match the information on the unit tag. Commercial transfusion identification tagging systems use a separate wristband with special numbers to be attached to the patient specimen and any units prepared on the basis of that specimen. This system can be useful to ensure correct patient identification, and bar-code features and handheld scanners provide even greater accuracy.

Once issued for transfusion, blood products may be returned to the transfusion service for storage if they are not going to be used immediately. Unmonitored refrigerators in patient care areas should never be used for storage of blood products. Reissuing of blood products from the transfusion service is permitted if the closure has not been entered and the unit has not exceeded the upper or lower temperature conditions for that product (1° C to 10° C for RBCs). RBCs, if not stored in a monitored refrigerator, should be returned to the transfusion service within 30 minutes to allow reissue.

SECTION 3
COMPATIBILITY TESTING SPECIAL TOPICS

URGENT REQUIREMENT FOR BLOOD AND BLOOD COMPONENTS

In urgent transfusion situations, the patient's physician must look at the risks of transfusing uncrossmatched or partially crossmatched blood versus a delay in providing blood as compatibility testing is completed. If the blood is released before the completion of testing, the patient's record must contain the physician's signed statement indicating the clinical situation was urgent and required release of uncrossmatched blood.[4] Provision must be made by the transfusion service to expedite the release of blood in cases of life-threatening hemorrhage before completion of the usual compatibility tests. The transfusion service personnel would issue uncrossmatched group O RBCs if the patient's ABO group is unknown. D-negative blood is also provided if the D type is unknown. D-negative RBCs are critical if the patient is a woman of childbearing age.

TABLE 9.8	Urgent Requirement for Blood and Blood Components

- Release signed by physician
- Tag on donor unit indicating emergency release: compatibility or infectious disease testing was not completed at the time of issue
- Patient name and identifiers
- Donor unit number(s), ABO and D phenotype, expiration date
- Retain segments from units for crossmatching
- Name of person issuing units

If possible, a pretransfusion sample and recent transfusion history are highly desirable. However, obtaining such a sample is complicated if the patient received donor units that were ABO compatible (eg, group O, D-negative) but not identical at another facility. Because the chaotic atmosphere of an emergency situation increases the likelihood of making errors such as mislabeling or obtaining suboptimal specimens, personnel responsible for obtaining the blood bank sample must remain focused on the task of proper identification of the patient and acquisition of an adequate specimen.

After the specimen is in the blood bank, the most important test to complete is ABO and D phenotyping so that ABO- and Rh-compatible blood can be issued. The recipient's past records should also be consulted at the outset to provide a check on the ABO and D phenotype and to acquaint personnel with knowledge of any antibodies. Records alone (without current typing) may not be used as a basis for issuing blood. While these procedures are being performed, only group O, D-negative RBCs or group AB plasma should be issued. If group O, D-negative RBCs are in short supply, they should be reserved preferentially for emergency release to women younger than or of childbearing age. Group O, D-positive RBCs may be substituted for emergency release to men and to women older than childbearing age. When the phenotype is determined and confirmed, ABO-identical blood products should be issued. If an antibody is noted in the record, and if time permits, the RBC products should be screened for the corresponding antigen before being issued.

The second most important test to complete is the antibody screen. Crossmatching may be initiated simultaneously. If a positive reaction is noted at any step of the antibody screen, antibody identification procedures and antiglobulin crossmatches (on the issued units and additional ones) should be initiated at once. The patient's physician must be advised of the problem. Further transfusion should be delayed, if possible, until the problem is identified and safe units can be provided, but the patient's physician must make this decision. "The risk that the transfused unit might be incompatible may be judged to be less than the risk of depriving the patient of oxygen-carrying capacity."[9]

The AABB *Standards*[4] stipulate that detailed records be kept of the emergency release of blood products. These records must include the patient's full name, unique identifiers, ABO and D phenotype, list of all issued units, name of the person who issued them, and name of the physician who requested emergency release of blood (Table 9.8). The AABB *Standards* and the FDA *Code of Federal Regulations* (606.151) require that the physician sign a release. Although this step can wait until after the emergency, the physician should understand that it is his or her ultimate responsibility. In addition, the tag or label on each unit that was issued uncrossmatched must include a conspicuous indication that the unit was issued that way. Segments must be pulled from the donor bags as soon as possible before they are issued and must be placed in tubes labeled with the donor unit number for subsequent crossmatching.

During the acute emergency, the blood bank personnel should "stay ahead" by crossmatching additional RBC units, preparing platelets, and thawing cryoprecipitate and frozen plasma in anticipation of need by (and in consultation with) the team caring for the patient. If the patient dies as a result of the emergency, remaining compatibility testing may be waived or abbreviated at the discretion of the transfusion service physician. Testing should be complete enough to show that the death was unrelated to the transfusion of uncrossmatched blood.

In times of urgent transfusion, the blood bank personnel and the emergency staff must be operating as one team to provide the best patient care.

SELECTION OF BLOOD PRODUCTS AFTER NON-GROUP-SPECIFIC TRANSFUSION

After transfusion of blood products that were not ABO and Rh identical, as in an emergency situation, when can the patient begin to receive ABO and Rh type-specific blood? When the blood bank receives a sample for phenotyping, the patient can receive transfusions of ABO and Rh type-specific blood.[7] Because group O RBC units contain minimal amounts of anti-A and anti-B, the switch to ABO-identical RBCs is low risk to the patient. If passively acquired anti-A and anti-B are demonstrated in the patient's reverse grouping, transfusion with RBCs lacking the corresponding ABO antigen is recommended.[7] Passively acquired ABO antibodies may demonstrate after the transfusion of large volumes of blood, as in a massive transfusion. The patient may have a positive DAT due to this phenomenon. In addition, small children and infants can demonstrate passively acquired ABO antibodies after transfusion.

Regarding the D phenotype of blood products, D-negative RBCs should be selected in the following situations:

- D phenotype is not known
- Patient is a female of childbearing age
- Patient is demonstrating anti-D or has a previous history of anti-D

PRETRANSFUSION TESTING FOR NON–RED BLOOD CELL PRODUCTS

Plasma: blood component prepared from whole blood that contains only the plasma portion of whole blood and is frozen after separation

Platelets: a concentrate of platelets separated from a single unit of whole blood; should contain a minimum of 5.5×10^{10} platelets

Cryoprecipitate: blood component recovered from a controlled thaw of fresh frozen plasma; the cold-insoluble precipitate is rich in coagulation factor VIII, von Willebrand factor, factor XIII, and fibrinogen

Apheresis platelets: apheresis procedure in which the platelets are removed from a donor and the remaining red cells and plasma are returned

Granulocyte concentrates: blood component collected by cytapheresis; contain a minimum of 1.0×10^{10} granulocytes

Plasma, platelets, and **cryoprecipitate** contain almost no red cells and do not need to be crossmatched. **Apheresis platelets** and especially **granulocyte concentrates** may contain red cells, but they need to be crossmatched only if the unit contains more than 2 mL of red cells.[4]

The serum or plasma of the donors of non–red cell products has been thoroughly screened for antibodies by the blood centers. Therefore a repeat antibody screening and ABO and D phenotype for these products by the transfusing facility are not required. Products containing a large volume of plasma must be selected on the basis of ABO serum compatibility with the recipient. Cryoprecipitate and platelets may be transfused with combinations of ABO-compatible units and units that are not ABO compatible if the cumulative transfused volume is not large. For example, a group A recipient may receive a mixture of group A and group O platelets for transfusion. The transfusion of platelets with the same ABO phenotype as the patient may increase platelet survival rates in vivo.

In the transfusion of plasma, the D antigen is not important for compatibility because Rh antigens are found only on the red cells and are absent from plasma products. ABO antibodies are more important in the transfusion of plasma. Unlike the ABO antibodies, anti-D is not a non–immune-stimulated red cell antibody.

BLOOD INVENTORY MANAGEMENT

Each transfusion service requires a blood inventory of ABO- and Rh-compatible units to meet the hospital's routine needs and emergency situations while minimizing blood component expiration dates. This section describes some strategies used to improve inventory utilization.

Surgical Blood-Ordering Practices

Surgical ordering practices will have an impact on the component outdate rates. When donor units are crossmatched for surgical procedures, the units' shelf-lives are shortened if the surgeon does not use the blood in surgery. These units could have been available for other patient needs.

To aid in better practices for blood utilization, many transfusion services have used statistical measures of average blood use for certain surgical procedures in their own facility to develop a blood strategy for scheduled surgery. A list of all surgical procedures performed in the facility is first drawn up, and then actual usage figures for each procedure are compiled. The average number of blood units used is then determined. The surgeons, anesthesiologists, and blood transfusion physicians agree on this number

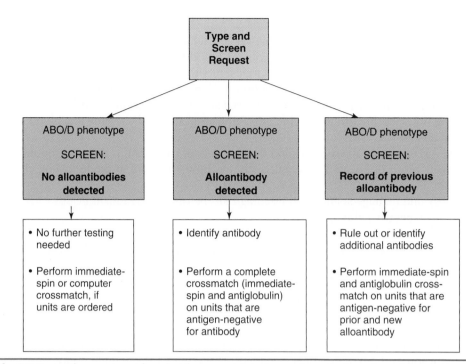

Fig. 9.7 Type and screen request flow chart for appropriate testing requirements of samples and the selection of the crossmatch procedure.

as the standard blood order for the stated procedure. For example, a procedure for a total hip replacement is determined to require a preoperative order of 5 units of RBCs. Such a list is called the *Maximum Surgical Blood Order Schedule (MSBOS)*. The MSBOS may also be used as a guide for the number of autologous units the patient may donate before surgery.

Type and Screen Protocols

If the average use for a particular surgical procedure is less than 1 unit of RBCs, many transfusion services decide that these are the cases where only a type and screen (T/S) is performed (unless clinically significant antibodies are found).[7] If blood is subsequently needed, the T/S specimen is retrieved. Donor units are crossmatched by the immediate-spin or computer crossmatch technique. Some institutions initially perform only a T/S on all preoperative patients and crossmatch (immediate-spin or computer) only when the blood is ordered. This policy allows greater inventory availability. The physician must be able to trust that blood is always issued quickly if the T/S protocol is used. If clinically significant antibodies are or were ever present, antigen-negative units should be identified and reserved or crossmatched.

These approaches are intended to conserve blood inventory by not "tying up" excess numbers of units unlikely to be transfused. Sufficient blood supply to cover unexpected needs must be readily available, although units may not be crossmatched until the time of issue. A flow chart for T/S testing decision making is outlined in Fig. 9.7.

INTRODUCTION TO PATIENT BLOOD MANAGEMENT

What Is Patient Blood Management?

Patient blood management (PBM) is a patient-centered, multidisciplinary, evidence-based approach to using blood products.[7] PBM identifies patients at risk of transfusion and provides a management plan to reduce or eliminate the risk of anemia and the need for allogeneic transfusion. Subsequently, the strategy also reduces the inherent risks associated with transfusion, blood inventory pressures, and the rising costs associated with transfusion.

Blood management is a collaborative effort between blood centers and hospital partners to enhance management of the blood supply and improve the availability of products for the community. The concepts of patient blood management developed due to advances in medical science and technology, which are changing the way blood is used. Many surgical procedures that required blood transfusions in the past no longer require transfusion due to less invasive surgical methods. In addition to technology, more information is now available that supports a "less is more" mentality, which means patients who are in need of blood may not need as many units as previously thought. The changing times are breathing new life into PBM programs and enabling less blood usage by hospitals.

PBM has expanded in scope beyond the surgical approach and is now a component of the patient's overall hospital experience. PBM is now indicated in the following clinical situations[7]:
1. Identify and manage anemia and bleeding risks before any treatment begins
2. Use intraoperative blood recovery in surgical procedures
3. Review how blood products are used and provide feedback to physicians
4. Employ strategies during intensive care and postoperative care that decrease need for transfusions
5. Provide education on PBM to health care providers

What Is the Rationale for Patient Blood Management?

The driving forces for the PBM movement include the risk of clerical errors, errors in patient identification, the threat of a new transfusion-transmitted pathogen, evidence of transfusion and adverse patient outcomes, shrinking of the eligible donor pool, and increased health care costs.[10]

In 2011, more than 13.5 million RBC transfusions were provided in U.S. hospitals. The associated cost for the transfusions was estimated at $10 billion.[12]

Allogeneic blood transfusion has been accepted as a lifesaving measure. However, the risks of transfusion, both infectious and noninfectious, are of concern to clinicians. Recent research on allogeneic blood transfusions has demonstrated a direct association between the use of blood products and the frequency of perioperative complications. These conditions included an increased risk of myocardial infarction, infection, transfusion-associated circulatory overload (TACO), or transfusion-related acute lung injury (TRALI). These events were linked to a prolonged stay in intensive care units and/or in the hospital and to an increased mortality.[11] Concerns relative to the safety, efficacy, and supply of allogeneic blood require careful consideration in transfusion practices. As a result, PBM's strategy to address anemia and decrease bleeding with reduced transfusions and improved patient outcomes has become a timely topic in transfusion medicine. Scan the QR code to read more about PBM.

CHAPTER SUMMARY

This chapter emphasizes that the process of compatibility testing extends beyond the boundaries of the transfusion service. The procedure begins and ends with the most important individual in the process: the recipient of the transfusion. Responsibilities of blood bank personnel include evaluating, monitoring, and following transfusion procedures and policies to meet the needs of these patients.

Process of Compatibility Testing

Patient:	✓	Accurate identification Two independent identifiers are required for pretransfusion samples.
Patient:	✓	Proper sample collection and handling Label each blood sample tube in patient's presence.
Patient:	✓	Review of past blood bank records Has the patient been transfused or pregnant within the previous 3 months?
Patient:	✓	ABO and D type, antibody screen, crossmatch ABO and D typing results on a current sample must be compared with previous blood bank records, if available.
Donor:	✓	ABO and D type, antibody screen, and infectious disease testing

Donor:	✓	Double-check of unit's ABO and D typing label
Patient:	✓	Tagging, inspecting, and issuing blood products
Patient:	✓	Accurate reidentification and monitoring of transfusion

Crossmatch Procedure

The crossmatch procedure combines serum or plasma from the recipient with red cells from the donor.

- **Compatible crossmatch:** No agglutination and no hemolysis at any phase of testing. Donor unit can be transfused.
- **Incompatible crossmatch:** Hemolysis or agglutination at any phase of testing. Donor unit is not acceptable for transfusion.

Crossmatch Types

- **Serologic crossmatch:** Uses procedures to demonstrate ABO incompatibility and clinically significant antibodies to red cell antigens. There are two types of serologic crossmatches: immediate-spin for ABO compatibility and antiglobulin for clinically significant antibodies.
- **Computer crossmatch:** Uses computer to make the final check of ABO compatibility in the selection of appropriate donor units. Recipient cannot possess clinically significant antibodies in the current or any previous sample.

Urgent Requirement for Blood and Blood Components

In emergency situations, group O RBCs are issued uncrossmatched if the patient's ABO group is unknown. D-negative blood is also provided if the D type is unknown, especially if the patient is a woman of childbearing age.

Selection of Blood Products after Non-Group-Specific Transfusion

When the blood bank receives a sample and the phenotype is determined, the patient can receive transfusions specific for the patient's ABO and Rh phenotype. This recommendation holds as long as no passively acquired ABO antibodies are present in the reverse grouping.

Pretransfusion Testing for Non–Red Blood Cell Products

- Frozen plasma, platelets, and cryoprecipitate contain almost no red cells and do not need to be crossmatched.
- Apheresis platelets and especially granulocyte concentrates may contain red cells, but they need to be crossmatched only if the unit contains more than 2 mL of red cells.

Blood Inventory Management

The MSBOS is a list of blood component requirements for scheduled surgery that is based on statistical measures of average blood use for certain surgical procedures in a facility. If the average use for a particular surgical procedure is less than 1 unit of RBCs, the pretransfusion order is a T/S unless clinically significant antibodies are found. If blood is subsequently needed, the T/S specimen is used to crossmatch units by the immediate-spin or computer crossmatch technique.

Patient Blood Management

PBM is the timely use of safe and effective medical and surgical techniques designed to prevent anemia and decrease bleeding in an effort to improve patient outcome.

CRITICAL THINKING EXERCISES

Exercise 9.1

A 60-year-old woman with anemia is admitted to the hospital. Her hematocrit is 17%, and she has been experiencing subtle gastrointestinal bleeding over many weeks. Her physician requests 4 units of RBCs for transfusion. The patient phenotypes as group AB, D-positive. Her antibody screen is negative on the sample drawn in the emergency department, but her records indicate a previously detected anti-E. Only 3 group AB, D-positive RBC units are available in the blood bank's inventory. The blood bank's inventory contains RBC donor units of all ABO and D types.

1. What ABO phenotype should be selected for the fourth donor unit? State your reasons for this choice.
2. What type of crossmatches should be performed?
3. Is any additional screening required on the donor units before crossmatching?

Exercise 9.1 Additional Testing

After antigen screening of the 4 units of RBCs for the E antigen, one of the group AB, D-positive units is E-positive.

4. How many donor units should be screened to find the 4 units ordered plus 2 more units to hold in reserve for the patient?

Exercise 9.1 Additional Testing

Having located 6 E-negative donor units, you perform crossmatches on the units. One of the units is incompatible in the antiglobulin phase (2+ reactivity). The physician is becoming insistent on beginning the transfusion because the patient is having some shortness of breath.

5. How do you respond to the physician's request?
6. List several reasons to explain the incompatible donor unit.
7. What additional testing do you perform?

Exercise 9.1 Additional Testing

Antibody identification testing reveals no detectable antibodies, and the autologous control is negative. Additional testing revealed a positive DAT on the donor unit.

8. What is the usual transfusion service policy on donor units with a positive DAT?

STUDY QUESTIONS

1. What test detects serologic incompatibility between donor RBCs and recipient serum?
   a. antibody screen
   b. crossmatch
   c. DAT
   d. autologous control

2. What incompatibilities are detected in the antiglobulin phase of a crossmatch?
   a. IgM alloantibodies in recipient's serum
   b. ABO incompatibilities
   c. IgG alloantibodies in recipient's serum
   d. room-temperature incompatibilities

3. What tests are included in compatibility testing?
   a. blood typing of recipient
   b. antibody screening of recipient
   c. crossmatch
   d. all of the above

4. One group B, D-positive unit of RBCs is received in the transfusion service. What repeat testing is required on this donor unit?
   a. ABO typing only
   b. ABO and D typing
   c. ABO, D, and weak D typing
   d. ABO and D typing; antibody screen

5. What ABO and D types are selected for RBC units issued to a patient in emergency release?
   a. group O, D-positive
   b. group O, D-negative

c. group A, D-positive

d. group AB, D-negative

6. What antibodies are detected in the immediate-spin crossmatch?

   a. Rh antibodies

   b. high-titer, low-avidity antibodies

   c. ABO antibodies

   d. Kell antibodies

For questions 7 and 8, use the following information. Current pretransfusion testing on John Smith reveals a negative antibody screen with a previous history of anti-K. He is group A, D-positive.

7. Which of the following crossmatch procedures is performed to identify compatible units?

   a. immediate-spin crossmatch

   b. electronic crossmatch

   c. antiglobulin crossmatch

   d. none of the above

8. Given the following inventory, which donor unit should be selected for crossmatching?

   a. group A, D-positive, K+k+

   b. group A, D-negative, K–k+

   c. group O, D-positive, K+k–

   d. group O, D-negative, K+k–

9. What information is required by AABB Standards for a labeled blood sample for the blood bank?

   a. name

   b. name, unique identification number, date of collection

   c. name, unique identification number, date of collection, physician name

   d. two independent identifiers

10. Which of the following products is crossmatched with the recipient if the unit contains greater than 2 mL of RBCs?

   a. granulocyte concentrates

   b. plasma

   c. platelets

   d. cryoprecipitate

11. A patient who phenotypes as group AB, D-negative requires 1 unit of plasma. Which of the following units of plasma would be best for transfusion?

   a. group A, D-negative

   b. group B, D-positive

   c. group AB, D-positive

   d. group O, D-negative

12. A donor's RBC phenotype gave the following results when checked in the transfusion service. The donor unit was labeled group A, D-negative. What is the next step?

Red Blood Cells Tested with:		
Anti-A	Anti-B	Anti-D
4+	0	3+

   a. transfuse as a group A, D-negative

   b. transfuse as a group A, D-positive

   c. discard the unit

   d. notify the collection facility

13. An antiglobulin crossmatch is performed with a donor RBC unit. The antiglobulin crossmatch result is a 2+ agglutination reaction. What is the most likely explanation for this result?
    a. recipient's RBCs are demonstrating polyagglutination
    b. recipient's RBCs have a low-frequency antigen
    c. recipient possesses an IgG alloantibody
    d. recipient possesses a cold autoantibody

14. A recipient's antibody screen is negative; however, the recipient is incompatible with the selected donor unit. Select a possible explanation for these results.
    a. recipient RBCs possess a high-frequency antigen
    b. recipient has a warm autoantibody
    c. recipient possesses an antibody to a low-frequency antigen
    d. recipient RBCs possess a cold autoantibody

True or False

____ 15. The computer crossmatch is easily implemented in the blood bank and does not require validation.

____ 16. A crossmatch detects most errors in the identification of antigens on patient's red cells.

____ 17. A crossmatch demonstrating a 2+ agglutination is interpreted as compatible.

____ 18. An immediate-spin crossmatch of a D-positive recipient with a D-negative donor unit is usually incompatible.

____ 19. The computer crossmatch requires two ABO and D phenotypes on the recipient.

____ 20. A crossmatch prevents the immunization of the recipient to blood group antigens.

____ 21. A type and screen protocol provides a mechanism to increase the number of uncrossmatched donor units in inventory.

____ 22. The only component that requires crossmatching is a unit of RBCs.

____ 23. Group O plasma is considered the universal donor of plasma products.

____ 24. A good practice for recipient's sample is to label with full name, a second unique identifier, date collected, and some means of identifying the phlebotomist.

____ 25. If a patient has been pregnant within the last 3 months before transfusion, the pretransfusion sample must be no more than 3 days old at time of intended transfusion.

Answers to Study Questions can be found on page 387.

(e) Additional student resources, including review questions, a laboratory manual, and case studies, can be found on the Evolve website.

REFERENCES

1. Guy LR, Huestis DW, Wilson LR: *Technical methods and procedures*, ed 4, Chicago, 1966, AABB.
2. Oberman HA: The crossmatch. A brief historical perspective, *Transfusion* 21:645, 1981.
3. Spraycar M, editor: *Stedman's medical dictionary*, ed 26, Baltimore, 1995, Williams & Wilkins.
4. Levitt J, editor: *Standards for blood banks and transfusion services*, ed 29, Bethesda, MD, 2014, AABB.
5. Roback JH, editor: *Technical manual*, ed 17, Bethesda, MD, 2011, AABB.
6. Butch SH, Oberman HA: The computer or electronic crossmatch, *Transfus Med Rev* 11:256, 1997.
7. Fung MK, editor: *Technical manual*, ed 18, Bethesda, MD, 2014, AABB.
8. Poole J, Daniels G: Blood group antibodies and their significance in transfusion medicine, *Transfus Med Rev* 21:58, 2007.
9. Vengelen-Tyler V, editor: *Technical manual*, ed 12, Bethesda, MD, 1996, AABB.
10. Hoffmann A, Farmer S, Shander A: Five drivers shifting the paradigm from product-focused transfusion practice to patient blood management, *The Oncologist* 16(Suppl 3):3, 2011.

11. Gombotz H: Patient blood management: a patient-orientated approach to blood replacement with the goal of reducing anemia, blood loss and the need for blood transfusion in elective surgery, *Transfus Med Hemother* 39:67, 2012.
12. Shander A, Hoffmann A, Ozawa S, et al.: Activity-based costs of blood transfusion in surgical patients at four hospitals, *Transfusion* 50:753, 2010.
13. *Guidance for Industry: "Computer Crossmatch" (Computerized Analysis of the Compatibility between the Donor's Cell Type and the Recipient's Serum or Plasma Type)*, April 2011. http://www.fda.gov/ BiologicsBloodVaccines/GuidanceComplianceRegulatoryInformation/Guidances/default.htm Accessed January 2016.

10

BLOOD BANK AUTOMATION FOR TRANSFUSION SERVICES

CHAPTER OUTLINE

LEARNING OBJECTIVES

On completion of this chapter, the reader should be able to:

1. Compare and contrast the forces driving the move to automation in the transfusion service.
2. Identify the potential benefits and challenges associated with change to automation.
3. Define the characteristics of an ideal instrument for blood bank testing.
4. Evaluate a vendor, base technology, and instrument for desired features.
5. Compare and contrast gel technology and solid-phase red cell assays.
6. Compare and contrast the automated platforms available for the transfusion service.
7. Select an automated platform for a transfusion service.
8. Interpret SPRCA and gel technology assays.

INTRODUCTION TO AUTOMATION IN IMMUNOHEMATOLOGY

Automation in immunohematology is not a new concept. In larger blood donor centers, automated blood bank systems have performed donor unit testing for many years. Until more recently, automation was practical only for these donor centers because no technology was available to address the needs of the hospital transfusion services. Advances in test technologies and robotics are opening up new opportunities for automation to meet the requirements of hospital transfusion services and medium-sized blood banks. Instruments are available for handling lower sample volumes and more individualized testing requests. Gel technology and solid-phase red cell assays can be performed on automated platforms. Consequently, automation is more feasible for immunohematology testing performed in multiple settings. Facilities have a selection of instruments to meet their needs. In context with other coincidental driving forces, the time is optimal for medium-sized blood centers and hospital transfusion services to move forward toward automation. As automated platforms are investigated as a potential tool for the improvement of laboratory services, the selection of the appropriate automation platform becomes key in achieving this goal. Targeting the appropriate automated blood bank platform has become a major pursuit for these laboratories.

 A component of the process in the selection of an automated system is an understanding of the answers to the following questions highlighted in this chapter:

- What are the forces driving the trend toward automation in the blood bank?
- What are the benefits and barriers in the adoption of an automated system?

- What are the characteristics of an "ideal" instrument for the blood bank?
- What are the major differences between fully automated and semiautomated blood bank systems?
- What automated technology is available to meet the laboratory's needs?

FORCES DRIVING THE CHANGE TO AUTOMATION

Although other disciplines within the clinical laboratory have been operating in an automated mode for many years, incentives to change to automated testing in the blood bank have received significant attention only more recently. Besides the availability of technology for automated systems, many other factors have been cited as stimulants in the movement toward automation of the blood bank. The movement toward an automated immunohematology laboratory has been attributed to the following contributing external forces[1]:

- Financial environment encouraging new economies
- Pressures to operate more efficiently; trend toward consolidation of hospitals and blood banks
- Higher testing volumes as a result of consolidation
- Compliance with increased regulations
- Standardization of testing and technology within the blood bank
- Shortage of skilled technologists attributed to the presence of fewer training programs in operation and the increase of opportunities in other professional careers
- Reduction in staff positions
- Spectrum of automated systems, with technology capable of automating the reading of reactions
- Increased use of blood bank computer software programs in transfusion services

The combined effect of all of these factors has propelled blood banks, plasma centers, and hospital transfusion services of all sizes to pursue the evaluation of blood bank automation.

BENEFITS AND BARRIERS OF AUTOMATED INSTRUMENTS

In the investigation of any new process, both the positive and the negative aspects of automation need to be taken into consideration. An awareness of the potential benefits and challenges can assist in the planning and implementation of the automated platform.[2]

Potential Benefits

Many potential benefits accompany the switch to automation. These benefits include, but are not limited to the following items.

Opportunity for Reduction in Operating Costs

With the prevalent pressures of cost containment, a major goal in the adoption of an automated system is to save operating funds. These savings may originate from laboratory expenses in labor, reagents and supplies, and biohazardous waste disposal. Labor costs represent a significant portion of laboratory expenses. Laboratory managers are concerned with controlling this cost. The implementation of automation allows a review of staffing pictures, with the potential to decrease the number of full-time equivalent positions for optimal operations. Automation also provides the opportunity to cross-train technologists more readily between the blood bank and other areas of the clinical laboratory, potentially generating economies in labor. The adoption of automation provides opportunities for standardization of all facilities within a health care network. Avoidance of needless waste of reagents and potential savings in this area are achieved with the more efficient usage. Generally, less biohazardous waste is generated, which decreases the volume of disposal waste and its accompanying costs.

Opportunity to Redesign Work Processes and Support Systems

As automated technology is considered, the laboratory is provided an opportunity to question and examine work processes and identify areas for improvement. With an automated system, workflow may be conducive to reengineering with the potential for batch testing. Batch processing of samples saves time, materials, and reagents. More efficient workplace configurations for the workload may also be possible with automated technology. Current staffing configurations may be reviewed and reconfigured in a manner that optimizes use of staff members. Automation reduces hands-on time for the technologist, freeing staff to perform other functions such as the preparation of customized blood products and compliance activities. The concept of work process redesign provides the tools for the successful implementation of these changes.[3]

Opportunity for Increased Productivity

An obvious benefit of automation is the increase in productivity. Testing capacity is increased. Turnaround times for testing are consistent and reliable. Technologists are free to perform other tasks. Automation technology can also be used in the laboratory as a mechanism to generate new revenue growth by adding new business.

Opportunity to Enhance Total Quality

Although saving and generating money are positive motivations for automated technology, the opportunity to improve total quality of testing is a top priority for any laboratory. Tube agglutination tests are associated with limitations related to sample identification, manual reagent and sample dispensing, subjective interpretation, and manual recording of results. Human errors and variations in technique are uncontrollable factors in the overall quality. Automated technology systems containing positive identification with bar coding, automated reagent and sample dispensers, automated readers, and computer interfaces for data generation and documentation eliminate these unpredictable sources of errors. Consequently, through the elimination of variability in the testing process, the end product possesses better precision and accuracy. In addition, the standardization of the automated systems enhances the laboratory's compliance with regulatory bodies.

Potential Challenges

The utopian viewpoint previously discussed is not free of its negative points. Several challenges may be encountered during the transition period.

Concerns among Staff Members

Any change to an existing system generates apprehension for the individuals who operate within it. Although managers may tout the efficiencies of the automated technology, the staff members may view the new instrument as a job replacement. The apprehension of possible position elimination among staff members is an item to be addressed. Involving staff members in the decision-making process and discussing their concerns are keys to the acceptance of the automated technology within the laboratory. Implementation of the automation requires thorough staff training for confidence and competence with the new technology, the operation of the selected instrument, and the computer software and interface.

Cost Justification Issues

The investment in the automated technology requires an initial capital investment for equipment purchases. Because laboratories must make a valid business case before committing to the significant capital investment, management should develop a capital investment plan for presentation to the administration. The plan sets a realistic budget and outlines ways to justify the investment with labor savings, improved efficiency, increased capacity, and improvement in the quality of operations. If the purchase of equipment is undesirable, the laboratory may consider other contractual configurations with the automation suppliers that preclude an initial capital investment.

Automation Implementation Issues

In any work process redesign, the startup of the operation requires an investment of time to accomplish validation protocols, conduct training, and get procedures in order. This step requires good planning because status quo testing is ongoing in a parallel manner. The transition time requires extra staffing coverage to allow the completion of training and validation.

CHARACTERISTICS OF AN IDEAL INSTRUMENT FOR THE BLOOD BANK

If available technology had no limitations, the "ideal" instrument would possess a proven track record with the ability to automate testing, sampling, and data handling. Plapp and Rachel[4] presented some characteristics of the ideal blood grouping analyzer that meet these handling criteria. The automation ideals suggested by Plapp and Rachel,[4] plus other important criteria, are outlined as follows:

1. Criteria important in the automation of testing include:
   - **Random-access** operating mode to accommodate STAT testing
   - Simultaneous multiple analyses to increase **throughput**
   - Extensive testing menu
   - Automated reader for reactions
   - Automatic reagent dispensing and reagent recognition
   - Precision pipetting
   - No excessive **preventive maintenance**
2. Criteria important in the automation of sample handling include:
   - Clot detection
   - Liquid detection
   - Positive identification link between sample tube and test results—bar-code reading of specimen labels
   - Direct closed-tube sampling of whole blood to reduce infectious disease risks
   - Automated sampling of red cells and plasma with precision and negligible carryover
   - Multiple sample tube acceptance
3. Criteria important in the automation of data handling include:
   - Flexible software for blood banks
   - Automatic comparison of current and previous test results to flag discrepancies
   - **Laboratory information system (LIS) interface** capabilities
   - Automatic update of patient files in the LIS

Random-access: system devices or workstations are used for multiple occurrences of a given laboratory operation within the automated procedure

Preventive maintenance: maintenance that maximizes the duration of the equipment or facility, decreases "downtime," and avoids unnecessary costly repairs

Throughput: productivity of a machine, procedure, process, or system over a unit period

Laboratory information system (LIS) interface: allows the direct transfer of test results between the automated test system and an LIS, reducing errors commonly caused by manual transcriptions

SECTION 2

SELECTION OF AUTOMATION TO MEET LABORATORY NEEDS

When considering the switch from manual to automated testing, it is important first to identify the appropriate automation for the facility and how much is needed. The philosophy of "one size fits all" is incorrect. After an evaluation of the automation goals of the facility and the completion of a needs assessment, the laboratory's needs should be compared with the characteristics of the analyzers on the market. In the evaluation of the available systems, several items should be considered, as discussed next.[5]

VENDOR ASSESSMENT

A thorough investigation of the automation vendors is vital to learn what they can do. In considering an automation partner, the laboratory should determine the level of the vendor's automation experience and the vendor's proven record for implementation and customer support. A list of reputable users can be informative. These laboratories can be consulted for information on their experiences with the instrumentation and the vendor.

When selecting an automation partner, a laboratory should also ascertain its requirements in terms of customer support, training, and service. The amount and availability of customer service and technical support are important factors. Is there a guaranteed response time for technical consultation? Is there an adequate training program for the new instrument? Is there customer service available to diagnose instrument problems and a guaranteed on-site supply of essential replacement parts? Important considerations in the selection of an automation vendor are summarized in Table 10.1.

BASE TECHNOLOGY ASSESSMENT

The foundation of any automated platform begins with a proven technology. The reliability and accuracy of the base technology require investigation. Is the technology proven in

TABLE 10.1	Checklist for Vendor Assessment

- Automation experience
- Record of installations
- Customer service
- Training programs
- Technical support—rapid response time
- Preventive maintenance programs
- Instrument validation and performance verification guides

TABLE 10.2	Checklist for Base Technology

- Assay performance
- Technology lends itself to automation
- Total turnaround time
- Workload capacity
- Direct costs for reagents and equipment
- Ease of performance
- Ability to cross-train technologists

terms of desired assay performance? Is the technology easy to use with stable reactions? Does the technology lend itself to automation? Does the technology possess the appropriate test repertoire to meet desired needs? Other considerations in the selection of the appropriate base technology are outlined in Table 10.2.

INSTRUMENT ASSESSMENT

Automation should make it easier to do things the right way and more difficult to do the wrong things.[5] In the assessment of an instrument's performance, the adaptability, availability, and cost effectiveness of the automated platform are important factors to evaluate.

Clinical laboratories must operate in terms of efficiency and economy of effort. Rapid turnaround times for selected samples and the ability to accommodate large-volume batch testing contribute to overall operational efficiency. Instrument maintenance requirements should have a minimal impact on instrument operation. The amount of hands-on time required by the user and the workload flexibility contribute to economy of effort. The user should be able to load a STAT sample efficiently. The instrument should also be able to meet the testing profile requirements of the clinical facility. The instrument's ability to interface with the existing LIS and the level of difficulty and required time and effort to link the two should be thoroughly investigated before purchase. The amount of training required for employees to gain confidence with the new system and the physical plant requirements to accommodate the new analyzer should also be considered.

In addition to demonstrating efficiency and economy of effort, clinical laboratories must operate in a cost-effective manner. Before the purchase of the automated platform, all of the associated immediate and long-term expenses require accounting. Beyond the capital cost of the analyzer itself lies the annual price tag for the operation of the instrument. Items that require attention include the following:
- Costs associated with reagents and disposable items
- Costs for the linkage of the analyzer to blood bank computer software and LIS
- Costs for replacement parts
- Costs to keep equipment in working condition
- Costs for training personnel
- Costs for physical plant modifications to accommodate the analyzer

Table 10.3 provides a checklist for the assessment of blood bank instruments. With so many choices of analyzers, laboratory professionals need to call on their collective management and technical expertise to make the right choice for the future of their institutions. Evaluating the vendor and base technology in conjunction with the instrument provides valuable tools for targeting blood bank automation.

TABLE 10.3 Checklist for Assessment of Instrument	
Item 1. Installation	**Item 3. Test Repertoire**
• Power requirements • Space and drainage requirements • Waste disposal • Heat output • Delivery • Installation assistance	• ABO/Rh phenotyping • Antibody screening/identification • Crossmatch • Direct antiglobulin test • User-defined testing profiles • Accuracy/reproducibility of test results • Errors in ABO/Rh typing • Rate of no type determined • Operator interpretation of unresolved tests
Item 2. Operation and Specifications	
• 24-hour continuous availability • Password-level access controls • Startup/shutdown and maintenance • Instrument throughput • Sample tube capacity • STAT capability • Supported bar-code types • Range of sample types • Range of sample tube sizes • Pediatric sample capability • Minimum sample volume • Liquid-level detection of samples and reagents • Clot detection • Hemolyzed, icteric, and lipemic samples • Carryover • Reagent capacity • Reagent volumes monitored • Reagent waste • Reagent preparation	**Item 4. Maintenance and Reliability**
	• Daily and weekly maintenance • Typical downtime • Maintenance contract • Ambient temperature requirements • Service representative response time • Diagnostic online service
	Item 5. Data Management
	• Windows-based software • Password access to instrument software • Bidirectional interface • Ability to configure screen and reports • Relevant information stored with results • Remote access to database

SECTION 3

AUTOMATED TESTING TECHNOLOGY AND SYSTEMS

Automated testing systems have been developed for solid-phase, gel technology, and microtiter plates. These systems can perform ABO and Rh phenotyping, antibody detection and identification, and crossmatching. The automation presented here is current at the time of publication.

AUTOMATED SYSTEMS FOR SOLID-PHASE RED CELL ADHERENCE ASSAYS

SPRCAs are manufactured by Immucor (Norcross, GA) under the trade name Capture-R Ready-Screen and Capture-R Ready ID. Capture technology is also referred to as SPRCA. The automated instruments that support this technology include Galileo, Galileo ECHO (Fig. 10.1), and NEO (Fig. 10.2). In addition, the Capture Workstation provides a means to perform a manual version of the Capture-R procedure (Fig. 10.3). The automated instruments use microplates and microwell strips to perform various predefined assays, including hemagglutination assays and SPRCAs, which are described subsequently.

Hemagglutination Assays

Hemagglutination assays are used for testing the following:
• ABO and D antigen phenotype
• Antigen typings
• Immediate-spin crossmatch

Hemagglutination assays performed in microplates use the same principle as tube agglutination but in a smaller medium. Bar-coded patient samples, reagents, and microtiter

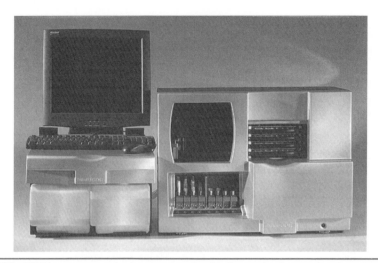

Fig. 10.1 ECHO. ECHO is an automated, microplate-based, solid-phase technology—a bench-top instrument. (Courtesy Immucor, Norcross, GA.)

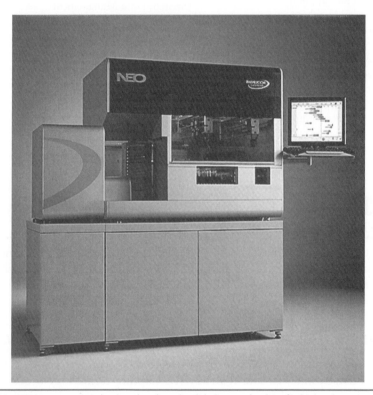

Fig. 10.2 NEO. NEO is an automated, microplate-based, solid-phase technology for high-volume testing. (Courtesy Immucor, Norcross, GA.)

plates provide a means of ensuring positive identification and system verification. After sample and reagent pipetting, the plate is automatically centrifuged and then read by the instrument's camera reader. Agglutination is a positive reaction and is visualized as a button of agglutinated cells. A negative reaction shows no red cell button (Fig. 10.4). Grading and interpretations are made by the instrument, which appear on the computer monitor. The reactions and interpretations must be verified by the operator before releasing results. ABO forward and reversed discrepancies are flagged, and a weak D test can be automatically ordered for D-negative sample results.

The immediate-spin crossmatch can also be performed by automated solid-phase hemagglutination methods and has the advantage of bar-code technology to enhance

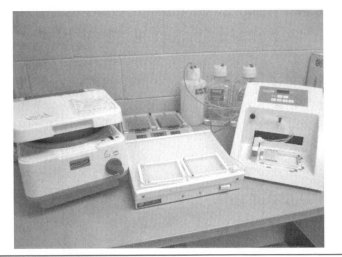

Fig. 10.3 Manual capture workstation for SPRCA.

Results - Group

Sample ID	Interp.	Flags	Mono Ctrl	Anti-A	Anti-B	Anti-D1	Anti-D2	A1 Cells	B Cells
R28786	0 Pos		0	0	0	3+	3+	4+	3+
			◯	◯	◯	●	●	●	●

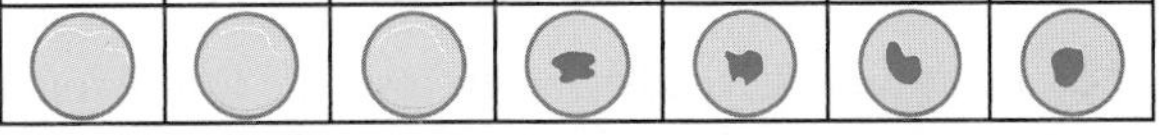

Fig. 10.4 Results and interpretation of an ABO/Rh phenotype. In the hemagglutination test, agglutination is a positive reaction, and no agglutination is a negative reaction. This sample's result is group O, D-positive. (Courtesy Immucor, Norcross, GA.)

patient and donor sample identification and verification. If online with the hospital information system, historical test results can also be checked for ABO/Rh and antibody history results. This technology is especially helpful when performing the computer (electronic) crossmatch.

Solid-Phase Red Cell Adherence Assays

Recall from Chapter 3 that SPRCA technology uses microplate test wells with immobilized reagent red cells or antibodies. The major advantages of solid-phase technology include standardization and stable, defined endpoints, leading to more objective and consistent interpretations of agglutination reactions.

SPRCAs are performed for the following tests:
- Antibody screen
- Antibody identification
- Direct antiglobulin test
- Weak D test
- IgG crossmatch

For SPRCA assays, the antigen or antibody is immobilized to the bottom and sides of the microplate wells. In a direct test, the antibody is fixed to the wells. Antigen-positive red cells from donor or patient sources adhere to the sides and bottom of the wells. Antigen-negative red cells from donor or patient sources settle to the bottom of the well and form a red cell button after centrifugation.

Capture-R Ready-Screen and Capture-R Ready ID are configured as indirect tests. Red cell membranes are bound to the microtiter wells. For antibody screen and identification procedures, pretreated wells are purchased that have red cell membranes bound to the surface of polystyrene microtiter plates as shown in Fig. 10.5. The antigen configurations vary with the lot, similar to standard reagent red cells.

Capture microstrips:

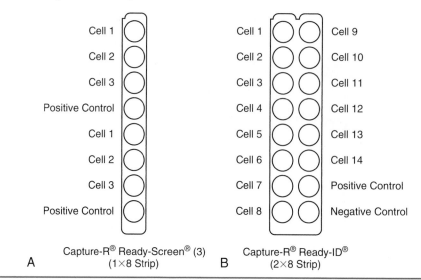

A   Capture-R® Ready-Screen® (3)
(1×8 Strip)

B   Capture-R® Ready-ID®
(2×8 Strip)

Fig. 10.5 Capture Ready-Screen and Ready-ID. Capture Ready-Screen and Ready-ID precoated test wells for antibody screen **(A)** and panel Capture microstrips **(B)** are purchased with red cell membranes preattached to the wells. Pooled and two-cell, three-cell, and four-cell screens are available. Several panel options are also available that provide different antigen configurations, such as D-positive and D-negative panels. (Courtesy Immucor, Norcross, GA.)

For a Capture-R Ready-Screen test, the following steps outline the procedure:

Capture-R Ready-Screen Procedure

1. The first step in testing is the addition of the specially formulated low-ionic-strength saline (LISS) reagent followed by the patient serum.
2. Unknown patient or donor serum is allowed to react at 37° C for a predetermined time.
   This step allows for the capture of IgG antibodies from the patient or donor serum to the red cell membranes.
3. A washing step removes unbound IgG antibodies. Red cells with bound antibodies remain.
4. To detect bound antibody, an IgG-coated indicator red cell is added.
5. The microtiter strips are centrifuged and examined. Centrifugation allows the cells to adhere to the antibody that may be attached to the red cell membrane.

In a positive indirect test, the indicator cells adhere to the sides and bottom of the well. Therefore adherence is a positive reaction. A positive reaction is indicative of a positive antibody screen result. If the cells pellet to the bottom of the well in a tightly packed button, antibodies either were not present or were not specific for the antigen on the well, and the reaction is interpreted as negative. Fig. 10.6 depicts the procedural steps for a Capture-R Ready-Screen test in a pictorial fashion.[6-8] SPRCAs can be used for both indirect and direct antiglobulin tests. An example of antibody screen and antibody identification results and interpretation using the Capture assay system is provided in Fig. 10.7.

SPRCAs use IgG-specific technology to detect clinically significant antibodies and allow processing of hemolyzed, rouleaux, lipemic, or icteric samples. Results are stable for 2 days. Controls are performed on each run to validate the test procedure.

A Capture-R Select Modified assay is available for the immobilization of red cells to the microtiter wells. This assay may be used for antibody screening, selected red cell panels, autologous controls, direct antiglobulin test (DAT), crossmatch, or weak D testing. In this assay, red cells used may be patient cells for a direct antiglobulin test, patient or donor cells for a weak D test, or donor cells for IgG crossmatch. Scan the QR code to SPRCA assays.

AUTOMATED SYSTEMS FOR SOLID-PHASE RED CELL ASSAYS

The TANGO infinity™ and the TANGO optimo™ from BioRad Laboratories, Inc. (Hercules, CA) combine Erythrotype® S and Solidscreen® II with state-of-the-art instrumentation

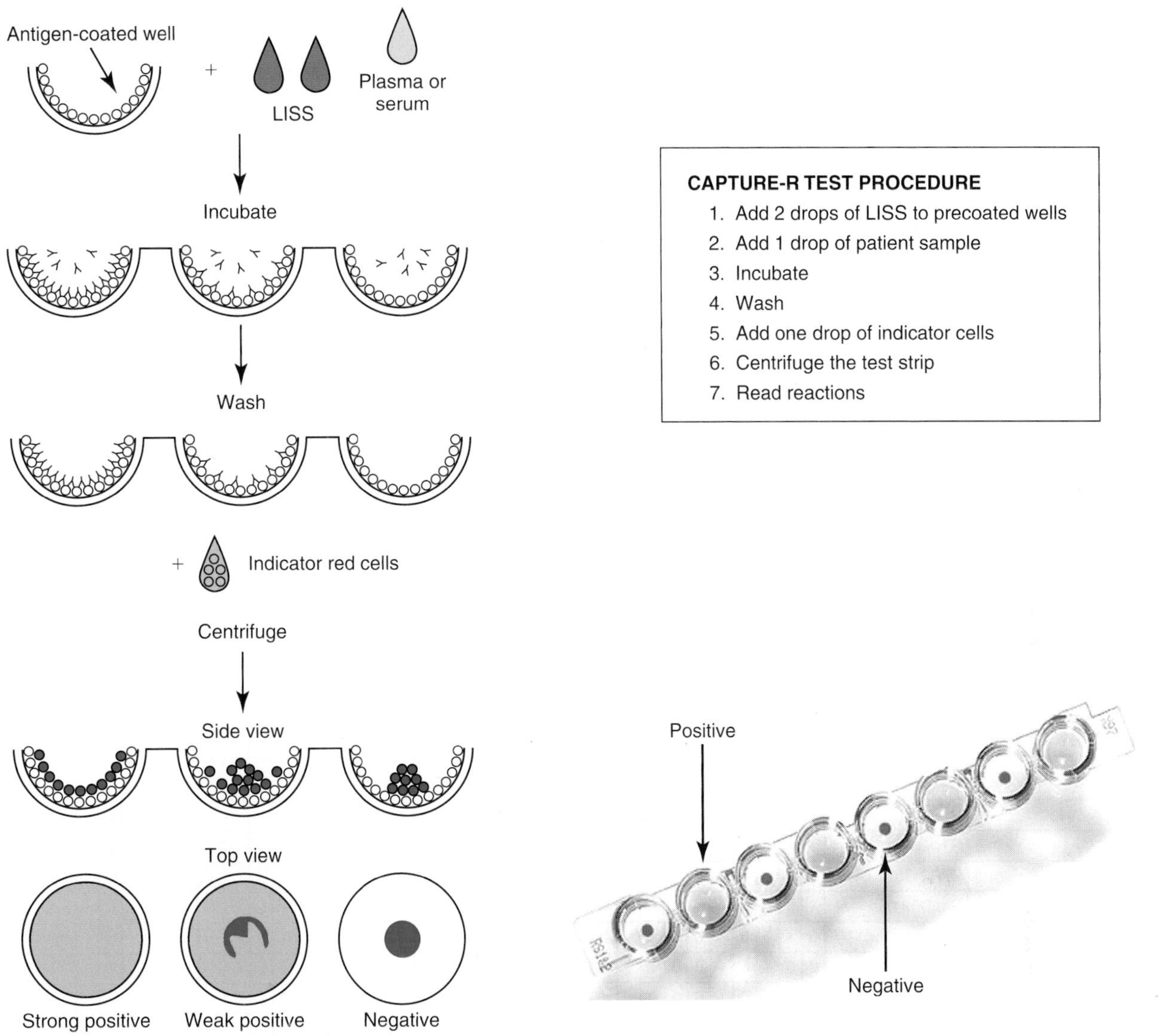
Antigen-coated well
+
LISS
Plasma or serum
Incubate
Wash
+
Indicator red cells
Centrifuge
Side view
Top view
Strong positive
Weak positive
Negative
CAPTURE-R TEST PROCEDURE
1. Add 2 drops of LISS to precoated wells
2. Add 1 drop of patient sample
3. Incubate
4. Wash
5. Add one drop of indicator cells
6. Centrifuge the test strip
7. Read reactions
Positive
Negative

Fig. 10.6 Reactions and interpretation of SPRCA. (Courtesy Immucor, Norcross, Ga.)

to provide laboratories with outstanding productivity, reliability, and lean automation. The TANGO infinity™ and the TANGO optimo™ are automated, random-access systems for blood group serology assays (antibody screen, antibody identification, direct antiglobulin test, IgG crossmatch, weak D, and ABD/Kell red cell phenotype). Similar to the Immucor Capture system, microtiter wells are designed to accommodate either antiglobulin tests or hemagglutination tests (Fig. 10.8).

Solidscreen® II Technology

Solidscreen® II is a solid-phase assay for antiglobulin testing. Unlike the Capture R Technology, the Bio-Rad method uses intact red cells rather than red cell stroma in the solid-phase assays. Red cells are not adhered to the wells. The wells in this assay are precoated with Protein A, a component of the cell wall of *Staphylococcus aureus,* which has a high affinity for the Fc portion of most immunoglobulin classes.[9] The instrument pipettes LISS (MLB2), plasma (or serum), and test erythrocytes into wells coated with Protein A. The wells are incubated at 37° C and then washed with phosphate buffered saline (PBS) to remove any unbound immunoglobulin. After washing, the instrument adds IgG antihuman globulin (AHG) and centrifuges the strip. If antibody was bound to its corresponding antigen during incubation, the IgG AHG Fab portion will bind to the antibody on the red

Results - Screen

Sample ID	Interp.	Flags	Screen 1	Screen 2	Screen 3	Pos Ctrl
R28786	Positive		4+	4+	0	4+

Results - Ready ID

Sample ID	Interp.	Flags	R-ID 1	R-ID 2	R-ID 3	R-ID 4	R-ID 5	R-ID 6	R-ID 7	R-ID 8
R28786	Complete	*	4+	4+	4+	4+	0	0	0	0

Sample ID	Interp.	Flags	R-ID 9	R-ID 10	R-ID 11	R-ID 12	R-ID 13	R-ID 14	Pos Ctrl	Neg Ctrl
R28786	Complete	*	0	0	0	0	0	4+	4+	0

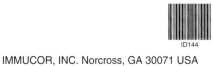

CAPTURE-R READY-ID
Master List

ID144

IMMUCOR, INC. Norcross, GA 30071 USA
US LICENSE NO: 886
LOT NO: ID 144
EXPIRES 2011/08/30

NAME _____
NO. R28786 _____
INSTITUTION _____
BLOOD GROUP _____
ANTIBODY IDENTITY _____
TECH _____ DATE _____

CELL	Special Type	Donor	D	C	c	E	e	V	Cʷ	K	k	Kpᵃ	Kpᵇ	Jsᵃ	Jsᵇ	Fyᵃ	Fyᵇ	Jkᵃ	Jkᵇ	Leᵃ	Leᵇ	P₁	M	N	S	s	Luᵃ	Luᵇ	Xgᵃ	CELL	PATIENT'S TEST RESULTS
1		RzR1 A3481	+	+	0	+	+	0	0	0	+	0	+	0	+	+	+	+	+	0	0	+	0	+	+	0	+	+	1	4+
2		R1wR1 B3785	+	+	0	0	+	0	+	+	+	0	+	0	+	0	+	+	+	0	+	0	+	0	+	0	+	+	2	4+
3		R2R2 C3723	+	0	+	+	0	0	0	0	+	0	+	0	+	0	+	+	0	+	+	+	0	0	0	0	+	+	3	4+
4		Ror D691	+	0	+	0	+	+	0	0	+	0	+	0	+	0	+	+	+	0	+	+	+	0	+	0	0	+	4	4+
5		r'r E766	0	+	+	0	+	0	0	0	+	0	+	0	+	+	+	0	+	0	+	0	+	+	+	0	0	+	0	5	0
6		r"r F792	0	0	+	+	+	0	0	+	+	0	+	0	+	+	+	+	+	0	0	+	+	+	0	+	0	+	6	0
7		r'r E831	0	+	+	0	+	0	0	0	+	0	+	0	+	0	+	+	0	+	0	+	0	+	0	0	0	+	7	0
8		rr G483	0	0	+	0	+	0	0	+	+	0	+	0	+	0	+	0	+	0	0	+	+	+	+	0	0	+	8	0
9		rr H1281	0	0	+	0	+	0	0	0	+	0	+	0	+	+	0	+	+	0	+	+	0	+	0	+	0	+	9	0
10	Yt(b⁺)	rr H347	0	0	+	0	+	0	0	0	+	0	+	0	+	+	0	+	0	+	0	+	+	+	+	0	+	0	10	0
11		rr V163	0	0	+	0	+	0	0	0	+	0	+	0	+	0	+	+	0	W	+	+	+	+	0	+	0	+	11	0
12		rr N3073	0	0	+	0	+	0	0	0	+	+	0	+	0	+	+	+	+	0	+	+	0	+	0	0	0	+	12	0
13		rr G964	0	0	+	0	+	0	0	+	+	0	+	0	+	0	+	+	0	0	+	+	+	0	+	+	+	+	13	0
14	Di(a⁺)	R1R1 B7587	+	+	0	0	+	0	0	0	+	0	+	0	+	0	+	+	0	0	+	+	0	0	+	0	+	+	14	4+
15		POSITIVE CONTROL	/	/	/	/	/	/	/	/	/	/	/	/	/	/	/	/	/	/	/	/	/	/	/	/	/	/	/	PC	4+
16		NEGATIVE CONTROL	/	/	/	/	/	/	/	/	/	/	/	/	/	/	/	/	/	/	/	/	/	/	/	/	/	/	/	NC	0

Rh - Hr columns: D C c E e V Cʷ; Kell: K k Kpᵃ Kpᵇ Jsᵃ Jsᵇ; Duffy: Fyᵃ Fyᵇ; Kidd: Jkᵃ Jkᵇ; Lewis: Leᵃ Leᵇ; P: P₁; MN: M N S s; Lutheran: Luᵃ Luᵇ; Xg: Xgᵃ

* Indicates those antigens whose presence or absence may have been determined using only a single example of a specific antibody.

NOTES:
An antigen designated with a 'w' represents a weakened expression of the antigen that may or may not react with all examples of the corresponding antibody.

426-17

PATIENT'S SERUM ANTIBODY SCREEN LOT		
I	4+
II	4+
III	0
IV	

Fig. 10.7 Capture Ready-Screen and Ready-ID test results and interpretation. Panel results show wells 1 to 4 and 14 as positive reactions. These results are transferred to the panel below, which can be interpreted by ruling out the negative reactions. As with tube testing methods, it is important that the correct panel lot number be chosen. Interpretation by ruling out demonstrates an anti-D. (Courtesy Immucor, Norcross, GA.)

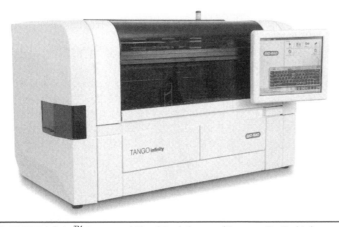

Fig. 10.8 TANGO Infinity™ Automated Blood Bank System. (Courtesy Bio-Rad Laboratories, Inc.)

cell. When spun, the Fc portion of the IgG AHG will attach to the Protein A layer at the bottom of the well, yielding a smooth monolayer of red cells—a positive reaction. If no antibody has been bound to red cells during incubation, no IgG AHG is attached and, after centrifugation, a compact cell button will indicate a negative reaction. The instrument reads and interprets the results. Fig. 10.9 illustrates this procedure.

Erytype® S Technology

The TANGO infinity® and the TANGO optimo™ use Erytype® S microplate wells/ strips for hemagglutination assays. ABD (forward and reverse) typing, plus C, c, E, e, and Kell red cell antigen phenotypes, may be determined on these strips, Wells are precoated with dried monoclonal antisera.[10] The instrument pipettes the sample, centrifuges, reads, and interprets the results. The Erytype® S ABD + A_1, B procedure is outlined in Fig. 10.10.

AUTOMATED SYSTEMS FOR GEL TECHNOLOGY ASSAYS

Gel technology assays are manufactured by Ortho Clinical Diagnostics (Raritan, NJ) under the trade name ID-MTS Gel Test. In the gel test, the gel particles combined with diluent or reagents are predispensed into specially designed microtubes manufactured in plastic cards. The gel card is approximately the size of a credit card and contains six microtubes. Each microtube consists of an upper reaction chamber and a section that contains predispensed gel and reagents. The gel acts as the medium to separate agglutinated red cells from unagglutinated red cells. A foil strip is present on the top of the gel card to prevent spillage or drying of microtube contents. The six-microtube configuration of the gel card allows for possible sample batch testing (ie, more than one patient sample can be tested in one gel card). Because this technology is suitable for automation, blood bank instrumentation is available for the performance of gel testing.

> The gel test is a hemagglutination reaction. The red cells migrate through the gel matrix to separate agglutinated from unagglutinated red cells.

Two major categories of gel cards are licensed for blood bank testing. Specific reagent antibody is incorporated into the gel:
- Cards for ABO and D phenotype and other Rh antigens (C, c, E, e)
- AHG cards (anti-IgG and anti-IgG, –C3d) for indirect antiglobulin test (IAT) (antibody screen, antibody identification, and compatibility testing) and DAT

To perform a gel test, measured volumes of red cells and plasma/serum are added to the reaction chamber of the microtube. The reaction chamber allows red cell sensitization to occur during the incubation of an IAT. The centrifugation step allows time for red cells to contact antisera and gel particles. Centrifugation also separates positive and negative agglutination results. In positive reactions, agglutinated red cells are trapped in the gel at various levels, depending on the agglutination strength and size of the agglutinates. In negative reactions, unagglutinated red cells pass through the gel and form a button on the bottom of the microtube.[11]

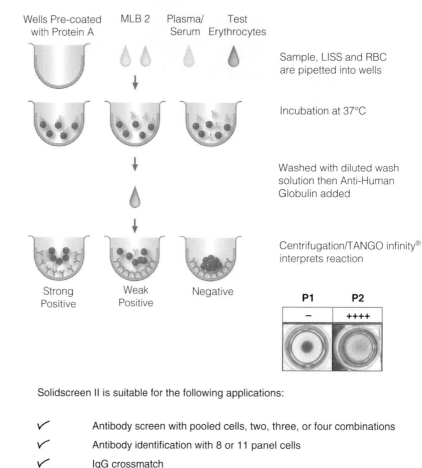

Solidscreen® II Test Principle

Solidscreen II is suitable for the following applications:

✓   Antibody screen with pooled cells, two, three, or four combinations

✓   Antibody identification with 8 or 11 panel cells

✓   IgG crossmatch

✓   Enzyme-treated red cells for antibody screen and identification

✓   Auto control

✓   Antibody titration

✓   Direct antiglobulin test

✓   Anti-D (RH1) blend for weak D and partial D tests

Fig. 10.9 Solidscreen® II technology. (Courtesy Bio-Rad Laboratories, Inc.)

Gel technology is applied in antibody screening as follows:

Gel Test Antibody Screen

1. Add 50 μL of 0.8% suspension of reagent screening cells to the microtubes of the anti-IgG gel cards.
2. Add 25 μL of patient serum or plasma to the microtubes.
3. Incubate the gel card at 37° C for a predetermined time and centrifuge.
4. After centrifugation, the test results are read and graded. No washing step is required for antiglobulin testing. No IgG-sensitized red cells are required.

Larger agglutinates are trapped at the top of the gel microtubes and do not travel through the gel during the centrifugation process. Smaller agglutinates travel through the gel microtubes and may be trapped in either the top or the bottom half of the microtubes. Unagglutinated screening cells travel unimpeded through the length of the microtube and form a red cell button at the bottom after centrifugation (Fig. 10.11).

The ID-MTS Gel Test procedure for the phenotyping of A, B, and D antigens is outlined in Fig. 10.12.[12] The gel cards incorporate anti-A, anti-B, and anti-D antibodies within the gel matrix. The patient's red cells are added to the cards. Centrifugation begins immediately after addition of patient red cells. Scan the QR code to learn more about gel test assays.

Erytype® S Test Principle

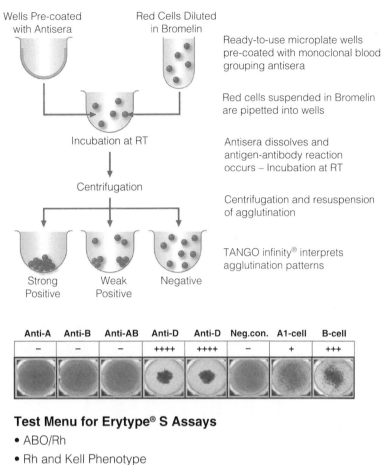

Ready-to-use microplate wells
pre-coated with monoclonal blood
grouping antisera

Red cells suspended in Bromelin
are pipetted into wells

Antisera dissolves and
antigen-antibody reaction
occurs – Incubation at RT

Centrifugation and resuspension
of agglutination

TANGO infinity® interprets
agglutination patterns

Anti-A	Anti-B	Anti-AB	Anti-D	Anti-D	Neg.con.	A1-cell	B-cell
−	−	−	++++	++++	−	+	+++

Test Menu for Erytype® S Assays

- ABO/Rh
- Rh and Kell Phenotype
- ABO donor confirmation
- Rh donor confirmation

Fig. 10.10 Example of Erytype® S assay. (Courtesy Bio-Rad Laboratories, Inc.)

Advantages of using the gel test include standardization of technique, stable reactions, and increased sensitivity over the traditional antiglobulin test; a no-wash antiglobulin test; and use of small quantities of reagents and samples.

The automated instrument that supports the gel technology is the ORTHO ProVue as shown in Fig. 10.13. ORTHO ProVue has been qualified for use with ID-MTS Gel Test gel cards and diluents and Ortho 0.8% Reagent Red Blood Cells.[13] The following tests are supported by the ORTHO ProVue:
- Direct agglutination tests: ABO forward and reverse grouping, D antigen typing, Rh phenotyping, immediate-spin crossmatch
- DATs: Anti-IgG DAT, anti-IgG, and –C3d DAT
- IATs: Antibody screen, antibody identification, and IAT crossmatch

Following the completion of the tests, the gel card is read by a camera, and the results are graded according to the reading algorithms built into the software. A printout of the results is provided by the ORTHO ProVue. An example of a printout screen is provided in Fig. 10.14. The ORTHO ProVue is equivalent to the standard manual method for both the direct agglutination test and DAT and IAT using the ID-MTS Gel Test.[13]

In August 2015, Ortho Clinical Diagnostics obtained 510(k) clearance for the ORTHO VISION™ Analyzer, a highly interactive, fully automated analyzer for transfusion medicine laboratories (Fig. 10.15).[14] The ORTHO VISION™ Analyzer for Ortho ID-MTS™ Column Agglutination Technology is now commercially available in the United States and Puerto Rico. For more information, check the vendor's website.

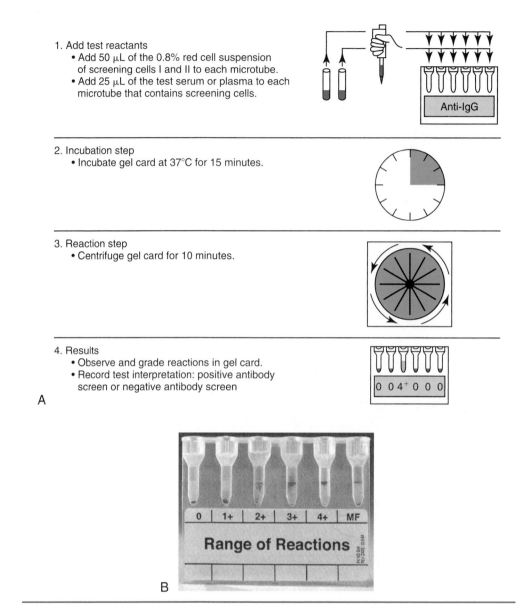

1. Add test reactants
   • Add 50 µL of the 0.8% red cell suspension of screening cells I and II to each microtube.
   • Add 25 µL of the test serum or plasma to each microtube that contains screening cells.

Anti-IgG

2. Incubation step
   • Incubate gel card at 37°C for 15 minutes.

3. Reaction step
   • Centrifuge gel card for 10 minutes.

4. Results
   • Observe and grade reactions in gel card.
   • Record test interpretation: positive antibody screen or negative antibody screen

0 0 4⁺ 0 0 0

A

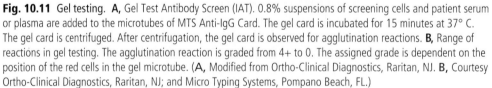

| 0 | 1+ | 2+ | 3+ | 4+ | MF |

Range of Reactions

B

Fig. 10.11 Gel testing. **A,** Gel Test Antibody Screen (IAT). 0.8% suspensions of screening cells and patient serum or plasma are added to the microtubes of MTS Anti-IgG Card. The gel card is incubated for 15 minutes at 37° C. The gel card is centrifuged. After centrifugation, the gel card is observed for agglutination reactions. **B,** Range of reactions in gel testing. The agglutination reaction is graded from 4+ to 0. The assigned grade is dependent on the position of the red cells in the gel microtube. (**A,** Modified from Ortho-Clinical Diagnostics, Raritan, NJ. **B,** Courtesy Ortho-Clinical Diagnostics, Raritan, NJ; and Micro Typing Systems, Pompano Beach, FL.)

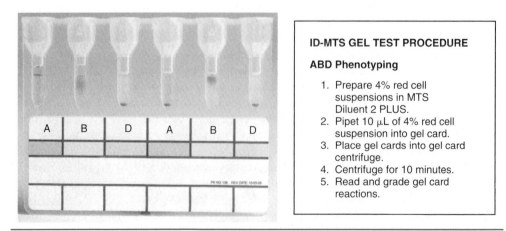

| A | B | D | A | B | D |

ID-MTS GEL TEST PROCEDURE

ABD Phenotyping

1. Prepare 4% red cell suspensions in MTS Diluent 2 PLUS.
2. Pipet 10 µL of 4% red cell suspension into gel card.
3. Place gel cards into gel card centrifuge.
4. Centrifuge for 10 minutes.
5. Read and grade gel card reactions.

Fig. 10.12 ID-MTS Gel Test procedure for the detection of A, B, and D antigens. (Courtesy ID-MTS Interpretation Guide, Ortho Clinical Diagnostics, Raritan, NJ.)

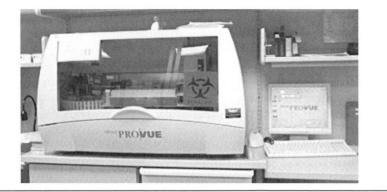

Fig. 10.13 ORTHO ProVue® instrument.

Results by sample

Date: 4/28/2011 12:30:28 PM
Batches: 666-702
Template: TX pin

Samples	A	B	D	Ctl	A1Cel	B Cell	Group	Rh	Cell 1	Cell 2	XIAT	XIS
1111802053A	4+	-	4+	-	-	4+	A	Pos	-	-		

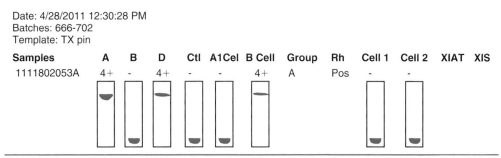

Fig. 10.14 Example of sample results for ABO and D typing and antibody screen on the ORTHO ProVue.

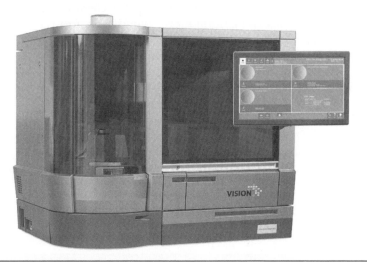

Fig. 10.15 ORTHO VISION™ Analyzer for Ortho ID-MTS™ Column Agglutination Technology. (Courtesy Ortho-Clinical Diagnostics, Raritan, NJ.)

CHAPTER SUMMARY

- Advances in test technologies and robotics are opening up new opportunities for automation to meet the requirements of hospital transfusion services and medium-sized blood banks.
- Automated testing systems have been developed for the detection of antigen–antibody reactions in immunohematology testing.
- The test system's computer may be interfaced with a laboratory's information system for reporting results.
- The benefits of automation in the transfusion service include opportunities for reduction in operating costs, redesign of work processes and support systems, increased productivity, and increased quality.

- The challenges of automation implementation include staff concerns, justification of investment costs, and issues associated with implementation.
- A thorough investigation of automation vendors is vital to learn what they can do for the transfusion service.
- The foundation of any automated platform begins with a proven technology. The reliability and accuracy of the base technology requires investigation.
- In the assessment of an instrument's performance, the adaptability, availability, and cost effectiveness of the automated platform are important factors to evaluate.
- Automated testing systems have been developed for solid-phase, gel technology, and microtiter plates. These systems can perform ABO and Rh phenotyping, antibody detection, and identification and crossmatching.

CRITICAL THINKING EXERCISES

Exercise 10.1

The transfusion service at JHM Hospital has been asked to implement the electronic crossmatch to reduce turnaround time. The lead technologist has been assigned the task of investigating the various automated technologies currently available.

What important criteria should be considered when deciding which automated testing system to bring on board to accommodate the electronic crossmatch procedure?

Exercise 10.2

A small remote hospital is having difficulty staffing the transfusion service section due to the lack of experience and hesitancy of many of the staff techs who work in other sections of the laboratory. An automated platform for the blood bank area is being considered to work around this issue.

How could an automated system help in this circumstance?

Exercise 10.3

A blood bank using the ECHO found a discrepant result on a donor sample that was tested for weak D. Prior donor records showed the result as weak D-positive, whereas current testing was weak D-negative. A review of the records indicated that previous testing was performed in the tube before implementing the automated system.

What are possible causes of these differing results, and how should the problem be resolved?

STUDY QUESTIONS

1. Which of the following statements is true regarding interpretation of SPRCA results?
   a. Grading reactions are based on a 1-to-4 grading scale where 4+ is a strong positive.
   b. A tight button of cells on the bottom of the well would be interpreted as a positive reaction.
   c. Hemagglutination assay results are interpreted the same as SPRCA results.
   d. An evenly distributed layer of cells on the well surface is a negative reaction.

2. What are the indicator cells used in SPRCA assays?
   a. IgM-coated red cells useful in determining the presence of ABO antibodies
   b. cells used to agglutinate IgG antibodies to form a pellet in the well after centrifugation
   c. IgG-coated red cells that cross-link with IgG antibodies attached to the well
   d. check cells that are added to negative reactions to validate the washing step

3. In the gel test, what is a button of cells at the bottom of the well called?
   a. 4+ positive reaction
   b. 1+ positive reaction
   c. negative reaction
   d. invalid reaction

4. Which method is used in the automated Immucor and Bio-Rad systems for ABO and D phenotype?
   a. solid-phase red cell adherence assay (SPRCA)
   b. enzyme-linked immunosorbent assay (ELISA)
   c. reverse-passive hemagglutination (RPHA)
   d. hemagglutination in a microwell

5. Where can false-negative reactions occur in both the gel and solid-phase testing?
   a. failing to centrifuge
   b. not mixing reagent red cells sufficiently
   c. incubation time was too short
   d. all of the above

6. Mixed-field reactions were observed in the ID-MTS Gel Test for ABO and D phenotype when the test was automated. What is the most likely cause of this observation?
   a. improper pipetting technique
   b. the use of contaminated reagents
   c. transfusion of group O cells to an A or B patient
   d. centrifugation error

7. After centrifugation using the ID-MTS Anti-IgG gel cards, a layer of agglutinated cells was observed at the top of two of the three screening cell microtubes. What should be done next?
   a. repeat the test
   b. proceed to an antibody identification panel
   c. perform a DAT to determine whether the patient has an autoantibody
   d. verify the negative reaction with check cells

8. What tests are performed with the MTS Monoclonal A/B/D Grouping Gel Card?
   a. typing A, B, and D antigen
   b. antiglobulin crossmatches
   c. typing Rh system antigens
   d. direct antiglobulin tests

9. What test uses the Capture-R Select microwell strips?
   a. direct antiglobulin test
   b. antiglobulin testing of selected panel cells
   c. weak D test
   d. all of the above

10. Select the method that uses the principle of sieving to separate larger agglutinates from smaller agglutinates in Ag-Ab reactions.
    a. gel technology
    b. solid-phase
    c. microplate
    d. none of the above

True or False

_____ 11. Bar-code technology is used in automated instruments to ensure positive sample identity.

_____ 12. LIS interfaces link the automated test system with a laboratory information system for reporting results.

_____ 13. Automation should make it easier to do things the right way and more difficult to do the wrong things.

_____ 14. When selecting an automation partner, a laboratory does not need to determine its requirements in terms of customer support, training, and service.

_____ 15. Rapid turnaround times for selected samples and the ability to accommodate large-volume batch testing contribute to overall operational efficiency.

_____ 16. Vendors of automation for the transfusion service require prior approval from the Food and Drug Administration (FDA).

_____ 17. Vendor assessment, base technology, and instrument assessment are important considerations in the selection of an automated system.

Answers to Study Questions can be found on page 387.

Additional student resources, including review questions, a laboratory manual, and case studies, can be found on the Evolve website.

REFERENCES

1. Paxton A: Blood banks step up move to automation, *CAP Today* 13(10):1, 28–32, 34, 1999.
2. Wilde M: Automation a simple solution to do more with less, *Adv Med Lab Prof* 9:6, 1997.
3. South SF: *Automation and work process redesign*, Raritan, NJ, 1999, Ortho-Clinical Diagnostics.
4. Plapp FV, Rachel JM: Automation in blood banking, *AJCP* 98(Suppl 1):17, 1992.
5. Johnson SM, Aller RD: Weeding out the wrong coagulation analyzer, *CAP Today* 14:46, 2000.
6. Capture-R Select, Solid Phase System for the Immobilization of Human Erythrocytes (package insert), Immucor, Norcross, GA.
7. Capture-R Ready Screen and Capture-R Ready ID (package insert), Immucor, Norcross, GA.
8. Sinor L: Advances in solid phase red cell adherence methods and transfusion serology, *Transfus Med Rev* 6:26, 1992.
9. Solidscreen II (package insert). *Bio-Rad*. www.bio-rad.com. Accessed December 2011.
10. Erytype ABD+Rev.A₁, B (package insert). *Bio-Rad*. www.bio-rad.com. Accessed December 2011.
11. *ID-Microtyping System interpretation guide*, Raritan, NJ, 2004, Ortho-Clinical Diagnostics.
12. MTS Monoclonal A/B/D Grouping Card (package insert), *Ortho Clinical Diagnostics*. www.orthoclinical.com. Accessed October 2015.
13. Casina TS, Weiland D, Howard P, et al.: AP108: Evaluation of a fully automated system for gel testing, *Transfusion* 43(Suppl):166A, 2003.
14. ORTHO VISION™ Analyzer. http://www.orthoclinical.com/en-us/Pages/HomeNew.aspx. Accessed October 2015.

ADVERSE COMPLICATIONS OF TRANSFUSIONS

11

CHAPTER OUTLINE

LEARNING OBJECTIVES

On completion of this chapter, the reader should be able to:

1. Describe the hemovigilance model and its role in improving transfusion safety.
2. List common signs and symptoms of adverse transfusion reactions.
3. Distinguish between acute and delayed transfusion reactions and provide examples.
4. Compare and contrast immune-mediated and non–immune-mediated red cell destruction.
5. Describe the distinguishing features of the following transfusion reactions: febrile, urticarial, anaphylactic, transfusion-related acute lung injury, and transfusion-associated graft-versus-host disease.
6. Discuss the causes and clinical features of bacterial contamination of blood products.
7. Describe the clinical features of transfusion reactions caused by circulatory overload and patients at risk of this transfusion reaction.
8. Describe the mechanisms and prevention of transfusion hemosiderosis, citrate toxicity, and posttransfusion purpura.
9. Provide direction to medical personnel performing the transfusion in the event of a reported adverse reaction.
10. List initial tests performed in the transfusion service on a receipt of a patient sample after a reaction.
11. Identify additional testing that might be required in the investigation of transfusion reactions and the rationale for selecting these tests.
12. Describe the required documentation and reporting in the investigation of a transfusion reaction.
13. Interpret the results of transfusion reaction cases.
14. Perform a transfusion reaction workup.

Transfusion safety measures are incorporated at all steps of the blood collection, donor unit processing, and transfusion protocols. Despite careful pretransfusion testing and patient monitoring, noninfectious complications of transfusions occur and are not always preventable. Many systems and procedures have been designed to reduce the risk of adverse complications of blood transfusions. This chapter provides an overview of the proposed mechanisms, risks, and preventive measures associated with complications of blood transfusions.

SECTION 1
OVERVIEW OF ADVERSE REACTIONS TO TRANSFUSION

HEMOVIGILANCE MODEL

An **adverse transfusion reaction** is "an undesirable response or effect in a patient temporarily associated with the administration of blood or blood component."[1] Statistically, noninfectious complications of transfusions pose a greater risk to patients than infectious diseases.[2] Table 11.1 summarizes the U.S. Food and Drug Administration (FDA) reportable transfusion fatalities for combined fiscal years 2009 to 2013.[2]

The Hemovigilance Model under the National Healthcare Safety Network (NHSN) was developed with the cooperation of the AABB and the Centers for Disease Control and Prevention (CDC) to track, analyze, and ultimately improve transfusion outcomes. This confidential, voluntary reporting system collects data from participating hospitals that report to the CDC on a monthly basis. The CDC publishes these results to assist facilities in quality improvement activities, collaborative research, and recognition of trends. The contents of this chapter follow the case definition criteria for adverse reactions of blood transfusion used in the hemovigilance model, which is based on International Society of Blood Transfusion (ISBT) definitions.[3] Scan the QR code to review Biovigilance Component Adverse Reactions – Case Definition Exercises.

RECOGNITION OF A TRANSFUSION REACTION

Clinical signs and symptoms of a complication of transfusion (Table 11.2) may be associated with more than one type of reaction, and early recognition and evaluation are important for the best outcome. Transfusion reactions may occur as an **acute reaction** (immediately or within 24 hours) or a **delayed reaction** (>24 hours). In patients who are anesthetized or medicated, clinical symptoms may not be as obvious.

Reactions are further classified as either **immune-mediated reactions** or **non–immune-mediated reactions,** meaning that the recognition of foreign proteins and cells

Adverse transfusion reaction: undesirable response by a patient to the infusion of blood or blood products

Acute reaction: reaction occurring within 24 hours of transfusion

Delayed reaction: reaction occurring more than 24 hours after transfusion

Immune-mediated reactions: reactions involving antigen–antibody complexes, cytokine release, or complement activation

Non–immune-mediated reactions: reactions that may be due to the component transfused, the patient's underlying condition, or the method of infusion

Rigors: a sudden feeling of cold with shivering accompanied by a rise in temperature, often with copious sweating, especially at the onset or height of a fever

TABLE 11.1	Categories of Transfusion Complications from FDA DATA: Combined Fiscal Years 2009 to 2013[2]	
TRANSFUSION COMPLICATION		**FREQUENCY OF MORTALITY**
Transfusion-related acute lung injury (TRALI)		38%
Transfusion-associated circulatory overload (TACO)		24%
Hemolytic transfusion reactions due to non-ABO		15%
Hemolytic transfusion reactions due to ABO incompatibilities		7%
Microbial infections		10%
Anaphylactic reactions		5%

TABLE 11.2	Clinical Signs Indicative of a Transfusion Reaction[4]

- Fever ≥1° C increase or >38° C
- Chills and rigors
- Respiratory distress: wheezing, coughing, dyspnea, cyanosis
- Hypertension or hypotension
- Pain: abdominal, chest, flank or back, infusion site
- Skin manifestations: urticaria, rash, flushing, edema
- Jaundice or hemoglobinuria
- Nausea or vomiting
- Abnormal bleeding
- Oliguria or anuria

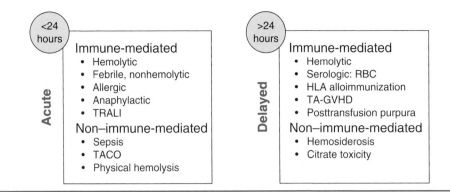

Fig. 11.1 Categories of transfusion reactions. *TACO,* Transfusion-associated circulatory overload; *TRALI,* transfusion-related acute lung injury; *RBC,* red blood cell; *HLA,* human leukocyte antigen; *TA-GVHD,* transfusion-associated graft-versus-host disease.

by the immune system may or may not be involved. In a nonimmune reaction, the component given, the method of transfusion, or the patient's underlying condition may be the cause of the reaction. Fig. 11.1 presents the categories of reactions to be discussed further in this chapter.

SECTION 2
CATEGORIES OF TRANSFUSION REACTIONS

HEMOLYTIC TRANSFUSION REACTION

A hemolytic transfusion reaction is the destruction of transfused red cells that results in intravascular or extravascular hemolysis or a combination of both. Hemolytic reactions are classified as acute or delayed, and both types may stem from immune or nonimmune causes.

Acute Hemolytic Transfusion Reaction

An acute hemolytic transfusion reaction (AHTR) is the rapid destruction of red cells during, immediately after, or within 24 hours after a transfusion of red cells. The clinical presentation of an AHTR ranges in severity from fever to death. Signs and symptoms associated with an acute hemolytic reaction include fever, chills, pain or oozing at the infusion site, back or flank pain, hypotension, epistaxis (nosebleed) hemoglobinuria, disseminated intravascular coagulation (DIC), oliguria, anuria, and renal failure.[1]

Multiple simultaneous clinical events contribute to the degree of severity resulting from the destruction of red cells. The interaction of preformed antibodies with red cell antigens, usually an ABO incompatibility, is the immunologic basis for AHTR.

Events in an immune-mediated AHTR are shown in Fig. 11.2.

> Severe symptoms of an AHTR can occur after the infusion of as little as 10 mL of incompatible blood.[4]

Pathophysiology of Acute Hemolytic Reactions

The first event in an immune-mediated AHTR is the interaction of red cell antibodies with respective red cell antigens. This antigen–antibody complex formation initiates the clinical sequence of events associated with hemolysis. Characteristics of both the red cell alloantibody and the corresponding antigen are major determinants for the course and severity of a hemolytic transfusion reaction. Preformed antibodies in the recipient interact with the transfused red cells to create the most severe hemolytic reactions.

The concentration or titer of the red cell alloantibody also influences the extent and severity of an AHTR. Higher concentrations of circulating antibody in a transfusion recipient are more likely to produce severe clinical manifestations. The density (number of antigens per red cell) and distribution of the targeted red cell antigens also influence the severity of an AHTR. Scattered surface antigens bind fewer antibody molecules per red cell and are less likely to initiate severe hemolytic episodes. In contrast, antigens that are clustered together on the red cell surface increase the chances for the activation of the classical pathway of complement.

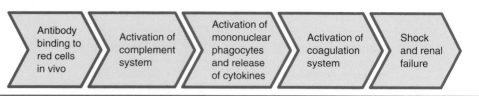

Fig. 11.2 Events in an immune-mediated AHTR.

Red cell stroma: red cell membrane that remains after hemolysis

Serotonin: potent vasoconstrictor liberated by platelets

Histamine: compound that causes constriction of bronchial smooth muscle, dilation of capillaries, and decrease in blood pressure

Bradykinin: potent vasodilator of the kinin family

Kinins: group of proteins associated with contraction of smooth muscle, vascular permeability, and vasodilation

Haptoglobin: plasma protein that binds free hemoglobin and carries the molecule to the hepatocytes for further catabolism

Ischemia: decreased supply of oxygenated blood to an organ or body part

ABO antibodies of the IgM class readily activate the classical pathway of complement, leading to the potential for intravascular hemolysis (destruction of the transfused red cells within the vascular component). Intravascular hemolysis releases free hemoglobin and **red cell stroma** into the plasma. ABO antibodies of the IgG class less commonly activate the complement pathway but can interact with Fc receptors of mononuclear phagocytes, effecting phagocytosis and cellular activation. In an AHTR, complement functions in three capacities: opsonization, anaphylatoxin generation, and red cell lysis.

- *Opsonization* occurs because the membrane-bound complement products are cleared by mononuclear phagocytic cells.
- *Anaphylatoxins,* potent inducers of inflammation, are liberated into the plasma. These products act on mast cells, smooth muscle, and neutrophils. C5a acts on smooth muscle to effect contraction with an overall net effect of vascular dilation and bronchospasm. C3a and C5a also cause vasoactive amine (**serotonin** and **histamine**) release by mast cells and basophils and effect degranulation of neutrophils. The net effect of the systemic release of serotonin and histamine is increased vascular permeability. **Bradykinin**, a potent vasodilator and one of the plasma **kinins**, is generated to increase vasodilation and hypotension. In addition, antigen–antibody complex deposition and thrombus formation contribute to the vascular compromise observed in the kidneys.[4]
- *Red cell lysis* is the final outcome in complement activation after the assembly of the membrane attack complex. Liberated hemoglobin is bound by plasma haptoglobin. When the hemoglobin-binding capacity of plasma **haptoglobin** is exceeded, hemoglobinemia and hemoglobinuria are detectable. Free hemoglobin released into the bloodstream has cytotoxic and inflammatory effects.[5]

Antigen–antibody-complement complexes may initiate the coagulation and fibrinolytic systems. DIC is often associated with an AHTR. The cardinal signs of DIC include the consumption of clotting factors (particularly fibrinogen, factor V, and factor VIII) and platelets, with resulting diffuse, uncontrolled microvascular bleeding. DIC causes bleeding into organs and microvascular thromboses, which may produce multiple organ dysfunction and failure. The microvascular thrombi promote tissue **ischemia** and release of tissue factor, encouraging the activation of more thrombin. Hemostatic profiles of patients in DIC demonstrate low platelet counts, decreased fibrinogen levels, and increased fibrin degradation products (specifically plasma D-dimers). Fibrin degradation products compete with thrombin and thus slow down clot formation by preventing the conversion of fibrinogen to fibrin.

With the release of anaphylatoxins, vasoactive amines, kinins, and cytokines into the circulation as consequences of intravascular red cell destruction, the patient may present with shock. Shock is an abnormal condition of inadequate blood flow to the body's peripheral tissues, with life-threatening cellular dysfunction.

Renal failure caused by a severe AHTR is a multifactorial event and is most prominent in an untreated AHTR.[4] Contributing factors to renal failure include systemic hypotension, reactive renal vasoconstriction, and deposition of intravascular thrombi whose cumulative effects compromise the renal cortical blood supply. The release of norepinephrine in a physiologic reaction to the hypotension and shock produces vasoconstriction observed in the kidneys and lungs. The developing renal ischemia may be transient or advance to acute tubular necrosis and renal loss.

In summary, the transfusion of ABO-incompatible blood may be lethal due to the events of shock, DIC, and renal failure. In the majority of patients who receive ABO-incompatible blood, DIC is mild or undetectable and renal failure does not develop. Three important factors determine the outcome of the incompatible transfusion[6]:

1. Potency of the recipient's anti-A or anti-B in plasma
2. Volume of incompatible blood transfused
3. Rate of transfusion

Most fatalities are associated with the transfusion of more than 200 mL of blood. However, volumes as low as 30 mL have been implicated in fatalities.

Prevention of Acute Hemolytic Transfusion Reactions

Clerical and misidentification errors that lead to the transfusion of ABO-incompatible red blood cell (RBC) units continue to be the most common cause of AHTRs.[4] Misidentification of the patient, incorrect sample collection, and incorrect or missed entry of test results occur because of failure to follow standard operating procedures when collecting, testing, and transfusing units of blood. Table 11.3 presents data relative to errors contributing to an AHTR. Awareness of these potential errors is important in preventing the serious consequences of AHTRs.

Delayed Hemolytic Reaction

As outlined in the previous section, an AHTR in a transfusion recipient may produce serious clinical consequences. These reactions are usually associated with the transfusion of ABO-incompatible red cells. In contrast, delayed hemolytic transfusion reactions (DHTRs), with symptoms appearing after 24 hours, are caused by a secondary immune response.

In a DHTR the recipient has been immunized after red cell exposure from prior transfusions or pregnancy. Normally, pretransfusion testing detects clinically significant antibodies. However, the antibody may have been below detectable levels when pretransfusion testing was performed. In some cases, the antibody may have been missed in error or not detected because of the sensitivity of the test method. In rare cases, an antibody to a low-frequency antigen may not have been detected because the antigen may not have been demonstrating on the screening cells.

The first detectable sign of a delayed hemolytic reaction may be an inadequate increase of posttransfusion hemoglobin levels, a rapid decrease back to pretransfusion levels, or an unexplained appearance of spherocytes. Newly identified red cell alloantibodies demonstrating between 24 hours and 28 days after transfusion provide definitive criteria for an immune-mediated DHTR.[1] Posttransfusion alloantibody formation has been reported in approximately 1% to 1.6% after RBC transfusions, excluding Rh system antibodies.[4] Blood group antibodies associated with delayed hemolytic reactions include antibodies in the Rh (particularly anti-C and anti-E), Kidd, Duffy, Kell, and MNS blood group systems.[6]

TABLE 11.3 Errors Contributing to Acute Hemolytic Transfusion Reactions	
ERRORS KNOWN TO CAUSE AHTR	**CONTRIBUTING FACTORS CAUSING ERRORS**
• Collection of blood from the incorrect patient • Incorrect labeling of blood samples • Misidentification of sample at blood bank • Issuance of wrong unit from blood bank • Transfusion of blood to incorrect patient • Aliquoting a patient sample to improperly labeled test tube	• Insufficient segregation of units • Preprinted sample labels • Patients with similar or identical names • Sequential patient identifiers • Verbal and STAT orders • Manual issuance of blood • Simultaneous processing of specimens from multiple patients • Tested the correct sample but recorded results on the wrong patient record • Overriding computer error messages

Data from Sazama K: Reports of 355 transfusion-associated deaths: 1976 through 1985, *Transfusion* 30:583–590, 1990.

Pathophysiology of Delayed Hemolytic Reaction

The hemolytic potential and rapid production of the implicated alloantibody influence the clinical course of the transfusion reaction.[4] The most constant clinical signs of a DHTR are fever and fall in hemoglobin concentration, Jaundice, appearing day 5 after transfusion, and hemoglobinuria are other clinical features of DHTRs. Red cells, sensitized with either immunoglobulin or complement, are removed from the circulation by the mononuclear phagocyte system. The macrophages, located in the spleen, are probably most active in this mechanism, although Kupffer cells of the liver also participate.

These mononuclear phagocytes also generate cytokines that mediate the systemic effects often associated with AHTRs. Cytokines are protein hormones involved in cell-to-cell communication. The combined effects of these cytokines include fever, hypotension, activation of T cells and B cells, and activation of endothelial cells to express procoagulant activity. AHTRs and DHTRs are compared in Table 11.4. The table provides additional information on laboratory testing, management, and prevention of these transfusion reactions.

Non–Immune-Mediated Mechanisms of Red Cell Destruction

For a transfusion reaction in a patient experiencing hemoglobinemia and hemoglobinuria, the initial focus is to investigate the possibility of an immune-related response. When alloantibodies are not implicated, an investigation into the nonimmune mechanisms of red cell destruction should be initiated. This process necessitates examination of the segments or remaining blood from the unit in question, with careful questioning of personnel regarding the transfusion process itself. If a hemolyzed donor unit is accidentally transfused, the

TABLE 11.4	Acute Versus Delayed Hemolytic Transfusion Reactions	
	ACUTE HEMOLYTIC	**DELAYED HEMOLYTIC**
Clinical Signs and Symptoms	• Immediate or within 24 hours posttransfusion • Fever, chills, flushing, pain at site of infusion, tachycardia, tachypnea, lower back pain • Hemoglobinemia, hemoglobinuria, hypotension	• >24 hours to 28 days posttransfusion • Fever: temperature increase ≥1° C (or 2° F) with or without chills • Unexplainable decrease in hemoglobin and hematocrit • Jaundice and hemoglobinuria
Major Complications	• DIC, renal failure, shock, mortality	• Anemia
Causes	• ABO incompatibility • Complement activation	• Anamnestic response to red cell antigen • Alloantibody not demonstrating or missed pretransfusion

Clinical Laboratory Tests	• Clerical check and visual inspection of posttransfusion sample
	• DAT: positive or negative
	• Repeat ABO testing
	• Tests for hemolysis:
	  • ↑ Plasma-free hemoglobin
	  • ↑ Serum bilirubin
	  • ↓ Haptoglobin
	  • Hemoglobinuria
		• DAT: positive
		• Posttransfusion antibody screen: positive
		• ↓ Hemoglobin and hematocrit
		• Tests for hemolysis:
		  • ↑ Plasma-free hemoglobin
		  • ↑ Serum bilirubin
		  • ↓ Haptoglobin
		  • Hemoglobinuria

Management	• Treat hypotension and DIC • Maintain renal blood flow	• Identify antibody(ies) • Provide antigen-negative donor units
Prevention	• Avoid clerical and misidentification errors • Design systems to decrease chances of technical error	• Check of patient records • Recently transfused or pregnant have sample drawn within 3 days of transfusion

DIC, Disseminated intravascular coagulation; *DAT,* direct antiglobulin test; ↑, increased levels; ↓, decreased levels.

recipient receives free hemoglobin and red cell stroma. The red cell stroma may stimulate complement activation and a procoagulant state.

Examples of the causes of non–immune-mediated red cell hemolysis include the following:

- Exposure of red cells to extreme temperatures (>50° C or <0° C)
  Exposure to extreme temperatures may produce hemolysis of red cells. The use of malfunctioning or unregulated blood-warming devices or warming during refrigerated storage may lead to hemolyzed units. RBC units stored frozen without additive cryo-protectants induce the hemolysis of the units.
- Improper deglycerolization of an RBC unit on thawing
  A simple test to prevent this complication of transfusion is to observe the supernatant of a red cell suspension for evidence of hemolysis after the deglycerolization has been completed.
- Mechanical destruction of red cells
  Small-bore needles, mechanical valves, excessive pressure, and blood salvage equipment have been linked with nonimmune hemolysis of red cells.
- Incompatible solutions
  The only solution that may be added to a donor unit is physiologic saline (Fig. 11.3). Blood mixed with nonphysiologic solutions such as half-strength saline, 5% dextrose in 0.18% saline, Ringer's lactate, and medications may cause osmotic rupture of the red cells. Exceptions to normal saline can be made if they have been approved by the FDA or documentation is available to show that the addition is safe and does not adversely affect the blood and blood component.[4]
- Transfusion of bacterially contaminated blood products
- Intrinsic red cell defect attributable to a clinical condition
  Certain clinical disease states may be responsible for hemolysis unrelated to the transfusion, including sickle cell disease, thermal burns, glucose-6-phosphate dehydrogenase deficiency, and paroxysmal nocturnal hemoglobinuria.

> Thermal damage, mechanical damage, osmotic destruction, and bacterial contamination are nonimmune mechanisms that can generate a hemolytic episode in a transfusion recipient.

DELAYED SEROLOGIC TRANSFUSION REACTIONS

The term delayed serologic transfusion reaction (DSTR) describes an anamnestic response after transfusion with no signs of hemolysis.[7] In addition to immune-mediated acute or delayed hemolytic transfusion reaction, a delayed serologic reaction should be considered

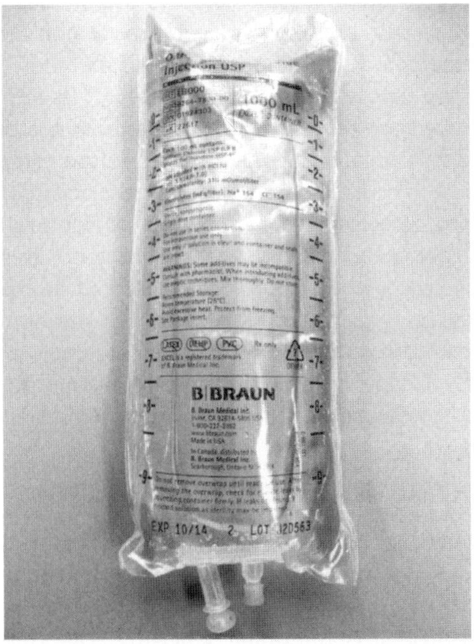

Fig. 11.3 0.9% saline. No medications or solutions other than 0.9% sodium chloride injection (USP) should be administered with blood components through the same tubing.

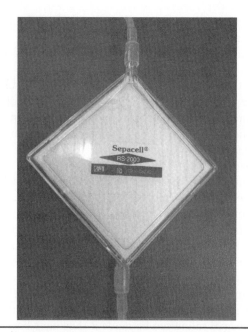

Fig. 11.4 Leukocyte removal filter. Removing leukocytes before storage reduces the cytokines and leukocytes in blood components, which can cause febrile transfusion reactions.

if an antibody develops between 24 hours and 28 days after transfusion, even though there is an adequate, maintained hemoglobin response.[1] A newly identified antibody or a positive direct antiglobulin test (DAT) would confirm the diagnosis of this type of reaction. Blood group antibodies associated with delayed serologic reactions may go unrecognized because most patients do not undergo red cell antibody screening after transfusion unless additional units are requested.[8]

FEBRILE NONHEMOLYTIC TRANSFUSION REACTIONS

The febrile nonhemolytic transfusion reaction is a commonly observed adverse effect of transfusion. Because the presenting clinical features are similar to an AHTR, a careful investigation is necessary to rule out hemolysis. A febrile nonhemolytic reaction is typically manifested by a temperature elevation of ≥1° C above 37° C occurring during or shortly after transfusion (up to 4 hours after transfusion).[4] In addition to fever, chills, rigors, headache, and vomiting may present. These transfusion reactions are nonthreatening, but may be accompanied by considerable discomfort for the recipient.

The most common cause is transfused cytokines or the action of cytokines generated by the recipient in response to transfused leukocytes.[1] In addition to cytokines, antibodies to donor white blood cells have been implicated in the reaction.[4] Prestorage leukocyte reduction of platelets and RBC units decreases the frequency of febrile reactions (Fig. 11.4).[9] It also has been suggested that premedication with acetaminophen may be beneficial in avoiding febrile nonhemolytic reactions.[10] A summary of febrile nonhemolytic transfusion reactions appears in Table 11.5. The table provides additional information on laboratory testing, management, and prevention of this transfusion reaction.

ALLERGIC AND ANAPHYLACTIC TRANSFUSION REACTIONS

Allergic reactions to transfusion range in clinical severity from minor urticarial effects to fulminant anaphylactic shock and death. The cause of these reactions derives from soluble allergens present in donor plasma. These reactions are more commonly associated with the transfusion of blood products containing a plasma component, and symptoms may occur within seconds or minutes of the start of the transfusion.[1]

TABLE 11.5   Febrile Nonhemolytic Transfusion Reactions

Clinical Signs and Symptoms	• Fever: temperature increase ≥1° C (or 2° F) above 37° C • Other symptoms: chills, rigors, headache and vomiting
Major Complications	• Nonthreatening • Significant discomfort to the recipient
Causes	• Antibody to donor WBCs • Cytokines released by WBCs during blood product storage
Clinical Laboratory Tests	• DAT: negative • No visible hemolysis
Management	• Antipyretics: acetaminophen
Prevention	• Prestorage leukocyte reduction of blood products

WBC, white blood cell; DAT, direct antiglobulin test.

Urticarial Response

In the classic type I hypersensitivity response, preformed IgE antibodies in the recipient react with the allergen (plasma protein), which activates mast cells. Mast cell activation results in degranulation and the release of histamine, proteases, and chemotactic factors. Symptoms commonly include urticaria (hives) and pruritus (itching).

Anaphylactic Response

More severe anaphylactic reactions sometimes have life-threatening outcomes. Mast cell degranulation has been triggered by non-IgE mechanisms. In this reaction, the recipient exhibits the symptoms of urticaria and **angioedema** in the majority of cases.[4] In addition, severe hypotension, shock, and loss of consciousness can present with respiratory involvement (dyspnea and wheezing). Approximately 30% of these patients will present with gastrointestinal symptoms such as nausea, vomiting, diarrhea, and cramping.[4] Cardiovascular symptoms may also be present.

Angioedema: rapid swelling of the dermis, subcutaneous tissue, mucosa, and submucosal tissues

Allergic transfusion reactions progressing beyond the urticarial response may occur in IgA-deficient patients. In IgA-deficient patients, severe anaphylactic reactions occur if they have made an antibody to the IgA immunoglobulin and receive plasma components. It may be necessary for IgA antibody–deficient patients with antibodies to IgA to receive IgA-deficient plasma from the rare donor registry or washed red cell and platelet components to avoid these reactions. Severe reactions may require treatment with methylprednisolone, prednisone, or epinephrine.[1]

Two or more of the following signs or symptoms, observed within 4 hours of transfusion, are definitive characteristics of an allergic reaction[1]:
• Urticaria (hives)
• Pruritus (itching)
• Maculopapular rash
• Generalized flushing
• Localized angioedema
• Edema of the lips, tongue, and uvula
• Erythema and edema of the periorbital area
• Conjunctival edema
• Respiratory distress. bronchospasm
• Hypotension

Treatment of mild allergic transfusion reactions with antihistamines is usually adequate, and transfusions can be resumed once symptoms have dissipated. "Signs and symptoms suggestive of mild allergic reactions need not be reported to the blood bank or transfusion service."[11] In patients with prior allergic reactions to transfusions, premedication with antihistamines 30 minutes before transfusion may be beneficial. Table 11.6 summarizes and compares different issues relative to allergic transfusion reactions.

TABLE 11.6	Allergic Transfusion Reactions	
	URTICARIAL	**ANAPHYLACTIC**
Clinical Signs and Symptoms	• Hives and itching within 15–20 min of transfusion	• Rapid onset and severe wheezing, coughing, dyspnea, bronchospasm, respiratory distress, vascular instability • No fever
Major Complications	• None	• Shock • Loss of consciousness • Mortality
Causes	• Recipient antibodies to foreign plasma proteins or other substances such as drugs or food consumed by blood donor	• Associated with genetic IgA deficiency in recipient who possesses IgG complement-binding anti-IgA antibodies
Clinical Laboratory Tests	• DAT: negative • No visible hemolysis	• DAT: negative • No visible hemolysis • Perform IgA antigen and anti-IgA testing
Management	• Transfusion interrupted • Antihistamine administered	• Transfusion terminated • Epinephrine and similar drugs administered • Oxygen administered and open airways maintained
Prevention	• Premedication with antihistamine, if patient history reveals repetitive reactions • May necessitate washed cellular products	• Plasma-containing products from IgA-deficient donors • Washed red cell and platelet products

DAT, Direct antiglobulin test.

Transfusion-Related Acute Lung Injury

Transfusion-related acute lung injury (TRALI) can be a life-threatening or fatal transfusion reaction. In fact, TRALI is currently the leading cause of mortality from transfusion.[2] TRALI is a clinical syndrome whose diagnosis relies on the assessment of clinical symptoms. This reaction has many overlapping symptoms with transfusion-related sepsis, circulatory overload, and anaphylactic reactions, which require rule out by medical personnel. Respiratory distress and pulmonary edema may occur during transfusion or within 6 hours. Symptoms include fever (1 to 2° C increase), chills, severe hypoxemia, dyspnea, nonproductive cough, new-onset bilateral pulmonary edema, tachycardia, and hypotension.[4] Specific criteria for diagnosing acute hypoxia associated with acute lung injury after transfusion are defined by respiratory measurements along with a chest x-ray showing bilateral infiltrates.[1]

The exact mechanism of lung injury in TRALI has not been determined.[12] The current proposed model states that TRALI occurs from the result of two hits: one from the recipient's underlying medical condition and the second from the transfusion itself (Fig. 11.5). Recipient-related risk factors contribute to the development of TRALI (ie, medical condition of patient).

In addition, transfusion risk factors contribute to the development of TRALI (ie, plasma from a donor with a pregnancy history, anti–human leukocyte antigen [HLA], anti–human neutrophil antigens [HNA], and biologic response molecules). Plasma from female multiparous donors repeatedly exposed to fetal HLA antigens may generate a wide variety of HLA antibodies and neutrophil antibodies. The presence of anti-HLA class II antibodies are strong predictors of TRALI risk.

The mechanism is associated with the infusion of antibodies to leukocyte antigens, which activates neutrophils in the pulmonary microvasculature. The activated neutrophils cause pulmonary epithelial damage, capillary leakage, and pulmonary edema. Transfused donor antibodies to class I and class II HLA antigens and neutrophil antigens have been

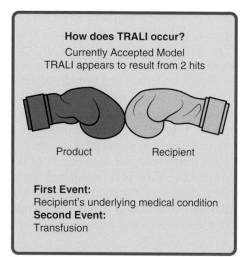

Fig. 11.5 What causes TRALI? TRALI may result from an interaction between the recipient's underlying condition and the event of transfusion.

TABLE 11.7	Transfusion-Related Acute Lung Injury
Clinical Signs and Symptoms[4]	• Fever (1–2° C increase) • Chills • Hypoxia • Dyspnea (shortness of breath) • Cyanosis (bluish discoloration of skin) • Nonproductive cough • New onset bilateral pulmonary edema • Hypotension • Acute onset within 6 hr of blood transfusion
Major Complications	• Severe and dramatic presentation • Can be fatal
Causes	• Interaction of recipient-related risks and transfusion event • Donor with pregnancy history, anti-HLA, anti-HNA
Clinical Laboratory Tests	• DAT: negative • No visible hemolysis • WBC antibody screen in donor and recipient • Chest x-ray
Management	• Respiratory support
Prevention	• Avoid use of plasma components from multiparous women who have HLA antibodies

HLA, Human leukocyte antigen; *DAT*, direct antiglobulin test; *WBC*, white blood cell.

implicated as the most probable cause of TRALI. Because multiparous women are more likely to have antibodies associated with TRALI, an effort to reduce the risk by using male donors for plasma products has decreased the fatalities reported to the FDA.[13]

AABB Standard 5.4.1.2, the TRALI risk mitigation standard, was effective April 1, 2014.[11] The standard stated that "[p]lasma and whole blood for allogeneic transfusion shall be from males, females who have not been pregnant, or females who have been tested since their most recent pregnancy and results interpreted as negative for HLA antibodies." This standard was implemented to reduce the incidence of TRALI as a complication of transfusion. Table 11.7 provides a summary of the important concepts of TRALI.

TRANSFUSION-ASSOCIATED GRAFT-VERSUS-HOST DISEASE

Transfusion-associated graft-versus-host disease (TA-GVHD) is a rare but highly lethal complication of transfusion; it is associated with a 90% mortality rate.[4] This immune reaction is mediated by immunocompetent donor lymphocytes in cellular blood components.

Symptoms can occur 3 to 30 days after transfusion and include maculopapular rash, fever, nausea, diarrhea, pancytopenia, and elevated liver function tests.[1,4] After the transfusion of donor lymphocytes to a recipient who is immunologically incompetent or closely HLA similar, the donor lymphocytes engraft and mount an immune response against the host tissues. Because the host is unable to destroy the transfused cells, the donor lymphocytes proliferate and respond to unshared histocompatibility antigens in the host. TA-GVHD is only rarely successfully treated; therefore identifying patients at risk and providing irradiated blood products is essential. Table 11.8 lists indications for irradiated components.

Immunocompromised patients and recipients who are receiving blood products from donors that share similar HLA phenotypes are at high risk of developing TA-GVHD and should receive blood products that have been irradiated at specific doses required by AABB standards.[11] Irradiation eliminates the ability of leukocytes to replicate and mount an immune response. Leukocyte reduction of the blood component is *not* sufficient to avoid TA-GVHD. Table 11.9 summarizes the important concepts regarding TA-GVHD.

BACTERIAL CONTAMINATION OF BLOOD

A serious and potentially fatal adverse complication of transfusion is secondary to bacterial proliferation in donor units during storage. The transfusion of small amounts of bacterially contaminated blood can be fatal or cause serious morbidity.[14] The major sources of the bacterial contamination include the following:

• Donor has asymptomatic bacteremia at time of donation

TABLE 11.8   Indications for Irradiated Components

INDICATED	NOT INDICATED
Intrauterine transfusions	Patients with HIV
Premature, low-birth-weight infants	Full-term infants
Congenital immunodeficiencies	Nonimmunosuppressed patients
Hematologic malignancies	
HLA-matched components	
Directed donations from related donors	
Granulocyte components	
Newborns with erythroblastosis fetalis	

HIV, Human immunodeficiency virus.
Data from Fung MK, editor: *Technical manual*, ed 18, Bethesda, MD, 2014, AABB.

TABLE 11.9   Transfusion-Associated Graft-Versus-Host Disease

Clinical Signs and Symptoms	• Onset 3–30 days posttransfusion • Fever, erythematous maculopapular rash, abnormal liver function, diarrhea, pancytopenia
Major Complications	• Marrow aplasia and hemorrhage • 90% mortality rate
Cause	• Transfused immunocompetent T lymphocytes mount immunologic response against recipient
Clinical Laboratory Tests	• Confirmation by HLA typing to demonstrate a disparity between donor lymphocytes and recipient tissues
Management	• Unresponsive to medical intervention
Prevention	• Irradiation of blood products before transfusion in at-risk recipients • Gamma irradiation (25 Gy) to prevent blast transformation of donor lymphocytes[11]

HLA, Human leukocyte antigen.

- Rare bacterial infection that can survive in storage conditions recommended for RBCs and platelet components
- System failure: pinhole in blood collection set, testing error, not following standard operation procedure (SOP)

Bacterial endotoxins, generated during the storage period, result in a dramatic clinical picture on transfusion of the contaminated blood product. Transfusion recipients may experience shock rapidly. Fatalities attributed to transfusion of contaminated blood are more common after platelet transfusions.[2]

Efforts to reduce the possibility of a bacterially contaminated product have evolved. Current mitigations in place to assist in the contamination of blood components include:

- Closed sterile system of collection bags for use in collection and blood product manufacturing
- Attention during the donor phlebotomy process to scrub arm at and around the venipuncture site
- Diversion of the skin plug, generated during phlebotomy, into a sample diversion pouch
- Donor health check before donation
- Postdonation information provided to donors to report any health issues after donation
- Requirement for methods to limit and to detect or inactivate bacteria in all platelet components[11]

Any contaminating bacteria in the donor unit that are unable to survive at 4° C die after several days of storage. However, organisms capable of growth at 4° C find an ideal environment for their perpetuation. Gram-negative bacteria such as *Yersinia enterocolitica, Serratia liquefaciens,* and *Pseudomonas fluorescens* can thrive under these conditions and promote transfusion reactions. In addition, *Listeria monocytogenes,* a gram-positive bacterium, can thrive at cold temperatures and utilize iron as a growth requirement.[15] Gram-positive and gram-negative organisms have also been linked to platelets stored at 20° C to 24° C. These organisms include bacteria from *Staphylococcus* and *Streptococcus* species, *Bacillus cereus; Klebsiella, Serratia,* and *Enterobacter* species; and *Escherichia coli.*[4,16]

The clinical symptoms of bacterial contamination mimic AHTR, including fever, chills, headache, hypotension, shock, muscular pain, vomiting, and diarrhea. The number of infused organisms influences the symptomatic presentation and the clinical outcome. Treatment of the reaction must be initiated before confirmation of the cause to prevent a fatal outcome. Broad-spectrum antibiotic therapy is provided to the recipient.[1] Blood cultures from the patient and the blood bag are obtained. Transfusion service personnel perform visual checks of all donor units at the time of issue. The individual inspecting the donor unit should be alert for any visible discoloration, clots, cloudiness, or hemolysis.

TRANSFUSION-ASSOCIATED CIRCULATORY OVERLOAD

Transfusion-associated circulatory overload (TACO), as a category of adverse complications of transfusion, is defined by the CDC as "infusion volume that cannot be effectively processed by the recipient either due to high rate and/or volume of infusion or an underlying cardiac or pulmonary pathology."[1] Patients older than 70 years old and infants are at greatest risk.[4] Recent FDA data from 2009 to 2013 showed that TACO is now the second cause of mortality from transfusion.[2] This complication of transfusion is considered with new onset or exacerbation of three or more of the following symptoms within 6 hours after completion of transfusion[1]:

- Acute respiratory distress (dyspnea, orthopnea, cough)
- Elevated brain natriuretic peptide (BNP)
- Elevated central venous pressure (CVP)
- Evidence of left heart failure
- Evidence of positive fluid balance
- Radiographic evidence of pulmonary edema

Patients with compromised cardiac and pulmonary status poorly tolerate rapid elevations in total blood volume and are more susceptible to TACO. Suggested intervention strategy when TACO is suspected includes[17];

1. Stop transfusion or infusion of other fluids
2. Stabilize patient
3. Contact physician and notify blood bank
4. Provide respiratory support (eg, supplemental oxygen, ventilatory assistance)
5. Administer diuretics where not contraindicated
6. Perform blood bank investigations to rule out other adverse effects (eg, hemolysis, sepsis, TRALI, etc.).

Transfusion candidates susceptible to TACO should receive RBC units, not whole blood. The units should be administered at a slower rate in small-volume aliquots. Infusions of large volumes of plasma should be avoided. Refer to Table 11.10 for a summary of a TACO transfusion reaction.

TRANSFUSION HEMOSIDEROSIS

Thalassemia: inherited disorder causing anemia because of a defective production rate of either α or β hemoglobin polypeptide

Hemosiderosis is a condition that results from the accumulation of excess iron in macrophages in various tissues. Iron overload is a potential complication in patients undergoing long-term transfusions, such as patients with **thalassemia** and sickle cell disease with persistent hemolysis. In transfusion hemosiderosis, iron intake (250 mg/unit) exceeds the daily iron excretion (1 mg/day) with the subsequent deposition of excess iron in the liver, heart, and kidney. When patients have received more than 100 transfusions, iron deposition may interfere with the function of the liver, heart, or endocrine glands. Prevention of iron toxicity through the use of iron chelators such as deferiprone or deferoxamine allows the body to bind and excrete excess iron through the urine and feces.[4]

CITRATE TOXICITY

The transfusion of large quantities of citrated blood in a relatively short time frame introduces the risk of citrate toxicity for the transfusion recipient. Citrate, which is present in the formulation of the anticoagulants used in the blood collection process, binds ionized calcium. Excess citrate may be toxic to patients receiving large volumes in massive transfusion situations or in patients with impaired liver function for the metabolism of the citrate. Citrate toxicity is a possible adverse event in the transfusion of preterm infants with severe hepatic or renal insufficiency. Removing the additive-containing plasma may be beneficial in these patients. Injections of calcium chloride or calcium gluconate negate the toxic effects.[4]

TABLE 11.10	Transfusion-Associated Circulatory Overload
Clinical Signs and Symptoms[4]	• Acute respiratory distress (dyspnea, cough) • ↑Brain natriuretic peptide • ↑Central venous pressure • Left heart failure • Positive fluid balance • Radiographic evidence of pulmonary edema • Acute onset within 6 hr of blood transfusion
Major Complications	• Acute pulmonary edema
Causes	• Transfusion of large volumes of blood component and fluids • High flow rates
Clinical Laboratory Tests	• Rule out TRALI • Chest x-ray
Management	• Respiratory support • Administer diuretics when possible
Prevention	• Infusions of large volumes of plasma avoided • Transfuse only RBC units • Transfuse blood at slower rate

↑, increased levels.

POSTTRANSFUSION PURPURA

In posttransfusion purpura (PTP), the patient's platelet count plummets 5 to 12 days after the transfusion of blood or blood products containing platelets. Generalized purpura and an increased probability of bleeding episodes follow. This complication is an anamnestic response to a previous sensitization with the high-incidence platelet antigen, HPA-1a, which has a 98% frequency in the population. Antigen-negative individuals are at risk of developing PTP. HPA-1a–negative women are sensitized through multiple pregnancies and respond with the immune production of anti–HPA-1a. This platelet-specific alloantibody destroys not only the transfused HPA-1a platelets, but also the patient's HPA-1a–negative platelets. The mechanism for the concomitant destruction of the autologous platelets with transfused platelets has not been determined. Treatment of PTP includes plasmapheresis, exchange transfusion, and use of intravenous immunoglobulin (IVIG).[4] Scan the QR code to listen to transfusion reaction podcasts by the Blood Bank Guy.

SECTION 3
EVALUATION AND REPORTING A TRANSFUSION REACTION

INITIATING A TRANSFUSION REACTION INVESTIGATION

Protocols for the initiation of a transfusion necessitate that the transfusionist carefully check all the identifying information and document informed patient consent before the infusion of the blood product. This information is documented in the transfusion record with the date and time of the start of the transfusion.[11] In addition to verifying identification, the transfusionist records the patient's pretransfusion vital signs, including temperature, blood pressure, pulse, and respiration rate. The transfusionist should remain with the patient for the first few minutes of the infusion to detect any indications of acute hemolysis, anaphylaxis, or bacterial contamination. After the first 15-minute period, the patient should be observed and the vital signs should be recorded. Clinical personnel should continue to observe the patient periodically throughout the transfusion and 4 to 6 hours after completion to detect febrile or pulmonary reactions to the blood administration.[4]

If an adverse reaction is suspected, the following procedure is performed:
- The transfusion should be stopped; reidentification of the patient and the transfused component is initiated.
- The transfusion service and the patient's physician are notified immediately of the suspected reaction.
- An intravenous line is maintained (for administration with blood) with normal saline or a solution approved by the FDA.
- The physician evaluates the patient to determine any clinical intervention and potential medical management.
- If signs and symptoms of possible AHTR, anaphylaxis, TRALI, transfusion-induced sepsis, or other serious complications are seen, a postreaction blood sample is sent to the transfusion service for evaluation. This specimen must be properly labeled and forwarded to the transfusion service with the blood bag, the administration set, the attached intravenous solutions, and all related forms and labels. In some cases, the first voided postreaction urine is collected for possible evaluation.
- If the presenting clinical signs and symptoms are indicative of urticarial or circulatory overload, the transfusion service does not need to evaluate any postreaction blood and urine samples.[4]

An outline of transfusion reaction instructions to medical personnel is provided in Fig. 11.6.

Any suspected transfusion reaction becomes a high priority in the transfusion service. On receipt of the postreaction clinical materials, the transfusion service personnel perform the following steps (Fig. 11.7):

1. Clerical check for any errors in identification
Patient's sample and blood component are checked for any errors relating to identification. If such an error is discovered, notification is provided to the medical personnel

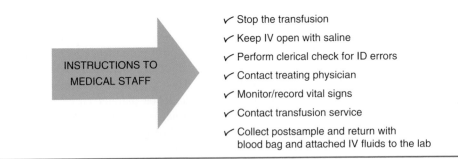

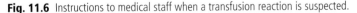

Fig. 11.6 Instructions to medical staff when a transfusion reaction is suspected.

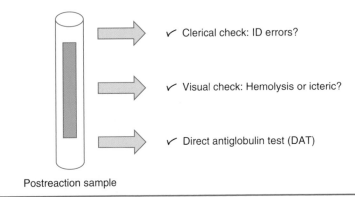

Fig. 11.7 Postreaction workup. Initial investigation to determine whether a hemolytic transfusion reaction is occurring.

handling the transfusion reaction. All records are double-checked to determine whether another potential transfusion recipient is at risk because of this error. The source of the error is evaluated in light of the overall transfusion process to determine where the system failed.

2. Visual check for hemolysis or icterus

Because red cells immediately release free hemoglobin into the plasma during intravascular hemolysis, the postreaction sample is evaluated for any evidence of hemolysis or **icterus** and is compared with the pretransfusion sample, if available in the laboratory. Any pinkish or reddish discoloration suggests the presence of free hemoglobin. If a transfusion has occurred over a 3- to 4-hour period, icterus may be noted as the degradation of free hemoglobin to bilirubin progresses. Bilirubin levels usually peak at 5 to 7 hours after a hemolytic event.

Icterus: pertaining to or resembling jaundice

3. DAT

To check for a serologic incompatibility, a DAT is performed on a postreaction (preferably anticoagulated) sample. A microscopic DAT is performed by some laboratories because the ratio of donor to recipient cells is small. If the postreaction sample is positive, a recipient alloantibody may have sensitized the transfused red cells. A positive DAT from a transfusion reaction appears as a mixed field with the transfused red cells demonstrating agglutination and the autologous red cells remaining unagglutinated. If the transfused red cells have experienced a rapid clearance, the DAT may be negative at the time of sample collection. Comparison of the postreaction sample with the DAT performed on the pretransfusion sample is helpful in evaluating the transfusion reaction.

4. Other serologic tests are performed, as needed

Additional Laboratory Testing in a Transfusion Reaction

Depending on the results of the aforementioned testing, further laboratory testing may be performed (Table 11.11). The extent of the additional testing is in part at the discretion

TABLE 11.11	Additional Testing in a Transfusion Reaction Investigation
TEST	**REASON**
ABO/D phenotyping	Errors in patient or sample identification
Antibody screen	Newly detected antibodies
Crossmatch	Serologic compatibility
Hemoglobin/hematocrit	Therapeutic effectiveness
Haptoglobin	Hemolytic process
Bilirubin	Hemolytic process
Urine hemoglobin	Hemolytic process
Inspection of donor unit	Nonimmune hemolysis or bacterial contamination
Gram stain and blood culture	Bacterial contamination

of the physician in charge of the transfusion service and preestablished policies for the investigation of a transfusion reaction.[11] According to AABB *Standards*, "[T]here must be a process for evaluation for suspected nonhemolytic transfusion reactions including, but not limited to, febrile reactions, possible bacterial contamination, and TRALI."[11] A review and interpretation by the medical director is also required. Additional laboratory testing that may follow the initial investigation includes any combination of the following analyses:

- TEST: ABO testing of pretransfusion and posttransfusion patient samples, along with a reconfirmation of the ABO of the donor unit
  REASON: Any discrepancies of typing confirm an error in sample or patient identification; if an error in the patient's sample has occurred, an investigation of another potential clerical error affecting another patient should be initiated.
- TEST: Parallel testing of pretransfusion and posttransfusion patient samples for antibody detection
  REASON: The use of additional enhancement techniques in the antibody screen may be helpful in the detection of a weakly reactive antibody. Polyethylene glycol or enzyme techniques may provide additional information in the workup. If a new antibody is detected, antibody identification procedures are performed. A previously undetected antibody, now evident in the posttransfusion sample, is indicative of a possible anamnestic immune response after the recent transfusion exposure. The donor unit transfused to the recipient is checked for the presence of the antigen.
- TEST: Repetition of crossmatch using pretransfusion and posttransfusion patient samples
  REASON: The recommended crossmatch procedure includes both the immediate-spin and the antiglobulin crossmatch phases. Check to see if results differ.
- TEST: Frequent checks of hematologic status
  REASON: Hemoglobin and hematocrit values are evaluated after transfusion for expected therapeutic elevations of 1 g/dL hemoglobin and 3% hematocrit for each RBC unit transfused.[4]
- TEST: Analysis of haptoglobin levels on both the pretransfusion and the posttransfusion patient samples
  REASON: Haptoglobin is a plasma protein with the sole function of binding free hemoglobin and carrying the molecule to hepatocytes for further catabolism. During a hemolytic process, haptoglobin levels decrease in plasma because haptoglobin–hemoglobin complexes are formed. Free hemoglobin, released during intravascular red cell destruction, is excreted into the urine after exceeding the plasma haptoglobin-binding capacity.
- TEST: Examination of returned donor unit and administration tubing for abnormal appearance or hemolysis
  REASON: If bacterial sepsis is suspected, Gram stain and culture of the donor unit may be performed.

- **TEST:** Other postreaction testing
  REASON: Other postreaction testing may include bilirubin, IgA levels, and HLA and granulocyte antibody detection.

RECORDS AND REPORTING OF TRANSFUSION REACTIONS AND FATALITIES

Hemovigilance Component

Facilities that elect to participate in the hemovigilance component of the NHSN are required to use case definition criteria in reporting reactions.[3] The reactions are also assessed as definitive, probable, or possible on whether they meet the defined criteria. The severity of the reactions is graded on a scale of 1 to 4, where 1 is least severe and 4 is death. The relationship of the reaction to the transfusion is also assessed as definitive, probable, or possible. These reporting guidelines allow for consistency and thus more accurate evaluation and assessment of data collected by the participating facilities. Case definition criteria are outlined in Table 11.12.

Records

Records of patients who experience an adverse reaction to a transfusion remain indefinitely in the transfusion service.[11] Cases of transfusion-transmitted disease and bacterial contamination must also be reported to the blood collection facility. These records serve as a determining factor in the prevention of future reactions. For example, a patient with a history of a previous clinically relevant alloantibody, currently not demonstrable in the antibody screen test, would require a transfusion with antigen-negative donor units.

FDA-Reportable Fatalities

Fatalities attributable to transfusion must be reported as soon as possible by telephone, express mail, or electronic means to the director of the FDA Office of Compliance, Center for Biologics Evaluation and Research, followed by a written report within 7 days.[13] The formal report includes medical and laboratory documentation and an autopsy report.

TABLE 11.12	Case Definition Criteria for Hemovigilance Reporting
CRITERIA	**DEFINITIONS**
Signs and symptoms	*Definitive:* Conclusive *Probable:* Evidence in favor *Possible:* Evidence indeterminate
Laboratory/radiology	*Definitive:* Conclusive *Probable:* Evidence in favor *Possible:* Evidence indeterminate
Severity (graded)	*Grade 1:* Nonsevere *Grade 2:* Severe—requires medical intervention or prolongation of hospitalization or both *Grade 3:* Life-threatening; major intervention needed to prevent death *Grade 4:* Death as a result of adverse transfusion reaction
Relationship to transfusion (imputability)	*Definitive:* Conclusive *Probable:* Evidence in favor *Possible:* Evidence indeterminate

Data from NHSN manual: biovigilance component protocol hemovigilance module, August 2014. *Guidelines and procedures for monitoring hemovigilance.* http://www.cdc.gov/nhsn/bio.html. October 2015

CHAPTER SUMMARY

The major immune-mediated and non–immune-mediated adverse complications of transfusion are summarized in the following table:

Adverse Complications of Transfusion

	CAUSE	SIGNS AND SYMPTOMS	CLINICAL TESTS
Immune-mediated			
Hemolytic	Acute: ABO incompatibility Delayed: Primary or secondary alloimmunization	Fever, chills, pain, hypotension Unexplained decrease in hemoglobin	Positive DAT, eluate, serum antibody, elevated plasma hemoglobin or bilirubin
Febrile nonhemolytic	Recipient leukocyte antibodies, transfused cytokines	Fever, chills, rigors	Rule out hemolysis, test for HLA antibodies
Urticarial	Plasma allergen	Rash, hives, flushing	None, responds to symptomatic treatment
Anaphylactic	Anti-IgA in IgA-deficient recipient	Respiratory distress, hypotension	IgA antibody
TRALI	Donor WBC antibodies	Hypoxemia	Bilateral infiltrates in chest x-ray
Posttransfusion purpura	Anti–HPA-1a or other platelet antibody	Thrombocytopenia (↓20% of pretransfusion count)	Anti–HPA-1a antibody
TA-GVHD	Immunocompetent donor lymphocytes to susceptible host	Fever, rash, diarrhea	Abnormal liver dysfunction test, WBC chimerism
Non–immune-mediated			
Hemolytic	Mechanical or chemical trauma to unit	Fever, chills, pain, hypotension	Check blood administration needles, fluid, blood warmers
TACO	Volume overload secondary to rapid, high volume infusion	Respiratory distress, pulmonary edema, cardiac failure	Underlying cardiac or pulmonary pathology
Bacterial infection	Donor septicemia or contamination during phlebotomy	Fever, chills	Gram stain, culture of unit

CRITICAL THINKING EXERCISES

Exercise 11.1

An inexperienced nurse from an outpatient facility calls the transfusion service to report a transfusion reaction. The transfusion recipient is complaining of shortness of breath and chills. The nurse is seeking advice on the appropriate procedure.
1. What instructions should be provided to the nurse?
2. What documentation should be returned to the transfusion service?
3. What immediate procedures should be performed in the laboratory to initiate the transfusion reaction investigation?

Exercise 11.2

Seven days after the transfusion of 5 RBC units, a patient demonstrates a 5 g/dL decrease in hemoglobin and is mildly jaundiced. No evidence of bleeding is identified.
1. What tests would provide evidence for a delayed transfusion reaction?
2. What is the rationale for the test selection?

Exercise 11.3

A 55-year-old man was admitted to the emergency department after a motor vehicle accident. The patient is hemorrhaging from a lacerated spleen and requires emergency surgery. Pretransfusion testing determined that the patient's phenotype is group A, D-negative with a negative antibody screen. Crossmatches with RBC units were compatible by the immediate-spin crossmatch. During surgery, the patient receives 6 units of group A, D-negative RBCs and 4 units of group A frozen plasma. Three days later, during the first 15 minutes of a subsequent RBC transfusion using a blood-warming device, the patient developed fever and chills.

1. Based on the information provided, propose three possible explanations of the cause of the transfusion reaction.
2. Determine a strategy for the evaluation of the transfusion reaction to rule in or rule out any possible mechanism.

Exercise 11.4

Refer to the table in the Chapter Summary.
1. Outline possible preventive measures for each of the reactions listed.
2. Describe the category of patients most likely to experience each reaction.

STUDY QUESTIONS

1. A patient experiences chills and fever, nausea, flushing, and lower back pain after infusion of 150 mL of blood. What action should be taken to rule out an acute hemolytic transfusion reaction?
   a. perform a DAT and visually compare pretransfusion and posttransfusion serum samples
   b. measure serum haptoglobin on prereaction and postreaction samples
   c. repeat crossmatches on prereaction and postreaction samples
   d. perform Gram stain and culture of the unit

2. Select the type of transfusion reaction that presents with dyspnea, severe headache, and peripheral edema occurring soon after transfusion.
   a. hemolytic
   b. TRALI
   c. TACO
   d. anaphylactic

3. What is a common cause of a febrile nonhemolytic transfusion reaction?
   a. recipient is allergic to the donor's plasma proteins
   b. donor unit is cold
   c. donor unit has a positive DAT
   d. recipient has antibodies to the donor's HLA antigens

4. What plasma protein functions to bind hemoglobin after intravascular hemolysis?
   a. albumin
   b. haptoglobin
   c. transferrin
   d. C-reactive protein

5. Which of the following adverse complications of transfusion is prevented by the irradiation of blood components?
   a. TRALI
   b. hyperkalemia
   c. febrile
   d. TA-GVHD

6. Which of the following characteristics is associated with a delayed serologic transfusion reaction?
   a. hives and wheals
   b. hemosiderosis
   c. positive antibody screen in posttransfusion sample
   d. ABO incompatibility between donor unit and recipient

7. What blood group system antibodies are more commonly associated with delayed hemolytic transfusion reactions?
   a. Rh
   b. ABO
   c. MNS
   d. Lewis

8. A patient has experienced two febrile nonhemolytic reactions after RBC transfusion. What is the preferred blood component if future transfusions are necessary?
   a. leukocyte-reduced RBCs
   b. irradiated RBCs
   c. cytomegalovirus-negative RBCs
   d. group O, D-negative RBCs

9. Which of the following patient histories might suggest future transfusions with saline-washed RBCs?
   a. history of multiple red cell alloantibodies
   b. history of congestive heart failure
   c. IgA-negative recipient with anti-IgA antibodies
   d. history of transfusion-associated sepsis

10. What is the cause of transfusion-induced hemosiderosis?
    a. excess citrate
    b. HPA-1a antigen
    c. iron overload
    d. circulatory overload

11. What laboratory test is useful to detect clerical errors of sample identification in an acute transfusion reaction investigation?
    a. ABO typing
    b. antibody screen
    c. crossmatch
    d. DAT

12. What microorganism grows well at 4° C and may result in a transfusion-transmitted sepsis?
    a. *Staphylococcus aureus*
    b. *Yersinia enterocolitica*
    c. *Staphylococcus epidermidis*
    d. *Bacillus cereus*

13. What is the expected therapeutic effect in the recipient's hematocrit after the transfusion of 1 unit of RBCs?
    a. increase of 0.5%
    b. increase of 1%
    c. increase of 2%
    d. increase of 3%

14. What is the usual cause of an anaphylactic reaction to transfusion?
    a. anti-IgA in an IgA-deficient recipient
    b. anti-IgG in an IgA-deficient recipient
    c. IgA deficiency
    d. IgG deficiency

15. Which of the following events is associated with a precipitous decrease in a recipient's platelet count after a transfusion?
    a. circulatory overload
    b. posttransfusion purpura
    c. citrate toxicity
    d. factor VIII deficiency

16. When evaluating a possible delayed hemolytic reaction, what is the best sample to use for bilirubin determination?
    a. 6 hours posttransfusion
    b. 12 hours posttransfusion
    c. 24 hours posttransfusion
    d. 48 hours posttransfusion

17. In a delayed serologic or hemolytic transfusion reaction, what is the typical result of the DAT?
    a. negative
    b. weak positive, mixed field
    c. positive with C3 only
    d. negative if serum antibody screen is negative

18. Which type of transfusion reaction will be prevented by the use of plasma from only male donors for transfusion?
    a. febrile
    b. TRALI
    c. allergic
    d. TACO

19. Premedication with diphenhydramine (Benadryl) is a common procedure when administrating platelets to patients undergoing frequent transfusions. Which type of transfusion reaction does this medication prevent?
    a. allergic
    b. TRALI
    c. febrile nonhemolytic reactions
    d. TACO

20. What is the usual cause of posttransfusion purpura after transfusion of platelets?
    a. HLA antibodies in the donor unit
    b. HLA antibodies made by the recipient
    c. anti–HPA-1a made by the recipient
    d. febrile reactions secondary to cytokines in the unit

21. Five days after a transfusion, a patient returned to his physician for postsurgical blood tests. It was noted that the hemoglobin value decreased from 11 mg/dL to 9 mg/dL during that time. The patient had not experienced any symptoms. To rule out a delayed hemolytic transfusion reaction, what test should be performed?
    a. DAT on current sample, elution if positive
    b. antibody screen on the current sample
    c. blood smear to check for spherocytes
    d. all of the above

22. According to AABB *Standards,* what type of transfusion reaction does not have to be reported to the blood bank?
    a. febrile
    b. TACO
    c. TRALI
    d. allergic

Answers to Study Questions can be found on page 387.

Ⓔ Additional student resources, including review questions, a laboratory manual, and case studies, can be found on the Evolve website.

REFERENCES

1. NHSN manual: biovigilance component protocol hemovigilance module: *Guidelines and procedures for monitoring hemovigilance.* August 2014. http://www.cdc.gov/nhsn/pdfs/biovigilance/bv-hv-protocol-current.pdf. Accessed October 2015.
2. Food and Drug Administration: *Fatalities reported to FDA following blood collection and transfusion: Annual summary for fiscal year 2013*, Rockville, MD, 2013, CBER Office of Communication, Outreach, and Development. http://www.fda.gov/biologicsbloodvaccines/safetyavailability/reportaproblem/transfusiondonationfatalities/ucm391574.htm. Accessed October 2015.
3. National Healthcare Safety Network: *Hemovigilance module: adverse reaction case definition exercises, July 2009.* Centers for Disease Control and Prevention. http://www.cdc.gov/nhsn/PDFs/slides/bio/Adverse-Reactions_Final_March2013.pdf. Accessed October 2015.
4. Fung MK, editor: *Technical manual,* ed 18, Bethesda, MD, 2014, AABB.
5. Wagener FA, Eggert A, Boerman OC, et al.: Heme is a potent inducer of inflammation in mice and is counteracted by heme oxygenase, *Blood* 98:1802, 2001.
6. Klein HG, Anstee DJ: *Mollison's blood transfusion in clinical medicine*, ed 12, West Sussex, UK, 2014, Wiley Blackwell.
7. Ness PM, Shirey RS, Thoman SK: The differentiation of delayed and serologic and delayed hemolytic transfusion reactions: incidence, long-term serologic findings, and clinical significance, *Transfusion* 30:688, 1990.
8. Schonewille H, van de Watering LMG, Brand A: Additional red cell alloantibodies after blood cell transfusion in a nonhematological alloimmunized patient cohort: Is it time to take precautionary measures? *Transfusion* 46:630, 2006.
9. Pagliano JC, Pomper GJ, Fisch GS, et al.: Reduction of febrile but not allergic reactions to RBCs and platelets after conversion to universal prestorage leukoreduction, *Transfusion* 44:16, 2004.
10. Ezidiegwu CN, Lauenstein KJ, Rosales LG, et al.: Febrile non-hemolytic transfusion reactions: Management by premedication and cost implications in adult patients, *Arch Pathol Lab Med* 128:991, 2004.
11. Levitt J: *Standards for blood banks and transfusion services*, ed 29, Bethesda, MD, 2014, AABB.
12. Shaz BH: Bye-bye TRALI: By understanding and innovation, *Blood* 123:22, 2014.
13. Food and Drug Administration: *Code of federal regulations, 21 CFR 606.170*, Washington, DC, 2011, US Government Printing Office (revised annually).
14. Qureshi R: *Introduction to Transfusion Science Practice*, ed 6, Manchester, UK, 2015, British Blood Transfusion Society.
15. Guevara RE, Tormey MP, Nguyen DM, et al.: *Listeria monocytogenes* in platelets. A case report, *Transfusion* 46:305–309, 2006.
16. Brecher ME, Hay SN: Bacterial contamination of blood components, *Clin Micro Review* 18:195–204, 2005.
17. Andrzejewski C: Understanding TACO: What is it and what can we do to reduce the risk? *AABB Audioconference*, April 7, 2015. AABB.

12

HEMOLYTIC DISEASE OF THE FETUS AND NEWBORN

CHAPTER OUTLINE

LEARNING OBJECTIVES

On completion of this chapter, the reader should be able to:

1. Discuss the etiology of hemolytic disease of the fetus and newborn (HDFN).
2. Contrast the metabolism of bilirubin in the fetus versus bilirubin in the newborn.
3. Correlate the tests included in an initial prenatal workup with their significance in predicting HDFN.
4. Distinguish clinically significant and insignificant antibodies in terms of causing HDFN.
5. Explain the primary value of performing antibody titration, and state what results are considered significant.
6. Outline the intervention procedures used in the diagnosis and management of HDFN.
7. Explain the role of cordocentesis and fetal genotyping in the prediction of HDFN.
8. List the tests routinely performed on cord blood cells when HDFN is suspected, and discuss possible sources of error when performing each test.
9. Compare and contrast the clinical and laboratory findings in ABO HDFN versus HDFN caused by anti-D.
10. Discuss the composition, eligibility criteria, and principle of Rh immune globulin (RhIG).
11. Explain the principle, interpretation, and significance of a positive rosette test for fetomaternal hemorrhage.
12. Outline the principle, interpretation, and significance of the Kleihauer–Betke acid elution.
13. Evaluate laboratory test results on postpartum samples, and determine whether RhIG should be administered.
14. Given the fetomaternal hemorrhage results, calculate the dose of RhIG.
15. Explain the selection of blood for an intrauterine transfusion or exchange transfusion with regard to ABO and D phenotype.
16. List the special considerations that must be met when selecting blood for exchange transfusion, and explain the purpose of each requirement.

Hemolytic disease of the fetus and newborn (HDFN), also known as **erythroblastosis fetalis,** is a disorder of the fetus or newborn in which fetal and newborn red cells are destroyed by maternal IgG antibodies. These antibodies, directed against fetal antigens, cross the placenta, sensitize fetal red cells, and shorten red cell survival. This premature red cell destruction results in disease varying from mild anemia to death in utero. The transfusion service plays a critical role in the prediction, diagnosis, treatment, and prevention of this potentially life-threatening disease. The terms **prenatal, antenatal,** and **antepartum** refer to the time before delivery when testing is done to prevent or predict HDFN. **Neonatal** testing involves testing the newborn up to 28 days after delivery. The **perinatal** period extends from 28 weeks of gestation to 28 days after delivery.

SECTION 1
ETIOLOGY OF HEMOLYTIC DISEASE OF THE FETUS AND NEWBORN

During pregnancy, the placenta functions as the site of oxygen, nutrient, and waste exchange. In addition, the placenta serves as a barrier between maternal and fetal circulations. This barrier limits the number of fetal red cells entering the maternal circulation during pregnancy and reduces the chances of antibody production during pregnancy. ABO incompatibility between mother and child can also provide additional protection against immunization. Intravascular hemolysis of ABO-incompatible fetal red cells by maternal anti-A or anti-B reduces exposure to fetal cells carrying foreign antigens. At the time of delivery, when the placenta is separated from the uterus, a significant number of fetal red cells escape into the maternal circulation (known as **fetomaternal hemorrhage** [FMH]). In addition to delivery, immunization can result from fetal red cell exposure after amniocentesis, spontaneous or induced abortion, **cordocentesis,** ectopic pregnancy, or abdominal trauma. Fetal red cells carrying antigens that are different from the mother (paternal antigens) can stimulate an active immune response in the mother, which results in the production of IgG antibodies.

In a subsequent pregnancy, the IgG antibodies cross the placental barrier by an active transport mechanism. The antibodies bind to the fetal antigens, which ends in red cell destruction by macrophages in the fetal liver and spleen. Hemoglobin liberated from the damaged red cells is metabolized to indirect bilirubin. The indirect bilirubin is transported across the placenta, conjugated by the maternal liver, and harmlessly excreted by the mother (Fig. 12.1, *A*). As red cell destruction continues, the fetus becomes increasingly anemic. The fetal liver and spleen enlarge as erythropoiesis increases in an effort to compensate for the red cell destruction. Immature red cells (erythroblasts) are released into the fetal circulation (which explains the term erythroblastosis fetalis). If this condition is left untreated, cardiac failure can occur, accompanied by **hydrops fetalis,** or edema and fluid accumulation in fetal peritoneal and pleural cavities. The greatest threat to the fetus is cardiac failure resulting from uncompensated anemia.

After delivery, the infant faces a different challenge. Red cell destruction continues with the release of indirect bilirubin. In utero, indirect bilirubin is conjugated in the maternal liver and excreted. However, the newborn liver is deficient in glucuronyl transferase (the liver enzyme needed to conjugate indirect bilirubin). As indirect bilirubin is released, it binds to albumin and circulates harmlessly. When the binding capacity of the albumin is exceeded, indirect bilirubin binds to tissues, which results in jaundice. In particular, it may bind with tissues of the central nervous system (CNS) and cause permanent brain damage (kernicterus), resulting in deafness, mental retardation, or death (Fig. 12.1, *B*).

SECTION 2
OVERVIEW OF HEMOLYTIC DISEASE OF THE FETUS AND NEWBORN

Three important factors must be present for HDFN to occur:
1. *The red cell antibody produced by the mother must be of the IgG class.* IgG is the only immunoglobulin capable of crossing the placental barrier. This active transport across

---

Erythroblastosis fetalis: also called hemolytic disease of the fetus and newborn

Prenatal: time period before birth

Antenatal: time period before birth

Antepartum: period between conception and onset of labor, used with reference to the mother

Neonatal: time period within the first 28 days after birth

Perinatal: period extends from 28 weeks of gestation to 28 days after delivery

Fetomaternal hemorrhage: escape of fetal cells into the maternal circulation, usually occurring at the time of delivery

Cordocentesis: procedure that punctures the umbilical vein at the point of placental insertion and aspirates a sample of fetal blood

Hydrops fetalis: edema in the fetus

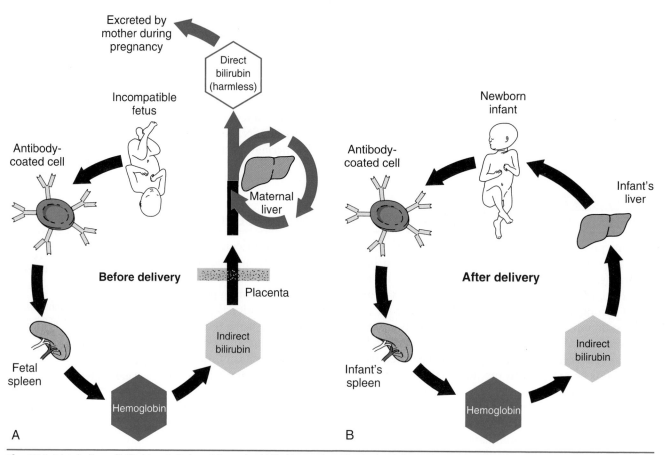

Fig. 12.1 Metabolism of bilirubin. **A,** Before delivery, fetal bilirubin, produced by the breakdown of sensitized red cells in the fetal spleen, is safely metabolized by the maternal liver. **B,** After delivery, the newborn's liver does not produce glucuronyl transferase and cannot convert bilirubin to an excretable form. As a result, the excess bilirubin collects in tissues and causes brain damage. (From Ortho Diagnostics: Blood group antigens and antibodies as applied to hemolytic disease of the fetus and newborn, Raritan, NJ, 1968, Ortho Diagnostics.)

the placenta is determined by the fragment, crystallizable, or Fc portion of the immunoglobulin molecule. IgM antibodies such as anti-Le[a], anti-Le[b], anti-M, anti-N, and anti-P1 have not been implicated in HDFN.[1]

2. *The fetus must possess an antigen that is lacking in the mother.* The gene for the antigen is inherited from the father. If the father is known to be homozygous for the gene, 100% of the children inherit the gene and are at risk for HDFN. If the father is known to be heterozygous, only 50% of the children may inherit the gene and are at risk.

3. *The antigen must be well developed at birth.* Blood group antigens such as Lewis, P1, and I are not well developed at birth. Antibodies to these antigens are not expected to cause HDFN because the antigen is not available to bind with the maternal antibody. HDFN is often classified into three categories based on antibody specificity: Rh (D), ABO, and other antibodies. These categories are described in the following section.

Rh HEMOLYTIC DISEASE OF THE FETUS AND NEWBORN

The D antigen of the Rh blood group system is a potent immunogen. Anti-D is responsible for the most severe cases of HDFN. In most cases, D-negative women become alloimmunized or sensitized at delivery in the first pregnancy with a D-positive baby. The first pregnancy rarely demonstrates clinical signs of HDFN. After production of anti-D, subsequent D-positive fetuses are affected to varying degrees (Fig. 12.2). In some cases, the maternal anti-D binds to fetal D-positive red cells and causes a positive direct antiglobulin test (DAT) and minimal, if any, signs of red cell destruction. Moderately affected infants develop signs of jaundice and corresponding elevations in bilirubin levels during the first few days of life. Severely affected D-positive infants, in whom rapid red cell

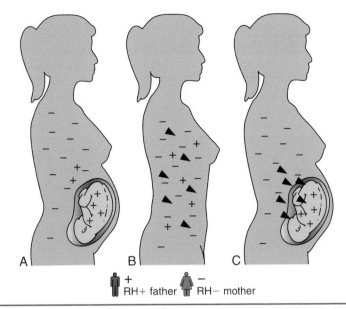

+
RH+ father   RH− mother

Fig. 12.2 Illustration of Rh (D) HDNF. **A,** During the first pregnancy involving an Rh (D)-negative mother and Rh (D)-positive fetus, fetal red cells will circulate in mother prenatal and postnatal. **B,** Between pregnancies, mother can mount an immune response to the fetal red cells and form anti-D. **C,** The next Rh (D)-incompatible pregnancy will be affected by the maternal IgG antibodies crossing the placenta and entering fetal circulation. Rh (D)-positive fetal red cells will become sensitized and destroyed by the maternal anti-D. (From Kee JL, et al: *Pharmacology*, ed 8, St. Louis, 2015, Elsevier.)

destruction occurs, experience anemia in utero and develop jaundice within hours of delivery. Exchange transfusion may be necessary to reduce bilirubin levels to prevent kernicterus after delivery.

The introduction of **Rh immune globulin (RhIG)** in 1968 dramatically reduced the incidence of Rh HDFN. Before the implementation of RhIG prophylaxis, 16% of ABO-compatible D-negative mothers with a D-positive infant became immunized. ABO-incompatible D-negative mothers with a D-positive infant had a ≤2% immunization rate.[2–4] HDFN caused by anti-D continues to occur in about 6.7 of 1000 live births in the United States. This rate likely reflects the failure to administer RhIG prophylaxis, inadequate prenatal care, or antenatal sensitization before RhIG administration at 28 weeks' gestation.[5]

Rh immune globulin (RhIG): commercially available human-source gamma globulin consisting of high-titered anti-D that is used in preventing alloimmunization to the D antigen

ABO HEMOLYTIC DISEASE OF THE FETUS AND NEWBORN

ABO antibodies are more commonly involved in newborn red cell destruction than are anti-D. Most cases are subclinical and do not necessitate treatment. Some infants may experience mildly elevated bilirubin levels and some degree of jaundice within the first few days of life. Based on the number of infants who develop jaundice, HDFN caused by ABO incompatibility occurs in 1 in 125 newborn infants.[4] These cases can usually be treated with **phototherapy.** Possible explanations for the mild red cell destruction despite high levels of maternal antibody include the following:

Phototherapy: treatment of elevated bilirubin or other conditions with ultraviolet light rays

- Presence of A or B substances in the fetal tissues and secretions that bind or neutralize ABO antibodies, which reduces the amount of ABO antibody available to destroy fetal red cells
- Poor development of ABO antigens on fetal or infant red cells
- Reduced number of A and B antigen sites on fetal or infant red cells

ABO HDFN occurs most frequently in group A or B babies born to group O mothers. In 15% of all pregnancies in white people, the mother is group O and her infant is group A or B. However, clinical presentation of HDFN is rare.[4] Group O individuals are more likely to have higher titers of IgG ABO antibodies compared with other ABO groups. In contrast to HDFN caused by anti-D, ABO incompatibility often affects the first pregnancy because of the presence of naturally occurring ABO antibodies. In Table 12.1, the clinical and laboratory findings in HDFN caused by ABO incompatibilities and anti-D are compared.[6]

TABLE 12.1	Comparison of ABO and Rh Hemolytic Disease of the Fetus and Newborn	
	ABO HDFN	**RH HDFN**
Clinical Findings		
Jaundice	Mild to moderate	Moderate to severe
Edema	No	Mild to severe
Serologic Results		
ABO and D type	Mother: O	Mother: D-negative
	Baby: A or B	Baby: D-positive
Direct antiglobulin test	Negative or weakly positive	Positive
Antibody	Anti-A, anti-B, anti-A,B	Anti-D
Hematology Results		
Anemia	Mild	Moderate to severe
Reticulocyte count	Mild increase	Greatly increased
Morphology	Spherocytes	Macrocytes, hypochromia
Nucleated RBC	Mild increase	Greatly increased
Chemistry Results		
Bilirubin	Mild increase, peaks at 24–48 hr after birth	Moderate to severe

HDFN, Hemolytic disease of the fetus and newborn; *RBC*, red blood cell.
Data from McKenzie SB: *Textbook of hematology*, ed 2, Baltimore, MD, 1996, Williams & Wilkins.

ALLOANTIBODIES CAUSING HEMOLYTIC DISEASE OF THE FETUS AND NEWBORN OTHER THAN ANTI-D

Any IgG antibody is capable of causing HDFN if the fetal red cells possess the antigen and the antigen is well developed at birth. Anti-c and anti-K are the next most common antibodies to cause HDFN after anti-D.[7] Less commonly reported antibodies include anti-E, anti-k, anti-Kp[a], anti-Kp[b], anti-Js[a], anti-Js[b], anti-Jk[a], anti-Fy[a], anti-Fy[b], anti-S, anti-s, and anti-U. Antibodies to low-frequency antigens, such as Js[a] and Kp[a], may not be detected when using screening or panel cells. If evidence of HDFN is present, testing paternal red cells with the mother's serum may demonstrate a positive reaction not detected with reagent red cells. Agglutination reaction with paternal cells would provide a clue to the presence of an antibody to a low-frequency antigen, and further testing with selected cells could be used to identify the specificity.

SECTION 3
PREDICTION OF HEMOLYTIC DISEASE OF THE FETUS AND NEWBORN

Prenatal or antepartum testing serves the following two purposes:
- To identify D-negative women who are candidates for RhIG (see Section 5 "Prevention of Hemolytic Disease of the Fetus and Newborn")
- To identify women with antibodies capable of causing HDFN, which helps assess potential risk to the fetus

Prenatal testing should be performed in the first trimester and should include ABO and D phenotyping. Testing the mother for weak D antigen is not required according to AABB standards.[8] However, a recent College of American Pathologists survey revealed that the standard of practice in the United States for laboratory testing for weak D phenotype varies.[9]

Most laboratories will test blood samples from donors with a D phenotype method intended to detect and interpret a weak D phenotype as D-positive. In other laboratories blood samples from patients, including pregnant women, are tested by methods to avoid detection of the weak D phenotype and are interpreted as D-negative to prevent alloimmunization and Rh hemolytic disease of the newborn.

TABLE 12.2	Prenatal Testing: Recommended Tests to Identify Women at Risk of Hemolytic Disease of the Fetus and Newborn
Initial Prenatal Visit	ABO/D (weak D test is optional) Antibody screen for IgG antibodies If antibody screen is positive, identify antibody Antibody titration for IgG antibodies to establish baseline
Follow-up Visits (if IgG antibody was identified)	Selected reagent red cell panel should be run to exclude other clinically significant antibodies Perform antibody titration in parallel with initial sample at 2- to 4-week intervals
26–28 Weeks' Gestation	Confirm D typing Repeat antibody screen[15]: • Before RhIG therapy in D-negative • In third trimester if patient was transfused or has a history of unexpected antibodies

RhIG, Rh immune globulin.
From Judd WJ: Practice guidelines for prenatal and perinatal immunohematology, revisited, *Transfusion* 41:1445, 2001.

An antibody screen using separate screening cells to detect clinically significant IgG alloantibodies is performed. If the antibody screen is positive, antibody identification should be performed. Laboratory testing of the paternal red cells for homozygosity or heterozygosity for the corresponding red cell antigen can predict future risk of HDFN. If the father is homozygous, 100% of the offspring will be at risk versus 50% of the offspring if he is heterozygous. Women with clinically significant IgG antibodies require careful management to monitor risk to the fetus. Table 12.2 outlines recommended laboratory testing to identify women at risk of HDFN.

MATERNAL HISTORY

An accurate obstetric and transfusion history is essential in predicting the course of a sensitized pregnancy. For a woman with a history of HDFN secondary to anti-D, a subsequent D-positive fetus has a much greater chance of being affected. A history of a previously affected infant can be useful in predicting the prognosis for future pregnancies.

ANTIBODY TITRATION

Antibody titration can be helpful in decisions regarding the performance and timing of procedures such as amniocentesis, ultrasound, color Doppler ultrasonography, and cordocentesis. Methods for determining the titer vary by institution, and the critical value for the potential of fetal anemia is usually established in each laboratory. The baseline antibody titer should be determined during the first trimester, and the specimen should be frozen for future testing. Testing should be repeated at 4- to 6-week intervals thereafter. A titer rising by two dilutions or greater is generally considered a significant change.[7] To ensure the validity of a rising titer, successive titrations should be performed using the same methods and test cells. Some facilities use a scoring method that combines titer and agglutination strength for the endpoint value. Titration methods are discussed in the AABB *Technical Manual* and should be carefully validated and used consistently at each facility.[7]

> Testing previously frozen samples in parallel with the current specimen ensures that any change in the titer is not the result of technical variables.

Critical titers for anti-D and other Rh system antibodies should be determined by each facility's medical director and is usually 16 or 32 at the antihuman globulin (AHG) phase.[7] The critical titer for anti-K is generally lower because of the K-antigen presence on early red cell precursors.[10] Once the critical value is met, assessments for the possibility of fetal anemia must be undertaken using amniocentesis or middle cerebral artery Doppler ultrasound. Refer to Fig. 12.3 for an explanation of the titration technique and Fig. 12.4 for an example. Scan the QR code for more information on antibody titration.

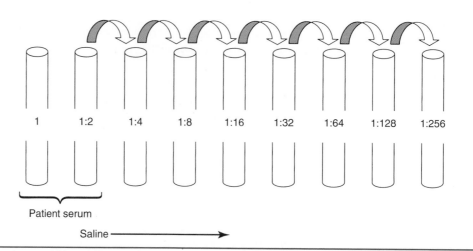

Fig. 12.3 Twofold serial dilutions of the serum containing the antibody are prepared with saline as the diluent. An equivalent volume of saline is first added to tubes 1:2→1:256. The same volume of serum is then added to tube 1 and 1:2. The 1:2 tube is mixed well. The equivalent volume of serum is transferred from the 1:2 to 1:4 tube continuing to the last tube, changing pipette tips to prevent carryover. The red cell selected for testing is usually homozygous. Testing uses the antiglobulin technique with anti-IgG. The titer is reported as the reciprocal of the highest dilution that gives a 1+ reaction.

Sample	Dilution Strength								
	1:1	1:2	1:4	1:8	1:16	1:32	1:64	1:128	1:256
#1	2+	2+	1+	(1+)	0	0	0	0	0
#2 (4 weeks later)	3+	3+	2+	1+	1+	(1+)	0	0	0

Fig. 12.4 Example of parallel testing for monitoring antibody increases during pregnancy. Sample #1 titer is reported as "8." Sample #2 titer is reported as "32." In this example, the increase of two tubes is noted (fourfold increase) and is considered to be significant.

ULTRASOUND TECHNIQUES

Over the past 20 years, investigators have studied ultrasound to indirectly screen for fetal anemia due to concerns about amniocentesis complications. The only validated tool for fetal anemia prediction is middle cerebral artery Doppler ultrasound.[11] Anemic fetuses have increased cardiac output, decreased blood viscosity, and thus increased flow velocity. Fetal anemia caused by hemolysis of red cells during pregnancy can be detected by ultrasound techniques, specifically color Doppler ultrasonography, which can be used to measure blood flow velocity.[10] Evaluation of the peak systolic velocity in the middle cerebral artery of the fetus with color Doppler ultrasonography can determine the severity of fetal anemia without invasive procedures. Before the development of color Doppler ultrasonography, the severity of HDFN was measured by amniocentesis, which is described next.

AMNIOCENTESIS

Amniocentesis: process of withdrawal of amniotic fluid by aspiration for the purpose of analysis

Liley graph: graph used to predict severity of HDFN during pregnancy by evaluation of the amniotic fluid

One measure of red cell destruction and the severity of HDFN is the level of bilirubin pigment found in amniotic fluid. Amniotic fluid is obtained by **amniocentesis,** or the insertion of a needle through the mother's abdominal wall and uterus and extraction of fluid from the amniotic sac. The aspirated fluid is scanned spectrophotometrically from 350 to 700 nm. The change in optical density (ΔOD) above the baseline at 450 nm is a measure of the bilirubin pigments (Fig. 12.5).

The ΔOD is plotted on the **Liley graph** according to gestational age, from 27 to 40 weeks (Fig. 12.6, *A*). This graph defines three zones to estimate the severity of HDFN. The upper zone correlates with severe HDFN and fetal death, the lower zone indicates a mildly affected or unaffected fetus, and the middle zone correlates with moderate disease and necessitates repeat testing to establish a trend. A graph similar to the Liley graph includes four zones and begins at 14 weeks of gestation (Fig. 12.6, *B*).[12]

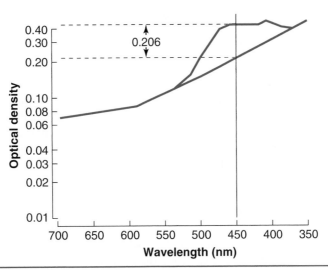

Fig. 12.5 Plot taken at 35 weeks of the optical density (absorbance) reading of amniotic fluid from a woman immunized to the D antigen. The difference between the baseline optical density at the 450-nm wavelength and the reading of the amniotic fluid is measured. In this case the result is 0.206. The change in optical density or ΔOD is plotted on a Liley graph to determine the correct course of treatment according to the period of gestation. (From Mollison PL, Engelfriet CP, Contreras M: *Blood transfusion in clinical medicine,* ed 9, London, UK, 1993, Blackwell Scientific.)

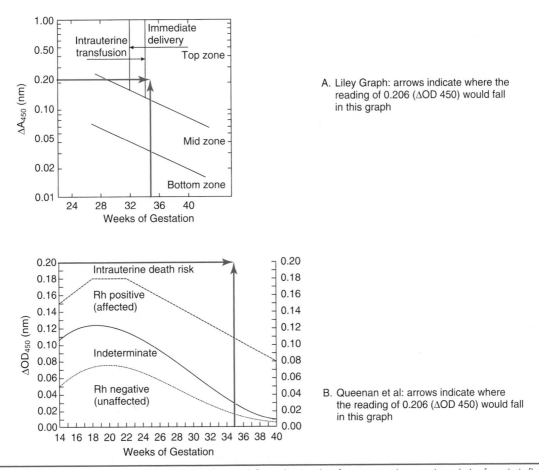

Fig. 12.6 Liley graph and Queenan et al modification. **A,** Liley graph for evaluating data from spectrophotometric analysis of amniotic fluid. The change in optical density at 450 (ΔOD 450) and weeks of gestation are plotted to estimate the severity of HDFN. A reading of 0.206 at 35 weeks correlates with severe HDFN, which may necessitate immediate delivery. **B,** Modification by Queenan et al of the Liley graph to include four zones beginning at 14 weeks of gestation. (From McCullough J: *Transfusion medicine,* ed 2, Philadelphia, PA, 2005, Saunders.)

Respiratory distress syndrome: inability to maintain stable pulmonary alveolar structures, caused by low levels of surfactant, lecithin, and other pulmonary lipids in premature infants

Lecithin/sphingomyelin (L/S) ratio: ratio of lecithin to sphingomyelin that indicates lung maturity

Based on amniotic fluid analysis, three alternatives exist:

1. Allow the pregnancy to continue to term.
2. Perform intrauterine transfusion (see Section 6 "Treatment of Hemolytic Disease of the Fetus and Newborn").
3. Induce early labor.

If labor is induced, fetal lung maturity must be determined to avoid **respiratory distress syndrome.** Lecithin and phosphatidylglycerol are biochemical components of surfactant, a mixture of phospholipids that allows the exchange of gases in the lungs. A **lecithin/sphingomyelin (L/S) ratio** of greater than 2:1 is generally considered evidence of lung maturity.

CORDOCENTESIS

Cordocentesis is a useful diagnostic and therapeutic technique. Using an ultrasound-guided needle, the umbilical vein is punctured near the point of placental insertion. A fetal blood sample is aspirated, which can be used to measure hematologic (hemoglobin/hematocrit) or biochemical (bilirubin) variables directly. Before testing, the specimen must be determined to be fetal and not maternal in origin. This distinction is made by measuring fetal hemoglobin. Red cell genotyping by molecular methods can be performed to determine the presence of an antigen on the fetal red cells if the mother has an IgG antibody. The fetal mortality rate associated with this technique is reported to be between 1% and 2%.[7] In cases of severe HDFN, cordocentesis also can be used for direct intravascular transfusion to the fetus (see Section 6 "Treatment of Hemolytic Disease of the Fetus and Newborn").

FETAL GENOTYPING

Molecular typing of fetal DNA can be performed on maternal plasma during the second trimester.[13,14] Fetal genotyping for blood groups, particularly the D antigen, can assist in predicting the risk that the antibody present during pregnancy could cause HDFN. The prediction of fetal genotype could potentially avoid amniocentesis or cordocentesis if the fetus lacks the antigen for the maternal antibody.

SECTION 4
POSTPARTUM TESTING

After delivery, it is desirable to collect a sample of cord blood from newborns when there is a risk of HDFN. The specimen should be properly labeled and can be stored for 7 days. The sample can remain available for testing if the mother is D-negative or if the newborn develops signs or symptoms of HDFN. Cord blood should be washed several times before testing to avoid false-positive test results because of contamination with Wharton's jelly, a gelatinous substance found in the umbilical cord. Cord blood samples collected using a needle and a syringe avoid contamination with Wharton's jelly, eliminating the need for additional washing.[7]

POSTPARTUM TESTING OF INFANTS AND MOTHERS

D Testing

All infants born to D-negative mothers should be tested for the D antigen, including a test for weak D antigen.[8] D-negative mothers whose infants are found to be D-positive (including weak D-positive) are candidates for RhIG therapy (see Section 5 "Prevention of Hemolytic Disease of the Fetus and Newborn").

Testing for the D antigen on the cord cells or newborn's blood sample must be performed and interpreted carefully. In cases of HDFN, the baby's red cells may have a positive DAT, which can lead to false-positive or false-negative D-testing results. To ensure the validity of a D-positive test result, it is essential to include appropriate Rh controls. In cases where the mother is demonstrating anti-D in her serum and HDFN is suspected, the fetal red cells may type as D-negative. This false-negative D result may be due to a **blocking phenomenon,** where the D antigen sites are blocked by antibody. An elution

Blocking phenomenon: D antigen phenotype on cord blood may be falsely negative, if the cells are heavily coated with maternal anti-D; usually associated with D-positive cord blood and maternal anti-D

performed on the fetal red cells demonstrates anti-D. Washing the cells several times with warm saline and retesting are suggested.[7] A false-positive D typing may occur if the weak D test is performed on red cells that are coated with antibodies. Antibodies coating the cells when testing for weak D should be suspected if the Rh control and anti-D are positive at the antiglobulin phase.

A diagnosis of HDFN is based on medical history, physical examination of the newborn, and results of laboratory testing on both the mother and the infant. Table 12.3 lists the tests that should be performed on the maternal and cord blood (or newborn's sample) to determine whether RhIG is needed and in cases of suspected HDFN.[10]

ABO Testing

When ABO phenotyping is performed on newborns, only the ABO forward grouping is tested because ABO antibodies are not yet produced. ABO reverse-grouping results can lead to misinterpretation or delays because of discrepancies. In addition, it is important to follow the manufacturer's directions carefully because ABO antigens might not be fully developed and might demonstrate weaker results than expected in an adult.

> ABO typing on cord blood and newborn samples should include forward grouping only.

Direct Antiglobulin Test

The DAT must be performed carefully because the result may be weak, especially in cases of ABO HDFN. In cases of a positive DAT, performing an elution is optional unless there are clinical indications or if the mother's antibody has not been identified.[10] If a maternal sample is unavailable, testing the eluate may be useful to confirm HDFN and determine the cause.

If the maternal antibody screen is negative and the DAT is positive, ABO incompatibility should be suspected. ABO HDFN can be confirmed by performing an elution. The eluate should be tested against groups A_1, B, and O cells (screening cells) using an antiglobulin technique. Positive results with group A_1 or B cells (or both) and negative results with the screening cells are indicative of ABO HDFN. If the eluate is negative with all red cells, an antibody to a low-frequency antigen should be suspected. The maternal serum or eluate from the baby's red cells should be tested against the paternal red cells.

Intrauterine Transfusions

ABO and D phenotypes and DATs should be interpreted with extreme caution in newborns who have received intrauterine transfusions. Because group O, D-negative blood

TABLE 12.3	Testing at Delivery (Postpartum Testing)	
BLOOD SAMPLE	**TEST**	**INDICATION**
Maternal	ABO/D typing	To determine whether RhIG is needed For pretransfusion testing or suspected ABO HDFN Weak D test is not required if test for D is negative
	Antibody screen	If transfusion is necessary or HDFN is suspected
	Antibody ID	If screen is positive
	Fetal screen (rosette)	If mother is D-negative and baby is D-positive
	Kleihauer–Betke	If fetal screen (rosette) is positive, to determine dosage of RhIG
Cord or Infant	ABO/D typing	To determine whether RhIG is needed for the mother or if ABO HDFN is suspected
		Weak D test is required if test for D is negative
	DAT	Performed routinely or in suspected cases of HDFN
	Elution	If DAT is positive; test eluate against A cells, B cells, panel cells, or paternal cells, as indicated if HDFN is suspected

RhIG, Rh immune globulin; HDFN, Hemolytic disease of the fetus and newborn; DAT, direct antiglobulin test.

is used for intrauterine transfusions, cord blood test results may be misleading. Depending on the number of transfusions, the infant may phenotype as group O, D-negative or demonstrate weak mixed-field reactions with ABO and anti-D antisera. The DAT likewise may be falsely negative or only weakly positive.

SECTION 5
PREVENTION OF HEMOLYTIC DISEASE OF THE FETUS AND NEWBORN

As discussed previously, the production of IgG antibodies (particularly anti-D) can have life-threatening consequences for the fetus. Once a woman is alloimmunized and produces antibodies, the condition cannot be reversed. Therefore accurate testing must ensure that alloimmunization in women of childbearing age is prevented whenever possible. RhIG is available and prevents alloimmunization in D-negative mothers exposed to D-positive red cells. RhIG was developed during the early 1960s and licensed for administration in 1968. Since its introduction, there has been a dramatic decrease in the incidence of HDFN caused by anti-D. Before the use of RhIG, 16% of ABO-compatible D-negative mothers with a D-positive infant became immunized. The formation of anti-D during gestation was reduced to less than and equal to 2% with postpartum administration only.[7]

RhIG is a concentrate of IgG anti-D prepared from pools of human plasma. The product is given to D-negative women at 28 weeks of gestation (antepartum) and again within 72 hours of delivery (postpartum) of a D-positive infant. A D-negative woman must not have produced anti-D. Different preparations of RhIG are available for either intravenous or intramuscular administration. RhIG suppresses the immune response after exposure to D-positive fetal red cells and prevents the mother from producing anti-D. The mechanism of antibody suppression is not clearly understood, but it may involve the removal of D-positive cells by macrophages causing the release of cytokines that suppress the immune system response.[7] Antepartum and postpartum criteria for RhIG administration are outlined in Table 12.4.

TABLE 12.4	Decision Matrix for Rh Immune Globulin Administration	
TEST RESULTS	RhIG?	CONSIDERATIONS
Antepartum RhIG Administration		
Mother: D-positive	No	RhIG not indicated
Mother: D-negative	Yes	Weak D test is optional
Mother: D-negative; anti-D in serum	No	Review patient history to ensure anti-D is not from RhIG administration and is immune anti-D
Postpartum RhIG Administration		
Mother: D-positive Cord: D-negative	No	RhIG not indicated
Mother: D-negative Cord: D-negative	No	Perform weak D test on cord cells
Mother: D-negative Cord: D-positive	Yes	Calculate dose
Mother: D-positive Cord: D-positive	No	RhIG not indicated
Mother: D-negative Cord: D-negative Anti-D in mother's serum	No*	Check records to verify that anti-D is not from antepartum RhIG administration

RhIG, Rh immune globulin
*Consider blocking phenomenon, where the baby's D-positive red cells are blocked by maternal anti-D, giving a false-negative result.

ANTEPARTUM ADMINISTRATION OF Rh IMMUNE GLOBULIN

Antepartum administration of RhIG reduces the formation of anti-D during gestation to 0.1% compared with 1.5% with postpartum administration only.[7] The American College of Obstetricians and Gynecologists recommends an initial dosage of RhIG to unsensitized D-negative mothers at 28 weeks. Indications for additional doses of RhIG during pregnancy include invasive procedures such as amniocentesis, cordocentesis, intrauterine transfusions, inversion of a breech fetus, or abdominal trauma.[7]

Criteria for antepartum administration include D-negative mothers when the fetus is either D-positive or unknown. A D-negative mother whose infant is known to be D-negative or has been previously immunized to D is not a candidate for RhIG. D-positive mothers are also not candidates for RhIG. Weak D testing is not required. Mothers with red cells that are clearly weak D-positive should be considered D-positive and not receive RhIG.[7]

As mentioned previously, all women should be phenotyped for ABO and D antigens and tested for alloantibodies during the first trimester of pregnancy. If the antibody screen is negative in initial testing, it is recommended that the screen be repeated before RhIG therapy is administered to D-negative prenatal patients.[15] Other alloantibodies (eg, anti-K, anti-E) should *not* prevent a woman from receiving RhIG. RhIG does not prevent immunization of antibodies other than D.

POSTPARTUM ADMINISTRATION OF Rh IMMUNE GLOBULIN

Cord blood from infants born to D-negative mothers should be tested for the D antigen, including the test for weak D.[7] A nonimmunized D-negative woman who delivers a D-positive infant should receive a full dose of RhIG within 72 hours of delivery. If the delivering hospital has a verified record of a negative antibody screen during the current pregnancy, the screen does not need to be repeated before administration of postpartum RhIG. When the antibody screen is repeated at delivery, results must be interpreted with caution. A weak antibody to D may be detected because of prenatal administration of RhIG. If a check of the patient's history reveals administration of RhIG at 28 weeks, a full postpartum dose of RhIG still should be administered. Differentiating between active and passive anti-D by titration is not necessary.[7]

Screening for Fetomaternal Hemorrhage

A full 300-µg dose of RhIG provides protection for up to 15 mL of D-positive red cells (approximately 30 mL of fetal whole blood). If a woman experiences FMH exceeding 30 mL of D-positive fetal red cells, it is essential that she receive more than one dose of RhIG. All postpartum RhIG candidates should have a postpartum specimen tested for significant FMH.[4]

The most frequently used method to screen for FMH at the present time is the rosette test (Fig. 12.7). In this method, a suspension of the maternal red cells (containing D-negative maternal red cells and a small number of D-positive fetal red cells) is incubated with anti-D. During incubation, anti-D binds to the D-positive fetal red cells. The suspension is washed thoroughly, and D-positive indicator red cells are added, which bind to the anti-D and form a rosette around the D-positive fetal red cells. The blood suspension is placed on a slide and examined microscopically for the appearance and number of rosettes. Appropriate positive and negative controls should be run concurrently to ensure valid test results. A positive test indicates significant FMH and the potential need for more than one dose of RhIG. The rosette test detects a bleed of only 10 mL.[7] Because the rosette assay is a screening test only, a method to quantify the number of fetal red cells should be performed.

The fetal cells must be D-positive and the mother must be D-negative for the rosette test to be valid. A false-positive result can occur if the mother is weak D-positive. A false-negative result can occur if the fetus is positive for weak D. Scan the QR code for more information.

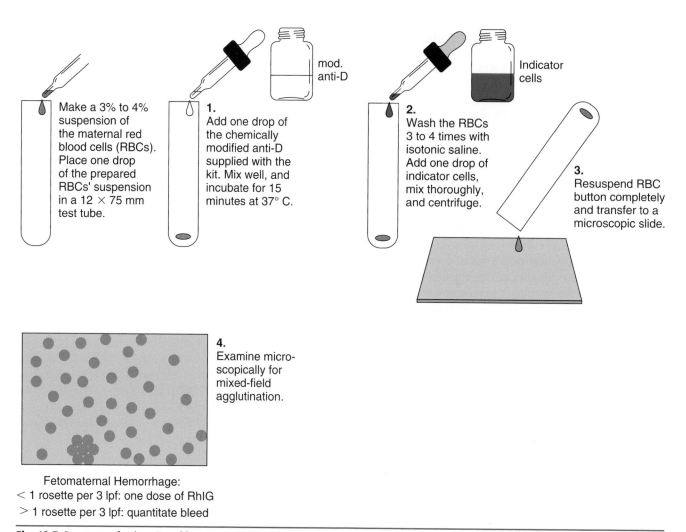

4.
Examine micro-
scopically for
mixed-field
agglutination.

Fetomaternal Hemorrhage:
< 1 rosette per 3 lpf: one dose of RhIG
> 1 rosette per 3 lpf: quantitate bleed

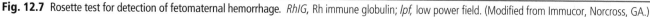

Fig. 12.7 Rosette test for detection of fetomaternal hemorrhage. *RhIG*, Rh immune globulin; *lpf*, low power field. (Modified from Immucor, Norcross, GA.)

Quantifying Fetomaternal Hemorrhage

In patients with a positive rosette test, a quantitative test such as the Kleihauer–Betke test or flow cytometry is performed to calculate the dose of RhIG. Flow cytometry measures fetal hemoglobin or D-positive red cells or both.[16] Kleihauer–Betke acid elution is based on the fact that fetal hemoglobin is resistant to acid elution and adult hemoglobin is not. A blood smear is prepared from a postpartum maternal sample and exposed to an acid buffer. Hemoglobin from adult red cells leaches into the buffer and leaves only stroma, whereas the fetal red cells retain their hemoglobin. Smears are washed, stained, and examined under oil immersion. Adult red cells appear as "ghosts," and fetal cells appear pink (Fig. 12.8). Results are reported as the percentage of fetal red cells (number of fetal red cells divided by total red cells counted).

The volume (in milliliters of whole blood) of the FMH uses the percentage of fetal red cells counted or determined by flow cytometry. This percentage is multiplied by the mother's blood volume. The mother's blood volume can be calculated based on her height and weight or the average of 5000 mL used. Because a full dose of RhIG protects against 30 mL of whole blood, the volume of FMH is divided by 30 to determine the number of doses of RhIG. Fig. 12.9 provides an example.

To obtain a whole number, if the number to the right of the decimal point is less than 0.5, one rounds down. If the number to the right of the decimal is greater than or equal to 0.5, one rounds up. Because the accuracy and precision of this method are poor, a safety margin should be provided to ensure adequate protection by adding one dose of RhIG to the final number calculated.

The fetal screen (rosette test) is a screening or qualitative test, whereas the Kleihauer–Betke and flow cytometric methods are quantitative tests for determining dosage of RhIG.

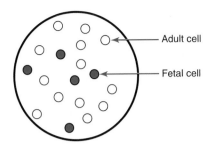

Fig. 12.8 Acid elution test for determination of hemoglobin F. After staining, fetal red cells appear dark pink, and adult cells appear as pale ghost cells. Fetal hemoglobin resists acid elution and remains intact, whereas the adult red cells lose the hemoglobin and do not take up the stain.

	Steps	Explanation	Example
1.	Estimate the volume of fetal blood in maternal circulation	Determine the percentage of fetal cells counted in 2000 total cells Percentage of fetal cells × maternal blood volume = fetal whole blood (mL)	16 fetal cells/2000 = 0.008 0.008 × 5000 = 40 mL of fetal whole blood
2.	Calculate how many vials are needed: each 300-μg dose of RhIG protects against a **30** mL whole blood bleed	Divide the mL of fetal whole blood by **30**	40/30 = 1.3
3.	Round up or down to obtain a whole number	Round the calculated dose **up** if ≥ 0.5 following decimal point or **down** if < 0.5	1.3 →1 (rounded down)
4.	Add 1 vial of RhIG to calculated dose to provide a safety margin	Calculated dose + 1	1 →2 (add one)

Fig. 12.9 Calculating the dosage of RhIG. (From Fung MK, editor: *Technical manual*, ed 18, Bethesda, MD, 2014, AABB.)

SECTION 6
TREATMENT OF HEMOLYTIC DISEASE OF THE FETUS AND NEWBORN

IN UTERO TREATMENT

Intrauterine transfusions are given to correct anemia in utero and prevent potential heart failure. Intrauterine transfusions historically have been administered by the intraperitoneal route. In an intraperitoneal transfusion, a needle is inserted into the mother's abdomen and into the peritoneal cavity of the fetus. The red cells are infused into the peritoneal cavity and absorbed into the fetal circulation through the lymphatics. Drawbacks of this procedure include the inability to perform the procedure before 25 weeks and variable absorption of red cells (particularly in hydropic fetuses). More recently cordocentesis has been used to provide direct intravascular transfusion into the umbilical vein. Benefits of this procedure include the ability to obtain blood-for-blood typing, DAT, antigen typing, hemoglobin, hematocrit, and bilirubin.

Blood for intrauterine transfusion should be:
- Group O, D-negative
- Red blood cells (RBCs) collected within 7 days
- Irradiated to prevent graft-versus-host disease
- Cytomegalovirus (CMV)-reduced-risk: CMV seronegative or leukocyte reduced
- Hemoglobin S–negative

Red cells with a hematocrit of 75% to 80% are used to avoid volume overload. Group O, D-negative is used because the ABO and D typing of the fetus is usually not known. If the mother has an alloantibody, the blood selected should be negative for the corresponding antigen. Fresh blood is necessary to ensure longer viability, higher 2,3-diphosphoglycerate (for release of oxygen to the tissues), and lower potassium (to avoid cardiac arrhythmias). Irradiation is necessary to prevent graft-versus-host disease in the fetus. Donor red cells are crossmatched using the maternal serum.

POSTPARTUM TREATMENT

Phototherapy

Phototherapy is performed as an initial treatment for hyperbilirubinemia. Exposure of newborns to fluorescent blue light in the 420- to 475-nm range can successfully treat physiologic jaundice and mild cases of HDFN, particularly ABO HDFN. When exposed to light, bilirubin undergoes photoisomerization to form photobilirubin. These isomers of bilirubin are carried by the plasma to the liver and are excreted in the bile without the need for conjugation. Cases of hyperbilirubinemia that fail to respond to phototherapy require exchange transfusion.

Exchange Transfusion

As mentioned previously, newborns with HDFN are at risk of anemia and hyperbilirubinemia. If left untreated, elevated levels of indirect bilirubin can result in damage to the CNS. Exchange transfusion that involves the replacement of one to two whole blood volumes is primarily used to treat excessively high levels of unconjugated bilirubin.

Exchange transfusion accomplishes the following:
- Corrects anemia without expanding blood volume
- Removes a sensitized newborn's red cells and replaces them with antigen-negative cells
- Reduces the level of bilirubin to prevent kernicterus
- Reduces the level of maternal antibody

Many variables enter into the decision to perform exchange transfusion. A bilirubin level of 18 to 20 mg/dL historically has been used as the level at which kernicterus is a serious risk and exchange transfusion is necessary. However, complications such as low birth weight, sepsis, acidosis, or signs of CNS deterioration can affect the threshold level and indicate the need for exchange at levels much less than 20 mg/dL. For these reasons, premature infants may require exchange transfusions at lower bilirubin levels and more often than do full-term infants. Many physicians consider the rate of increase in the bilirubin level to be a better predictor of the need for exchange transfusion.[7]

Selection of Blood and Compatibility Testing for Exchange Transfusion

Before the initial exchange transfusion, infant cells must be tested to determine the ABO and D phenotype. Repeat ABO and D typing is not necessary for the remainder of the infant's hospital admission.[8] Serum or plasma from the infant or the mother may be used for the antibody screen. Maternal serum is used most commonly because it is readily available and has a high concentration of antibodies. If the antibody screen is positive, the RBCs for transfusion must lack the antigen corresponding to the maternal antibody and be crossmatch compatible by the antiglobulin technique. If maternal serum is not available, the newborn's serum or an eluate from the newborn's red cells can be used for antibody detection and compatibility testing.

Many institutions simplify the procedure of selecting blood for exchange transfusion by using group O, D-negative RBCs for all exchange transfusions, but this is not always necessary. If the mother and the infant are ABO identical, type-specific RBCs can be used.

Fresh frozen plasma (FFP) is used to reconstitute the RBCs to a hematocrit between 45% and 60%.[7] Plasma must be ABO compatible (or group AB) with the RBCs. FFP restores albumin and coagulation factors. Additional requirements for CMV-seronegative blood and irradiation are commonly due to the immunocompromised status of newborns. Hemoglobin S–negative blood should be provided to avoid any possibility of intravascular sickling.[7] Table 12.5 summarizes the criteria to consider when selecting blood for exchange.

Fresh frozen plasma (FFP): blood component prepared from whole blood that contains only the plasma portion of whole blood and is frozen after separation to retain labile factors

TABLE 12.5 Selection of Blood for Exchange Transfusion

- Group O (or ABO-compatible) D-negative blood
- RBCs <7 days old, resuspended in group AB FFP
- CMV-reduced-risk components: CMV-seronegative donors or leukocyte reduced
- Irradiated blood
- Hemoglobin S–negative blood
- Blood lacks antigen corresponding to maternal antibody
- Compatible crossmatch with maternal serum or eluate prepared from newborn's red cells

RBCs, Red blood cells; *FFP*, fresh frozen plasma; *CMV*, cytomegalovirus.

CHAPTER SUMMARY

HDFN is prevented, monitored, and treated with the help of tests performed in the laboratory. Understanding the physiology of HDFN is important in choosing the correct tests to perform and detecting early indicators of hemolytic disease. Important points to remember when performing these tests are outlined.

1. HDFN occurs when:
   - Fetal red cells, carrying antigens inherited from the father, stimulate the mother to produce IgG antibodies.
   - Maternal IgG antibodies destroy fetal red cells.
2. Hemolytic processes can cause the following:
   - In utero, red cell destruction can cause severe anemia, which can proceed to heart failure and possibly death.
   - After delivery, red cell destruction continues with the increase of bilirubin, causing jaundice and possible damage to the CNS (kernicterus).
3. HDFN can be caused by ABO, Rh, or other IgG antibodies:
   - ABO HDFN is the most common type of HDFN and occurs most commonly in group O mothers who deliver group A or B babies.
   - HDFN caused by anti-D is the most severe type of HDFN; it occurs in D-negative women with anti-D who deliver D-positive infants.
   - Any IgG antibody can cause HDFN if the child inherits the antigen from the father, and the red cell antigen is well developed on the fetal red cells. Anti-c and anti-K are most frequently reported after anti-D.
4. Laboratory tests to predict, prevent, or monitor HDFN before delivery include:
   - ABO/D phenotype and antibody screen are performed on the mother.
   - D-negative mothers should receive prenatal RhIG.
   - Titration of the maternal antibody can be helpful in deciding when to perform diagnostic and invasive procedures.
   - Spectrophotometric analysis of the amniotic fluid and use of the Liley graph can aid in predicting the severity of HDFN.
5. After delivery, HDFN is monitored, prevented, and treated by:
   - Cord blood testing determines whether a D-negative mother should receive postpartum RhIG.
   - RhIG dosage is determined by the fetal screen (rosette) and Kleihauer–Betke test performed on the mother.
   - If HDFN is suspected, ABO and D phenotype and DAT should be performed; hemoglobin and bilirubin levels should also be closely monitored.
   - Depending on the severity of HDFN, treatment can begin in utero or after delivery.
   - After delivery, exchange transfusion is used to correct anemia, remove sensitized red cells, and reduce levels of maternal antibody and bilirubin.
   - Blood for exchange and intrauterine transfusion should be less than 7 days old, irradiated, CMV negative, hemoglobin S negative, and negative for the antigen corresponding to the maternal antibody. Group O, D-negative RBCs resuspended in AB plasma are used most often.

CRITICAL THINKING EXERCISES

Exercise 12.1

R.T. was seen by her OB-GYN for her initial visit at 9 weeks of gestation. This is her first pregnancy.

1. What tests should be run for her initial prenatal workup?

Exercise 12.1 Additional Testing

Results of prenatal testing indicate R.T. phenotypes as group A, D-negative with a negative antibody screen.

2. Does R.T. need any additional laboratory testing during her pregnancy?
3. If so, what tests are needed, and when should the testing be performed?

Exercise 12.1 Additional Testing

R.T. was seen again by her OB-GYN at 28 weeks. Her antibody screen is repeated and is negative. Based on these test results, she received a 300-μg dose of RhIG. R.T. delivered a healthy 6 lb 4 oz boy 12 weeks later.

4. What testing, if any, needs to be performed at the time of delivery?

Exercise 12.1 Additional Testing

Results of the cord blood from R.T.'s infant indicate phenotype of group A, D-positive with a negative DAT.

5. Is R.T. a candidate for postpartum RhIG?
6. What additional test needs to be performed on R.T. before RhIG is given?

Exercise 12.2

J.M. is seen at the outpatient clinic for her first prenatal visit at 15 weeks of gestation. Obstetric history indicates one ectopic pregnancy (no RhIG given) and one full-term pregnancy (RhIG given). The last child required phototherapy. Results of prenatal testing indicate group O, D-negative with a positive antibody screen.

1. What additional testing needs to be performed?

Exercise 12.2 Additional Testing

An antibody panel identifies anti-D. Parallel titers were performed on the sample from 15 weeks and 20 weeks of gestation. The following results were obtained:

	Dilution Strength								
Sample	1:1	1:2	1:4	1:8	1:16	1:32	1:64	1:128	1:256
#1 (15 weeks)	2+	2+	2+	1+	1+	0	0	0	0
#2 (20 weeks)	3+	3+	2+	2+	1+	1+	1+	+w	0

2. What is the purpose of performing antibody titration?
3. Are the results shown in the table significant, and how is this reported?
4. Why is parallel testing recommended for antibody titrations?

Exercise 12.2 Additional Testing

Amniocentesis performed at 24 weeks shows a ΔOD of 0.10.

5. Using the Liley graph, what outcome might be expected for this pregnancy given this result and the patient history?

Exercise 12.2 Additional Testing

J.M. continues to be closely monitored throughout her pregnancy. She delivered a 4 lb 10 oz girl at 37 weeks. Results of cord blood testing were as follows:

Anti-A	Anti-B	Anti-D	Weak D	D control	DAT
3+	0	0	2+	2+	2+

The hemoglobin is 13 g/dL; bilirubin is 5.2 mg/dL.
6. What is the ABO and D phenotype interpretation?
7. What additional tests are necessary to resolve the D typing?
8. Does this infant have HDFN? If so, what is the cause? Use laboratory data to support your conclusions.

Exercise 12.2 Additional Testing
The following evening, J.M.'s infant has a bilirubin value of 17.4 mg/dL. An exchange transfusion is requested.
9. What ABO and D blood type should be selected, and how should it be tested?
10. What are the special requirements for blood selected for exchange transfusion?

Exercise 12.3
B.W. was seen by her OB-GYN at 10 weeks of gestation with her first pregnancy. Results of her prenatal workup indicate she is group O, D-negative with a negative antibody screen. Repeat testing at 28 weeks continues to indicate a negative antibody screen, and she is given 300 µg of RhIG. The pregnancy proceeds normally, and she delivers a 7 lb 2 oz boy at 39 weeks of gestation. Results of cord blood tests are as follows:

Anti-A	Anti-B	Anti-D	Weak D	Weak D control	DAT	Mother's Sample Screen cells
3+	0	0	1+	1+	1+	Weak positive

Infant hemoglobin is 17.3 g/dL, and bilirubin is 0.6 mg/dL.
1. Does this infant have HDFN? If so, what is the most probable cause?
2. What could be causing the positive screen result? How would you confirm?

Exercise 12.3 Additional Testing
An elution is performed. The eluate is tested against A_1, B, and O reagent red cells, incubated at 37° C, and tested at the AHG phase:

	A_1	B	O
Eluate	1+	1+	Negative

3. What do these results indicate?
4. What type of treatment would be recommended for this infant?
5. Is B.W. a candidate for postpartum RhIG? If so, are any additional tests necessary?

Exercise 12.3 Additional Testing
A fetal screen performed on B.W. yields a positive result.
6. What test needs to be performed and why?

Exercise 12.3 Additional Testing
A Kleihauer–Betke stain is performed on B.W.'s postpartum specimen to quantify the amount of FMH. There were 19 fetal cells counted in a total of 2000 cells.
7. How many doses of RhIG should B.W. receive?

Exercise 12.4
M.K., a 26-year-old mother of two, is admitted to labor and delivery. No prenatal records are available. The antibody screen is positive at the AHG phase.

Anti-A	Anti-B	Anti-D	D control	Weak D	Weak D control	A_1 cells	B cells	Interpretation
0	4+	0	0	0 ✓	0 ✓	4+	0	?

The antibody identification is performed, and a weak anti-D is identified.
Cord blood test results follow:

Anti-A	Anti-B	Anti-D	D control	DAT	Interpretation
0	0	3+	0	0 ✓	?

DAT, Direct antiglobulin test; ✓, check cells reacted.
1. Based on these results, is M.K. a candidate for postpartum RhIG?

STUDY QUESTIONS

1. What item listed is not an objective for performing an exchange transfusion?
   a. decrease the level of maternal antibody
   b. reduce the level of indirect bilirubin
   c. provide platelets to prevent disseminated intravascular coagulation
   d. provide compatible RBCs to correct anemia

2. What is the greatest danger to a fetus affected by HDFN before delivery?
   a. kernicterus
   b. anemia
   c. hyperbilirubinemia
   d. hypertension

3. How many milliliters of whole blood from an FMH is covered with a 300-μg dose of RhIG?
   a. 10 mL
   b. 15 mL
   c. 30 mL
   d. 50 mL

4. What is the time frame for RhIG administration after delivery?
   a. 6 hours
   b. 48 hours
   c. 72 hours
   d. 96 hours

5. What is the name of an often-fatal condition characterized by general edema that results from anemia?
   a. kernicterus
   b. disseminated intravascular coagulation (DIC)
   c. erythroblastosis fetalis
   d. hydrops fetalis

6. What is the mechanism for HDFN occurrence?
   a. maternal antigens react with fetal antibodies
   b. fetal antibodies react with maternal antibodies
   c. maternal antibodies react with fetal antigens
   d. fetal antigens react with maternal antigens

7. What is the greatest danger to the newborn affected by HDFN postpartum?
   a. kernicterus
   b. anemia
   c. conjugated bilirubin
   d. low L/S ratio

8. Which of the following women should receive postpartum RhIG?

Mother's ABO/D phenotype	Mother's antibody screen	Newborn's ABO/D phenotype
a. A, D-negative	Negative	O, D-positive
b. O, D-negative	Negative	A, D-negative
c. A, D-positive	Negative	B, D-negative
d. B, D-negative	Immune anti-D	B, D-positive

9. Which of the following antibodies carries no risk of HDFN?
   a. anti-Le^a
   b. anti-C
   c. anti-K
   d. anti-S

10. Which of the following is *not* a characteristic of ABO HDFN?
    a. may occur in first pregnancy
    b. usually treated with phototherapy
    c. strongly positive DAT
    d. most frequent in babies born to group O mothers

11. Which of the following requirements is important when selecting blood for exchange transfusion to avoid high levels of potassium?
    a. irradiated blood
    b. CMV-negative blood
    c. leukocyte-reduced blood
    d. blood less than 7 days old

12. A mother is group A, D-negative with anti-D in her serum. Which of the following units should be selected for an intrauterine transfusion?
    a. group O, D-negative
    b. group O, D-positive
    c. group A, D-negative
    d. group A, D-positive

13. Select the statement that is true regarding the rosette test.
    a. performed on a cord blood sample
    b. used to screen for FMH
    c. a quantitative test used to calculate the volume of FMH
    d. an acid elution used to estimate the volume of FMH

14. Which of the following tests is *not* necessary when testing a cord blood sample?
    a. ABO
    b. D
    c. DAT
    d. antibody screen

15. What is the principle of the Liley method for predicting the severity of HDFN?
    a. resistance of fetal hemoglobin to acid elution
    b. ratio of lecithin to sphingomyelin
    c. change of optical density of amniotic fluid measured at 450 nm
    d. direct bilirubin evaluation of a cord blood sample

16. A titer was performed on a prenatal sample from a D-negative woman with anti-D. The sample was tested 4 weeks later in parallel with a current sample. The following results were obtained:

	1:1	1:2	1:4	1:8	1:16	1:32	1:64	1:128	1:256
Week 24:	2+	1+	1+	0	0	0	0	0	0
Week 28:	3+	2+	2+	2+	1+	1+	0	0	0

How would the titer results be interpreted?
    a. an intrauterine transfusion is necessary
    b. early induction of labor should be considered
    c. color Doppler ultrasonography should be considered
    d. RhIG should be administered

17. A group A, D-negative mother demonstrating anti-D antibodies delivered a group O, D-negative baby with a positive DAT (2+), elevated bilirubin (18 mg/dL), and low hemoglobin (8 g/dL). Which is the most probable explanation for these test results?
    a. ABO hemolytic disease of the newborn
    b. hemolytic disease of the newborn with a false-negative D typing due to blocking antibodies
    c. large fetomaternal hemorrhage causing discrepancy in the blood type
    d. prenatal RhIG administration

18. How would you interpret the appearance of spherocytes in a baby's blood smear after delivery?
    a. ABO HDFN
    b. HDFN caused by anti-D
    c. HDFN caused by other IgG antibodies
    d. normal physiologic anemia detected in newborns

19. What is the purpose for the irradiation of blood selected for an exchange transfusion?
    a. prevent formation of HLA antibodies
    b. prevent sepsis from bacterial contamination
    c. prevent graft-versus-host disease
    d. prevent transmission of viruses

20. What bleed is detected by the rosette test used for screening for a fetomaternal hemorrhage?
    a. 5 mL
    b. 10 mL
    c. 20 mL
    d. 30 mL

21. A Kleihauer–Betke stain performed on a postpartum blood sample demonstrated 10 fetal cells in a field of 2000. What is the estimated blood volume of the fetomaternal hemorrhage expressed as whole blood?
    a. 25 mL
    b. 30 mL
    c. 45 mL
    d. 100 mL

22. A rosette test performed on a D-negative mother who delivered a D-positive baby demonstrated two rosettes per three fields observed. What is the correct course of action?
    a. submit the sample for a Kleihauer–Betke test
    b. recommend two vials of RhIG
    c. suggest that RhIG is not necessary because records indicate that the mother received prenatal RhIG
    d. recommend one vial of RhIG because it is below the cutoff for the fetal screen

23. What is the principle of the Kleihauer–Betke test?
    a. fetal hemoglobin resists acid elution
    b. adult hemoglobin resists acid elution
    c. fetal red cells lose hemoglobin under alkaline conditions
    d. adult red cells accept dye under alkaline conditions

24. Results of a Kleihauer–Betke test determine there was a fetomaternal hemorrhage of 35 mL of whole blood during delivery. What is the correct dosage of RhIG?
    a. one vial
    b. two vials
    c. three vials
    d. four vials

25. A weakly reactive anti-D test was identified in a postpartum sample from a D-negative woman who gave birth to a D-positive baby. What is the most likely cause?
    a. immune anti-D produced from exposure during the first pregnancy
    b. immune anti-D produced from exposure during the current pregnancy
    c. antenatal RhIG given
    d. error in antibody identification or D typing

Answers to Study Questions can be found on page 387.

ⓔ Additional student resources, including review questions, a laboratory manual, and case studies, can be found on the Evolve website.

REFERENCES

1. Reid ME, Lomas-Francis C, Olsson ML: *The blood group antigen facts book*, ed 3, San Diego, CA, 2012, Elsevier Academic Press.
2. Bowman JM: The prevention of Rh immunization, *Trans Med Rev* 2:129, 1988.
3. Bowman JM: Controversies in Rh prophylaxis: Who needs Rh immune globulin and when should it be given? *Am J Obstet Gynecol* 151:289, 1985.
4. Klein HG, Anstee DJ: *Mollison's blood transfusion in clinical medicine*, ed 12, Oxford, UK, 2014, Wiley-Blackwell.
5. Eder AF: Update on HDNF: New information on long standing controversies, *Immunohematology* 22:188, 2006.
6. McKenzie SB: *Textbook of hematology*, ed 2, Baltimore, MD, 1996, Williams & Wilkins.
7. Fung MK: *Technical manual*, ed 18, Bethesda, MD, 2014, AABB.
8. Levitt JL: *Standards for blood banks and transfusion services*, ed 29, Bethesda, MD, 2014, AABB.
9. Sandler SG, Roseff S, Dorman RE, et al.: for the CAP Transfusion Medicine Resource Committee. Policies and procedures related to testing for weak D phenotypes and administration of Rh immune globulin/Results and recommendations related to supplemental questions in the comprehensive transfusion medicine survey of the College of American Pathologists, *Arch Pathol Lab Med* 138:620–562, 2014.
10. Judd WJ: Practice guidelines for prenatal and perinatal immunohematology, revisited, *Transfusion* 41:1445, 2001.
11. Tarsa M, Kelly TF: Managing a pregnancy with antibodies: A clinician's perspective, *Immunohematology* 24:52, 2008.
12. McCullough J: *Transfusion medicine*, ed 2, Philadelphia, PA, 2005, Saunders.
13. Faas BHW, et al.: The detection of fetal RhD-specific sequences in maternal plasma, *Lancet* 352:1196, 1998.
14. Finning K, Martin P, Summers J, et al.: Fetal genotyping for the K (Kell) and Rh, Cc, and E blood groups on cell-free fetal DNA in maternal plasma, *Transfusion* 47:2126, 2007.
15. Judd WJ, Johnson ST, Storry JR: *Judd's methods in immunohematology*, ed 3, Bethesda, MD, 2008, AABB.
16. Radel DJ, Penz CS, Dietz AB, et al.: A combined flow-cytometry-based method for fetomaternal hemorrhage and maternal D, *Transfusion* 48:1886, 2008.

13

DONOR SELECTION AND PHLEBOTOMY

CHAPTER OUTLINE

LEARNING OBJECTIVES

On completion of this chapter, the reader should be able to:

1. Describe the required donor registration information and state its requirements.
2. Distinguish between the terms donor eligibility and donation suitability.
3. Provide rationale for Blood Donor Educational Materials.
4. Compare the donor medical history criteria intended for protecting the donor with questions that protect the recipient.
5. Analyze health history examples that could cause a permanent, indefinite, or temporary deferral.
6. List the physical examination criteria for allogeneic blood donation.
7. Apply the physical examination guidelines to potential blood donor situations.
8. Determine eligibility status of donors when common medications and recent vaccines are part of the donor history.
9. Select eligible donors based on registration information, and identify donors for deferral.
10. List possible adverse donor reactions and the appropriate treatment.
11. Compare and contrast allogeneic and autologous donor criteria.
12. List various forms of autologous donations.
13. Describe the apheresis procedure, the donor requirements, and the products that can be collected.
14. Discuss the reason for directed donation and the donor criteria.
15. Define therapeutic phlebotomy and the clinical conditions for its use.

Blood centers and transfusion services are responsible for providing an adequate and safe blood supply to the patients they serve. Criteria for acceptable blood donors are established by the U.S. Food and Drug Administration (FDA) through the *Code of Federal Regulations* (CFR), guidance documents, or memoranda to the industry. The AABB, a voluntary accrediting agency, has established guidelines for blood donation, which are written in the *Standards for Blood Banks and Transfusion Services*. In an effort to provide uniformity and clarity for determining the eligibility criteria for volunteer blood donors, the AABB Donor History Questionnaire (DHQ) was developed. This document meets FDA requirements for donor screening, and an updated version can be found on the FDA and AABB websites.[1,2]

Maintaining an adequate blood supply begins with educating the public about the need for volunteer donations. After recruiting donors, the safety of the blood supply depends on thorough and accurate donor screening and processing or testing of each unit collected. This chapter discusses donor screening, and the next chapter discusses the testing performed on donated blood.

> The current donor history questionnaire and related materials are available from the AABB website at http://www.aabb.org/tm/question naires/Pages/dhqaabb.aspx.

SECTION 1
DONOR SCREENING

The screening of each donor can be divided into four phases: registration, educational materials, health history interview, and physical examination. The screening process includes information on the donation process and potential adverse consequences of blood donation. In addition, a questionnaire is provided to the donor to assess any risky behaviors, medications, travel, and other factors with potential impact to donor and recipient safety. A physical examination of the donor is included with parameters set for blood donation.

Two phrases are used in the donation process: donor eligibility and suitability of the donation. The donor's eligibility is the determination that the donor is qualified to donate blood and blood components. The suitability of the donation means a determination of whether the donation is acceptable for transfusion or for further manufacturing use.

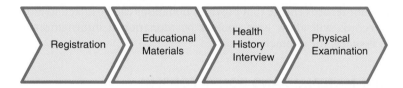

Registration → Educational Materials → Health History Interview → Physical Examination

BLOOD DONORS

Who are the people who generously donate their blood for others? Let's look at some facts related to blood donors. Only about 5% of U.S. general population donate blood every year.[3] In addition, 40,000 units of blood are needed every day in the United States and Canada.[4] Data from a Healthy People 2010 report indicated that 18- to 24-year-olds donated blood at a rate slightly exceeding 8% compared with less than 2% for those aged 65 and older in 2001.[5] In the evaluation of racial diversity within the donor pool, whites donated blood at a rate of 7%, which was at least twice the rates for blacks, Hispanics, and Asians. The report also indicated that years of education had a positive influence on blood donation. Individuals aged 25 years and older who had at least some college donated blood at a rate of 7.9% compared with 1.8% of those who had not completed high school. Blood donors are a totally volunteer force, supplying more than 15 million pints of blood for transfusion per year.[4] Scan the QR codes for more information about blood donation.

DONOR REGISTRATION AND DONOR IDENTIFICATION

The donor registration process includes documenting information that fully identifies the donor on an individual donation registration record. Questions regarding name changes or nicknames are important for correct identification. Registration should also include prescreening for donor eligibility status. With the exception of first-time donors, access to past donation history, usually through computerized databases, allows the staff to confirm that:
- Donor information is correct
- Sufficient time has passed since the last donation
- The donor has not been deferred from a donation based on previous history questions or test results

Correct identification of the donor is essential to prevent collection from someone who is not qualified and to ensure that the donor can be contacted with test results or other relevant information. Donation records include the following:

- Donor's full name
- Permanent address and contact information (obtain a *postal* address for the donor that is good for 8 weeks)
- Date of birth (donor must be at least 16 years old; if the state considers 16-year-olds to be minors, parental consent is required)
- Gender
- Date of last donation
  - Eight weeks must elapse between whole blood donations.
  - Sixteen weeks must elapse after a two-unit RBC collection.
  - Four weeks must elapse after infrequent plasmapheresis.
  - Two days or more must elapse after plasmapheresis, plateletpheresis, or leukapheresis.

Additional useful information includes the following:

- Unique identification number: such as Social Security number or driver's license number
- Positive identification: usually entails photo identification
- Race: can be useful in selecting donor units for patients requiring certain phenotypes
- Intended use of the donation: **allogeneic donation, directed donation, autologous donation,** or **apheresis donation**

These special donation processes are described later in this chapter.

Why does the blood center need this accurate donation record?

- Accurate donor records ensure that previous donations can be linked to any given donor.
- Accurate records will allow easy contact postdonation if information regarding test results necessitates the contact.

Allogeneic donation: donation for use by the general patient population

Directed donation: donation reserved for use by a specific patient

Autologous donation: donation by a donor reserved for the donor's later use

Apheresis donation: donation of a specific component of the blood; parts of the whole blood that are not retained are returned to the donor

EDUCATIONAL MATERIALS AND DONOR CONSENT

Before donating, all prospective donors must be given educational materials describing the donation process and donor eligibility. Donor educational materials must contain risk factors for relevant transfusion-transmitted infections (RTTIs). In addition to human immunodeficiency virus (HIV) and acquired immunodeficiency syndrome (AIDS), information regarding risks of other infectious diseases transmitted by blood transfusion are now included in educational materials. The signs, symptoms, and high-risk behaviors associated with the disease must be included (Fig. 13.1).

Prospective donors should be given ample opportunity to read the material, ask questions, and understand that they are excluded from donating blood if they have experienced any of the signs or symptoms described. Information regarding the tests performed on the donor blood and state requirements for reporting positive test results to government agencies must be made available. This preinterview material also describes the possible side effects and risks associated with the donation process. Donor centers need policies for the communication of this information to donors who are not fluent in English, are illiterate, or who have other physical disabilities.

Informed Consent or Donor Acknowledgement

Before donation, the donor must sign a written informed consent to allow blood to be collected and used. The blood center is required to provide the donor with a written statement of understanding to be read and signed by the donor. The establishment would be required to use procedures to assure that the donor understands the material provided, and the donor is asked to read and sign a statement that shows an understanding of all the donor information presented, including what high-risk behaviors are included. The donor is also asked if he or she has additional questions. The donor is informed about the infectious disease tests to be run on the blood and notification if testing indicates that the blood donation presents a risk for transmitting disease; the donor's name is then placed on a list to defer future donations. If units are to be used for reasons other than transfusion, such as research, informed consent must address this as well.

Blood Donor Educational Materials:
MAKING YOUR BLOOD DONATION SAFE

Thank you for coming in today! This information sheet explains how **YOU** can help us make the donation process safe for yourself and patients who might receive your blood. **PLEASE READ THIS INFORMATION BEFORE YOU DONATE! If you have any questions now or anytime during the screening process, please ask blood center staff.**

ACCURACY AND HONESTY ARE ESSENTIAL!
Your **complete honesty** in answering all questions is very important for the safety of patients who receive your blood. **All information you provide is confidential.**

DONATION PROCESS:
To determine if you are eligible to donate we will:
– Ask questions about health, travel, and medicines
– Ask questions to see if you might be at risk for hepatitis, HIV, or AIDS
– Take your blood pressure, temperature, and pulse
– Take a small blood sample to make sure you are not anemic
If you are able to donate we will:
– Cleanse your arm with an antiseptic. **(If you are allergic to iodine, please tell us!)**
– Use a new, sterile disposable needle to collect your blood

DONOR ELIGIBILITY – SPECIFIC INFORMATION
Why we ask questions about sexual contact:
Sexual contact may cause contagious diseases like HIV to get into the bloodstream and be spread through transfusions to someone else.
Definition of "sexual contact":
The words "have sexual contact with" and "sex" are used in some of the questions we will ask you, and apply to any of the activities below, whether or not a condom or other protection was used:
1. Vaginal sex (contact between penis and vagina)
2. Oral sex (mouth or tongue on someone's vagina, penis, or anus)
3. Anal sex (contact between penis and anus)

HIV/AIDS RISK BEHAVIORS AND SYMPTOMS
AIDS is caused by HIV. HIV is spread mainly through sexual contact with an infected person OR by sharing needles or syringes used for injecting drugs.

DO NOT DONATE IF YOU:
– **Have AIDS or have ever had a positive HIV test**
– Have ever used needles to take drugs, steroids, or anything not prescribed by your doctor
– Are a male who has had sexual contact with another male, even once, since 1977

– Have ever taken money, drugs, or other payment for sex since 1977
– Have had sexual contact in the past 12 months with anyone described above
– Have had syphilis or gonorrhea in the past 12 months
– In the last 12 months have been in juvenile detention, lockup, jail, or prison for more than 72 hours
– Have any of the following conditions that can be signs or symptoms of HIV/AIDS:
  • Unexplained weight loss or night sweats
  • Blue or purple spots in your mouth or skin
  • Swollen lymph nodes for more than one month
  • White spots or unusual sores in your mouth
  • Cough that won't go away or shortness of breath
  • Diarrhea that won't go away
  • Fever of more than 100.5° F for more than 10 days
Remember that you CAN give HIV to someone else through blood transfusions even if you feel well and have a negative HIV test. This is because tests cannot detect infections for a period of time after a person is exposed to HIV. **If you think you may be at risk for HIV/AIDS or want an HIV/AIDS test, please ask for information about other testing facilities. *PLEASE DO NOT DONATE TO GET AN HIV TEST!***

Travel to or birth in other countries
Blood donor tests may not be available for some contagious diseases that are found only in certain countries. If you were born in, have lived in, or visited certain countries, you may not be eligible to donate.

What happens after your donation:
To protect patients, your blood is tested for hepatitis B and C, HIV, certain other infectious diseases, and syphilis. If your blood tests positive, it will not be given to a patient. You will be notified about test results that may disqualify you from donating in the future. **Please do not donate to get tested for HIV, hepatitis, or any other infections!**

Thank you for donating blood today!
(Donor Center Name)
(Telephone Number)

Fig. 13.1 Blood Donor Educational Materials (version 1.3, May 2008). (Courtesy AABB, Bethesda, MD.)

HEALTH HISTORY INTERVIEW

The health history assessment is performed on a document called the DHQ. The document is used to protect both the donor during the donation process and the patient receiving the blood. Questions are asked in an environment that provides confidentiality and encouragement to answer truthfully. Self-administered interview formats have been shown to yield more information regarding HIV high-risk behavior.[6] The interviewer should document and evaluate all responses to determine suitability for donation.

Although the use of the DHQ (Fig. 13.2) developed by AABB and approved by the FDA is recommended, **medical directors** have the option to add questions as appropriate for their center, based on demographics or questions not addressed by the FDA. These questions must be placed at the end of the DHQ.

Medical direktors: designated physicians responsible for the medical and technical policies of the blood bank

Full-Length Donor History Questionnaire

		Yes	No	
Are you				
1.	Feeling healthy and well today?	❑	❑	
2.	Currently taking an antibiotic?	❑	❑	
3.	Currently taking any other medication for an infection?	❑	❑	
Please read the Medication Deferral List.				
4.	Are you now taking or have you ever taken any medications on the Medication Deferral List?	❑	❑	
5.	Have you read the educational materials?	❑	❑	
In the past 48 hours				
6.	Have you taken aspirin or anything that has aspirin in it?	❑	❑	
In the past 6 weeks				
7.	Female donors: Have you been pregnant or are you pregnant now? (Males: check "I am male.")	❑	❑	❑ I am male
In the past 8 weeks have you				
8.	Donated blood, platelets, or plasma?	❑	❑	
9.	Had any vaccinations or other shots?	❑	❑	
10.	Had contact with someone who had a smallpox vaccination?	❑	❑	
In the past 16 weeks				
11.	Have you donated a double unit of red cells using an apheresis machine?	❑	❑	
In the past 12 months have you				
12.	Had a blood transfusion?	❑	❑	
13.	Had a transplant such as organ, tissue, or bone marrow?	❑	❑	
14.	Had a graft such as bone or skin?	❑	❑	
15.	Come into contact with someone else's blood?	❑	❑	
16.	Had an accidental needle-stick?	❑	❑	
17.	Had sexual contact with anyone who has HIV/AIDS or has had a positive test for the HIV/AIDS virus?	❑	❑	
18.	Had sexual contact with a prostitute or anyone else who takes money or drugs or other payment for sex?	❑	❑	
19.	Had sexual contact with anyone who has ever used needles to take drugs or steroids, or anything not prescribed by their doctor?	❑	❑	
20.	Had sexual contact with anyone who has hemophilia or has used clotting factor concentrates?	❑	❑	
21.	Female donors: Had sexual contact with a male who has ever had sexual contact with another male? (Males: check "I am male.")	❑	❑	❑ I am male
22.	Had sexual contact with a person who has hepatitis?	❑	❑	
23.	Lived with a person who has hepatitis?	❑	❑	
24.	Had a tattoo?	❑	❑	
25.	Had ear or body piercing?	❑	❑	
26.	Had or been treated for syphilis or gonorrhea?	❑	❑	
27.	Been in juvenile detention, lockup, jail, or prison for more than 72 hours?	❑	❑	
In the past 3 years have you				
28.	Been outside the United States or Canada?	❑	❑	
From 1980 through 1996,				
29.	Did you spend time that adds up to three (3) months or more in the United Kingdom? (Review list of countries in the U.K.)	❑	❑	
30.	Were you a member of the U.S. military, a civilian military employee, or a dependent of a member of the U.S. military?	❑	❑	

Fig. 13.2 Donor History Questionnaire (version 1.3, May 2008). (Courtesy AABB, Bethesda, MD.)

		Yes	No	
From 1980 to the present, did you				
31.	Spend time that adds up to five (5) years or more in Europe? (Review list of countries in Europe.)	❑	❑	
32.	Receive a blood transfusion in the United Kingdom or France? (Review list of countries in the U.K.)	❑	❑	
From 1977 to the present, have you				
33.	Received money, drugs, or other payment for sex?	❑	❑	
34.	Male donors: had sexual contact with another male, even once? (Females: check "I am female.")	❑	❑	❑ I am female
Have you **EVER**				
35.	Had a positive test for the HIV/AIDS virus?	❑	❑	
36.	Used needles to take drugs, steroids, or anything <u>not</u> prescribed by your doctor?	❑	❑	
37.	Used clotting factor concentrates?	❑	❑	
38.	Had hepatitis?	❑	❑	
39.	Had malaria?	❑	❑	
40.	Had Chagas' disease?	❑	❑	
41.	Had babesiosis?	❑	❑	
42.	Received a dura mater (or brain covering) graft?	❑	❑	
43.	Had any type of cancer, including leukemia?	❑	❑	
44.	Had any problems with your heart or lungs?	❑	❑	
45.	Had a bleeding condition or a blood disease?	❑	❑	
46.	Had sexual contact with anyone who was born in or lived in Africa?	❑	❑	
47.	Been in Africa?	❑	❑	
48.	Have any of your relatives had Creutzfeldt-Jakob disease?	❑	❑	
Use this area for additional questions		Yes	No	

Fig. 13.2, cont'd

An abbreviated DHQ for qualified frequent donors has been approved by the FDA for use in a few blood centers.[6] This abbreviated questionnaire is intended to improve the donation process for frequent donors, as well as maintain safety of the blood supply.

Questions generally can be divided into two categories: questions intended to protect the donor and questions intended to protect the recipient. An explanation of some of the questions from the DHQ follows (see Fig. 13.2).

Donor Deferrals

There are several categories for the referral of a donor. Donors may be deferred indefinitely, permanently, or temporarily based on medical history or prior tests. An *indefinite deferral* is sometimes due to current regulatory requirements that may change in the future. For example, a donor states that he lived in England for 1 year between 1980 and 1996. A *permanent deferral* is required based on a high-risk behavior or a positive test result. Donors with permanent deferrals are not expected to ever regain eligibility, even if rules or testing technologies change. Examples of permanent deferrals for donors include the medication etretinate (Tegison), a confirmed positive test for hepatitis B surface antigen (HBsAg), and reactive nucleic acid tests for hepatitis C virus or HIV during reentry testing. Table 13.1 lists current indefinite and permanent deferrals. A *temporary deferral* is recommended if the donor would be eligible at a specific time in the future. An example of a temporary deferral is potential contact with hepatitis from body piercing, tattoos, or living with a person with symptomatic viral hepatitis, which necessitates a 12-month deferral. The temporary deferral allows for viral screening tests to detect a developing antibody or the presence of the virus.

Check the current edition of AABB *Standards* for updated donor deferrals since the publication of this book.

TABLE 13.1	Conditions for Indefinite or Permanent Deferral

- History of viral hepatitis after eleventh birthday
- Confirmed positive test for hepatitis B surface antigen
- Reactive test to antibodies to hepatitis B core on more than one occasion
- Present or past clinical or laboratory evidence of infection with hepatitis C virus, human T-cell lymphotropic virus, or HIV
- History of babesiosis or Chagas disease
- Family history of CJD
- Recipient of dura mater or human pituitary growth hormone
- Risk of vCJD
- Use of a needle to administer nonprescription drugs

HIV, Human immunodeficiency virus; *CJD,* Creutzfeldt-Jakob disease; *vCJD,* variant Creutzfeldt-Jakob disease. Data from Fung MK, editor: *Technical manual,* ed 18, Bethesda, MD, 2014, AABB.

Questions for Protection of the Donor

Properly trained blood bank personnel are required to ask specific questions to determine donor eligibility, such as questions regarding general health, previous surgeries, heart and lung disease, bleeding problems, cancer, and pregnancy. Donors with cold or influenza symptoms, headache, or nausea should be temporarily deferred. Donors who are currently pregnant or have been pregnant in the past 6 weeks are also deferred. The medical director of the facility must evaluate donors with a history of cancer because there are no U.S. federal regulations or professional standards that address donor eligibility regarding cancer.[7]

Deferring donors for any reason should be handled tactfully. Donors should be provided with a full explanation of the reason for the deferral and information on whether they can donate in the future.

Questions for Protection of the Recipient

Donors are thoroughly questioned regarding possible exposure to diseases that could be transmitted through the blood supply. Transmissible diseases, medications, vaccinations, and high-risk activities are carefully evaluated to protect recipients of blood transfusions from risks. The list of donor questions in this category is updated frequently to reflect current knowledge of bloodborne pathogen and medication issues.

Transfusion-Transmissible Infections

Although viral marker testing has increased the safety of the blood supply, questions to determine potential exposure to certain transmissible diseases are also necessary. Many viral markers may be below detectable limits on donation, and an available screening test may not currently exist for some bloodborne diseases, such as malaria or Creutzfeldt-Jakob disease (CJD). Questions regarding potential exposure through travel may be the only method to prevent transmission through the blood supply.

Transmissible spongiform encephalopathies are degenerative brain disorders caused by prions, which are believed to be infectious proteins. Two forms of transmissible spongiform encephalopathies include classic CJD and variant Creutzfeldt-Jakob disease (vCJD). Both forms are potentially transmitted by blood transfusion. Because there are no current tests to screen donors, donor history questions are critical to avoid transmission. Current deferral criteria for vCJD and CJD as directed by the FDA can be found on the FDA's website.[8] The FDA document outlines the research and current restrictions regarding residing in the United Kingdom, France, and other countries in Europe. In addition, receipt of human pituitary growth hormone, history of familial CJD, or dura mater transplant has been associated with transmission of CJD.

Malaria, Chagas disease, leishmaniasis, and babesiosis are parasitic infections that can be transmitted through transfusion. Malaria is caused by several species of the protozoan genus *Plasmodium.* Chagas disease is endemic in South and Central America and is caused by the parasite *Trypanosoma cruzi. Leishmania* species are transmitted by the sandfly (*Phlebotomus* species) and have been reportedly found in personnel stationed in Iraq. Infected deer ticks in the northeastern United States can spread the parasite *Babesia microti,* which causes babesiosis. An important method of screening for these diseases is

TABLE 13.2 Deferral Periods for Potential Transfusion-Transmitted Infections

INFECTIOUS DISEASE	HEALTH HISTORY DEFERRAL
Malaria (*Plasmodium* spp.)	History of malaria: 3 years Lived in endemic area(s) for 5 consecutive years: 3 years from departure Travel to endemic area: defer for 1 year from departure
Babesiosis (*Babesia microti*)	History of babesiosis: indefinite deferral
Chagas disease (*Trypanosoma cruzi*)	History of Chagas disease: indefinite deferral
Leishmaniasis	Travel to Iraq: defer for 1 year from departure
vCJD	Received blood transfusion in United Kingdom from 1980 to present Lived ≥3 months in United Kingdom from 1980 to 1996 Lived ≥5 years in Europe from 1980 to present Member of U.S. military, a civilian military employee, or a dependent of a member of U.S. military from 1980 to 1996
CJD	Family history of CJD, dura mater transplant, human pituitary-derived growth hormone: indefinite deferral

CJD, Creutzfeldt-Jakob disease; *vCJD*, variant Creutzfeldt-Jakob disease.
Data from Fung MK, editor: *Technical manual*, ed 18, Bethesda, MD, 2014, AABB.

TABLE 13.3 Medications Commonly Accepted for Blood Donation

- Hypnotics used at bedtime
- Blood pressure medications (if patient is free of side effects and cardiovascular symptoms)
- Over-the-counter bronchodilators
- Decongestants
- Oral contraceptives
- Replacement hormones
- Weight-reduction drugs
- Mild analgesics
- Vitamins
- Tetracyclines and other antibiotics taken for acne

by questioning donors regarding travel or immigration from endemic areas. A summary of deferrals related to travel is presented in Table 13.2.

Medications

Certain medications may cause deferrals based on the nature of the disease process for which they are being used, not because of the drug's properties. Antibiotics, anticonvulsants, anticoagulants, insulin, and antiarrhythmic drugs are prescribed for conditions that generally exclude donors. Medications such as finasteride (Proscar), dutasteride (Avodart), isotretinoin (Accutane), etretinate (Tegison), and acitretin (Soriatane) can cause birth defects if present in high levels and transfused to a pregnant woman. Aspirin and aspirin-containing medications inhibit platelet function. For this reason, donors who are the only source of platelets for a patient (eg, apheresis donors) are deferred for 2 days. Commonly used medications that are acceptable for donation are listed in Table 13.3. Medications requiring deferrals are listed in Table 13.4. Scan the QR code to refer to the AABB's Medication Deferral List for more information on various medications.

Vaccines

Donors receiving vaccinations that are prepared from toxoids or killed organisms do not require deferral if the donor is free of symptoms. With the exception of receiving an intranasal live attenuated flu vaccine, the use of attenuated viral and bacterial vaccines

TABLE 13.4   Medication Deferrals

MEDICATION	PRIMARY USE	DEFERRAL
Finasteride (Proscar)	Benign prostatic hyperplasia	1 month
Finasteride (Propecia)	Male baldness	1 month
Dutasteride (Avodart, Jalyn)	Benign prostatic hyperplasia	6 months
Isotretinoin (Accutane, Amnesteem, Claravis, Sotret)	Severe acne	1 month
Acitretin (Soriatane)	Severe psoriasis	3 years
Etretinate (Tegison)	Severe psoriasis	Indefinite deferral
Warfarin (Coumadin)	Prevention of blood clots	1 week
Bovine insulin	Diabetes	Indefinite deferral
Aspirin and piroxicam (Feldene)	Nonsteroidal antiinflammatory	2 days after last dose for platelet donors
Clopidogrel (Plavix), ticlopidine (Ticlid)	Prevention of blood clots	14 days for platelet donors
Hepatitis B immune globulin	Exposure to hepatitis B	1 year

Data from Fung MK, editor: *Technical manual,* ed 18, Bethesda, MD, 2014, AABB.

TABLE 13.5   Temporary Deferrals

DEFERRAL TIME	REASON FOR DEFERRAL
2 weeks	Measles (rubeola) vaccine Mumps vaccine Polio (oral) vaccine Typhoid (oral) vaccine Yellow fever vaccine
4 weeks	German measles (rubella) vaccine Varicella-zoster (chickenpox) vaccine
6 weeks	Conclusion of pregnancy
12 months	Tattoos or permanent makeup (unless applied by a state-regulated facility with sterile needles and ink that is not reused) Mucous membrane or skin penetration exposure to blood Sexual contact with an individual at high risk for HIV Incarceration in a correctional institution for >72 hr Completion of therapy for syphilis Transfusion of blood, components, human tissue, plasma-derived clotting factor concentrates Human diploid cell–rabies vaccine after animal bite

HIV, Human immunodeficiency virus.

generally necessitates a temporary deferral, as indicated in Table 13.5. Recombinant vaccines, such as human papillomavirus vaccine, do not require deferral. A 12-month deferral is necessary if the donor was exposed to an animal that resulted in the need for a rabies vaccination.

High-Risk Activities

A 12-month deferral is necessary if a prospective donor has had a positive test for syphilis or has been treated for syphilis or gonorrhea.[9] The likelihood of transmitting syphilis through a transfusion is improbable. The potential high-risk behavior that makes transmission of other infectious diseases more likely is the main reason for deferral.

Questions regarding high-risk behavior associated with transmission of HIV are required. Donors must understand the activities that might be considered high risk, and they must be deferred if they are donating for the purpose of HIV testing. Alternative site testing should be offered to individuals seeking HIV testing. Donors must also be informed of local requirements and policies that necessitate notification to government agencies of the donor's HIV status. A 12-month deferral is required for donors who have had sexual contact with anyone who:

- Has used a needle to take drugs not prescribed by a physician
- Has taken clotting factor concentrates for a bleeding problem
- Has HIV/AIDS or has had a positive test for HIV

In addition, men who have had sex with other men since 1977 were permanently deferred until 2015. A recent draft guidance for industry issued by the FDA has recommended that this restriction be changed.[10,11,12] The FDA changed its policy from the indefinite deferral period established in 1977 to a 1-year deferral since sexual contact. Women who have had sexual contact with a man who has had sex with another man are deferred for 12 months. The donor's responses to these questions could lead to additional questions or to a temporary, indefinite, or permanent deferral from donating.

PHYSICAL EXAMINATION

General Appearance

The prospective donor should appear to be in generally good health. Donors should be deferred if alcohol or drug use is suspected.

Hemoglobin or Hematocrit Determination

Blood for the hemoglobin or hematocrit test is obtained from venipuncture or finger stick. For whole blood donation, recent FDA guidelines require that males have a minimum hemoglobin level of 13 g/dL (130 g/L) or minimum hematocrit of 39%.[13] The minimum hemoglobin level will remain at 12.5 g/dL (125 g/L) or the minimum hematocrit is 38% for females.[13] However, a variance will be possible for female donors to be permitted to donate at 12.0 g/dL if additional steps are taken to assure donor safety. This requirement ensures a sufficient hemoglobin level to allow the removal of a maximum of 525 mL, including samples drawn for testing, without harming the donor.

> The spun hematocrit is determined by centrifugation of a capillary tube filled with blood.

> Methods for determining the donor's hemoglobin include the copper sulfate method and spectrophotometric methods.

Temperature

Body temperature should not exceed 37.5° C (99.5° F).[14] An elevated temperature could indicate a possible infection in the donor, which could pose a danger to the recipient.

Blood Pressure

There are no specific AABB requirements for **systolic blood pressure** and **diastolic blood pressure** for donors. In the final ruling effective May 2016, FDA guidelines require blood pressure within FDA-established ranges: systolic 90 to 180 mm Hg and diastolic 50 to 100 mm Hg.[13] Blood pressure outside of these ranges must be evaluated by an onsite medical director.[15]

> **Systolic blood pressure:** contraction of the heart; the first sound heard while taking a blood pressure

Pulse

For whole blood donors, there are no specific requirements in the AABB standards. In the same FDA ruling effective in May 2016, the pulse measurement was added as an FDA requirement. The pulse should be between 50 and 100 beats per minute for source plasma donors according to FDA guidelines.[13]

> **Diastolic blood pressure:** filling of the heart chamber; the second sound heard while taking a blood pressure

Weight

A minimum weight of 110 pounds is now an FDA requirement. Whole blood donors can be asked their weight.[13] AABB standards permit collection of 10.5 mL of blood per kilogram (kg) of the donor's weight for each donation.[7] Donors weighing a minimum of 110 lb (50 kg) can tolerate a maximum withdrawal of 525 mL, including samples drawn for processing.

TABLE 13.6	Physical Examination Requirements
CRITERIA CHECKED	**ACCEPTABLE LIMIT**
Appearance	In good health
Hemoglobin	≥12.5 g/dL (125 g/L) Females 13.0 g/dL (130 g/L) Males
Hematocrit	≥38% Females ≥39% Males
Blood pressure	Systolic 90–180 mm Diastolic: 50–100 mm
Temperature	≤37.5° C (99.5° F)
Pulse	50–100 beats/minute
Weight	Minimum 110 lb (50 kg)
Age	Conform to applicable state law or >16 years

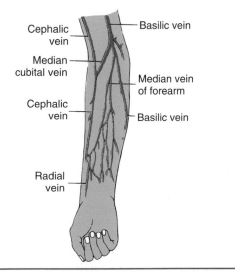

Fig. 13.3 Diagram of the arm showing the antecubital vein. This vein is the best for the donor's venipuncture and subsequent donation. (From Potter PA, et al: *Fundamentals of nursing*, ed 9, St. Louis, 2017, Elsevier.)

Donors who weigh less are not restricted from donating, but a proportionally smaller amount of blood should be removed. For example, a donor who weighs 100 lb (45 kg) can donate 473 mL. The physical examination criteria for blood donation are summarized in Table 13.6.

SECTION 2

PHLEBOTOMY

IDENTIFICATION

The donor's identity should be confirmed at each step of the donation process. The phlebotomist is often different from the person taking the donor's health history; therefore he or she needs to confirm the identity of the donor before beginning the venipuncture. Next, the antecubital area of both donor arms needs to be inspected. This inspection gives the phlebotomist the opportunity to select the arm with the best vein and to check for skin lesions and intravenous drug use (Fig. 13.3).

BAG LABELING

The primary bag used for blood collection, all attached satellite bags, sample tubes, and the donor registration form must be labeled with a unique identification number. The

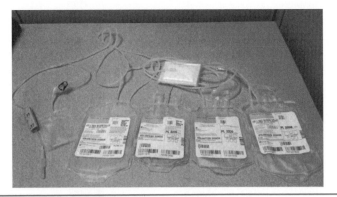

Fig. 13.4 Example of a collection bag with unique identification number labels. The bag set allows the collection of whole blood and has satellite bags for the manufacture of blood components.

PREPARING THE DONOR'S ARM FOR BLOOD COLLECTION

Step	Action
1	Apply tourniquet or blood pressure cuff; identify venipuncture site; then release tourniquet or cuff.
2	Scrub area at least 4 cm (1.5 inches) in all directions from the intended site of venipuncture (ie, 8 cm or 3 inches in diameter) for a minimum of 30 seconds with 0.7% aqueous solution of iodophor compound. Excess foam may be removed, but the arm need not be dry before the next step.
3	Starting at the intended site of venipuncture and moving outward in a concentric spiral, apply "prep" solution; let stand for 30 seconds or as indicated by manufacturer.
4	Cover the area with dry, sterile gauze until the time of venipuncture. After the skin has been prepared, it must not be touched again. Do not repalpate the vein at the intended venipuncture site.

Fig. 13.5 Proper antiseptic preparation of a donor's arm before phlebotomy is essential to preserve the sterility of the collection. (From Fung MK, editor:*Technical manual*,ed 18, Bethesda, MD, 2014, AABB.)

label consists of both numbers and letters readable by the phlebotomist and bar-codes used for computer scanning. The use of identical numbers allows the collected blood, prepared components, and blood samples used for testing to be traced back to the original donor registration record (Fig. 13.4).

ARM PREPARATION AND VENIPUNCTURE

Blood is usually drawn from the antecubital area. After an appropriate vein has been selected, the skin needs to be prepared for the venipuncture. Skin cannot be sterilized, but several methods are acceptable for disinfecting the drawing site.

The venipuncture site is scrubbed with a 0.7% aqueous scrub solution of iodophor compound to remove surface dirt and bacteria and begin germicidal action. Next, a preparation solution of 10% povidone-iodine is applied, beginning at the intended venipuncture site and continuing outward in a concentric spiral. The area is allowed to air-dry for 30 seconds before being covered with sterile gauze. For donors sensitive to these solutions, another method should be designated by the blood bank physician, such as chlorhexidine (ChloraPrep 2%) and 70% isopropyl alcohol (Fig. 13.5).[6]

A tourniquet or blood pressure cuff inflated to 40 to 60 mm Hg makes the vein more prominent for venipuncture. A 16-gauge needle attached to a primary blood bag is inserted into a large, firm vein free of skin lesions. The usual donation time for a unit of whole blood is 8 to 12 minutes. Units requiring more than 15 minutes draw time may not be suitable for the preparation of platelets, fresh frozen plasma (FFP), or cryoprecipitated antihemophilic factor (CRYO). Frequent mixing of the blood during donation with the

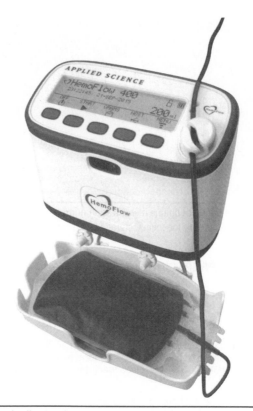

Fig. 13.6 Example of a blood collection device that monitors the blood volume drawn and time to complete collection. (Courtesy Applied Science, Inc., Grass Valley, Calif.)

anticoagulant/preservative in the bag is critical to avoid blood clots and can be performed manually or with a mechanical mixing device. A balance system or electronic scale is used to monitor the volume of blood drawn. Either before or after donation, two to four specimen tubes used for testing, along with the segments, are filled before the needle is removed. After the needle is removed, pressure is applied to the venipuncture site over the gauze and the arm is elevated (elbow straight). The needle is disposed of in an appropriate biohazard container (Fig. 13.6).

To prevent potential contamination with epidermal cells and potential bacteria entering the donor unit, AABB standards require the use of collection containers that divert the first 10 to 20 mL of blood into a "diversion pouch" when platelet products are to be prepared from whole blood donations (Fig. 13.7).[7]

ADVERSE DONOR REACTIONS

Donors usually tolerate the donation process, but adverse reactions do occur. Most reactions are vasovagal, which may include sweating, rapid breathing, dizziness, nausea, and syncope (fainting). Whether caused by the actual loss of blood or the sight or thought of donating blood, the tourniquet and needle are removed, and immediate treatment is initiated at the first sign of a reaction. Instructions for handling donor reactions, including procedures for emergency medical treatment, must be available to the staff as part of their training. Table 13.7 summarizes possible donor reactions and appropriate treatment.[16]

POSTDONATION INSTRUCTIONS AND CARE

The donor is given postphlebotomy care instructions as follows:
• Contact the donor center if there are any concerns regarding the safety of the blood or if you believe the blood should not be transfused.

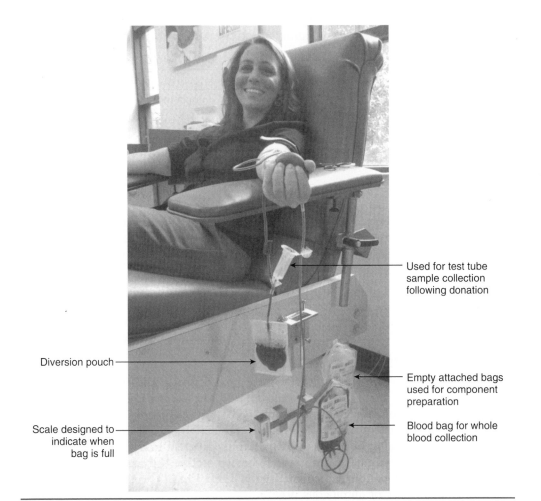

Used for test tube
sample collection
following donation

Diversion pouch

Empty attached bags
used for component
preparation

Scale designed to
indicate when
bag is full

Blood bag for whole
blood collection

Fig. 13.7 Diversion pouch. The sample diversion pouch automatically diverts the initial volume of whole blood into a pouch to reduce the incidence of bacterial contamination. The diverted blood is subsequently used for collection of test samples.

TABLE 13.7	Adverse Donor Reactions and Appropriate Treatment
SYMPTOMS	**TREATMENT**
Weakness, sweating, dizziness, pallor, nausea and vomiting	Remove needle and tourniquet; elevate legs above head; apply cold compresses to forehead and back of neck
Syncope (fainting)	Cold compresses on back of neck
Twitching, muscle spasms	Have donor cough
Hematoma	Apply pressure for 7–10 minutes; apply ice to area for 5 minutes
Convulsions	Call for help; prevent donor from falling from the donor chair or injuring himself or herself; ensure donor's airway is adequate
Cardiac difficulties	Begin cardiopulmonary resuscitation; call for emergency help

- Avoid smoking for 30 minutes; avoid alcohol until something has been eaten.
- Drink more fluids than usual in the next 4 hours.
- If dizziness or fainting occurs, lie down or sit with the head between the knees.
- Caution donors who work at certain occupations who will be returning to work immediately (involving heights, construction, or machine operators).
- Remove the bandage after a few hours.
- Inform the blood center if any symptoms persist.

TABLE 13.8	Advantages and Disadvantages of Autologous Donations	
ADVANTAGES	**DISADVANTAGES**
Prevention of transfusion-transmitted diseases	Inventory control
Prevention of alloimmunization	Preoperative anemia
Supplementing blood supply	Increased cost
Prevention of febrile and allergic reactions	High wastage
Reassurance of patient	Increased incidence of adverse reactions to donation

Postdonation fluid replacement begins in the donor room. Donors should not be released until checked by a staff member. Total fluid-volume replacement is usually restored within 72 hours of donation. Iron replacement takes substantially longer; a whole blood donor must wait 56 days to be eligible to donate again.

SECTION 3
SPECIAL BLOOD COLLECTION

AUTOLOGOUS DONATIONS

A voluntary donation of blood for use by the general patient population is called allogeneic. Any donation of blood reserved for the donor's own use at a later time is considered an autologous donation. Risk of disease transmission, transfusion reactions, or alloimmunization to RBCs, platelets, white blood cells, or plasma proteins is significantly reduced. Requirements for autologous donors are significantly different from the requirements for allogeneic donors and are described in the following section. Advantages and disadvantages of autologous donations are summarized in Table 13.8.

Three general types of autologous procedures exist: preoperative collection, normovolemic hemodilution, and blood recovery. Preoperative autologous donation is the most common and necessitates careful tracking and handling to ensure units are available for surgery. Each category is summarized in the following sections.

Preoperative Collection

In preoperative collection, the blood is drawn and stored before the anticipated transfusion. This procedure is used for stable patients scheduled for surgical procedures likely to necessitate blood transfusion. It is especially useful for patients with rare antibodies that make crossmatching allogeneic units difficult or for patients whose religious beliefs do not allow allogeneic transfusions. Patients being treated for bacteremia are ineligible to be autologous donors.

The preoperative blood collection process begins with a written order from the patient's physician. Informed consent must be obtained from the patient (donor), with written notification that all test results are released to the patient's physician. Criteria for donor selection do not include high-risk questions. The collecting facility's medical director establishes guidelines concerning the autologous donor's health for donation eligibility. Donors are not restricted by age; the ability of younger patients to donate is determined more by the size of the patient. For patients weighing less than 110 lb, the volume of blood collected and the amount of anticoagulant used should be proportionately less. The patient (donor) hemoglobin concentration should be no less than 11 g/dL. The hematocrit should be no less than 33%.[7] Blood collection should be completed more than 72 hours before surgery. In addition to the routine labeling of the blood bag, the name of the donor, the recipient name, identification number, the blood group, and the name of the hospital must be included along with the phrase "for autologous use only."[7]

The ABO and D phenotype must be determined at the collecting facility. If the blood is transfused outside the collecting facility, infectious disease testing must be performed before shipping.[6] At a minimum, the first unit shipped within each 30-day period must be tested.[17] A repeatedly reactive viral test does not necessarily mean that the unit is destroyed

with allogeneic units. With permission of the patient's physician and the receiving facility's transfusion service, autologous units can ship after a biohazard label has been affixed. Autologous units that are not used cannot be crossed over to the general inventory because they do not meet the same donation and testing requirements as allogeneic donations.

Special procedures must exist (either manual or computerized) to ensure that the units are located and transfused to the intended recipient. A system must exist to identify the units for transfusion to the recipient before any directed or allogeneic units are transfused. The extent of pretransfusion testing for autologous donations varies in individual facilities. Some facilities perform a crossmatch in addition to a check on ABO and D phenotyping.

Normovolemic Hemodilution

Normovolemic hemodilution involves removing one or more units of blood at the beginning of surgery. The blood removed is replaced with crystalloid or colloid solutions to restore fluid volume. The blood is stored for reinfusion during or at the end of surgery. This process is sometimes referred to as acute normovolemic hemodilution.

Blood Recovery

Blood recovery is the collection and reinfusion of shed blood. A medical device is used to collect shed blood from the operative field. The process can include collecting and directly reinfusing the blood using a device that washes, filters, and concentrates it. Washing does not remove bacteria; intraoperative blood collection should not be used if the operative field has bacterial contamination. Fig. 13.8 shows an intraoperative cell recovery instrument.

DIRECTED DONATIONS

The public's concern for the safety of the blood supply led to demands from potential recipients to choose their own donors. Although no substantial evidence exists that directed donations provide safer blood than allogeneic donations, most blood centers and hospitals participate in a directed-donor program. Donor requirements and testing must meet the same criteria as allogeneic donations. The donor collection, health history, and testing requirements are the same for directed donors as for routine blood donors. Policies regarding crossover to the general patient population, determination of the ABO phenotype before collection, additional fees, and time for unit availability vary among institutions. The 56-day interval between donations may be waived with the medical director's approval. Pretransfusion testing for directed donations follows the same protocols as allogeneic donations.

APHERESIS

Apheresis is a category of procedures in which whole blood is removed from a donor or patient, a component is separated by mechanical means, and the remainder of the blood is returned. The following terms describe the portion that is removed and the donor requirements:
- *Leukapheresis:* white blood cells are removed
  Collection of sufficient granulocytes for a therapeutic dose requires drugs or sedimenting materials be given to the donor before collection. Donor consent to the use of these treatments is required.
- *Plateletpheresis:* platelets are removed
  At least 48 hours must elapse between donations, and donors should not undergo plateletpheresis more than twice a week or more than 24 times in a rolling 12-month period.[7] Plateletpheresis donors must have a platelet count of at least 150,000 per μL before collection if the interval between donations is less than 4 weeks.
- *Plasmapheresis:* plasma is removed
  Collection of plasma by apheresis is designated as either frequent or infrequent. For an infrequent plasmapheresis program, donors do not donate more often than once every 4 weeks. The donor must weigh at least 110 lb. Plasmapheresis more often than once every 4 weeks necessitates that total plasma protein, IgG, and IgM levels be monitored at 4-month intervals.[18]
- *Red cell apheresis:* two units of RBCs are removed

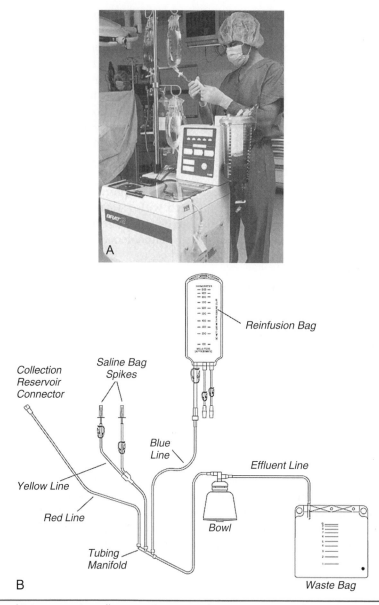

Fig. 13.8 A and B, Intraoperative cell recovery instrument. (**A** courtesy COBE Cardiovascular, Arvada, CO. **B** Image of the Haemonetics © blood processing disposable set is used by permission of Haemonetics Corporation.)

Therapeutic apheresis:
blood is removed from a patient and the portion that might be contributing to a pathologic condition is retained; the remainder is returned along with a replacement fluid such as colloid or fresh frozen plasma

Donors who meet certain criteria levels may have two units of RBCs removed by apheresis. Current FDA guidelines require donors to be larger and have higher hematocrit values than for single RBC donations.[19] For male donors, the minimum weight is 130 lb and the minimum height is 5 feet 1 inch; female donors must weigh at least 150 lb and be 5 feet 5 inches tall. Both male and female donors must also have a hematocrit of 40% or higher. Donors are also deferred for 16 weeks after a double RBC donation. Saline infusion is used to minimize volume depletion.[6]

These procedures are used with donors to collect a greater quantity of a specific component than can be obtained from single whole blood donations. The apheresis procedure in patients is used to treat various diseases (**therapeutic apheresis**) as described in more detail in a later chapter.

Apheresis was originally performed manually. The process involved removing a unit of whole blood, centrifuging it, removing the desired component, and returning the remaining blood before removing the next unit. At the present time, apheresis is routinely performed with a cell-separator machine (Fig. 13.9). Centrifugal force is used to separate the blood into components based on their specific gravity. The blood flows directly from the donor's arm into the centrifuge bowl, a specific component is removed, and the remainder

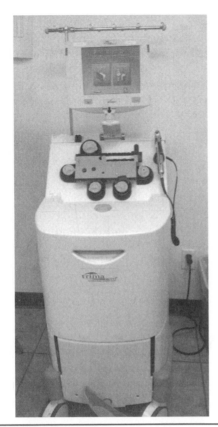

Fig. 13.9 Example of an apheresis machine.

of the blood is returned to the donor; all of this occurs within a closed system. Depending on the procedure and the equipment used, the process can take 30 minutes to 2 hours. The procedure can be performed by intermittent or continuous flow. An intermittent flow process involves one venipuncture; blood is removed, centrifuged, and returned in alternating steps. A continuous flow procedure necessitates a venipuncture in both arms; blood is removed from one arm, centrifuged, and returned in the other arm.

THERAPEUTIC PHLEBOTOMY

Therapeutic phlebotomy is performed to withdraw blood from a patient for medical reasons. Although the removal of blood does not cure the disease, it can help treat the patient's symptoms. Common indications for therapeutic phlebotomy include polycythemia, hemochromatosis, and porphyrias. Blood collected from donors with hereditary hemochromatosis, which is a disorder of iron metabolism, can be put into the blood supply if the blood center meets certain FDA criteria.[6] The FDA has permitted variances regarding labeling and frequency of collection. The service to the donor for phlebotomy must be free of charge, regardless of the donor's eligibility. Donor centers that provide this service are available on the FDA website.[20]

CHAPTER SUMMARY

- Careful donor selection by trained phlebotomy personnel is the most important element in ensuring a safe blood supply.
- Criteria for acceptable blood donors are established by the FDA through the CFR, guidance documents or memoranda to the industry, and AABB *Standards*.
- Registration and donor identification determine whether sufficient time has elapsed for donating and whether the donor was previously deferred.

- Donors must be informed of high-risk behavior and discouraged from donating if they have the potential of transmitting infection through the blood supply.
- Blood is not tested for certain diseases, such as malaria and CJD; therefore questions regarding exposure and travel are important for screening purposes.
- The safety of the donor and the recipient is an important element of the screening process, which includes medical history questions and a brief physical examination to determine eligibility.
- Arm preparation to avoid contamination with bacteria involves a two-step disinfecting procedure and a diversion pouch for collection of platelets, including whole blood from which platelets are made.
- Signs of adverse donor reactions during phlebotomy, although uncommon, must be recognized and responded to quickly.
- Postdonation instructions to the donor regarding concerns about the safety of his or her donation, activities to avoid, and the importance of increasing fluid intake complete the donation process.
- Special donations, such as autologous, directed, apheresis, and therapeutic phlebotomy, are important donor and patient services that necessitate unique policies and procedures.

CRITICAL THINKING EXERCISES

Exercise 13.1
A potential donor is questioned regarding her previous medical history, and she states that she has been living in an endemic malarial area for 1 year doing Peace Corps activities. She just returned last week.
1. Is this person eligible as a blood donor?
2. If not, how long must she wait?

Exercise 13.2
A potential donor has the following results on a physical examination:
Hemoglobin: 14 g/dL
Temperature: 98.9° F
Weight: 150 lb
   She states she has had aspirin for a headache that day and received hepatitis B immune globulin for a needle stick 3 months ago.
1. Is she eligible as a blood donor?
2. Is there a deferral time?

Exercise 13.3
A 15-year-old girl would like to donate blood for her relative. She weighs 108 lb. Her temperature and hemoglobin are within acceptable limits.
1. Is she an eligible directed donor?
2. If she were donating for herself for a planned surgery, could she donate?
3. What are some of the issues surrounding directed donations?

Exercise 13.4
An 18-year-old student donated for the first time at a blood drive at his high school.
1. Concerned that he may have contracted HIV before the donation, what instructions should he follow to prevent his unit from being transfused?
2. Why are questions regarding HIV important even when tests are performed to detect the virus?

Exercise 13.5
Research the FDA's Guidance for Industry: Recommendations for Donor Questioning, Deferral, Reentry and Product Management to Reduce the Risk of Transfusion-Transmitted Malaria (Updated August 2014). Locate the document on the FDA's website.

1. Define the following terms:
   a. Malaria-endemic area
   b. Malaria-endemic country
   c. Residence in a malaria-endemic country
   d. Travel to a malaria-endemic area
2. What are the recommended deferral periods for blood donation for residents of a malaria-endemic country and travelers to a malaria-endemic area?

STUDY QUESTIONS

For questions 1 through 12, determine the best course of action based on the information for potential whole blood allogeneic donors. Indicate whether you would:

A = Accept
TD = Temporarily defer (indicate when donor is eligible)
PD = Permanently or indefinitely defer

1. A 28-year-old woman; 112 lb; hemoglobin, 12.5 g/dL; miscarried 2 weeks ago

2. A 56-year-old man; 168 lb; hematocrit, 44%; took aspirin 4 hours ago for arthritis pain

3. A 35-year-old woman; 115 lb; temperature, 37° C; pulse, 75

4. A 17-year-old female high-school student; taking isotretinoin (Accutane) for acne

5. A 75-year-old male donor center volunteer; first-time blood donor; contracted hepatitis 20 years ago after surgery

6. A 22-year-old male; received tattoo while in the service 4 months ago, just before he returned from Iraq

7. A 65-year-old female; has instructions from physician to donate for upcoming surgery; had syphilis and was treated 40 years ago; hematocrit, 37%; temperature, 99° F

8. A 38-year-old male; received recombinant hepatitis B vaccine as a new employee 3 months ago

9. A 19-year-old male first-time donor; received human growth hormone 12 years ago

10. A 24-year-old female with a history of a positive test for hepatitis C from another blood center

11. A 52-year-old businessman who was a resident in England for 1 year in 1993

12. A 130-lb, 5-feet-1-inch female; hematocrit, 40%; would like to donate two RBC units by apheresis

13. Which of the following is a cause for temporary deferral of a whole blood donor?
    a. intranasal influenza vaccine
    b. antibiotics taken for acne
    c. oral polio vaccine 4 weeks ago
    d. rubella vaccine 2 weeks ago

14. A donor with a physician's request to donate for planned surgery in 3 weeks has a hemoglobin value of 10 g/dL. What is her eligibility status?
    a. permitted to donate as an autologous donor
    b. deferred because of low hemoglobin
    c. permitted to donate with the approval of the blood bank's medical director
    d. permitted to donate a smaller unit of blood

15. What is the maximum number of donations for plateletpheresis donors in the period of a year?
    a. 6
    b. 12
    c. 24
    d. 48

True or False

_____ 16. Viral marker tests are not required on autologous blood intended for use within the collection facility.

_____ 17. Autologous units may be given to other patients if they are not used for the patient who donated the units.

_____ 18. A unit donated therapeutically from a person with hereditary hemochromatosis cannot be used for transfusion purposes.

_____ 19. Donor centers are authorized to release positive test results to their state health department if the donor signs a consent form.

_____ 20. According to the FDA, prospective donors with a history of cancer are not permitted to donate blood.

Answers to Study Questions can be found on page 387.

Ⓔ Additional student resources, including review questions, a laboratory manual, and case studies, can be found on the Evolve website.

REFERENCES

1. AABB Blood Donor History Questionnaire. http://www.aabb.org/tm/questionnaires/Pages/dhqaabb .aspx. Accessed October 2015.
2. Full-Length Donor History Questionnaire Documents, Version 1.3, May 2008. http://www.fda.gov/ BiologicsBloodVaccines/BloodBloodProducts/ApprovedProducts/LicenseProductsBLAs/BloodDonor Screening/ucm164185.htm. Accessed October 2015.
3. Gillespie TW, Hillyer CD: Blood donors and factors impacting the blood donation, *Trans Med Review* 16:115, 2002.
4. America's Blood Centers. http://www.americasblood.org/about-blood/facts-figures.aspx. Accessed October 2015.
5. Healthy People 2010 Progress Review: *Medical Product Safety*, U.S. Department of Health and Human Services, November 5, 2003. http://www.healthypeople.gov/2010/data/2010prog/focus17/Med _Prod_Safety.pdf. Accessed October 2015.
6. Fung MK, editor: *Technical manual*, ed 18, Bethesda, MD, 2014, AABB.
7. Levitt J: *Standards for blood banks and transfusion services*, ed 29, Bethesda, MD, 2014, AABB.
8. U.S. Food and Drug Administration: *Guidance for industry: revised preventative measures to reduce the possible risk of transmission of Creutzfeldt-Jakob disease (CJD) and variant Creutzfeldt-Jakob disease (vCJD) by blood and blood products (May 2010)*, Rockville, MD, 2010, CBER Office of Communication, Outreach and Development.
9. U.S. Food and Drug Administration: *Memorandum: clarification of FDA recommendations for donor deferral and product distribution based on the results of syphilis testing (Dec. 12, 1991)*, Rockville, MD, 1991, CBER Office of Communication, Outreach and Development.
10. U.S. Food and Drug Administration: *Memorandum: revised recommendations for the prevention of human immunodeficiency virus (HIV) transmission by blood and blood products (April 23, 1992)*, Rockville, MD, 1992, CBER Office of Communication, Training Outreach and Development.

11. U.S. Food and Drug Administration: *Draft Guidance for Industry: revised recommendations for reducing the risk of human immunodeficiency virus transmission by blood and blood products (May 2015)*, Rockville, MD, 2015, CBER.

12. U.S. Food and Drug Administration: *Guidance for industry: revised recommendations for reducing the risk of human immunodeficiency virus transmission by blood and blood products (December 2015)*, Silver Spring, MD, 2015, CBER Office of Communication, Training Outreach and Development.

13. U.S. Food and Drug Administration: *Final Rule: requirements for blood and blood components intended for transfusion or for further manufacturing use (May 2015)*, Rockville, MD, 2015, CBER.

14. U.S. Food and Drug Administration: *Code of federal regulations*, 21 CFR 640.3(1). Washington, DC, 2011, U.S. Government Printing Office (revised annually).

15. AABB Audioconference: *Requirements for Blood and Blood Components Intended for Transfusion or for Further Manufacturing Use (August 26, 2015)*, Bethesda, MD, 2015, AABB.

16. Brecher ME, editor: *Technical manual*, ed 15, Bethesda, MD, 2005, AABB.

17. U.S. Food and Drug Administration: *Code of federal regulations*, 21 CFR 640.40(d), Washington, DC, 2010, U.S. Government Printing Office (revised annually).

18. U.S. Food and Drug Administration: *Code of federal regulations*, 21 CFR Part 640, Subpart G—Source Plasma, Washington, DC, 2010, U.S. Government Printing Office (revised annually).

19. U.S. Food and Drug Administration: *Guidance for industry: recommendations for collection of red blood cells by automated apheresis methods (January 30, 2001: Technical Correction February 2001)*, Rockville, MD, 2001, CBER Office of Communication, Training Outreach and Development.

20. U.S. Food and Drug Administration: *Guidance for industry: variances for blood collection from individuals with hereditary hemochromatosis (August 22, 2001)*, Rockville, MD, 2001, CBER Office of Communication, Training Outreach and Development.

CHAPTER OUTLINE

LEARNING OBJECTIVES

On completion of this chapter, the reader should be able to:

1. List the required tests performed on allogeneic and autologous donor blood.
2. Describe the enzyme-linked immunosorbent assay (ELISA) and chemiluminescent immunoassay.
3. Differentiate among sandwich, indirect, and competitive ELISA techniques.
4. Describe the principle of nucleic acid amplification technology for testing donor blood samples.
5. Compare and contrast internal and external controls in viral marker testing.
6. Compare and contrast test sensitivity with test specificity.
7. Compare and contrast the different viral markers for hepatitis screening.
8. Describe when cytomegalovirus screening is performed.
9. State the frequency of positive tests on blood donated for allogeneic transfusion.
10. Define look-back and the Food and Drug Administration (FDA) requirements with regard to hepatitis C virus and human immunodeficiency virus testing on blood donors.
11. State the reason for performing bacterial detection tests on plateletpheresis products.
12. Define transfusion-transmitted infection and relevant transfusion-transmitted infection and the evidence required to implement changes to the donor selection and testing process.

SECTION 1
OVERVIEW OF DONOR BLOOD TESTING

The laboratory testing of donor blood follows a careful donor screening process. The interview process with the prospective donor asks questions to identify someone who may potentially be at a higher risk for exposure to infectious agents. Some of these agents, such as malaria (*Plasmodium* genus) and prions (Creutzfeldt-Jakob disease [CJD], variant Creutzfeldt-Jakob disease [vCJD]) do not have Food and Drug Administration (FDA)–approved sensitive and/or specific donor screening tests to identify exposure. Malaria and prions screening is solely dependent on donor questioning, which determines acceptability or exclusion. Other infectious agents, such as hepatitis and human immunodeficiency virus (HIV), have blood tests that can identify donors with potential exposure. With each donation, the donor's blood undergoes testing for a battery of infectious agents to ensure the safety of the blood products. This screening process is critical to the blood transfusion process, because many blood components are administered to the recipient without undergoing treatment to inactivate any infectious agent. An infectious agent in the donor's blood not detected by the screening process would directly affect the recipient.

Before the distribution of blood components, a sample of donor blood is tested using tests licensed by the FDA. All testing must be performed in accordance with the manufacturer's instructions following specimen and quality control requirements. Test results must be recorded and maintained to ensure traceability to a specific donor unit or blood component. Test results are confidential and cannot be released to anyone without the donor's written consent. At time of donation, donors sign an informed consent form granting permission to release positive infectious disease test results to appropriate public health agencies if required by state or other laws.

REQUIRED TESTING ON ALLOGENEIC AND AUTOLOGOUS DONOR BLOOD

The goal of donor testing is to improve the safety of the blood supply. Tests can be divided into two categories:
1. Serologic testing to determine ABO and D phenotype and antibody screen
2. Infectious disease screening

The scope and characteristics of the testing will be modified as new tests are licensed and new regulatory requirements are imposed on the blood bank industry. The required testing performed on allogeneic donor blood at the present time is outlined in Table 14.1.[1,2]

With an autologous donation, the intended recipient is the blood donor. Autologous donations are phenotyped for ABO and D antigens and are tested for unexpected antibodies. Blood collection facilities are not required to perform infectious disease testing on autologous blood products that are not shipped. However, many facilities perform the infectious disease testing on these donor units and attach a biohazard label if any of the infectious disease test result is positive or reactive. Scan the QR code for a good overview of current infectious disease testing performed on donated blood.

A directed donation undergoes the same testing as an allogeneic donation.

TRANSFUSION-TRANSMITTED INFECTION AND RELEVANT TRANSFUSION-TRANSMITTED INFECTION

The FDA's final rule, Requirements for Blood and Blood Components Intended for Transfusion or for Further Manufacturing Use, provided the blood industry with definitions of transfusion-transmitted infection (TTI) and relevant transfusion-transmitted infection (RTTI).[3]

TTI is defined as a disease or disease agent that has two criteria:
1. Disease or disease agent that could be fatal or life threatening and potentially cause permanent damage of a body function or body structure requiring medical or surgical intervention.
2. Disease or disease agent may pose a risk of transmission by blood or blood components or by a blood byproduct manufactured from blood or blood components.

TABLE 14.1	Required Donor Blood Tests
TESTING FOR	**TESTING PERFORMED**
RBC antigens	ABO and D phenotype
Clinically significant RBC antibodies	Antibody screen
Hepatitis	HBsAg Anti-HCV Anti-HBc HCV NAT HBV DNA
HIV-1/2	Anti-HIV-1/2 HIV-1 RNA
HTLV-I/II	Anti-HTLV-I/II
Syphilis	Nontreponemal serologic test for syphilis (eg, rapid plasma reagin) or IgG or IgG + IgM antibody to *Treponema pallidum* antigens
WNV	WNV RNA
Trypanosoma cruzi (Chagas disease)	IgG antibody to *T. cruzi* (one-time testing for donor screening)

RBC, Red blood cell; *HBsAg,* hepatitis B surface antigen; *anti-HBc,* antibody to hepatitis B core; *anti-HCV,* antibody to hepatitis C virus; *HCV,* hepatitis C virus; *HIV,* human immunodeficiency virus; *HTLV,* human T-cell lymphotropic viruses; *WNV,* West Nile virus.

Incidence: the number of new disease cases that develop in a given period of time

Prevalence: the number of cases of a disease present in a particular population at a given time

Dengue fever: a mosquitoborne viral infection; the infection causes flulike illness and occasionally develops into a potentially lethal complication called severe dengue

Babesiosis: microscopic parasites that infect red blood cells and are spread by the bite of infected *Ixodes scapularis* ticks

Sometimes a TTI will also meet the definition of an RTTI. The FDA has defined the RTTI into two groups:

Group 1 lists 10 named TTIs: HIV, hepatitis B virus (HBV), hepatitis C virus (HCV), human T-lymphotropic virus (HTLV), syphilis, West Nile virus (WNV), Chagas disease, CJD, vCJD, and *Plasmodium* species (malaria).

Group 2 rules list criteria to identify other TTIs that present future risks to safety, purity, and potency of blood and blood components. Under these criteria, a TTI will be identified as an RTTI. To become an RTTI, donor screening measures have been developed and/or a screening test has been FDA licensed, approved, or cleared for testing. In addition, the disease or disease agent's **incidence** and/or **prevalence** is capable of affecting the donor population. Once a disease or disease agent meets the criteria of an RTTI, the FDA would issue guidance to address donor screening and any donor testing requirements for blood donation. Current examples of such TTIs include **dengue fever**, Zika virus, and **babesiosis**.

SECTION 2
SEROLOGIC TESTING OF DONOR UNITS

ABO AND D PHENOTYPE

In determination of the ABO group, red cells are tested with reagent anti-A and anti-B to detect the presence of A or B antigens. Serum or plasma is tested with reagent A_1 and B cells to detect anti-A or anti-B. Test methods used for the ABO phenotype include tube, microplate, solid-phase, and gel test. The results of ABO testing are compared with previous ABO results, if available. Red cell ABO testing results (forward typing) and serum ABO testing results (reverse typing) must agree for the ABO result to be valid. Discrepancies or mismatch between red cell and serum testing or with previous ABO determinations must be resolved before labeling the donor unit.

Routine D typing for donors involves testing with reagent anti-D. If the initial D antigen typing is negative, an additional test for weak D is performed. If the initial test or the test for weak D is positive, the unit is labeled Rh-positive. When tests for both D and weak D are negative, the unit is labeled Rh-negative. Test methods used for the D phenotype include tube, microplate, solid-phase, and gel test. AABB standards mandate weak D testing on donor blood.[4]

In donor collection facilities, ABO and D phenotype testing is often performed on automated equipment using methods such as solid-phase, microplate, or gel technology because of the large volume of donor samples tested on a daily basis.

ANTIBODY SCREEN

The antibody screen detects unexpected blood group antibodies in the donor's plasma. Anti-A and anti-B are not detected by this test. The antibodies considered most important are those clinically significant antibodies produced after exposure to foreign red cell antigens after transfusion or pregnancy. The method used to perform the antibody screen should detect clinically significant antibodies. Donor samples can be tested separately or in pools. The screening cells can be separate or pooled. Standard tube, gel technology, solid-phase, and microplate techniques are used in addition to automated techniques.

If a clinically significant antibody is detected, the donor's plasma and platelet components are not used for transfusion purposes. RBC products that have not been washed, frozen, or deglycerolized contain minimal amounts of the donor's plasma. If these blood products are used for transfusion, the antibody interpretation is required on the label of the RBC component.

SECTION 3
INFECTIOUS DISEASE TESTING OF DONOR UNITS

SEROLOGIC TESTS FOR SYPHILIS

Syphilis is a venereal disease caused by the spirochete bacterium *Treponema pallidum*. Although the most common method of transmission is direct sexual contact, at least one case of transmission has occurred through transfusion.[5] The FDA mandated donor testing for syphilis in the 1950s. This test was the first infectious disease screening performed on blood donations. Serologic testing for syphilis has been performed on donor samples for more than 60 years. The routine storage of RBCs at refrigerated temperatures limits the survival of *T. pallidum*, but platelets stored at room temperature could transmit the organisms. Donated blood can be tested by various methods, including rapid plasma reagin (RPR), hemagglutination tests, and the fluorescent treponemal antibody absorption test.

Rapid Plasma Reagin Test

The RPR test is a nontreponemal screening test and is not specific for antibodies to *T. pallidum*. This test detects reagin, an antibodylike substance in the blood directed against cardiolipin, a widely distributed lipoidal antigen. Cardiolipin antibodies routinely develop in individuals who have had untreated syphilis infection; however, they may also develop after the appearance of other infections. In an RPR test, the donor's serum is placed onto a card and mixed with cardiolipin-coated charcoal particles. The particles serve as an indicator by making the antigen–antibody reaction visible. This screening method results in many false-positive reactions. False-positive test results are associated with viral infections, pregnancy, malignant neoplasms, autoimmune diseases, and advanced age.[6]

Treponemal Tests for *Treponema pallidum* Antibodies

Many donor centers have converted their syphilis screening to tests that detect antibodies to *T. pallidum* and can be performed on automated instrumentation. Treponemal tests include the microhemagglutination assay and the *T. pallidum* particle assay.[6] The microhemagglutination assay is performed in microtiter plates for the detection of IgG and IgM antibodies to *T. pallidum*. The test uses sensitized sheep erythrocytes coated with *T. pallidum*. These red cells will agglutinate with the antitreponemal antibodies. The *T. pallidum* particle assay is based on agglutination with the same treponemal antigen bound to colored gelatin particles.[6] Automation has enhanced the value of the test by significantly reducing the time and labor needed to perform the assay.

Confirmatory Testing for Syphilis

Most positive screening tests for syphilis do not indicate an active syphilis infection. Biological false-positive results are commonly observed. Hemagglutination tests are positive in previously treated individuals because of the presence of the antibodies to *T. pallidum*. If either of the syphilis screening tests is reactive, a test for the specific antibody to *T. pallidum* is performed for confirmation. Fluorescent treponemal antibody absorption is the procedure of choice. This test is used to guide the management of donors and components. The FDA has permitted the release of donor units with reactive nontreponemal screening test results and negative treponemal confirmatory test results, provided that both test results are labeled on the donor unit.[7] A positive confirmatory test result defers the donor for at least 12 months.

PRINCIPLES OF VIRAL MARKER TESTING

Infectious disease testing involves a variety of methods. This section provides a general overview of the theory for serologic testing using enzyme-linked immunosorbent assay (ELISA) technology, chemiluminescence immunoassays, and nucleic acid testing (NAT). These methods are viewed as the state of the art in viral marker testing and are widely used to detect viral antigens and antibodies.

Sensitivity and Specificity

To enhance the understanding of viral marker testing, the concepts of assay sensitivity and specificity are first presented. All assays are designed to optimize both of these variables in performance.

Sensitivity is the ability of an assay to identify samples from infected individuals as positive.

$$\text{Sensitivity percentage} = \frac{100 \times \text{Number of positive individuals detected in an infected population}}{\text{Total number of infected individuals tested}}$$

Sensitivity can also be defined as:

$$\text{True Positives (TP)} / [\text{True Positives (TP)} + \text{False Negatives (FN)}]$$

Specificity is the ability of an assay to identify samples from noninfected individuals as negative.

$$\text{Specificity percentage} = \frac{100 \times \text{Number of negative individuals detected in a healthy population}}{\text{Total number of healthy individuals tested}}$$

Specificity can also be defined as:

$$\text{True Negatives (TN)} / [\text{True Negatives (TN)} + \text{False Positives (FP)}]$$

To provide a safe blood supply, viral marker screening tests are designed to have the highest possible sensitivity and to detect all infected donors. Testing is not yet 100% sensitive, but it is close. Sensitivity and specificity are inversely proportional; samples from noninfected donors may occasionally give a false-positive reaction. Because of this limitation, reactive samples must be retested, and confirmatory or supplemental testing must follow.

SEROLOGIC TESTING

Testing Process

A donor sample is tested for all viral markers. If the screening test is nonreactive, the test result is negative, indicating no evidence of infection. If the sample is reactive upon testing, it is called initially reactive. The sample is then repeated in duplicate. If both of the repeated tests are nonreactive, the test's final interpretation of the donor's sample is nonreactive or negative. If one or both of the repeated tests is reactive, then the final interpretation of the donor's sample is repeatedly reactive. FDA requires further testing on repeatedly reactive donor samples using FDA-approved confirmatory assays (if available).[7] A blood donation with a repeatedly reactive result on a screening test is not permitted for use in allogeneic transfusion. This rule applies despite the results of any confirmatory testing. As discussed earlier, syphilis is an exception to this policy.

Enzyme Immunoassays

ELISA technology, sometimes referred to as enzyme immunoassay (EIA), is used to detect the presence of small amounts of antigen or antibody. ELISA tests use a solid object such as a plastic bead in a tray or the well of a plastic microplate, coated with either antigen or antibody (Fig. 14.1). Although each test varies, the general principles of the test are the same. The **indirect ELISA** technique detects antibodies, whereas the **sandwich ELISA** technique detects antigen. **Competitive ELISA** can be used to detect antigen or antibody. Fig. 14.2 illustrates the principle of these ELISA techniques. Table 14.2 defines terminology commonly used in ELISA testing.

> Most of the serologic screening tests used to detect the antibody or antigen when testing donor blood are enzyme immunosorbent assays or chemiluminescent immunoassays.

Indirect ELISA: enzyme-linked immunosorbent assay (ELISA) technique used to determine the presence or quantity of an antibody; also called EIA

Sandwich ELISA: enzyme-linked immunosorbent assay (ELISA) technique used to determine the presence or quantity of an antigen

Competitive ELISA: enzyme-linked immunosorbent assay (ELISA) technique used to determine the presence or quantity of an antigen or an antibody; in this test, a lower absorbance indicates detection of the marker

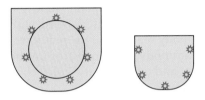

✳ = Antigen or antibody on the bead or well

Fig. 14.1 Enzyme-linked immunosorbent assay methodologies. Enzyme-linked immunosorbent assay tests are performed either in a microplate well *(right)* or in a tray containing wells with beads *(left)*. The well or the bead contains the antigen or antibody that combines with the antibody or antigen being detected (if present).

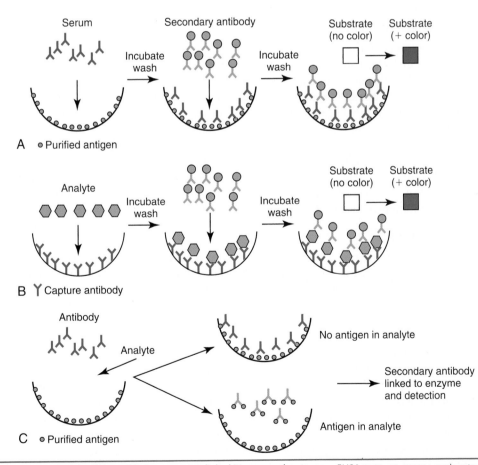

Fig. 14.2 Principle of the solid-phase enzyme-linked immunosorbent assay. ELISA tests use enzyme conjugates to detect the viral marker through a colored end product that is read spectrophotometrically. **A,** Indirect ELISA. **B,** Sandwich ELISA. **C,** Competitive ELISA. (From Roback JD, editor: *Technical manual*, ed 17, Bethesda, MD, 2011, AABB.)

TABLE 14.2	Enzyme-Linked Immunosorbent Assay Test Terms and Definitions
TERM	**DEFINITION**
Internal controls	Validation materials provided with assay kit
External controls	Reagents or materials that are not part of test kit used for surveillance of test performance
Cutoff value	Absorbance value unique to each test run that determines a positive or negative result; calculated from internal controls
Conjugate	Enzyme, usually horseradish peroxidase, labeled antibody or antigen
Substrate	Color developer, usually o-phenylenediamine

As an example of ELISA, hepatitis B surface antigen (HBsAg), a hepatitis viral marker, is detected using a bead or microplate (solid phase) coated with unlabeled antiserum against the antigen. An antibody, labeled with an enzyme, is used as an indicator of the antigen–antibody reaction. If the unknown serum contains the HBsAg, it binds to the solid-phase antibody. The indicator antibody binds to the HBsAg. A substrate is added to the test, and an enzymatic color change is measured with absorbance values.

Interpretation of the results obtained on completion of the sandwich or indirect ELISA test is summarized as follows:

• Specimens with absorbance values less than the cutoff value are considered nonreactive; further testing is not required.
• Specimens with absorbance values greater than or equal to the cutoff value are defined as initially reactive.

Chemiluminescent Immunoassays

Chemiluminescence is the emission of light from a chemical reaction. In chemiluminescence, an excited electron state is created by a chemical treatment of the luminescent compound. When the electrons move from this "excited" or more energetic state back to their more natural "relaxed" state, they release energy in the form of light.

Chemiluminescent labels can be attached to an antigen or an antibody, depending on the assay format. The light from the label is emitted in the form of a flash lasting 1 to 5 seconds. The highest intensity is used for the measurement. The detection device for analysis is a photomultiplier tube used to detect emitted light. Chemiluminescent immunoassays have the advantage of being stable, relatively nontoxic, and very sensitive. Reagent use is less than ELISA, and because the reactions are quick, turnaround time is faster. The principle of chemiluminescence is illustrated in Fig. 14.3.

Internal Controls

Viral marker testing is performed in donor testing facilities with "kits," which contain specific reagents for each assay, licensed by the FDA. Internal controls are the validation materials that accompany the licensed assay kit. These controls are used to demonstrate that the test performed as expected.

External Controls

The Clinical Laboratory Improvement Amendment (CLIA) regulations state that a positive and a negative control must be tested with each run of patient specimens. The same rule applies to donor testing. Controls provided by a test kit manufacturer are considered calibration material if they are used to calculate the cutoff value. If the negative control from the reagent kit is used to calculate the assay cutoff, a separate negative control, external to the test kit, needs to be included. External controls are not a component of the test kit. They can be purchased separately or are developed by the institution.

External control results not within the acceptable stated range may "invalidate" ELISA testing and necessitate that all samples be retested. The FDA has issued strict guidelines regarding the interpretation of reactive test results when the testing performed is invalid because of external controls.[8]

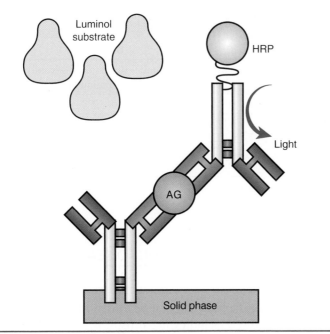
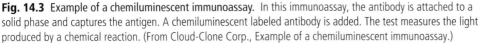

Fig. 14.3 Example of a chemiluminescent immunoassay. In this immunoassay, the antibody is attached to a solid phase and captures the antigen. A chemiluminescent labeled antibody is added. The test measures the light produced by a chemical reaction. (From Cloud-Clone Corp., Example of a chemiluminescent immunoassay.)

NUCLEIC ACID TESTING TECHNOLOGY

Nucleic acid amplification technology (NAT) for blood screening detects the presence of viral nucleic acid, DNA (deoxyribonucleic acid) or RNA (ribonucleic acid) in donation samples. The technique requires the extraction of nucleic acid from donor plasma followed by amplification to detect the viral genetic sequences. A specific RNA/DNA segment of the virus is targeted and amplified in vitro. The amplification step enables the detection of low levels of the virus in the original sample. It increases the amount of specific target to a level that is easily detectable. The presence of specific nucleic acid indicates the presence of the virus itself. The blood donation is likely to be infectious.

The advantage of NAT is the detection of very low numbers of viral copies in the bloodstream before the appearance of antibodies. The possibility of detecting the virus during the serologic window period—the period from time of infection to detection of antibody in serologic laboratory assays—is enhanced with NAT technology.[9]

These test systems were first introduced in 1999 for screening of HIV and HCV RNA.[10] Plasma samples were tested in minipools of 16 to 24 donors. The sensitivity of NAT allowed for the pooling of these donors. If a minipool NAT result was negative, all donations in that pool were considered negative for HIV and HCV RNA. A positive minipool NAT result required further separation of donor plasma samples to identify the source of the positive test. Donations nonreactive on additional testing were released for transfusion. Donations that reacted positive at the individual sample level were regarded as positive for the viral nucleic acid and could not be released for transfusion. Scan the QR code for a review of tests performed on donated blood.

Fully automated systems are now available for donor viral nucleic acid testing.[7] These systems use multiplex assay platforms that can detect HIV RNA, HCV RNA, and HBV DNA in a single reaction chamber. The FDA has approved the systems for testing individual samples (**ID-NAT**) or pools of 6 to 16 donor plasma samples (**MP-NAT**). The FDA requires permanent deferral for any donor who has a reactive result on NAT screen for HIV, HCV, or HBV using an individual (unpooled) sample.

The RNA viruses routinely tested using NAT technology are HIV, HCV, and WNV in addition to HBV, a DNA virus.[7] Polymerase chain reaction (PCR) testing and transcription-mediated amplification are two examples of testing procedures using NAT. Chapter 4 described the principle of the PCR test, and a source of information on current NAT and chemiluminescent viral marker screening for blood donors is provided in the QR code.

Because of its increased sensitivity, NAT has reduced the window period for detection of HIV to 9 days and the detection of HCV to 7.4 days.[7]

ID-NAT: individual donation (ID) screening—nucleic acid test (NAT)

MP-NAT: minipool (MP) screening—nucleic acid test (NAT)

TABLE 14.3	Hepatitis Viruses				
	A	**B**	**C**	**D**	**E**
Transmission	Enteric; oral and fecal	Parenteral; sexual; perinatal	Parenteral; sexual; perinatal	Parenteral; sexual; perinatal	Enteric; oral and fecal
Incubation (days)	15–50	60–150	14–300	30–50	21–42
Classification	Picornavirus	Hepadnavirus	Flavivirus	Satellite	Calicivirus
Nucleic acid	RNA	DNA	RNA	RNA	RNA
Donor Testing	No	Yes	Yes	No	No

RNA, Ribonucleic acid; *DNA,* deoxyribonucleic acid.

SECTION 4
TRANSFUSION-TRANSMITTED INFECTIOUS DISEASES AND DISEASE AGENTS

HEPATITIS

Hepatitis is inflammation of the liver that can be caused by bacteria, drugs, alcohol, toxins, and several different viruses, including hepatitis A, B, C, D, and E. Data from the U.S. Centers for Disease Control and Prevention (CDC) confirm that viral hepatitis B and C are the leading cause of liver cancer, with hepatitis C being the most common reason for liver transplantation. An estimated 4.4 million Americans have chronic hepatitis; most do not know they are infected.[11]

The hepatitis viruses are compared in Table 14.3. Hepatitis B and hepatitis C are transfusion-transmitted diseases and are linked to development of most posttransfusion hepatitis cases. Both viruses can establish prolonged carrier states in donors with accompanying viremia and absence of symptoms.

Hepatitis Viruses
Hepatitis A

Hepatitis A, also known as infectious hepatitis, is usually transmitted by fecal contamination and oral ingestion. The hepatitis A virus (HAV) circulates in the bloodstream only during the initial phase of infection, when an individual is usually too ill to donate; however, if blood is collected while the virus is circulating, it can be transmitted by transfusion. Because transfusion transmission is extremely rare, donated blood is not tested for hepatitis A antigen or antibody.

Hepatitis B

Originally called serum hepatitis, HBV was the first known hepatitis virus transmitted by blood transfusion. It can also be transmitted **parenterally,** by sexual contact, and **perinatally.** The rate of new HBV infections has declined by approximately 82% since 1991. The decline has been greatest among children born since 1991, when routine vaccination of children was first recommended.[11] See Fig. 14.4 for incidence of acute HBV from 1980 to 2013.

The serology and clinical patterns observed in hepatitis B infections are illustrated in Fig. 14.5. During HBV infection, the viral envelope material, the surface antigen or HBsAg, is detected in the blood before the antibody to the core antigen (anti-HBc) is produced. The FDA requires donor screening for HBsAg, anti-HBc, and HBV-DNA.

Hepatitis C

Posttransfusion hepatitis persisted after hepatitis B testing was implemented due to hepatitis C virus (HCV).[12] HCV is transmitted by the same modes as HBV. Recent data from the CDC indicate that approximately one-third of young (aged 18 to 30 years) intravenous drug users are HCV infected. Older and former intravenous drug users typically have a much higher prevalence (approximately 70% to 90%) of HCV infection, reflecting the increased risk of continued injection drug use.[11]

Parenterally: by routes other than the digestive tract, including needle stick and transfusion

Perinatally: exposure before, during, or after the time of birth

The window period for detection of HBV is estimated at 18.5 to 26.5 days with current testing using HBV DNA.[7]

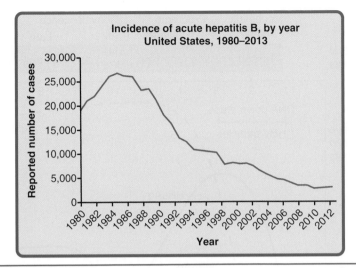

Fig. 14.4 Incidence of acute HBV by year in the United States, 1980 to 2013. (From Centers for Disease Control and Prevention: *CDC Viral Hepatitis*. http://www.cdc.gov/hepatitis.)

Hepatitis D

Although hepatitis D virus (HDV) is also transmitted by blood, the concurrent presence of HBV is necessary to cause disease. HDV is a defective virus found only in HBV carriers. Blood is not screened for HDV because testing for HBV is sufficient to avoid hepatitis D transmission.

Hepatitis E

Hepatitis E is spread in much the same way as hepatitis A, through an oral-fecal route. Therefore donated blood is not tested.

Hepatitis G

Hepatitis G virus (HGV) is a virus that might not even cause hepatitis. HGV is an RNA virus similar to, but distinct from, HCV. The transmission routes of hepatitis G are not well known other than through infected blood products. HGV was discovered in the mid-1990s. A flavivirus similar to HCV, HGV was originally found in a person with liver disease, which associated the virus with hepatitis.

Hepatitis Tests

To prevent the transmission of hepatitis by transfusion, five tests are currently performed on donor blood: HBsAg, total anti-HBc (IgM and IgG antibody), antibody to HCV (anti-HCV), and NAT to detect HCV RNA and HBV DNA.[7]

Hepatitis B Surface Antigen

Studies published in 1965 by Blumberg et al described an antigen in the blood of Australian Aborigines later named HBsAg.[13] HBV comprises intact viral particles and excess noninfectious forms of the antigen consisting of the outer surface of the virus. HBsAg is a protein on the surface of HBV. The presence of HBsAg indicates that an individual is infectious. The body normally produces antibodies to HBsAg as part of the normal immune response to infection. The period between exposure and the emergence of HBsAg is estimated at 30 to 38 days.[7] See Fig. 14.5 for the serology and clinical symptoms. Symptoms typically last several weeks but can persist for 6 months. HBsAg is the antigen used to make hepatitis B vaccine. Because of the large amount of HBsAg present, it is possible to test for the antigen directly. By the mid-1970s, donor screening for HBsAg was implemented. Enzyme and chemiluminescent immunoassays, described earlier in this chapter, are used to screen donors.

The HBsAg confirmatory assay uses the principle of specific antibody neutralization to confirm the presence of HBsAg. In the neutralization procedure, antibody to HBsAg is incubated with the donor's serum. If HBsAg is present in the serum, the antibody binds

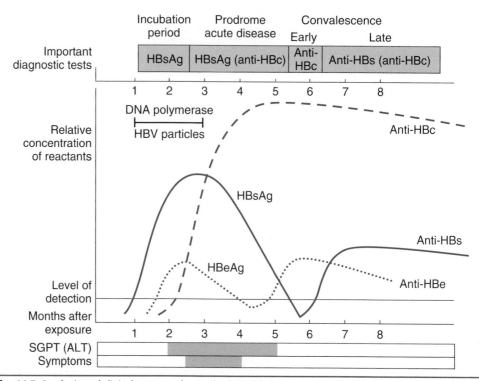

Fig. 14.5 Serologic and clinical patterns observed in hepatitis B. *HBsAg,* Hepatitis B surface antigen; *anti-HBc,* antibody to hepatitis B core; *HBV,* hepatitis B virus; *HBeAg,* hepatitis B e antigen; *anti-HBe,* antibody to hepatitis B e antigen; *ALT,* alanine aminotransferase; *SGPT,* serum glutamate pyruvate transaminase. (From Hollinger FB, Dreesman GR: In Rose RN, Friedman H, editors: *Manual of clinical immunology,* ed 2, Washington, DC, 1980, American Society for Microbiology.)

the antigen. The neutralized HBsAg is blocked from binding to the antibody-coated solid medium. If the neutralization causes the reaction to disappear or diminish by at least 50%, the original result is considered positive for HBsAg.[14]

Antibody to Hepatitis B Core

In 1986 anti-HBc and alanine aminotransferase (ALT) were added as **surrogate markers.** Anti-HBc is an antibody to the inner portion or core of the hepatitis B antigen. These antibodies generally appear after HBsAg is detected but before the manifestation of hepatitis symptoms (see Fig. 14.5). Anti-HBc can persist at detectable levels for many years after infection and has been demonstrated in individuals who have transmitted other types of hepatitis. No specific confirmatory test for anti-HBc exists. The FDA and AABB no longer require ALT testing. Anti-HBc was licensed and required by the FDA in 1991. Scan the QR code to read the CDC's information on the interpretation of hepatitis B serologic test results.

Surrogate markers: disease markers such as antibodies or elevations in enzymes that can be used as indicators for other potential infectious diseases; often used when direct testing is not available

Antibody to Hepatitis C Virus

In 1989 the existence of hepatitis C was demonstrated, and a test was developed and implemented for donor screening by 1990. Antibody to HCV (anti-HCV) is detectable by third-generation ELISAs and chemiluminescent assays approximately 10 weeks after infection.[14] After the ELISA test for anti-HCV was added to routine donor blood testing, the incidence of posttransfusion hepatitis dramatically decreased.[15]

A recombinant immunoblot assay (RIBA) was initially used as a supplemental test to determine the specificity of the antibody to HCV. However, as of 2013, RIBA is not available for a supplemental assay.[7] Positive results using NAT for HCV are approved by the FDA to confirm a reactive HCV antibody test.

Nucleic Acid Testing to Detect DNA of Hepatitis B Virus and RNA of Hepatitis C

In 1999 NAT for HCV RNA was initially implemented to screen donor blood in minipools of samples from 16 to 24 whole blood donations. The current recommended screening for DNA and RNA uses a minipool of 6 to 16 donor samples. Sensitive NAT techniques for HCV RNA even in pooled donor samples have reduced the window period for HCV detection to 7.4 days.[7] HBV DNA testing has reduced the window period for HBV detection to 18.5 to 26.5 days.

HUMAN RETROVIRUSES

Retroviruses contain reverse transcriptase, which allows the virus to copy its RNA onto DNA and to integrate this DNA into the DNA of the host cell. Three subfamilies of retroviruses exist: lentivirus (HIV types 1 and 2), oncornavirus or oncovirus (HTLV types I, II, and V), and spumavirus (no association with human disease).[16]

Fig. 14.6 illustrates the incidence of HIV infection in the United States. In 2014 the 50 states and six U.S. dependent areas estimated the rate of diagnosis of HIV infection was 16.6 per 100,000 persons for a total of 44,609 new cases. The estimated rates of diagnosis of HIV infection ranged from 0.0 per 100,000 in American Samoa, Guam, Republic of Palau, and the Northern Mariana Islands to 66.9 per 100,000 in the District of Columbia.[17]

Three tests are currently used as a screen for retroviruses in donated blood: antibody to HIV type 1 or type 2 (anti-HIV-1/2), NAT to detect HIV-1 RNA, and antibody to HTLV types I and II (anti-HTLV-I/II). The first donor screening test for HIV antibodies was implemented in 1985, followed by the anti-HTLV-I test in 1988. In 1992 the anti-HIV-1/2 test was licensed, with improved detection of early infection and an expanded range of detection to include HIV-2. This test was closely followed in 1996 by the HIV-1 p24 antigen test. This test detected HIV-1 infection six days earlier than the antibody screen and reduced the window period. New anti-HTLV-I/II antibody tests expanded the detection to include HTLV-II in addition to HTLV-I in 1997 to 1998. As stated previously, HIV-1

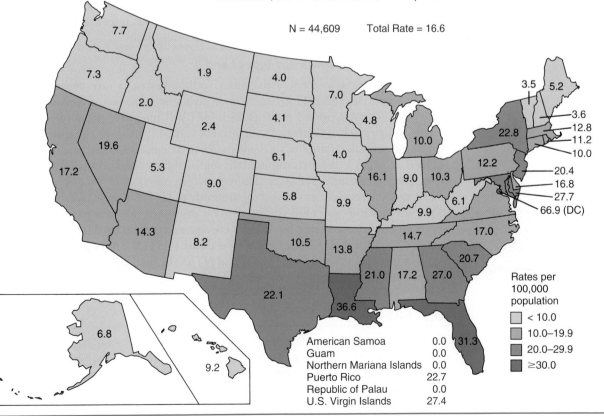

Fig. 14.6 Rates of diagnoses of HIV infection, 2014—50 states and six U.S. dependent areas. (From Centers for Disease Control and Prevention: *CDC HIV/AIDS*. www.cdc.gov/HIV.)

NAT was initially implemented in 1999 as investigational assays and received FDA licensure in 2002.[14] Screening tests for HIV are designed to possess high sensitivity to low-titer antibody and variant forms of the virus. This assay design concept is driven by the adverse outcome of missing even one truly infected individual in the donor population.

Human Immunodeficiency Virus Types 1 and 2

HIV-1 was the first virus designated as the causative agent of acquired immunodeficiency syndrome (AIDS) in 1984. The virus infects CD4-positive T lymphocytes (helper T cells). Viremia is first detectable in plasma 10 days to 3 weeks after infection.[14] Approximately 60% of acutely infected individuals develop a flulike illness during this phase. The disease enters a clinically latent stage on appearance of HIV-1 antibodies. The long incubation period before immunosuppression symptoms appear promotes the spread of the disease by sexual contact and exposure to blood products.

A second type of HIV, HIV-2, was discovered in 1985 and also causes AIDS. This form of the virus is more common in Africa than in the United States, and it appears to produce a less severe disease. Both forms of HIV are spread by sexual contact, perinatal breastfeeding, and parenteral exposure to blood.

Testing for the antibody to HIV-1 has been included in donor blood testing since 1985. In 1992, anti-HIV-2 was added to the requirements for donor testing. Most donor collection facilities use a combination test that detects anti-HIV-1 and anti-HIV-2. Because this test detects antibody, a 22- to 25-day window exists between the time a person is infected and the time the antibody is measurable.[18]

Nucleic Acid Testing for Ribonucleic Acid of Human Immunodeficiency Virus Type 1

In 1999 NAT for the RNA of HIV antigen type 1 was added to the test for anti-HIV required on all donor blood. The FDA and AABB no longer require HIV-1-antigen testing as long as licensed HIV-1 NAT is in place. With its increased sensitivity, the implementation of HIV RNA for donor testing has reduced the window period for HIV to 9 to 9.1 days for MP-NAT.[7] The HIV NAT has also reduced the number of false-positive tests with increased test specificity. A profile of HIV-1 infection with laboratory marker tests is presented in Fig. 14.7.[19] HIV RNA and the **Western blot** tests can be useful as confirmatory testing for a reactive HIV-1 antibody screening result.[7]

Western blot: test that separates and identifies viral antigens according to molecular weight using viral antibodies in an electrophoretic procedure

Human T-Lymphotropic Virus Types I and II

HTLV-I has been associated with adult T-cell leukemia, a rare neoplasm, and tropical spastic paraparesis and HTLV-I–associated myelopathy, a semiprogressive neurologic disease.[20,21] The first reported patients with HTLV-II infections showed an atypical T-cell variant of hairy cell leukemia. At the present time, HTLV-II is assumed to be associated with large granular lymphocyte leukemia[22] and leukopenic chronic T-cell leukemia.[23] HTLV-I and HTLV-II are transmitted through cellular blood products, breast milk, sexual contact, contaminated needles, and injection drug users.

In 1997, the requirement to test for antibody to HTLV-II was added to the requirement to test for antibody to HTLV-I. The two are combined into one assay. There is no FDA-approved confirmatory test for HTLV. However, the Western blot is commonly used as a supplemental test for confirmation of a positive HTLV antibody result. The screening assays detect IgG antibody to HTLV-I and HTLV-II. Scan the QR code for more information on the Western blot for HIV and HTLV confirmation.

WEST NILE VIRUS

WNV is a mosquitoborne flavivirus that manifests symptoms ranging from a mild febrile illness to encephalitis, coma, and death. WNV has been present in the United States since 1999. Before 2002 the human infection was generally believed to occur via infected mosquitoes. In 2002 transfusion transmission was identified as the cause of WNV infection in at least 21 people. The persistent low-level transmission of WNV by transfusion continued in 2003 and led to the implementation of nationwide donor screening for WNV using NAT in 2003.[7] In 2009 the FDA recommended NAT testing of individual donations rather than minipools

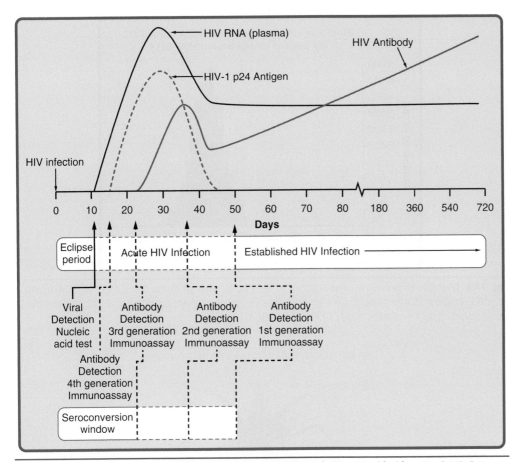

Fig. 14.7 Sequence of appearance of laboratory markers for HIV-1 infection. (Modified from Busch MP, Satten GA. Time course of viremia and antibody seroconversion following human immunodeficiency virus exposure. *Am J Med.* 1997;102(5B):117-124; with updated data from Fiebig EW, Wright DJ, Rawal BD, et al. Dynamics of HIV viremia and antibody seroconversion in plasma donors: implications for diagnosis and staging of primary HIV infection. *AIDS.* 2003;17(13):1871-1879; Owen SM, Yang C, Spira T, et al. Alternative algorithms for human immunodeficiency virus infection diagnosis using tests that are licensed in the United States. *J Clin Microbiol.* 2008;46(5):1588-1595; Masciotra S, McDougal JS, Feldman J, Sprinkle P, Wesolowski L, Owen SM. Evaluation of an alternative HIV diagnostic algorithm using specimens from seroconversion panels and persons with established HIV infections. *J Clin Virol.* 2011;52(Suppl 1):S17-22; and Masciotra S, Luo W, Youngpairoj AS, et al. Performance of the Alere Determine HIV-1/2 Ag/Ab Combo Rapid Test with specimens from HIV-1 seroconverters from the US and HIV-2 infected individuals from Ivory Coast. *J Clin Virol.* 2013;58(Suppl 1):e54-58.)

at times of increased geographic WNV activity. WNV ID-NAT prevents diluting the donor samples, which already contain a low concentration of the viral RNA load during that period. Data from the CDC describe the disease cases reported by week of illness onset from 1999 to 2014 (Fig. 14.8). As seen in this figure, outbreaks occur during the summer months.[24] In 2012 WNV transmission season was the most severe since 2003. In this outbreak, a total of 5674 human cases of WNV, including 286 deaths, were reported to the CDC. Of the total reported cases, 51% were neuroinvasive disease cases, including meningitis, encephalitis, or acute flaccid paralysis. According to AABB's WNV Biovigilance Network, 752 WNV-reactive donations were identified in 2012. Due to the unpredictable nature of annual outbreaks and the potential for cases of breakthrough transfusion transmissions, the AABB has suggested refinements of the criteria for transitioning from minipool to individual NAT testing.[25] Routine donor blood screening for WNV continues to improve blood safety.

CHAGAS DISEASE

Chagas disease, or American trypanosomiasis, is a disease endemic in Central and South America caused by the protozoan parasite *Trypanosoma cruzi*. Infection usually results after contact with feces of infected reduviid bugs. Transmission is also possible by transfusion.

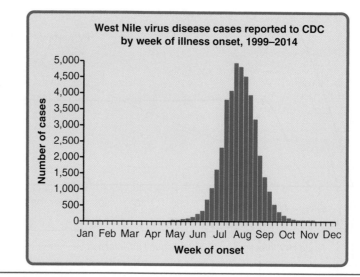

Fig. 14.8 West Nile virus disease cases reported to the CDC by week of illness onset, 1999 to 2014. (From ArboNET, Arboviral Diseases Branch, Centers for Disease Control and Prevention. http://www.cdc.gov/westnile/resources/pdfs/data/4-wnv-week-onset_1999-2014_06042015.pdf.)

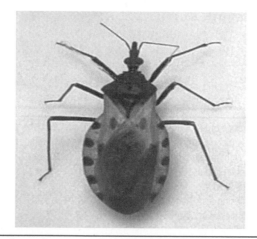

Fig. 14.9 Insect vector for Chagas disease. A reduviid bug, which, if infected, can transmit *T. cruzi*. (From Trivedi M, Sanghavi D: Knowledge deficits regarding Chagas disease may place Mexico's blood supply at risk, *Transfus Apher Sci 43(2):193-196*, 2010.)

Infected individuals can experience severe heart or intestinal problems, which usually occur many years after the initial infection (Fig. 14.9). The CDC estimates that more than 300,000 persons with *T. cruzi* infection live in the United States. These infected individuals acquired Chagas disease in endemic countries and not while residing in the United States.[26]

Because cases of transfusion-transmitted Chagas disease have been reported in the United States, some blood collection facilities with many immigrants from endemic areas perform an ELISA or chemiluminescent assay test to detect the antibodies to *T. cruzi*. The test is approved for screening donors of whole blood, plasma, and serum samples for cell, organ, and tissue donors (heart beating).[27] In response to the availability of a licensed test, multiple large blood-collecting facilities implemented testing in 2007. The rarity of donor seroconversion in the United States prompted one-time testing of blood donors. In 2010 the FDA issued guidance that recommended screening a U.S. blood donor once for *T. cruzi* infection.[7]

Malaria, Chagas disease, and WNV are referred to as infections transmitted by insect vectors.

Look-back: identification of persons who have received seronegative or untested blood from a donor subsequently found to be positive for disease markers

RECIPIENT TRACING (LOOK-BACK)

Look-back constitutes of a series of actions taken by a blood establishment when donor test results indicate infection with hepatitis, HIV, HTLV, WNV, or Chagas disease. These steps are performed on prior donations from that donor. These prior blood products were possibly donated during the window period of infection when screening tests were negative but infectious agent was present in the donor's blood. Immediate retrieval and quarantine of prior existing products from that donor shall occur within three calendar days of reactive HIV or HCV test results and within one week of reactive HBsAg, anti-HBc, or anti-HTLV screening tests.[7]

Look-back activities within the blood collection facility may include the following actions:

- Quarantine of prior collections from that donor that remain in inventory
- Notification of facilities (eg, hospitals, clinics) that received these products to quarantine prior collections
- Further testing of the donor, if not deceased
- Destruction or relabeling of potentially infectious prior collections
  Responsibilities of the transfusion service in the look-back process are as follows:
- Process to identify recipients, if appropriate, of blood or components from donors subsequently found to have, or be at risk for, relevant TTIs
- Notification, if appropriate, of the recipient's physician or recipient as specified in FDA regulations and recommendations[4]

ADDITIONAL TESTS PERFORMED ON DONOR BLOOD

Cytomegalovirus

Cytomegalovirus (CMV) is a widespread infection that can be transmitted through transfusion. Transmission occurs through the transfusion of intact white cells contained in cellular blood components. In most individuals, CMV infection is asymptomatic, but mononucleosislike symptoms are occasionally reported. For immunosuppressed patients, including premature infants, exposure to CMV may cause motor disabilities, mental retardation, and even death. In addition, CMV-seronegative recipients of organ or hematopoietic cell transplants are at increased risk of transfusion-transmitted CMV infection.[7]

Tests to detect antibody to CMV are not required for blood donors and are usually performed only on a portion of the blood collected. Units that test negative for CMV are set aside for intrauterine transfusion or blood replacement for premature infants and immunocompromised adults. CMV testing for antibodies can be performed by ELISA, latex agglutination, or hemagglutination.

CMV-reduced-risk blood products can also be achieved by leukocyte reduction because the virus resides within intact white cells. The estimated transmission of CMV by antibody negative is 1% to 2% compared with a 2% to 3% risk with leukocyte reduction.[7]

Testing for Bacterial Contamination of Blood Components

In March 2004 the AABB added a new testing requirement for bacterial contamination in apheresis platelets and platelet concentrates. This requirement was implemented because bacterial contamination is an important cause of transfusion morbidity and mortality. This testing is performed on the blood products rather than on the donor blood samples. Despite careful attention to phlebotomy techniques, blood processing, and storage requirements, it is impossible to eliminate the possible contamination with microbial organisms. Bacteria originating from the donor during phlebotomy or an unsuspected bacteremia can multiply more readily in blood components stored at room temperature.

Platelet components are stored at 20° C to 24° C to maintain their viability and function. These products provide an excellent environment for the growth of any bacteria. Normal skin flora account for the most common source of contamination isolated from platelet components. Severe transfusion reactions from bacterial contamination include fever, shock, and disseminated intravascular coagulation. Bacteria proliferate to a lesser extent in refrigerated RBCs.

Blood collection facilities have implemented measures for the reduction of bacteria in blood components at the time of collection. Careful attention in the preparation of the donor's arm before blood collection serves as an important check in the prevention of contamination. Another prevention measure diverts the first few milliliters of donor blood after phlebotomy into a pouch attached to the donor collection bag.

AABB standards require a check for bacteria detection in platelet components by FDA-approved methods.[4] The methods are culture based and require storage of platelet components for 24 hours before sampling. If negative culture results are obtained at 12 hours and 24 hours, the component is released for transfusion. If cultures become positive after 24 hours, the blood center should recall the unit. Positive cultures should be processed for identification of the organism. Donors should be notified if positive results are unrelated to skin contaminants.

EMERGING INFECTIOUS DISEASE AGENTS

Information on emerging infectious disease agents with potential concerns for the safety of blood products can be found on the AABB website at: http://www.aabb.org/tm/eid/Pages/eidpostpub.aspx. Fact sheets on each agent are presented with expert analyses of emerging infectious disease agents.

CHAPTER SUMMARY

Testing performed on blood samples from volunteer donors has increased from 1 infectious disease test to 11 tests within the last 20 years. These tests are also more specific and sensitive in detecting hepatitis, HIV, HTLV, WNV, and Chagas disease that could potentially be spread by transfusion. However, the safety of the blood supply continues to be a serious concern, and new testing methods and disease markers may be added in the future. The incorporation of NAT for HIV, HCV, WNV, and HBV detection has increased the ability to detect recently infected donors and decreased the window period. The following table summarizes the donor disease marker testing requirements currently mandated by regulatory agencies.

DONOR DISEASE MARKER TESTING

Disease	Marker Detected	Method
Hepatitis B	HBsAg IgG and IgM Anti-HBc HBV DNA	ChLIA or EIA ChLIA or EIA NAT
Hepatitis C	IgG Anti-HCV HCV RNA	ChLIA or EIA NAT
HIV	IgG and IgM Anti–HIV-1/2 HIV RNA	ChLIA or EIA NAT
HTLV	IgG Anti–HTLV-I/II	ChLIA or EIA
Syphilis	Nontreponemal test or IgG/IgM Anti-*T. pallidum*	Microhemagglutination or EIA
West Nile	WNV RNA	NAT
Chagas	IgG antibody to *T. cruzi*	ChLIA or EIA

HBsAg, Hepatitis B surface antigen; *Anti-HCV*, antibody to hepatitis C virus; *Anti-HBc*, antibody to hepatitis B core; *HIV*, human immunodeficiency virus; *HTLV*, human T-cell lymphotropic virus; *RPR*, rapid plasma reagin; *NAT*, nucleic acid amplification technology; *WNV*, West Nile virus; *ChLIA*, chemiluminescent assay; *EIA*, enzyme immunoassay.

CRITICAL THINKING EXERCISES

Exercise 14.1
A test for the HIV-1/2 antibody contains an external control that did not fall into the range required. What is the correct procedure for this problem? Why are external controls tested?

Exercise 14.2

A donor's sample tests positive with the hemagglutination test for syphilis. The confirmatory test is negative, and the donor's history indicates no high-risk behavior. The donor is 68 years old and donating an autologous unit for surgery. Can this autologous unit be used?

Exercise 14.3

On completion of hepatitis testing using the ELISA procedure, an acid is added to stop the color development of the conjugate substrate. On this particular day, a power failure results in equipment downtime, causing a delay. The acid is not added until 10 minutes past the allowable time. How might a delay in the addition of the acid affect the test results?

Exercise 14.4

A donor is identified with an anti-Fy^a in her serum. Can this donor's plasma be used for transfusion, or should it be discarded?

Exercise 14.5

Previous testing on a donor's computer record indicates CMV–antibody negative. The most recent donation demonstrates that antibodies are currently present.
1. Can the donor still donate?
2. Why has the CMV antibody test result changed?
3. What patients require the transfusion of CMV-reduced-risk blood products?
4. What alternatives exist in the provision of CMV antibody–negative blood?

STUDY QUESTIONS

1. Which disease has the highest potential for transmission through a transfusion?
   a. AIDS
   b. syphilis
   c. CMV
   d. hepatitis

2. Syphilis tests on donors are usually performed by which method or methods?
   a. RPR
   b. Venereal Disease Research Laboratory
   c. hemagglutination
   d. both a and c

3. What characteristic is associated with HTLV-I/II?
   a. an oncornavirus
   b. found in patients with tropical spastic paraparesis
   c. associated with adult T-cell leukemia
   d. all of the above

4. What marker demonstrates a previous exposure to hepatitis B that remains in convalescence?
   a. anti-HCV
   b. anti-HBc
   c. anti-HAV
   d. HBsAg

5. Which of the following is the confirmatory test for a positive anti-HIV screen?
   a. HIV RNA
   b. RIBA
   c. PCR
   d. Southern blot

6. Which of the following conditions requires a thorough donor history because it is not a routinely tested disease?
   a. syphilis
   b. Creutzfeldt-Jakob disease
   c. hepatitis C
   d. HTLV-I

7. Why is HAV transmission through a blood transfusion unusual?
   a. transmitted enterically
   b. an acute hepatitis
   c. not infective after 2 weeks
   d. all of the above

8. What is the donation status of a donor who is positive for HBsAg?
   a. temporarily deferred
   b. permanently deferred
   c. deferred if the antibody to HBc is also present
   d. deferred if ALT is elevated

9. Which of the following was a surrogate test for hepatitis and is no longer required?
   a. ALT
   b. CMV
   c. anti-HBc
   d. HBsAg

10. In a _____, a lower absorbance value indicates the detection of the viral marker.
    a. RIBA
    b. sandwich ELISA
    c. competitive ELISA
    d. Western blot

Answers to Study Questions can be found on page 387.

(e) Additional student resources, including review questions, a laboratory manual, and case studies, can be found on the Evolve website.

REFERENCES

1. AABB/America's Blood Centers/American Red Cross: *Circular of information for the use of human blood and blood components* (Nov 2013).
2. Food and Drug Administration: *Memorandum: West Nile Virus final guidance*, Rockville, MD, June 23, 2005, FDA.
3. U.S. Food and Drug Administration: *Final Rule: requirements for blood and blood components intended for transfusion or for further manufacturing use (May 2015)*, Rockville, MD, 2015, CBER.
4. Levitt J: *Standards for blood banks and transfusion services*, ed 29, Bethesda, MD, 2014, AABB.
5. Chambers RW, Foley HT, Schmidt PJ: Transmission of syphilis by fresh blood components, *Transfusion* 9:32, 1969.
6. Sena A, White BL, Sparling PF: Novel *Treponema pallidum* serologic tests: a paradigm shift in syphilis screening for the 21st century, *Clin Infect Dis* 51:700–708, 2010.
7. Fung MK, editor: *Technical manual*, ed 18, Bethesda, MD, 2014, AABB.
8. Food and Drug Administration: *Memorandum: Recommendations for the invalidation of test results when using licensed viral marker assays to screen donors*, Rockville, MD, January 3, 1994, Congressional and Consumer Affairs.
9. World Health Organization: *Screening donated blood for transfusion-transmissible infections*, WHO Department of Essential Health Technologies, WHO, 2010.
10. AABB: *Association bulletin No. 99-3: NAT implementation*, Bethesda, MD, February 8, 1999, AABB.
11. Centers for Disease Control and Prevention: CDC viral hepatitis. http://www.cdc.gov/hepatitis. Accessed November 2015.
12. Smith DM, Dodd RY, editors: *Transfusion transmitted infections*, Chicago, 1991, American Association of Clinical Pathologists.
13. Blumberg BS, Alter HJ, Visnich S: A "new" antigen in leukemia sera, *JAMA* 191:541, 1965.

14. Roback JD, editor: *Technical manual*, ed 17, Bethesda, MD, 2011, AABB.
15. Busch MP: Let's look at human immunodeficiency virus look-back before leaping into hepatitis C virus look-back, *Transfusion* 31:655, 1991.
16. Murray PR, Kobayashi GS, Pfaller MA, et al.: *Medical microbiology*, ed 3, St. Louis, 1997, Mosby.
17. Centers for Disease Control and Prevention: *CDC HIV/AIDS*. www.cdc.gov/HIV. Accessed November 2015.
18. Busch MP, Lee LL, Satten GA, et al.: Time course of detection of viral and serologic markers preceding human immunodeficiency virus type 1 seroconversion: implications for screening of blood and tissue donors, *Transfusion* 35:91, 1995.
19. Branson BM, et al.: *Laboratory testing for the diagnosis of HIV infection: Updated recommendations*, Centers for Disease Control and Prevention, June 27, 2014. http://stacks.cdc.gov/view/cdc/23447. Accessed November 2015.
20. McFarlin DE, Blattner WA: Non-AIDS retroviral infections in humans, *Annu Rev Med* 42:97, 1991.
21. Janssen RS, Kaplan JE, Khabbaz RF, et al.: HTLV-I-associated myelopathy/tropical spastic paraparesis in the United States, *Neurology* 41:1355, 1991.
22. Loughran TP Jr, Coyle T, Sherman MP, et al.: Detection of human T-cell leukemia/lymphoma virus, type II, in a patient with large granular lymphocyte leukemia, *Blood* 80:1116, 1992.
23. Sohn CC, Blayney DW, Misset JL, et al.: Leukopenic chronic T cell leukemia mimicking hairy cell leukemia: association with human retroviruses, *Blood* 67:949, 1986.
24. Centers for Disease Control and Prevention: *CDC West Nile Virus*. http://www.cdc.gov/westnile/statsmaps/cummapsdata.html. Accessed November 2015.
25. AABB: *Association Bulletin No. 13-02: West Nile virus nucleic acid testing – revised recommendations*, Bethesda, MD, June 28, 2013, AABB.
26. Centers for Disease Control and Prevention: *CDC Chagas disease*. http://www.cdc.gov/parasites/chagas/epi.html. Accessed November 2015.
27. AABB: *Association bulletin No. 06-08: Information concerning the implementation of a licensed test for antibodies to Trypanosoma cruzi*, Bethesda, MD, December 14, 2006, AABB.

15

BLOOD COMPONENT PREPARATION AND THERAPY

CHAPTER OUTLINE

LEARNING OBJECTIVES

On completion of this chapter, the reader should be able to:

1. Explain the benefits of component separation.
2. Define storage lesion, and list the elements that change during blood storage.
3. Compare anticoagulant and preservative solutions with regard to expiration and content.
4. Illustrate the steps in blood component preparation.
5. Given certain clinical conditions, state the blood component most appropriate for the patient's transfusion needs.
6. State the storage temperature and storage limits for each blood component.
7. Given laboratory quality control test measurements, determine which component products meet acceptable AABB standards and Food and Drug Administration (FDA) guidelines.

8. Explain the intent and activities of the FDA in regulating blood component preparation, storage, and distribution.
9. List the International Society of Blood Transfusion (ISBT 128) labeling requirements common to all blood components.
10. Discuss the importance of monitored storage equipment for blood components and the alarm requirements.
11. Describe essential aspects of safe blood administration.

The separation of **whole blood** into its parts, or **components,** allows for optimal storage of each part and the ability to provide appropriate therapy for patients. Each unit of whole blood can be separated into several components that can be transfused into patients, depending on their medical requirements. The separation of blood into components maximizes a limited resource and allows for a method of transfusing patients who require a large amount of a specific blood component. The availability of blood components permits patients to receive specific **hemotherapy** that is more effective and usually safer than the use of whole blood.

The primary goal of facilities that prepare components is to provide a product of optimal benefit to the recipient. All staff involved in the collection, testing, separation, labeling, storage, and distribution of blood and blood components must have an understanding of and adherence to Food and Drug Administration (FDA) **current Good Manufacturing Practices** (cGMPs). Regulations regarding cGMPs and blood product manufacture can be found in the FDA *Code of Federal Regulations*[1,2] and are written to optimize the "safety, purity, potency, quality, and identity" of blood products.

This chapter describes the preparation, labeling, and storage of blood components. A summary of the clinical indications for each component and general administration policies are also reviewed. Transfusion therapy specific for certain diseases and treatments are described in more detail in the next chapter. The component names presented in this chapter reflect the International Society of Blood Transfusion (ISBT 128) terminology[3] and are used in the 29th edition of the AABB *Standards for Blood Banks and Transfusion Services.* A detailed and updated description of product codes and terminology can be found on the International Council on Commonality in Blood Banking Automation website. Labeling requirements for blood products are described in more detail later in this chapter.

SECTION 1
BLOOD COLLECTION AND STORAGE

Blood is collected in a primary bag that contains an anticoagulant–preservative mixture. The entire blood collection set, including integrally attached satellite bags and tubing, is sterile and considered a **closed system.** Collecting blood in a closed system and using the integral satellite bags permit the maximal allowable storage time for all components. The sterile system becomes an **open system** when administration ports or other areas are exposed to air, and the allowable storage time is reduced because of potential bacterial contamination. Fig. 15.1 shows blood collection sets with integral satellite bags.

Anticoagulant–preservative solutions work together to prevent clotting and extend the storage of red cells. The volume of this solution in the primary collection bag is either 63 mL or 70 mL. The standard whole blood collection volume is 450 ± 45 mL or ±10% for blood collected in a bag containing 63 mL of anticoagulant or 500 ± 50 mL or ±10% for the larger volume bag containing 70 mL of anticoagulant–preservative solution. If collection is planned for less than 300 mL, the volume of anticoagulant–preservative solution should be reduced proportionately to ensure the correct anticoagulant–to–whole blood

Whole blood: blood collected from a donor before separation into its components

Components: parts of whole blood that can be separated by centrifugation; consist of red blood cells, plasma, cryoprecipitated antihemophilic factor (AHF), and platelets

Hemotherapy: treatment of a disease or condition by the use of blood or blood derivatives

Current Good Manufacturing Practices (cGMPs): methods used in, and the facilities or controls used for, the manufacture, processing, packing, or holding of a drug (including a blood product) to ensure that it meets safety, purity, and potency standards

Closed system: collection of blood in a sterile blood container

Open system: collection or exposure to air through an open port that would shorten the expiration because of potential bacterial contamination

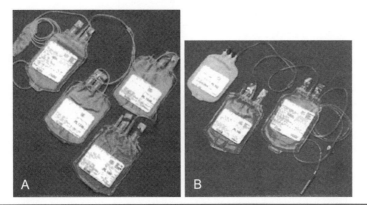

Fig. 15.1 Blood collection bags. **A,** Quad-bag system. **B,** Triple-bag system.

A unit labeled "Red Blood Cells Low Volume" is defined as RBCs prepared from:
- 300 to 404 mL of whole blood collected into an anticoagulant volume calculated for 450 ± 45 mL
- 333 to 449 mL of whole blood collected into an anticoagulant volume calculated for 500 ± 50 mL[4]

ratio. Reducing the anticoagulant may be necessary if a unit of blood is collected from an individual weighing less than 110 lb. Fig. 15.2 shows this calculation for the proportion of anticoagulant reduction, as well as the collection blood volume.

If the whole blood collection does not meet the volume requirements of the collection bag and the anticoagulant has not been adjusted, the RBCs prepared from the unit are labeled "Red Blood Cells Low Volume." Other components such as platelets, fresh frozen plasma (FFP), and cryoprecipitated AHF from low-volume units should be discarded.[4,5]

STORAGE LESION

Biochemical and morphologic (cell membrane shape) changes occur when blood is stored at 1° C to 6° C, which affects red cell viability and function. These changes are called the storage lesion. The biochemical changes that occur during storage of red cells are summarized in Fig. 15.3.

The purposes of the preservative solutions are to minimize the effects of the biochemical changes and to maximize the shelf life of the components. The storage limits and temperature criteria for each preservative solution are established by the FDA and are based on the blood container manufacturers' data to support that at least 75% of the original

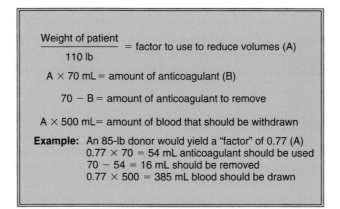

$$\frac{\text{Weight of patient}}{110 \text{ lb}} = \text{factor to use to reduce volumes (A)}$$

$$A \times 70 \text{ mL} = \text{amount of anticoagulant (B)}$$

$$70 - B = \text{amount of anticoagulant to remove}$$

$$A \times 500 \text{ mL} = \text{amount of blood that should be withdrawn}$$

Example: An 85-lb donor would yield a "factor" of 0.77 (A)
$0.77 \times 70 = 54$ mL anticoagulant should be used
$70 - 54 = 16$ mL should be removed
$0.77 \times 500 = 385$ mL blood should be drawn

Fig. 15.2 Calculation for adjusting anticoagulant and blood volume drawn. Donors who are below the acceptable weight limit can donate if the amount of blood and anticoagulant is adjusted.

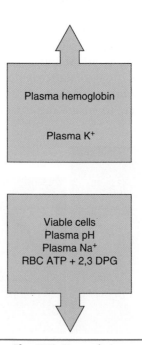

Plasma hemoglobin

Plasma K+

Viable cells
Plasma pH
Plasma Na+
RBC ATP + 2,3 DPG

Fig. 15.3 Storage lesion.

red cells remain in the recipient's circulation 24 hours after transfusion with less than 1% hemolysis.[5] Table 15.1 summarizes the function of the chemical elements in the preservative solutions.

Red cell glucose, adenosine triphosphate (ATP), and plasma pH decrease as red cells are stored. Storage also affects the level of red cell 2,3-diphosphoglycerate (2,3-DPG), which is important in the release of oxygen from hemoglobin. High levels of 2,3-DPG cause greater oxygen release, whereas lower levels increase the affinity of hemoglobin for oxygen. In red cells stored in citrate-phosphate-dextrose-adenine (CPDA-1) or additive solutions such as Adsol, 2,3-DPG levels decrease significantly. Following transfusion, stored cells regenerate ATP and 2,3-DPG to normal levels after about 12 to 24 hours.[5] Although the storage lesions seem significant, neonates may be the only group of patients requiring "fresh" RBC products.[6] RBC units for intrauterine transfusion and exchange transfusions are often fewer than 7 days old to maximize 2,3-DPG levels and to avoid high potassium and low pH levels.

> 2,3-DPG (2,3-disphos-phoglycerate) is also known as 2,3-BPG (2,3 bisphosphoglycerate).

ANTICOAGULANT–PRESERVATIVE SOLUTIONS

Anticoagulant–preservative solutions in the primary collection bag may be citrate-phosphate-dextrose (CPD), citrate-phosphate-2-dextrose (CP2D), or CPDA-1. Blood collected in CPD and CP2D is approved for storage for 21 days at 1° C to 6° C, whereas blood collected in CPDA-1 can be stored for 35 days at 1° C to 6° C. RBCs prepared from blood collected in CPDA-1 must have a hematocrit less than 80% to ensure sufficient plasma remains for red cell metabolism.[4] See Table 15.1 for chemical content and expiration limits of preservative solutions.

> ACD-A (anticoagulant citrate-dextrose A) is used in apheresis procedures with a shelf life of 21 days.

RED CELL ADDITIVE SOLUTIONS

Additive solutions (AS-1, AS-3, AS-5, or AS-7) are provided as an integral part of the collection bag system. After the whole blood is collected in CPD or CP2D and the plasma is separated from the RBCs, the additive solution bag is allowed to flow into the RBCs to enhance red cell survival and function. More plasma can be removed from the RBC units because the additive solution is added to maintain red cell metabolism during storage. The amount of additive solution is either 100 mL for a 450-mL whole blood collection or

TABLE 15.1	Anticoagulant-Preservative Composition: Purpose and Storage Limits
CHEMICAL	**PURPOSE**
Dextrose	Supports ATP generation by glycolytic pathway
Adenine	Acts as substrate for red cell ATP synthesis
Citrate	Prevents coagulation by chelating calcium, also protects red cell membrane
Sodium biphosphate	Prevents excessive decrease in pH
Mannitol	Osmotic diuretic acts as membrane stabilizer
RED CELL ANTICOAGULANT/PRESERVATIVE	**STORAGE LIMIT (DAYS)**
CPD/citrate-phosphate-dextrose	21
CP2D/citrate-phosphate-2-dextrose	21
CPDA-1/citrate-phosphate-dextrose-adenine	35
AS-1 (Adsol); AS-5 (Nutricel)/dextrose, adenine, mannitol, saline	42
AS-3 (Optisol)/dextrose, adenine, saline, citrate	42
AS-7 (SLOX)/dextrose, adenine, mannitol, saline, citrate, sodium bicarbonate	42

ATP, Adenosine triphosphate.

110 mL for a 500-mL collection. AS-1, AS-5, and AS-7 solutions contain mannitol along with saline, adenine, and dextrose. AS-3 contains additional sodium citrate and does not contain mannitol. AS-7 contains sodium bicarbonate in its formulation. These preservatives are designed to minimize hemolysis during storage to less than 1%.[5] The 100-mL additive solution must be added within 72 hours of the whole blood collection. In addition to extending the storage to 42 days from collection, the additive solution reduces the unit's red cell viscosity and improves the flow rate during administration because the hematocrit values of these units range from 55% to 65%.[5] Table 15.2 summarizes the storage limits, expiration limits, and quality control requirements for components.

TABLE 15.2	Storage Temperature, Expiration Limits, and Quality Control Requirements of Selected Blood Components		
COMPONENT	**STORAGE TEMPERATURE**	**EXPIRATION LIMITS**	**QUALITY CONTROL: MINIMUM REQUIREMENTS[4]**
Whole Blood	Storage: 1–6° C; Shipping: 1–10° C	CPD, CP2D: 21 days CPDA-1: 35 days	
RBCs	Storage: 1–6° C; Shipping: 1–10° C	CPD, CP2D: 21 days CPDA-1: 35 days AS-1, AS-3, AS-5, AS-7: 42 days	Hematocrit: ≤80% in CPDA-1 units
Frozen RBCs	≤–65° C	CPD, CPDA-1: 10 yr	None
RBCs, Deglycerolized or Washed (open system)	1–6° C	24 hr	Visual hemoglobin check; Method known to provide a ≥80% RBC recovery
Irradiated RBCs	1–6° C	28 days from irradiation or original outdate, whichever is first	Irradiator QC applied 2500 cGy/rad in center of unit
RBCs Leukocytes Reduced	1–6° C	Depends on anti-coagulant/ preservative	<5.0 × 10^6 residual leukocytes and 85% of original red cells retained
Plasma, Frozen Within 24 Hours After Phlebotomy (PF24)	≤–18° C	1 yr	None
Fresh Frozen Plasma	≤–18° C ≤–65° C	1 yr 7 yr	None
FFP, PF24, thawed	1–6° C	24 hr	None
Thawed Plasma	1-6° C	5 days from thawing	Not FDA-licensed product
Cryoprecipitated AHF	≤–18° C	1 yr	Factor VIII: ≥80 IU and ≥150 mg fibrinogen
Pooled Cryoprecipitated AHF (after thawing)	20–24° C	4 hr	Factor VIII: ≥80 IU and ≥150 mg fibrinogen times number in pool
Platelets	20–24° C with continuous agitation	5 days	≥5.5 × 10^10 platelets in 90% of units tested; pH ≥6.2
Pooled Platelets (open system)	20–24° C with continuous agitation	4 hr	None

TABLE 15.2 Storage Temperature, Expiration Limits, and Quality Control Requirements of Selected Blood Components—cont'd

COMPONENT	STORAGE TEMPERATURE	EXPIRATION LIMITS	QUALITY CONTROL: MINIMUM REQUIREMENTS[4]
Apheresis Platelets Leukocytes Reduced	20–24° C with continuous agitation	Open system: within 4 hr Closed system: 5 days	$<5.0 \times 10^6$ residual leukocytes in 95% of units; $\geq3.0 \times 10^{11}$ platelets in 90% of units tested; pH ≥6.2
Apheresis Granulocytes	20–24° C	24 hr	$\geq1.0 \times 10^{10}$ granulocytes in 75% of units tested

CPD, Citrate-phosphate-dextrose; *CP2D*, citrate-phosphate-2-dextrose; *CPDA-1*, citrate-phosphate-dextrose-adenine; *RBCs*, red blood cells; *AS*, additive solution; *FFP*, fresh frozen plasma; *CRYO*, cryoprecipitated antihemophilic factor; *PF24*, plasma frozen within 24 hours of phlebotomy; *QC*, quality control.
Source: Fung MK, editor: *Technical manual*, ed 18, Bethesda, MD, 2014, AABB.

PLATELET ADDITIVE SOLUTIONS

Platelet additive solution (PAS) is a buffered salt solution that replaces a portion of the plasma used to store platelets. PAS products have recently been approved for use in the United States.

PAS platelets are leukocyte-reduced apheresis platelets that are stored in a mix of 65% PAS and 35% plasma. The platelets can be stored up to 5 days at 20° C to 24° C with continuous agitation.[6,7]

PASs were developed to increase platelet viability during storage, minimize the amount of plasma in platelet products, and make more plasma available for other needs. Research suggests that PAS may reduce allergic transfusion reactions and enhance plasma recovery. Additionally, platelets stored in PAS appear to have equivalent value with the clinical outcome of bleeding compared with platelets stored in plasma. Scan the QR code to view a video on PASs.

REJUVENATION SOLUTION

Although the procedure is not routine, it may be necessary to restore 2,3-DPG and ATP levels in RBC units collected in CPD or CPDA-1 during storage or up to 3 days after expiration with a solution containing pyruvate, inosine, phosphate, and adenine. The rejuvenation solution extends the expiration date for freezing or transfusing the RBC unit, which may be necessary when a rare or autologous unit is involved. Rejuvenated RBCs require washing to remove the inosine before transfusion because it may be toxic to the recipient.[8]

PATHOGEN REDUCTION TECHNOLOGY

Recent innovations for the reduction of pathogens in blood components have been introduced for the treatment of plasma or for cellular blood components. Pathogen reduction is a postcollection manufacturing process. The process goal is to reduce the risk of certain transfusion-transmitted infections (TTIs) in components. Pathogen reduction technology uses ultraviolet (UV) irradiation and photosensitizers, which create damage to pathogen nucleic acids and prevents their replication and growth. The process reduces the infectivity of any residual pathogens in the blood components.[9]

Psoralen treatment is a specific pathogen reduction technology used to prepare pathogen-reduced, whole blood–derived pooled plasma; apheresis plasma; or apheresis platelets. Psoralen and UV light treatment inactivates a broad spectrum of viruses, as well as gram-positive and gram-negative bacteria, spirochetes, and parasites.[5]

SECTION 2
BLOOD COMPONENT PREPARATION

The facility's inventory requirements and the drawing location usually determine the number of satellite bags, or the "bag configuration," used for collecting blood from donors. The primary bag can have as many as four additional bags attached. Storage temperature and time constraints after collection also affect which components are to be prepared. For example, if platelets are to be prepared from a whole blood donation, the unit must not be allowed to cool below room temperature (20° C to 24° C). The platelets must be separated from whole blood within 8 hours. If platelets are not to be separated from the unit of whole blood, units are stored at 1° C to 6° C before component preparation.

Separation of components from the original whole blood unit is performed by centrifugation. Red cells move to the bottom of the collection bag because they are the heaviest component, whereas the platelets and plasma components remain on top. Variables that affect the yield of the product being prepared include speed of the centrifuge (revolutions per minute [RPM] or relative centrifugal force [g-force]) and length of time of centrifugation.

Each centrifuge used for preparing components is calibrated for optimal time and speed for each product made. Quality control measures are performed to evaluate the products and determine whether the centrifugation parameters are set for maximum product yield. A short centrifugation time at a low RPM is usually called a light spin, whereas a longer spin time at a higher RPM is called a heavy spin.

Steps in the preparation of RBCs, FFP, plasma, platelets, and cryoprecipitated AHF are outlined subsequently. This process varies according to the bag type and filter system the collection facility uses. Details regarding prestorage filtration are discussed in the sections addressing leukocyte reduction. The AABB *Technical Manual* provides detailed procedures for the preparation of blood components. Fig. 15.4 illustrates component separation.

- After the whole blood unit is centrifuged at a light spin, the platelet-rich plasma (PRP) is expressed or pushed through the attached tubing into an empty satellite bag. The RBCs remain in the original bag, and the tube between the plasma and red cells is heat sealed and cut.
- If collected in an additive system, the additive solution is added to the RBCs. Prestorage leukocyte reduction may be performed at this step. The RBCs are sealed and split from the remaining bags and refrigerated at 1° C to 6° C.
- The PRP unit is centrifuged again at a heavy spin, which causes the platelets to sediment to the bottom of the bag. All but about 50 to 70 mL of plasma is removed from the platelets. The additional plasma that remains with the platelets is required to maintain a pH of 6.2 or higher during the storage period. The platelets are sealed and allowed to "rest" for a period of at least 1 hour before they are stored on a rotator that maintains continuous gentle agitation. Platelet concentrates are stored at 20° C to 24° C for a maximum period of 5 days.
- The plasma that had been expressed into another empty attached bag can be processed further as:
  - FFP: Plasma frozen within 8 hours of collection and stored at or below −18° C for up to 1 year or stored at or below −65° C for 7 years with FDA approval. FFP contains all coagulation factors, including labile coagulation factors (factors V and VIII) and stable factors (ie, factor II, fibrinogen, ADAMTS13, etc.).[9]
  - Plasma frozen within 24 hours of phlebotomy (PF24): Contains similar coagulation factors as FFP, although labile factor VIII levels are reduced and factor V may be variable compared with FFP.[8] PF24 is stored at or below −18° C for up to 1 year. PF24 is referred to as FP24 in some literature.[6]
  - Recovered plasma for further manufacture, which is usually shipped to a fractionator for processing into derivatives such as albumin, immune globulin, and coagulation factor concentrates.
- If FFP will be processed further into Cryoprecipitated AHF, an empty satellite bag is left attached to the FFP and frozen with it. The FFP is thawed at 1° C to 6° C. A white precipitate forms, and the plasma and satellite bag are centrifuged (heavy spin). All but

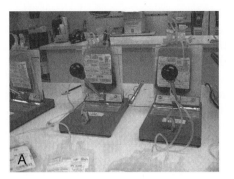

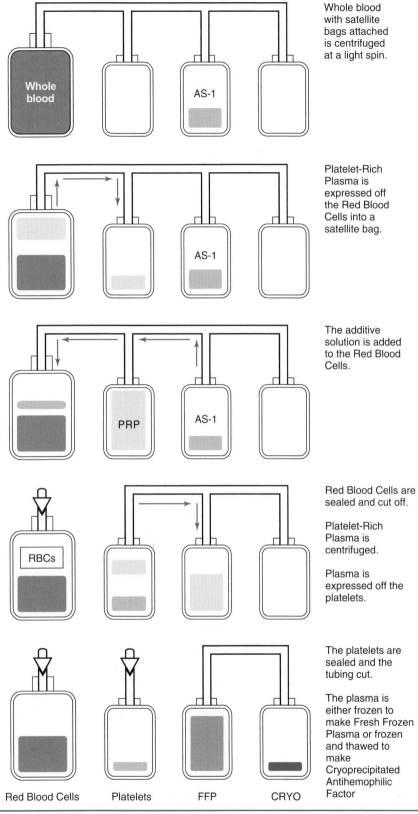

Whole blood with satellite bags attached is centrifuged at a light spin.

Platelet-Rich Plasma is expressed off the Red Blood Cells into a satellite bag.

The additive solution is added to the Red Blood Cells.

Red Blood Cells are sealed and cut off.

Platelet-Rich Plasma is centrifuged.

Plasma is expressed off the platelets.

The platelets are sealed and the tubing cut.

The plasma is either frozen to make Fresh Frozen Plasma or frozen and thawed to make Cryoprecipitated Antihemophilic Factor

Fig. 15.4 Component production. **A,** Component equipment used to express the plasma supernatant into a satellite bag during component production. **B,** Preparation of RBCs, FFP, cryoprecipitated AHF, and platelets from a whole blood unit. *AS,* Additive solution; *PRP,* platelet-rich plasma; *RBCs,* red blood cells; *FFP,* fresh frozen plasma; *CRYO,* cryoprecipitated antihemophilic factor. (**A,** Courtesy LifeSouth Community Blood Centers, Gainesville, FL.)

about 10 to 15 mL of the supernatant plasma is expressed into the empty satellite bag. The CRYO remains in the bag that originally contained the FFP. It is relabeled "Cryoprecipitated AHF," refrozen within 1 hour of thawing, and stored at or below −18° C for up to 1 year from the collection date. The plasma that is expressed into the satellite bag is used as recovered plasma or prepared into "Plasma Cryoprecipitate Reduced." This plasma is refrozen at −18° C or colder and has a 12-month expiration date. It is used primarily as a replacement solution for therapeutic plasmapheresis for the treatment of thrombotic thrombocytopenic purpura (TTP).[6]

WHOLE BLOOD

Whole blood is the unmodified component, drawn from a donor, which consists of erythrocytes, leukocytes, platelets, and plasma proteins with the anticoagulant–preservative solution. Whole blood is stored in a monitored refrigerator at 1° C to 6° C for 21 days if collected in CPD or for 35 days if collected in CPDA-1. Additive solutions cannot be added to whole blood to increase the storage period.

Before development of the technology involved in blood component preparation, whole blood was the only blood product available. In the 1960s, when plastic replaced glass as the collection medium, separation of whole blood into its components became possible. Availability of whole blood declined, and whole blood was replaced with RBCs. Problems associated with whole blood transfusions include circulatory overload in patients who require only oxygen-carrying capacity from RBCs. Viable platelets are lost, and labile coagulation factors decrease within the first 24 hours of storage. Whole blood must also be ABO identical to the patient, limiting its flexibility in inventory management and in emergency situations. Therefore whole blood has a limited use in most clinical situations.[6]

Indications for Use

Whole blood is indicated for patients who are actively bleeding and who have lost more than 25% of their blood volume.[6] The use of whole blood in massively bleeding patients may limit donor exposures if given in place of RBCs and plasma. Whole blood increases the hemoglobin by about 1 g/dL or the hematocrit by about 3%. Whole blood must be ABO identical to the recipient and crossmatched before administration. When whole blood is not available, RBCs administered with crystalloid solutions are usually effective in restoring both oxygen-carrying capacity and blood volume.[5] Reconstituted whole blood (RBCs reconstituted with group AB FFP from a different donor) is usually prepared for exchange transfusions in infants.

RED BLOOD CELL COMPONENTS

Indications for Use

RBCs contain hemoglobin, which transports oxygen through the bloodstream and to the tissues. RBC transfusions increase the mass of circulating red cells in situations where tissue oxygenation may be impaired by acute or chronic blood loss, such as in hemorrhage or anemia. Patients commonly requiring RBC transfusion therapy include (but are not limited to):
- Oncology patients undergoing chemotherapy or radiation therapy
- Trauma patients
- Patients undergoing cardiac, orthopedic, and other surgeries
- Patients with end-stage renal disease
- Premature infants and neonates
- Patients with sickle cell disease

The diseases and conditions that commonly necessitate component therapy are reviewed in the next chapter. Transfusing one unit of RBCs usually increases the hemoglobin by about 1 g/dL and increases the hematocrit by about 3% in the average 70-kg adult. RBCs necessitate crossmatching before issue.

RBCs are often modified into additional products needed for specific patient requirements. The following section summarizes the preparation, storage, and use of leukocyte-reduced, frozen and deglycerolized, washed, and irradiated RBCs.

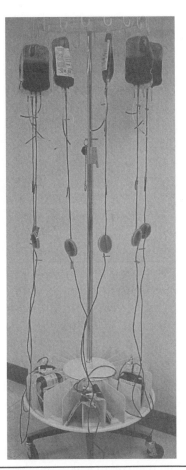

Fig. 15.5 Leukocyte reduction filter. RBC units are filtered before storage at the blood center for optimal effectiveness. (Courtesy LifeSouth Community Blood Centers, Gainesville, FL.)

Red Blood Cells Leukocytes Reduced

Leukocytes remaining in RBC units have been implicated in adverse transfusion reactions and immunization to leukocyte antigens. A reaction caused by leukocytes can be extremely uncomfortable for a patient, causing shaking chills or an increase in temperature, or both, soon after initiating the RBC transfusion. Intact or fragmented membranes and cytokines produced by leukocytes during RBC storage are responsible for febrile reactions.[5] Reduction in leukocytes *before* RBC storage is optimal because it reduces the leukocyte fragments and cytokines that increase during storage. The use of leukocyte-reduced RBCs has become standard practice in many hospitals. The use of leukocyte-reduced RBCs for trauma patients, who may not benefit from these more expensive products, remains controversial.

The standard 170-μm blood filter does not remove leukocytes. White blood cell removal is best accomplished by the use of commercially available leukocyte removal or leukocyte reduction filters. Filtration can be performed by the following procedures:

- Using inline filters integral to the collection set allows blood to be filtered before storage (Fig. 15.5). The inline filter is designed to remove leukocytes from whole blood without removing platelets. This filter provides a mechanism for manufacturing both red cell and platelet products that are leukocyte reduced before storage.
- Red cells that have been separated from the plasma can also be leukocyte reduced using inline filters. The manufacturer's instructions are followed regarding timing, priming with additive solutions, and the temperature of filtration.
- Sterile-connecting a leukocyte reduction filter to the RBCs and filtering before storage (Fig. 15.6).[10] FDA-approved sterile-connecting devices allow for the attachment of tubing from filters, from transfer pacts, and between units without creating an "open system."
- A bedside leukocyte reduction filter can be used when the unit is transfused. This system is least optimal because standardization of leukocyte removal is difficult to

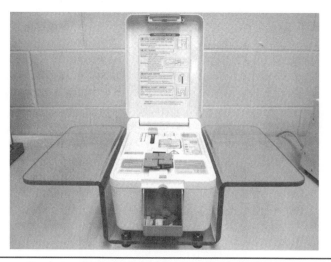

Fig. 15.6 Sterile connection device. Applications of sterile connection devices[5]:
- Addition of a bag while preparing components
- Pooling of components
- Preparation of pediatric units
- Addition of leukocyte reduction filter
- Removing samples for testing

attain. In addition, leukocyte fragments and cytokines that accumulate from storage are not removed, and the process has been associated with hypotensive transfusion reactions.[5]

In addition to preventing reactions, the removal of leukocytes reduces the danger of transfusion-transmitted cytomegalovirus (CMV) because this virus resides in the cytoplasm of white blood cells.[5] The removal of leukocytes does not prevent graft-versus-host disease (GVHD), which is a serious potential transfusion reaction for immunocompromised patients and patients who received units from blood relatives.

According to the AABB standards, leukocyte-reduced RBCs are prepared with a method known to retain at least 85% of the original RBCs and reduce the leukocyte number in the final component to less than 5.0×10^6 in each unit.[4]

Apheresis Red Blood Cells

Automated apheresis technology allows for the collection of one unit of RBCs and a second component such as platelets and plasma or two units of RBCs from one donor. The benefits to this method of red cell collection include the reduction of potential viral exposure to the recipient and reduction of pretransfusion viral marker testing and recruiting expenses.[5] Donor selection requirements differ from RBC collection with regard to donor weight and hematocrit. Donations can be collected every 16 weeks. Saline is used to replace the fluid lost to minimize volume depletion to the donor. The expiration date of the unit depends on the anticoagulant–preservative solution used. Apheresis red cells are drawn into acid-citrate-dextrose, which provides a 21-day storage limit. Depending on the instrument used, leukocyte reduction and the addition of an additive solution may be performed automatically by the instrument or manually using a sterile connection device.[5] This step increases the outdate to 42 days. To be labeled as "Apheresis Red Blood Cells Leukocytes Reduced," the method must be known to ensure a final component containing an average hemoglobin of greater than 51 g/dL (or 153 mL red cell volume).[4] Less than 5.0×10^6 residual leukocytes per unit is also required.[4] The double unit is placed in the inventory as two separate units, and the indications and dosage are comparable to single units of RBCs obtained from whole blood donations.

Frozen Red Blood Cells

RBCs can be frozen for long-term preservation to maintain an inventory of rare units or to extend the availability of autologous units. Freezing extends storage up to 10 years from

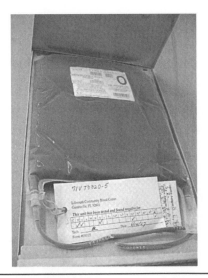

Fig. 15.7 Frozen RBCs. RBCs can be frozen for 10 years at −65° C or below to preserve rare or autologous units. (Courtesy LifeSouth Community Blood Centers, Gainesville, FL.)

collection when stored at or below −65° C. To prepare RBC units for freezing, glycerol is added as a **cryoprotective** agent to prevent cell dehydration and the formation of ice crystals, which causes cell hemolysis. Glycerol is slowly added to the unit for a final glycerol concentration of 40% weight per volume. The unit is transferred to a polyolefin or polyvinyl chloride bag and placed in a metal or cardboard canister to prevent breakage at low temperatures. Units can subsequently be stored at −65° C for up to 10 years from the date of collection (Fig. 15.7).[4]

Freezing can also be accomplished with a lower glycerol concentration if a liquid nitrogen freezer is used. This method is not as common for RBC storage. Glycerol concentration is approximately 20%, and the initial freezing temperature is −196° C (temperature of liquid nitrogen). Maximum storage temperature is −120° C for 10 years.[4]

Cryoprotective: solution added to protect against cell damage that occurs at or below freezing temperatures

Deglycerolized Red Blood Cells

Frozen RBCs are thawed, and the glycerol is removed by the process of deglycerolization. After thawing in a 37° C dry warmer or water bath, the unit is washed in a series of saline solutions of decreasing osmolarity. Saline solutions of 12% and 1.6%, followed by 0.9% normal saline that contains 0.2% dextrose, are used to draw the glycerol out of the cells. The dextrose in the 0.9% normal saline provides nutrients and supports posttransfusion red cell survival for 4 days of storage after deglycerolization. This process is usually performed on an instrument called a blood cell processor, which gradually adds preset saline volumes, mixes and centrifuges the cells, and removes supernatant automatically (Fig. 15.8). Because the process of glycerolization and deglycerolization involves entering the blood unit, the system is considered "open," and the product must be transfused within 24 hours. A visual check of the supernatant from the final wash is performed to ensure sufficient glycerol removal and minimal hemolysis.[5] The automated addition of glycerol to RBCs and removal from RBCs in a closed system is also available for RBC deglycerolization. RBCs prepared in this manner can be stored for 14 days at 4° C when suspended in AS-3.[5] Additional methods for quality control of deglycerolized RBCs are explained in more detail in the AABB *Technical Manual* Method Section.

Washed Red Blood Cells

Washing RBCs with normal saline may be indicated for patients who react to the small amount of plasma proteins that remain in a unit of RBCs. Reactions can be allergic, febrile, or anaphylactic. A patient with IgA deficiency and clinically significant anti-IgA requires washed RBCs if a transfusion is indicated. Washed RBCs may also be used in intrauterine or neonate transfusions.[9] Washing is accomplished with approximately 1000

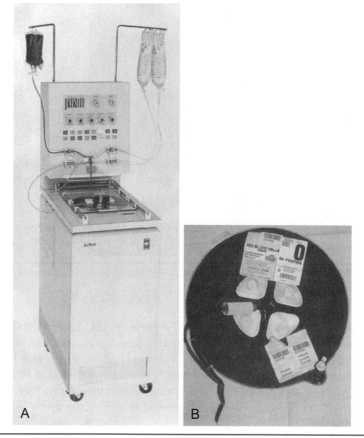

Fig. 15.8 Deglycerolization process. Blood cell processor **(A)** and washed RBCs **(B)**. The blood processor is used to wash RBC and platelet components. It is also used to deglycerolize thawed RBCs. (Courtesy COBE Cardiovascular, Arvada, CO.)

to 2000 mL of 0.9% saline using the automatic blood cell processor described for deglycerolizing frozen RBCs. Washing is associated with a loss of up to 20% of the original RBCs and is no longer considered an effective method of removing leukocytes.

Red Blood Cells Irradiated

Viable T lymphocytes in cellular blood components may cause transfusion-associated GVHD, which is fatal in more than 90% of affected patients.[5] Factors that determine a patient's risk for transfusion-associated GVHD include whether, and to what degree, the patient is immunodeficient and the degree of similarity between donor and recipient regarding human leukocyte antigens (HLAs). Gamma irradiation of cellular blood components prevents proliferation (multiplication) of the donor's T lymphocytes that cause transfusion-associated GVHD. RBCs that have been leukocyte reduced by filtration do not prevent GVHD because some leukocytes remain in the final product. AABB *Standards* require irradiation of cellular components (RBCs and platelets) if the donor unit is from a blood relative of the intended recipient or the donor unit is HLA-matched for the recipient.

Irradiation can be performed with a gamma irradiator (cesium-137 or cobalt-60 radioisotopes), linear accelerators, UV-A irradiation, and nonradioisotope equipment (x-rays). The required dose of irradiation is 2500 cGy/rad, or 25 Gy, in the middle of the canister, and the lowest dose should be 1500 cGy/rad. Periodic verification and documentation of dose delivery are required.[4]

Irradiation induces erythrocyte membrane damage that causes RBC units to have a higher plasma potassium level and a decrease in ATP and 2,3-DPG levels.[5] Cell activities that are not dependent on reproduction (notably platelet activation and oxygen delivery) are not significantly affected by irradiation. The expiration date of irradiated RBCs is

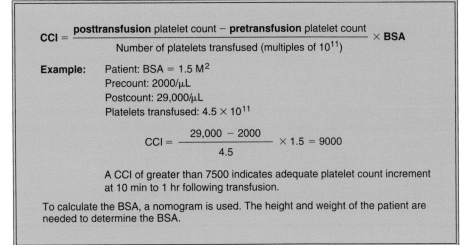

$$CCI = \frac{\textbf{posttransfusion} \text{ platelet count} - \textbf{pretransfusion} \text{ platelet count}}{\text{Number of platelets transfused (multiples of } 10^{11})} \times \textbf{BSA}$$

Example: Patient: BSA = 1.5 M^2
Precount: 2000/μL
Postcount: 29,000/μL
Platelets transfused: 4.5 × 10^{11}

$$CCI = \frac{29,000 - 2000}{4.5} \times 1.5 = 9000$$

A CCI of greater than 7500 indicates adequate platelet count increment at 10 min to 1 hr following transfusion.

To calculate the BSA, a nomogram is used. The height and weight of the patient are needed to determine the BSA.

Fig. 15.9 Platelet refractoriness and CCI. Platelet refractoriness may be due to immune or nonimmune causes. The CCI is used to calculate the effectiveness of platelet transfusions based on the number of platelets infused and the body surface area (BSA). *CCI,* Corrected count increment.

changed to 28 days after irradiation if the available shelf life exceeds 28 days. If the irradiated cells are not given to the originally intended recipient, they can be returned to the inventory and transfused to another patient.

PLATELET COMPONENTS

Indications for Use

Normal platelet function and adequate numbers of circulating platelets are essential for hemostasis. Functions of platelets include:
- Maintenance of vascular integrity
- Initial arrest of bleeding by formation of platelet plug
- Stabilization of the hemostatic plug by contributing to the process of fibrin formation
  Platelets are transfused to control or prevent bleeding associated with critically decreased circulating platelet numbers or functionally abnormal platelets.[9] Platelet transfusions are not usually effective or indicated for patients with destruction of circulating platelets caused by autoimmune disorders, such as idiopathic thrombocytopenic purpura, heparin-induced thrombocytopenia, or TTP. Patients requiring platelet transfusions typically include:
- Cancer patients undergoing chemotherapy or radiation therapy
- Recipients of hematopoietic progenitor cell transplants for a period after transplant
- Patients with postoperative bleeding
- Organ transplant patients (eg, liver transplants)
  Because transfused platelets normally circulate with a life span of only 3 to 4 days, frequent transfusion support is often necessary for patients using platelets. Evaluation of the effectiveness of platelet transfusions is important in determining whether the patient is **refractory,** or unresponsive to the platelet transfusions. The **corrected count increment** (CCI), outlined in Fig. 15.9, determines the increase in platelet count adjusted for the number of platelets infused and the size of the patient.[9] Platelet counts should be performed before transfusion and within 1 hour after transfusion. In a clinically stable patient, a CCI result of less than 5000/μL at 10 minutes to 1 hour posttransfusion may indicate a refractory state to platelet therapy. Table 15.3 lists conditions associated with refractoriness. Platelets do not require crossmatching before issue and should be ABO compatible with the recipient's red cells whenever possible.

Refractory: unresponsive to platelet transfusions; responsiveness is measured by posttransfusion platelet counts

Corrected count increment: relative increase in platelet count adjusted for the number of platelets transfused and the size of the patient

Platelets

Platelet concentrates prepared from a unit of whole blood, as described in the section on blood component preparation, contain at least 5.5 × 10^{10} platelets per unit and, under

TABLE 15.3	Conditions Causing Platelet Refractoriness or Poor Response to Platelet Transfusions
Immune	
HLA alloantibodies	
Platelet alloantibodies	
Autoantibodies	
Nonimmune	
Splenomegaly	
Medications	
Sepsis	
Active bleeding	
Disseminated intravascular coagulation (DIC)	
Fever	

optimal conditions, should elevate the platelet count by about 5000 µL in a recipient weighing 75 kg.[5] Platelets prepared from whole blood are also referred to as random donor platelets or platelet concentrates.

Pooled Platelets

To achieve a therapeutic dose, platelet concentrates are pooled for transfusion in adults. Pooling is accomplished by transferring the platelet concentrates into a transfer set, while being careful not to contaminate the ports. An approximate dose is 1 unit per 10 kg of patient body weight, yielding pools of 6 to 10 platelets. This platelet pooling method creates an "open system," which causes the expiration of the pooled product to change to 4 hours from the start of pooling. The pooled platelets should be stored at 20° C to 24° C with gentle agitation until transfusion. Platelets can also be pooled using a commercial prestorage pooling bag, which maintains an expiration date of the oldest component in the pool, up to 5 days.[5]

Units selected for pooling should be type specific or type compatible due to the presence of some RBCs in each unit. A unique pool number is placed on the final container, and all units present in the pool must be documented.

Apheresis Platelets

Plateletpheresis: collection of platelets by apheresis

Apheresis is an effective method of harvesting a therapeutic dose of platelets from one individual donor (Fig. 15.10). During **plateletpheresis,** whole blood is collected from a donor using automated apheresis equipment, which separates whole blood into components. The platelets are retained, and the remaining elements are returned. The product is also referred to as single-donor platelets. Plateletpheresis donors may donate as often as twice a week or 24 times a year with an interval of 48 hours between procedures. A unit of platelets prepared by apheresis should contain a minimum of 3.0×10^{11} platelets in 90% of the sampled units, which is about the same as a pool of 5 to 6 platelets prepared from whole blood. Quality control must also include the pH, which must be greater than or equal to 6.2 at the end of the allowable storage period.[4]

Platelets display class I HLA. Class I antigens refer to the A, B, and C antigens. Platelets also demonstrate platelet antigens that can elicit an immune response from a patient receiving frequent platelet components. Patients who have developed antibodies to HLA or platelet antigens usually require platelets matched for HLA antigens or crossmatched to achieve satisfactory increment. Locating HLA-matched donors from previously typed HLA plateletpheresis donors requires a large donor base. Identical HLA-A and HLA-B antigen matching from unrelated donors is rare (1 in 5000 to 20,000).[5] However, less-than-perfect matching may be sufficient to overcome the refractory state.

Platelets Leukocytes Reduced

Leukocyte reduction can be achieved using certain apheresis devices and leukocyte reduction filters designed for bedside and prestorage filtration. Leukocyte reduction is indicated

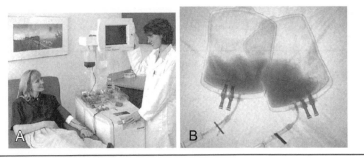

Fig. 15.10 Apheresis. **A,** Instrument used for apheresis procedures. **B,** Apheresis platelets. (Courtesy Baxter Healthcare Corp., Deerfield, IL.)

to prevent recurrent febrile nonhemolytic reactions and HLA alloimmunization for patients requiring long-term platelet support or eventual transplantation. As with leukocyte reduction in RBC products, leukocyte removal before storage also reduces cytokines and the potential febrile reactions they cause. Leukocyte-reduced platelets are also effective in preventing CMV infection.[5] Platelets collected by apheresis must have fewer than 5.0×10^6 leukocytes in 95% of the tested units.[4]

PLASMA COMPONENTS

Fresh Frozen Plasma (FFP), Plasma Frozen within 24 Hours of Phlebotomy (PF24)
Indications for Use

The process of coagulation involves a series of biochemical reactions that transform circulating plasma into an insoluble gel through conversion of fibrinogen to fibrin. This process requires certain plasma proteins or coagulation factors, phospholipids, and calcium. Impairment of the coagulation system can occur because of decreased synthesis of the coagulation factors or consumption of the factors. Defects in the plasma clotting factors may be due to congenital or acquired conditions.

FFP contains all the coagulation factors, including the **labile factors** V and VIII, which do not store well at temperatures greater than –18° C (Table 15.4).[5] PF24 may have reduced levels of factors V and VIII compared with FFP.[9] FFP and PF24 are indicated for the following situations[6]:

- Management of bleeding in patients who require coagulation factors II, V, X, or XI, when the concentrates are not available or are not appropriate
- Abnormal coagulation assays resulting from massive transfusion
- Management of patients anticoagulated with warfarin who are bleeding or require emergency surgery
- Replacement solution for therapeutic plasmapheresis for the treatment of TTP and hemolytic uremic syndrome (plasma cryoprecipitate reduced can also be used for these patients)
- Correction or prevention of bleeding complications in patients who have severe liver disease with multiple factor deficiencies
- Management of patients with disseminated intravascular coagulation when the fibrinogen level is less than 100 mg/dL
- Management of patients with rare specific plasma protein deficiencies

Units of FFP and PF24 are thawed before administration in a 30° C to 37° C water bath for approximately 20 to 30 minutes. Units should be placed in protective overwraps to prevent contamination of the administration ports or in a device that maintains the ports above water. Water baths with an agitator accelerate the thawing process. FDA-approved microwave ovens specially designed for plasma thawing also can be used by carefully following the manufacturer's instructions. Standard microwave ovens should never be used because they denature plasma proteins. After thawing, FFP is stored at 1° C to 6° C and should be transfused within 24 hours from thawing.

The dose of FFP or PF24 depends on the clinical situation and the underlying disease process. If coagulation factor replacement is necessary, the dose is 10 to 20 mL/kg (3 to

Labile factors: factors V and VIII, which are coagulation factors that deteriorate on storage

TABLE 15.4   Coagulation Factors and Their Sources

FACTOR NAME	INDICATION	SOURCE
Factor I, fibrinogen	Fibrinogen deficiency	Fibrinogen concentrate, cryoprecipitated AHF
Factor II, IX, X, prothrombin complex	Hemophilia B	Prothrombin complex concentrate
Protein C	Venous thrombosis, severe protein C deficiency	Protein C concentrate
Factor VIIa (recombinant)	Factor VII deficiency, hemophilia A or B with inhibitors	Recombinant factor VIIa concentrate
Activated prothrombin complex, factor II, IX, X (nonactivated), VII (activated)	Bleeding or prophylaxis before surgery for hemophilia A or B with inhibitors	Activated prothrombin complex concentrate
Factor VIII, antihemophilic factor	Hemophilia A, von Willebrand disease	Factor VIII concentrate, human and recombinant
Factor IX, Christmas factor	Hemophilia B	Factor IX concentrate, human and recombinant
Factor XI, plasma thromboplastin antecedent	Factor XI deficiency	Thawed plasma, FFP, PF24
Factor XIII, fibrin stabilizing factor	Factor XIII deficiency	Cryoprecipitated AHF or plasma
VWF, von Willebrand factor	von Willebrand disease	Factor VIII concentrate, cryoprecipitated AHF, FFP

FFP, Fresh frozen plasma; *PF24*, plasma frozen within 24 hours of phlebotomy.

6 units in an adult).[6] Crossmatching is not necessary, but the plasma should be ABO compatible with the patient's red cells.

If not transfused within 24 hours, the product should be relabeled as "thawed plasma" and stored at 1° C to 6° C for up to 5 days after thawing. Thawed plasma should not be used for replacement of labile coagulation factor VIII. Thawed plasma is not licensed by the FDA. However, it is an acceptable practice according to AABB *Standards* and the *Circular of Information for the Use of Human Blood and Blood Components*. Concentrations of all the coagulation factors have been shown to be comparable to FFP and clinically adequate for transfusion.[11,12]

> Plasma contains albumin, coagulation factors, immunoglobulins, and other proteins essential for metabolism.

> Plasma must be ABO compatible with the recipient's red cells.

Cryoprecipitated Antihemophilic Factor

Indications for Use

Cryoprecipitated AHF, also referred to as cryoprecipitate or CRYO, is the cold insoluble precipitate that forms when a unit of FFP is thawed between 1° C and 6° C. It contains, in a concentrated form, most of the coagulation factors that are found in FFP. These factors include:

- von Willebrand factor (vWF), which is needed for platelet adhesion to damaged endothelium
- Fibrinogen, which is cleaved into fibrin in the presence of thrombin to form a clot
- Factor VIII, the procoagulant activity factor that is deficient in hemophilia A
- Fibronectin
- Factor XII

Once separated from FFP, CRYO is refrozen within 1 hour of preparation and stored at −18° C or colder for up to 1 year from the date of collection.

The primary clinical uses of CRYO are as a supplement for patients with deficiencies of factor XIII and fibrinogen. Because viral inactivated factor VIII concentrates are currently available for patients with hemophilia A, von Willebrand disease, and factor VIII:C deficiency, CRYO is less commonly used for correcting or preventing bleeding in these patients. CRYO is the only concentrated fibrinogen product available and is used to treat patients with congenital or acquired fibrinogen defects. Dysfibrinogenemia, a condition in which fibrinogen is not functionally effective, is associated with severe liver disease.

Quality control of CRYO must demonstrate greater than 150 mg of fibrinogen and 80 international units (IU) of factor VIII per unit tested. In facilities that pool CRYO before freezing, the final unit shall have a minimum of 150 mg of fibrinogen and 80 IU of factor VIII times the number of components in the pool.[4]

Plasma Cryoprecipitate Reduced

After the removal of CRYO from FFP, the remaining plasma unit can be refrozen. The refreezing must occur within 24 hours of the thawing. The product is relabeled "Plasma, Cryoprecipitate Reduced" and is stored at –18° C or lower for 1 year from the date of collection. The CRYO-poor plasma (CPP) is used primarily in the treatment of TTP because it contains ADAMTS13, the protein that is reduced in TTP. Albumin and coagulation factors II, V, VII, IX, X, and XI remain in the same concentrations as in FFP. Once thawed for use, CPP has a 5-day expiration date and should be stored at 1° C to 6° C.

Cryoprecipitated Antihemophilic Factor (AHF), Pooled

Cryoprecipitated AHF is pooled into a transfer bag to achieve a therapeutic dose. The frozen units first must be thawed in a 30° C to 37° C water bath for up to 15 minutes, using overwraps to prevent contamination of the ports. The contents of bags can be rinsed with 10 to 15 mL of 0.9% sodium chloride while pooling. Pooled CRYO must be administered within 4 hours of first entry and should be stored at room temperature until transfusion. Dosage varies with the patient's condition, weight, and level of the factor requiring replacement. This formula is shown in Fig. 15.11. If large volumes of CRYO are to be administered, ABO-compatible units should be selected. Crossmatching is not indicated when issuing CRYO components. Coagulation factor levels and other laboratory studies are performed to determine the effectiveness and the need for repeat doses.

Cryoprecipitated AHF can also be pooled after separation from FFP at the collection facility. Units pooled by a closed system using a sterile collection device can be stored frozen for 1 year. After thawing, the closed-system pooled CRYO must be stored at 20° C to 24° C and used within 6 hours. If the CRYO was pooled in an open system, the product must be used within 4 hours. The number of units in the pool is indicated on the label, and the pooled product has a unique number. A record of the unit numbers contained in the pool must be maintained.

When thawing CRYO and FFP in a water bath, plastic overwraps prevent contamination of entry ports used for administration.

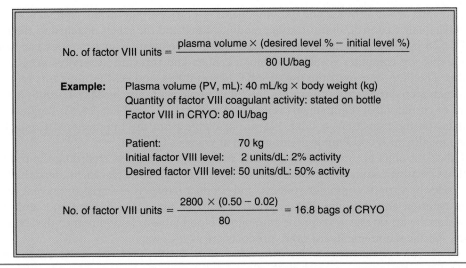

Fig. 15.11 Calculating the dose of CRYO concentrates. (From AABB/America's Blood Centers/American Red Cross/Armed Services Blood Program: *Circular of information for the use of human blood and blood components,* revised Nov 2014, Bethesda, MD, 2014.)

Fibrin Sealant from Cryoprecipitated Antihemophilic Factor

CRYO has also been used to prepare a topical hemostatic solution useful in controlling bleeding during surgery and various procedures. The solution contains 1 to 2 units of CRYO mixed with thrombin and is applied to the bleeding surface by layering, mixing, or spraying on the surgical field. Fibrinogen is converted to fibrin by the action of thrombin, which forms a clot to stop bleeding. Commercial products that are viral inactivated and have higher fibrinogen content are also available and have largely replaced the use of single CRYO units to prepare fibrin sealant.

APHERESIS GRANULOCYTES

Granulocytes are usually collected by apheresis techniques. Granulocyte transfusions are rarely used and limited to a small number of patients. This product contains leukocytes and platelets, as well as 20 to 50 mL of red cells. The number of granulocytes in each product equals or is greater than 1.0×10^{10}. Granulocytes deteriorate rapidly on storage and should be administered as soon as possible within 24 hours of collection. They are maintained at 20° C to 24° C without agitation until transfused. A standard blood infusion set should be used when administering granulocytes. Depth-type microaggregate filters and leukocyte reduction filters are not to be used because they remove granulocytes.

A crossmatch is usually required before transfusion because of red cell contamination at greater than 2 mL.[4] Granulocyte support is usually ongoing until the granulocyte count increases and the infection is cured. Because patients undergoing this therapy are severely immunosuppressed, irradiation of the product to prevent GVHD is important.

The preparation and use of this product is uncommon as a result of the following[6]:
- More effective antibiotics
- Recombinant growth factor that stimulates the bone marrow to produce leukocytes
- Adverse reactions associated with granulocyte transfusions
- Granulocytes are limited to patients with the following conditions:
  - Neutropenia (generally $<0.5 \times 10^9$/L or 500/µL)
  - Documented infections, especially gram-negative bacteria and fungi
  - Lack of response to antibiotics

SECTION 3
DISTRIBUTION AND ADMINISTRATION

LABELING

The labeling of whole blood and its components is a process that includes a final review of records, quality control, donor testing, modifications, and the labels attached to the unit. **ISBT 128** labeling is an international standard of labeling that incorporates bar-coded labels that are computer readable by blood centers and transfusion services around the world. The FDA approved the use of ISBT 128 in 2000, and AABB *Standards* required that each accredited facility convert to ISBT 128 implementation by May 1, 2008. A summary of current label requirements is included in Fig. 15.12 and Fig. 15.13. Progress and updates on the transition to ISBT 128 are available from the International Council on Commonality in Blood Banking Automation at www.iccbba.com.[3]

Labels on units are intended to provide sufficient information regarding the product without creating confusion. Standardization with regard to label placement, readability of bar codes by various computer systems, and product names is essential to prevent errors in transfusion and shipping. Required labels must be placed on the bag and cannot be substituted with tie tags (except for autologous blood labels). In addition to the standard label, specific requirements for other products are as follows:
- Irradiated components must have the name of the facility performing the irradiation.
- Pooled components must include the final volume, unique number assigned to the pool, and name of the facility preparing the pooled component.
- Autologous units must be labeled "For Autologous Use Only."

ISBT 128: International Society of Blood Transfusion (ISBT): recommendations regarding the uniform labeling of blood products for international bar-code recognition by computers

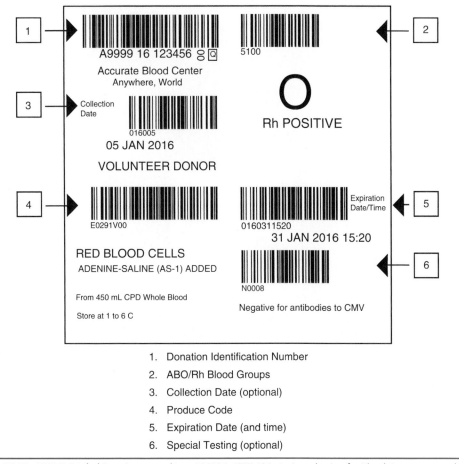

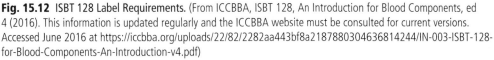

1. Donation Identification Number
2. ABO/Rh Blood Groups
3. Collection Date (optional)
4. Produce Code
5. Expiration Date (and time)
6. Special Testing (optional)

Fig. 15.12 ISBT 128 Label Requirements. (From ICCBBA, ISBT 128, An Introduction for Blood Components, ed 4 (2016). This information is updated regularly and the ICCBBA website must be consulted for current versions. Accessed June 2016 at https://iccbba.org/uploads/22/82/2282aa443bf8a21878803046368 14244/IN-003-ISBT-128-for-Blood-Components-An-Introduction-v4.pdf)

A facility receiving a unit of blood from another institution can place its own number on the unit; however, no more than two unique numeric or alphanumeric identification numbers should be visible on a blood component container. The original number must never be removed. The *Circular of Information* is referenced on the label as an important extension to component labels. This clear, concise guideline provides a description of each component, indications, and contraindications for use and information on dosage, administration, storage, side effects, and hazards. It is frequently updated and contains recent FDA guidelines.[9]

STORAGE AND TRANSPORTATION

Proper storage of blood components is important to maintain product potency and prevent bacterial growth. FDA and AABB guidelines define procedures for the calibration and maintenance of equipment designed for product storage, storage temperature limits, and monitoring parameters. Specifically, all refrigerators, freezers, and platelet incubators used for storing blood components must have the following:

- Recording devices to monitor the temperature at least every 4 hours
- Audible alarms to ensure a response 24 hours a day and an alarm set to signal the undesirable temperature *before* it is reached
- Alarm checks performed on a regular basis
- Emergency procedures for power failure and alarm activation
- Emergency power backup systems; continuous power source for alarms
- Use of calibrated thermometers checked against referenced thermometers
- Written procedures for all the preceding

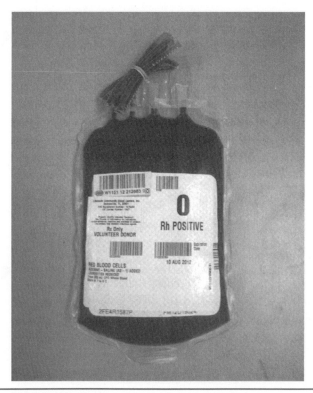

Fig. 15.13 Example of a labeled blood unit.
- Component name and unique identification that can be traced back to the blood donor.
- Manufacturer's name and registration number, license number if applicable.
- Expiration date and time if less than 72 hours.
- Amount of blood component and anticoagulant/preservative (within ±10%).
- Test results of ABO and Rh type (D type may be omitted for cryoprecipitated AHF). Selected tests such as CMV antigen or antibody identification can be indicated with a tie tag or label.
- Donor category: Paid, volunteer.
- Autologous units: "Autologous Use Only," name of the donor, blood group, hospital, and identification number. Autologous units that have reactive infectious disease markers require a biohazard label.
- Statements regarding recipient identification, reference to the circular of information, infectious disease risk, and prescription requirement. (Courtesy LifeSouth Community Blood Centers, Gainesville, FL.)

Appropriate storage temperatures for blood components are listed in Table 15.2. During storage, blood should be examined for evidence of hemolysis, abnormal coloring, or clots, any of which may indicate bacterial contamination.

Transportation of Blood Components

Whole blood or RBCs that are packaged for shipping must be maintained between 1° C and 10° C. Containers used for shipping must be validated periodically to ensure their effectiveness for shipping at wide ranges of outdoor temperatures (Fig. 15.14).[5]

Frozen units are shipped on dry ice. Because frozen products are brittle, they must be wrapped carefully. As dry ice evaporates, the extra space created allows the units to move about in the box and potentially break. Platelets must be maintained as close as possible to 20° C to 24° C during shipping. Discontinuation of the agitation of platelets during transportation should not exceed 24 hours.[4]

On receipt of a shipment of blood components, the temperature and appearance of the units must be observed and recorded (Table 15.5). Container closure and attached segments should also be inspected. Units that are received out of the designated temperature range must be evaluated for their suitability for transfusion. The shipping facility should be notified if the product is unacceptable. Questionable units should be quarantined until a responsible person determines the disposition. Shipping records, including details of problems and the outcomes, must be maintained.[4]

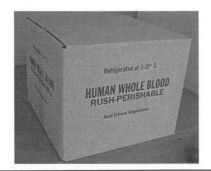

Fig. 15.14 Blood container for transporting blood products. (Courtesy LifeSouth Community Blood Centers, Gainesville, FL.)

TABLE 15.5 Checklist for Receiving Blood
✓ Temperature acceptable for component
✓ Appearance: clots, discoloration, hemolysis
✓ Container closure
✓ Attached segments intact: RBCs
✓ Expiration date and time
✓ Shipping list correct
✓ Intact labels

Units that are issued to an unmonitored area, such as a patient's room, are usually not accepted back into inventory unless a time limit is set or the units have been transported in an insulated cooler or container.[13] Validation of the acceptable time for returning an unmonitored unit of blood must be set by each facility. Only one unit is typically issued at a time, unless the transfusion requirement is urgent.

Appropriate training of staff involved in the shipping and transportation of blood and blood components, in both the hospital and the blood center setting, is essential for the maintenance of quality products. Policies and procedures for all aspects of component packaging, inspection, record keeping, and monitoring must be understood and followed carefully.

ADMINISTRATION OF BLOOD COMPONENTS

This section summarizes important aspects of blood administration that pertain to the components described earlier. A more detailed discussion can be found in the *Technical Manual* and the *Blood Transfusion Therapy: A Physician's Handbook*, both published by the AABB. Although laboratory personnel have limited involvement in blood administration, an understanding of the critical elements improves the communication between health care workers and the safety of the transfusion.

Requirements of safe blood administration include the following:
- *Positive identification* of the patient using two independent identifiers before transfusion is critical to avoid transfusion reactions that may be fatal.
- *A system to avoid and detect clerical errors* also contributes to avoiding serious reactions. Strict adherence to policies regarding identification numbers and mislabeled tubes should be followed.
- *Direct observation* of the patient should occur during the first 15 minutes after infusion begins and periodically until an appropriate time after the transfusion is completed.[4] Prompt intervention of a transfusion reaction is important in reducing its severity.
- *Only normal saline (0.9% USP)* should be administered with blood components. Hypotonic solutions such as 5% dextrose cause hemolysis in vitro. Ringer's lactate, which contains calcium, can initiate in vitro coagulation by reversing the action of citrate. The addition of medications to blood can cause hemolysis and mask adverse reactions.[9]

- *A 170- to 260-μm standard filter* must be used with all cellular and plasma components, even if leukocyte reduction of the product has been performed during preparation. The standard filter can be substituted with a bedside leukocyte reduction filter to prevent febrile reactions and HLA alloimmunization. They are specifically designed for either platelets or RBCs and cannot be interchanged.
- *Blood transfusion should be started before component expiration and completed within 4 hours* because of the risk of bacterial growth. If the patient's condition requires blood infusion to extend past 4 hours, the unit should be divided and kept in the blood bank refrigerator until needed.[4]
- *Documentation and record keeping* are essential. AABB *Standards* requires the following documentation with regard to a transfusion[4]:
  - Medical order for transfusion
  - Recipient consent
  - Name or type of component
  - Donor unit number or pool number
  - Date and time of transfusion
  - Pretransfusion and posttransfusion vital signs
  - Amount transfused
  - Identification of the transfusionist
  - Any adverse events possibly related to the transfusion

Adverse transfusion reactions can occur, regardless of how carefully the component was prepared, tested, crossmatched, and administered. If a transfusion reaction occurs, the transfusion must be discontinued immediately. The reporting of a reaction that occurs during or after administration is an important procedure that must be followed without deviation. Good communication between the transfusing personnel and the laboratory in the event of a reaction expedites its resolution and prevents further complications.

> Blood and blood components must be inspected before use for abnormal appearance such as excessive hemolysis, changes in color of blood bag compared with segments, floccular material, or cloudiness.

CHAPTER SUMMARY

- The receipt, preparation, and issue of blood components are guided by current cGMP regulations published and enforced by the FDA.
- Each blood product is prepared and stored to optimize its purity and potency at the time of transfusion.
- Quality control parameters are set by the FDA and AABB (outlined in Table 15.4).
- The following table provides an outline of component indications to prevent adverse transfusion reactions and for selected patient therapy.
- Selection of ABO-compatible red cells containing components and plasma is essential to prevent reactions and optimize component therapy and is summarized in the table that follows.[3]

SUMMARY OF BLOOD COMPONENT THERAPY

Component	Indications	Comments
Whole Blood	Increases red cell mass and plasma volume	Often available only for autologous units
Red Blood Cells (RBCs), Apheresis RBCs	Increase oxygen-carrying capacity in anemia, trauma, and surgery	Expiration varies with anticoagulant
Frozen/deglycerolized RBCs	Prolonged red cell storage for rare blood units and autologous storage	24-hour outdate after deglycerolization
Washed RBCs	Reduce plasma proteins to avoid allergic and anaphylactic reactions (IgA deficiency)	24-hour expiration after washing
Platelets and RBCs Leukocyte Reduced	Avoid febrile nonhemolytic reactions and prevent HLA alloimmunization, reduce CMV transmission	Prestorage filtration more effective in avoiding cytokines

Component	Indications	Comments
Irradiated RBCs and Platelets	Prevent GVHD in immunocompromised patients, HLA-matched platelets, or transfusions from a blood relative	Irradiation decreases shelf life of RBCs to 28 days
Platelets, Pooled Platelets	Bleeding caused by thrombocytopenia or thrombocytopathy	Pooling reduces expiration to 4 hours
Apheresis Platelets	Bleeding caused by thrombocytopenia or thrombocytopathy	May be HLA matched with recipient in cases of refractoriness
FFP, PF24	Replace stable and labile coagulation factors	Used in surgeries, trauma, and some factor deficiencies
Cryoprecipitated AHF (CRYO)	Contains fibrinogen, factors XIII and VIII, and von Willebrand factor	Treatment of von Willebrand disease, fibrinogen deficiency, and hemophilia A
Apheresis Granulocytes	Neutropenia with infection, unresponsive to antibiotics	Contains RBCs, must be ABO compatible

Recipient ABO	BLOOD COMPONENT		
	Whole blood	RBCs	Plasma products (Platelets, FFP, PF24)
A	A	A, O	A, AB
B	B	B, O	B, AB
AB	AB	AB, A, B, O	AB
O	O	O	O, A, B, AB

ABO-compatible CRYO is not required because of the small amount of plasma.
Compatibility testing is necessary for all products containing red cells, including granulocytes.

CRITICAL THINKING EXERCISES

Exercise 15-1
Is it possible to prepare CRYO and FFP from the same unit of whole blood? Explain your answer.

Exercise 15-2
A nonbleeding adult of average height and weight with chronic anemia is transfused with 2 units of RBCs. The pretransfusion hemoglobin is 7.0 g/dL.
1. What is the expected posttransfusion hemoglobin?
2. List several potential reasons for a failure of the patient's hemoglobin to increase after transfusion.

Exercise 15-3
A severely immunosuppressed adult patient has been transfused with 10 units of pooled platelets. The pretransfusion platelet count was 6000 µL.
1. What is the expected platelet count 1 hour from transfusion?
2. If the platelet count does not increase as expected, what are some potential causes?

Exercise 15-4
A unit of blood is released for a patient on the oncology floor. The nurse calls the blood bank 15 minutes later and reports that the patient has a visitor and does not want the transfusion until later that day. The nurse would like to hold the unit in the refrigerator on the floor because she is too busy to return it immediately. How do you respond?

Exercise 15-5

A 60-kg patient with hemophilia is going to surgery to have a small tumor removed. The physician requests enough Cryoprecipitated AHF to maintain the patient at 50% activity for surgery. The patient is currently at 15%. Determine how many units of Cryoprecipitated AHF will require pooling for surgery.

Exercise 15-6

A 70-lb child is scheduled for orthopedic surgery in 3 weeks. The physician requested that 2 units of autologous RBCs be drawn before surgery.

1. Determine the amount to be drawn and the anticoagulant adjustment to collect RBCs from this child.

On the day of surgery, the patient becomes ill and surgery is postponed. Because of the tight operating room schedule, the surgery cannot take place for 2 months.

2. Do the units need to be discarded and redrawn? Do any options exist?

The patient's older sister would like to be a donor for this patient. She meets the regular blood donor criteria and donates a unit of blood as a directed donor 1 week before the new surgery date.

3. What procedure is required before this unit can be made available to her sibling? Will the expiration date change?

4. If her sibling does not use the unit during surgery, can it be returned to regular inventory?

Exercise 15-7

A nurse is completing her shift in 1 hour and needs to start a transfusion and give the same patient an intravenous medication before she leaves. To expedite the process, she opts to give both through the Y-set she has prepared for the blood administration. She is not sure whether this protocol is allowed She calls the blood bank before obtaining the blood.

1. What should the blood bank personnel advise this nurse to do?

The nurse is in a hurry to start this transfusion and realizes that the intravenous solution she attached to the blood administration set is 2% dextrose instead of 0.9% saline.

2. Can the nurse proceed with this transfusion or should she wait for 0.9% saline? Why?

STUDY QUESTIONS

For questions 1 through 7, match the clinical condition to the component that would have the best therapeutic value. Components may be used more than once.

Patient Disease or Condition	Component
1. TTP patient undergoing therapeutic apheresis	a. Factor VIII concentrate
2. Fibrinogen deficiency	b. Cryoprecipitated AHF
3. Thrombocytopenia	c. RBCs, washed
4. Refractory platelet response	d. Plasma, cryoprecipitate reduced
5. Hemophilia A	e. Platelets
6. Sickle cell disease	f. Apheresis platelets, HLA-matched
7. IgA-deficient patient with anti-IgA	g. RBCs

For questions 8 through 15, match the correct expiration times on the right with the appropriate blood component on the left. Expiration times can be used more than once.

Component	Expiration times
8. RBCs, AS-1 added	a. 35 days
9. Washed RBCs	b. 28 days
10. Irradiated RBCs	c. 3 days

Component	Expiration times
11. RBCs collected in CPDA-1	d. 24 hours
12. Rejuvenated RBCs	e. 42 days
13. Frozen RBCs	f. 10 years
14. Deglycerolized RBCs	g. 21 days
15. RBCs collected in CPD	h. 1 year

16. What is the minimum amount of fibrinogen required in 1 unit of cryoprecipitated AHF?
    a. 150 mg
    b. 250 mg
    c. 80 IU
    d. 1000 mg

17. What fluid is administered with the transfusion of blood components?
    a. Ringer's lactate
    b. 5% dextrose
    c. 0.9% saline
    d. All of the above

18. Eight units of platelets were pooled in an open system without the use of a sterile connecting device. What is the new time of expiration of the pooled product?
    a. 2 hours
    b. 4 hours
    c. 6 hours
    d. 24 hours

19. What is the correct order of centrifugation in the preparation of platelets from a unit of whole blood?
    a. hard spin followed by hard spin
    b. light spin followed by light spin
    c. hard spin followed by light spin
    d. light spin followed by hard spin

20. What are minimum temperature and maximum storage time for a unit of frozen RBCs?
    a. –65° C for 5 years
    b. –85° C for 10 years
    c. –65° C for 10 years
    d. –80° C for 10 years

21. How many platelets must be obtained in a plateletpheresis in order to meet acceptance criteria?
    a. 5.5×10^{10}
    b. 3.3×10^{11}
    c. 5.0×10^{11}
    d. 3.0×10^{11}

22. How are sterile connecting devices used?
    a. connecting a leukocyte removal filter to RBCs
    b. preparing small aliquot transfusions for infants
    c. connecting platelets for pooling
    d. all of the above

23. What are the temperature limits for shipping RBCs?
    a. 1° C to 6° C
    b. 1° C to 10° C
    c. 2° C to 8° C
    d. 20° C to 24° C

24. The pH and platelet count of four bags of platelets were tested at the end of the allowable storage period. Which of the following results is an acceptable product?
    a. 5.5×10^9 and pH of 6.5
    b. 6.0×10^{10} and pH of 7.0
    c. 4.2×10^{11} and pH of 5.9
    d. 3.0×10^{10} and pH of 6.2

25. Although ABO compatibility is preferred, ABO incompatibility is acceptable for which of the following components?
    a. PF24
    b. cryoprecipitated AHF
    c. apheresis granulocytes
    d. apheresis platelets

Answers to Study Questions can be found on page 387.

Ⓔ Additional student resources, including review questions, a laboratory manual, and case studies, can be found on the Evolve website.

REFERENCES

1. Food and Drug Administration: *Code of federal regulations*, title 21 CFR parts 600–799. Washington, DC, 2010, US Government Printing Office (revised annually).
2. Food and Drug Administration: *Code of federal regulations*, title 21, CFR parts 210 and 211. Washington, DC, 2010, US Government Printing Office (revised annually).
3. ISBT-128. http://www.iccbba.org. Accessed December 2015.
4. Levitt J: *Standards for blood banks and transfusion services*, ed 29, Bethesda, MD, 2014, AABB.
5. Fung MK, editor: *Technical manual*, ed 18, Bethesda, MD, 2014, AABB.
6. King KE: *Blood transfusion therapy: a physician's handbook*, ed 10, Bethesda, MD, 2011, AABB.
7. AABB Association Bulletin #10-06-Information Concerning Platelet Additive Solutions (Updated table), November 22, 2010.
8. Biomet (Citra Labs). Rejuvesol Solution—Package Insert. October 2013. http://dailymed.nlm.nih.gov. Accessed December 2015.
9. AABB/America's Blood Centers/American Red Cross, Armed Services Blood Program: *Circular of information for the use of human blood and blood components*, revised Nov 2014, Bethesda, MD, 2014.
10. Food and Drug Administration: *Guidance for industry: use of sterile connecting devices in blood bank practices* (November 22, 2000), Rockville, MD, 2000, CBER Office of Communication, Outreach and Development.
11. Yazer MH, Cortese-Hassett A, Triulzi DJ: Coagulation factor levels in plasma frozen within 24 hours of phlebotomy over 5 days of storage at 1 to 6 C, *Transfusion* 48:2525, 2008.
12. Scott E, Puca K, Heraly J, et al.: Evaluation and comparison of coagulation factor activity in fresh-frozen plasma and 24 hour plasma at thaw and after 120 hours of 1 to 6° C storage, *Transfusion* 49:1584, 2009.
13. Chenoweth A: Revisiting the 30-minute rule (again!): how to return and reissue blood components safely, *AABB News* 14(2):4–5, 2012.

TRANSFUSION THERAPY IN SELECTED PATIENTS

CHAPTER OUTLINE

LEARNING OBJECTIVES

On completion of this chapter, the reader should be able to:

1. Describe the pathophysiology of acute blood loss and massive transfusion therapy.
2. Discuss the transfusion requirements and causes of bleeding during cardiac surgery.
3. Describe the unique hematologic problems and transfusion therapy issues associated with neonates.
4. Discuss the pathophysiology and transfusion needs of patients with sickle cell disease, thalassemia, and autoimmune disease.
5. Explain the transfusion requirements of oncology patients.
6. Compare and contrast hematopoietic progenitor cells collected from bone marrow, peripheral blood, and cord blood.

7. Describe the transfusion support issues unique to these transplants.
8. List the acquired and congenital disorders of hemostasis and the appropriate transfusion support for each type of disorder.
9. Compare and contrast the various applications of therapeutic apheresis and the conditions and diseases associated with its use.
10. Discuss the transfusion issues unique to patients with chronic renal disease and how the use of erythropoietin affects the need for RBC transfusions.
11. List several alternatives for transfusion of blood products and their application in patients with coagulation deficiencies, trauma patients, and oncology patients.

One of the benefits of blood component therapy is the ability to provide transfusion support for patients with many unique hematologic problems. For some patients, such as patients with sickle cell disease, the need for this support extends throughout their life. For others, it may be an urgent requirement resulting from surgery or trauma. By understanding the clinical conditions, laboratory professionals can appreciate the focus and urgency of laboratory testing and the value of the transfused blood components. Blood components, their therapeutic value, and the indications for their use were reviewed in the previous chapter. This chapter summarizes the pathophysiology of selected clinical conditions that commonly require transfusion support. These selected clinical conditions are complicated and multifaceted areas of concern for physicians. This chapter presents each topic in an introductory manner. For more detailed information, additional reading would be recommended.

SECTION 1
TRANSFUSION PRACTICES

MASSIVE TRANSFUSION

Rapid blood loss, or **hemorrhage,** initiates a series of complicated physiologic responses that involve the nervous, hormonal, and circulatory systems. Acute blood loss of greater

Hemorrhage: bleeding through ruptured or unruptured blood vessel walls

than 30% of the total blood volume may lead to hemorrhagic shock.[1] Characteristic signs and symptoms of hemorrhage that has progressed to hypovolemia are presented in Fig. 16.1.[2] Severe hemorrhage affects electrolyte metabolism and oxygen transport, which ultimately increases the heart rate and the stress on internal organs. Prolonged hypotension and extensive tissue damage can result in cardiac and renal failure. Disseminated intravascular coagulation (DIC) is a pathologic activation of the coagulation cascade that may be caused by hemorrhage, which would further complicate the ability to control bleeding.

The most important goal in treating acute blood loss is the restoration of blood volume through the control of hemorrhage and replacement of intravascular volume to prevent shock. Infusing sufficient fluid volume to maintain adequate blood flow and blood pressure for tissue oxygenation is critical. Initial symptoms that occur with blood loss are the result of volume depletion, not depletion of red cells. Immediate volume restoration with crystalloid or colloid solutions is usually recommended.[3] Other methods to control hemorrhagic shock include early transfusion of plasma, platelets, and red blood cells (RBCs) with minimal crystalloid use.[2]

The patient's vital signs, clinical situation, and hematocrit determine the requirement and urgency for RBC support. Fig. 16.1 lists priorities in acute blood loss.

RBC transfusions in trauma situations are usually urgent and of significant quantity. Adverse metabolic effects can occur from the transfusion of large quantities of stored blood over a short period. One blood volume exchanged within 3 to 4 hours can cause significant acute metabolic disturbances, such as citrate toxicity, hypothermia, and coagulation abnormalities. Coagulation abnormalities resulting in microvascular bleeding have been attributed to the dilution of platelets and coagulation factors occurring with two or three volume exchanges and the consumption of platelets and coagulation factors from extensive bleeding. Antifibrinolytics such as tranexamic acid may be administered to control bleeding.[3] Complications resulting from massive transfusion are summarized in Table 16.1.

Massive transfusion is defined as the replacement of one or more blood volumes within 24 hours whether in an infant or in an adult patient.[2] Average blood volume is estimated

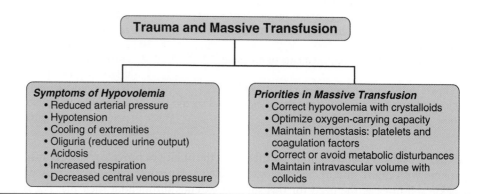

Fig. 16.1 Symptoms associated with hypovolemia and transfusion goals in treatment of trauma patients. (From Roback JD, editor: *Technical manual*, ed 17, Bethesda, MD, 2011, AABB.)

TABLE 16.1	Complications in Massive Transfusion	
PROBLEM	**CAUSES**	**TREATMENTS**
Microvascular hemorrhage	Dilution of coagulation factors and platelets Hypotension Consumption of coagulation factors Platelet consumption	Platelets Fresh frozen plasma to control defined deficiencies of coagulation factors Control hypotension
Citrate toxicity	Decrease in ionized calcium from anticoagulants in blood products	Slower infusion Calcium replacement if severe
Hypothermia	Rapid infusion of blood products	High-flow blood warmers

at 5000 mL, or about 10 units of whole blood, in a 70-kg adult. During massive transfusion, the blood products transfused in 24 hours approximate or exceed the recipient's original blood volume. At that point, the recipient's circulation contains almost entirely transfused blood and essentially no autologous blood. The original patient's sample no longer represents the circulating blood of the patient. The transfusion service physician should have a policy clearly in place dictating what is done under these circumstances and at what point a new "recipient" sample is required. Some policies indicate that the serologic immediate-spin crossmatch is eliminated for a time, and ABO-identical donor units are simply tagged and issued. If a computer crossmatch protocol was in place, this step would be unnecessary. When clinically significant antibodies are involved, all units issued must be negative for antigens, but an immediate-spin crossmatch still could be used.

The other consideration in massive transfusion is the availability of group O, D-negative blood and then of ABO-identical blood. When the blood group is established, group-specific blood should be transfused to protect the supply of group O, D-negative blood. Inventory management is critical during massive transfusion protocols. Blood bank staff are continuously monitoring and ordering to ensure an adequate blood inventory. However, if ABO-identical blood falls below the established critical inventory level, ABO-compatible blood may be used. In the case of group AB, A, or B recipients, group O RBCs may always be substituted. Group AB recipients could receive group A or group B but not both; group A is routinely used because of its greater availability in comparison to group B or AB. Refer to Table 16.2 for a review of these concepts.

ABO-identical blood should be issued after subsequent testing with a posttransfusion sample. This sample is tested to detect the presence of passive (free) ABO antibodies due to the massive transfusion. The safe point of switching the patient back to the original ABO phenotype is to evaluate if the levels of **passively transfused** anti-A, anti-B, or anti-A,B are sufficient to cause incompatibility with group A, B, or AB donors. In the selection of the D-antigen type, women of childbearing age who test negative for the D antigen should only receive D-negative blood. Other D-negative recipients may receive D-positive blood during massive transfusion protocols. However, approximately 50% to 70% of D-negative individuals subsequently develop anti-D, which sharply diminishes flexibility in a subsequent bleeding episode.[4] Scan the QR code to read a case report of massive transfusion.

Passively transfused: when an antibody is transferred to the recipient from the plasma portion of a blood product during transfusion

CARDIAC SURGERY

During cardiopulmonary bypass surgery, the patient's blood circulates through an oxygenating pump outside the patient's body. Extracorporeal circulation causes a decrease in platelet function and numbers. Coagulation factors are also decreased because of hemodilution and the cell salvage instrument. Hypothermia, transfusion of shed blood, thrombin-mediated activation, and residual heparin also affect hemostasis.[5] Table 16.3 summarizes risk factors unique to cardiac surgery that increase the need for component support perioperatively and postoperatively.

During and after surgery, heparin causes the activated partial thromboplastin time to be prolonged. The thrombin time confirms heparin excess. Treatment with a protamine sulfate, rather than fresh frozen plasma (FFP), corrects heparin excess.[3] FFP is usually indicated only for factor deficiency or massive transfusion from severe bleeding during

TABLE 16.2	ABO Compatibility for Whole Blood, Red Blood Cells, and Plasma Transfusions

RECIPIENT	DONOR		
ABO PHENOTYPE	WHOLE BLOOD	RED BLOOD CELLS	PLASMA
A	A	A, O	A, AB
B	B	B, O	B, AB
AB	AB	AB, A, B, O	AB
O	O	O	O, A, B, AB

TABLE 16.3   Risk Factors for Bleeding during Cardiac Surgery
• Time on pump
• Age of patient
• Previous cardiac surgery
• Type of surgery: valve replacement, CABG, or both
• Preoperative medications: aspirin and anticoagulant
• Heparin effect
• Hypothermia decreases platelet function

CABG, Coronary artery bypass graft.
From Despotis G, Eby C, Lubin DM: A review of transfusion risks and optimal management of perioperative bleeding with cardiac surgery, *Transfusion* 48:2S, 2008.

cardiac surgery. The effects of preoperative warfarin therapy also contribute to postoperative blood loss and transfusion requirements.[6]

A patient blood management approach in cardiac surgery was reported to reduce the number of RBC, FFP, and platelet transfusions.[7] Implementation of a meticulous surgical technique to reduce blood loss, more restrictive RBC transfusion threshold, and clinical management of the coagulation process for transfusion of platelets, plasma, or cryoprecipitate contributed to the reduction of transfusions.

NEONATAL AND PEDIATRIC TRANSFUSION ISSUES

Neonatal and pediatric transfusion issues are significantly different from transfusion issues for adults because of the small size, hemoglobin changes, and erythropoietin response in early infancy. Ill neonates are more likely to receive RBC transfusions than other hospitalized patients.[2]

Fetal red cells contain hemoglobin F, which has a higher affinity or ability to bind oxygen. This affinity is important during the intrauterine period because it enhances oxygen transfer from maternal red cells to fetal red cells. The switch from fetal to adult hemoglobin begins at about 32 weeks' gestation.[2] For this reason, preterm infants have a higher level of fetal hemoglobin than infants born at term. The change from fetal to adult hemoglobin occurs during the first few weeks of life, and the process causes a condition called physiologic anemia of infancy. In a full-term infant of normal birth weight, this change is well tolerated; however, treatment is often necessary in an infant born prematurely with low birth weight.

In addition to the shift in hemoglobin, the need for frequent laboratory tests contributes to the need for transfusions. **Iatrogenic blood loss** is the most common indication of transfusion in a preterm infant with low birth weight. Newborns do not compensate for hypovolemia as well as adults do.

Erythropoietin in adults is released from the kidneys in response to diminished oxygen delivery. This growth factor triggers the bone marrow to increase RBC production and release more erythrocytes into the circulation. Erythropoietin production in an infant is believed to be triggered in the liver, which is less responsive to low levels of oxygen. The lower level of response to low oxygen levels (hypoxia) protects the infant from generating an excess of red cells (polycythemia) during fetal life but does not allow an effective response to anemia in the immature infant.

The response of a newborn to hypothermia is also different from an adult's response. The metabolic rate, hypoglycemia, and acidosis can cause the temporary cessation of breathing, or apnea. Apnea may lead to hypoxia, hypotension, and cardiac arrest. For this reason, a monitored blood warmer is often used to administer RBCs, especially for exchange transfusions.

The ability to metabolize citrate and potassium is more difficult for newborns because of their immature liver and kidneys. For this reason, washed or fresh red cells are often indicated for newborns. Because potassium increases when blood is irradiated, washing irradiated RBCs is also recommended. The transfusion of fresh blood to maximize the level of 2,3-diphosphoglycerate (2,3-DPG), which decreases during storage, is also important in newborns because of their limited ability to compensate for hypoxia.

Iatrogenic blood loss: blood loss caused by treatment (eg, collection of samples for testing)

TABLE 16.4	Transfusion Issues Unique to Neonates

- Change from fetal to adult hemoglobin causing physiologic anemia of infancy
- Iatrogenic blood loss
- Decreased response of erythropoietin
- Low tolerance of hypothermia
- Greater risk of cytomegalovirus infection due to immature immune system
- Decreased ability to metabolize citrate and potassium
- Decreased ability to restore 2,3-DPG in older units

2,3-DPG, 2,3-Diphosphoglycerate.

In neonates, hemoglobin levels less than 13 g/dL during the first 24 hours of life initiates a clinical consideration of an RBC transfusion.[1] In addition, an ill neonate's loss of approximately 10% blood volume will trigger a transfusion evaluation. RBC transfusions are usually given in small volumes prepared from (pediatric) multiple-pack systems that allow preparation of several aliquots from a single donor unit. Infants do not form red cell antibodies during the first 4 months of age; therefore crossmatching is not indicated. Antigen-negative blood must be provided if a maternal red cell alloantibody is detected in infant's plasma or serum. Group O, ABO-identical, or ABO-compatible blood that is D-negative or the same as the infant's D type can be released during the first 4 months of age. However, before non–group O RBCs can be issued, testing of the infant's plasma or serum is required to detect passively acquired maternal anti-A or anti-B and should include an antiglobulin phase.[2]

Transfusion-transmitted cytomegalovirus (CMV) is a risk to preterm infants weighing less than 1200 g who are born to seronegative mothers or to mothers whose CMV status is unknown.[2] This risk is avoided by providing irradiated CMV antibody–negative blood to neonates. In addition, leukocyte reduction, using highly efficient leukocyte removal filters, is recommended because CMV resides within the white blood cell.[2]

Transfusion issues unique to infants are summarized in Table 16.4. Familiarity with these problems provides an understanding of the transfusion requirements for preterm newborns and infants.

Crossmatching of Infants Younger Than 4 Months Old

As stated, infants younger than 4 months old are unable to produce their own antibodies. Antibodies detected in the circulation of a newborn are maternal in origin. At 4 to 6 months of age, infants begin producing their own ABO antibodies and become capable of producing antibodies, if immunologically sensitized because of RBC transfusion.

Initial compatibility testing in an infant must include a pretransfusion ABO and D phenotype on a sample obtained from the neonate.[8] Because ABO antibodies are not present in an infant, performance of ABO reverse grouping is not required. ABO and D typing does not need to be repeated for the duration of the current admission or until the neonate reaches the age of 4 months, whichever is sooner. An initial antibody screen needs to be performed on either the infant's or mother's sample. If the antibody screen is negative, however, no crossmatches or repeat screens are needed during the current admission.

If the initial antibody screen is negative, it is unnecessary to crossmatch donor red cells for initial or subsequent transfusions.[8] In addition, the antibody screen does not need to be repeated for the duration of the current admission or until the neonate reaches the age of 4 months, whichever is sooner. If clinically significant maternal antibodies are found, the blood for transfusion needs to be antigen-negative or compatible in an antiglobulin crossmatch.[8] Crossmatching continues until maternal antibody is no longer detected in the infant's serum.

Donor centers customarily prepare pediatric units for infants by dividing a full unit of RBCs into sterile portions. The transfusing facility may subdivide these pediatric units further if necessary. The use of syringes for transfusions to infants is also a common practice. This method transfuses the same donor blood repeatedly to the infant if multiple transfusions are needed, limiting the exposures to undetected diseases and immunologic stimuli from donor blood.

TRANSPLANTATION

The transfusion service and blood bank provide support for transplantation of organs and hematopoietic progenitor cells (HPCs). This section describes the issues related to transplantation and transfusion requirements.

Organ Transplantation

Transfusion support for kidney, heart, lung, and liver transplants is varied because of the nature of the organ. Because of the complicated surgery on a vascular organ, liver transplantation can be associated with massive hemorrhage. Hemostatic problems are major complications of liver transplant because of the role the liver plays in the synthesis of factors and clearance of coagulation inhibitors. The preexisting liver disease also contributes to the excessive bleeding during the procedure. Historically, significant blood loss at the time of liver transplantation has been treated with large autologous transfusions of RBCs, FFP, platelets, and cryoprecipitate. Drugs are given along with the blood products to help correct metabolic and coagulation abnormalities. However, the trend in liver transplantation demonstrates a decreased blood loss and decreased usage of blood products.[9] There are even some reports of transplantation without the use of blood products. Operative techniques and drugs that minimize blood loss have contributed to minimizing transfusion requirements.

Heart and heart–lung transplants have similar product usage as cardiac surgery, outlined previously. Cardiopulmonary bypass can affect hemostasis secondary to hypothermia, heparin use, priming fluid used for the bypass instrument, and duration of surgery. A ventricular assist device (VAD), which is a relatively new therapeutic option for patients with end-stage heart failure awaiting heart transplant, can also contribute to the need for transfusion support during implantation and after surgery.[10] Platelet and hemostatic defects may be caused by the surface of the device and flow characteristics. Transfusions should be limited to leukocyte-reduced components to avoid sensitization and increase complications caused by human leukocyte antigen (HLA) antibodies.

Graft survival is enhanced with HLA-matched donor–recipient combinations, particularly if the recipient is demonstrating HLA antibodies. Graft survival of renal transplants is also improved with living donors. ABO compatibility is critical to the success of vascularized grafts, such as livers, kidneys, and hearts, but it is not essential in tissue grafts, such as bone, heart valves, skin, and cornea.

In the 1970s kidney allografts had a higher rate of survival if patients were given blood transfusions before undergoing renal transplantation. In the 1980s transfusion to induce tolerance in patients before kidney transplants was replaced by the use of cyclosporine for immunosupression.[4] Erythropoietin has also reduced the need for transfusion in patients with kidney disease. When RBCs are transfused, leukocyte-reduced products have decreased the alloimmunization to HLA antigens. When a potential kidney transplant recipient develops HLA antibodies, obtaining a compatible kidney becomes more challenging.

Table 16.5 provides a current estimate of average blood components transfused during transplant surgery.[11]

TABLE 16.5	Average Blood Components Transfused during Transplant Surgery		
ORGAN	**RBCs**	**PLATELETS**	**FFP**
Kidney	0–1	0	0
Heart	2–4	1	1–6
Liver (85%)	3	2	6–12
Liver (15%)	20	6	30

RBCs, Red blood cells; *FFP,* fresh frozen plasma,
Source: Sarkar RS, Philip J, Yadav P. Transfusion medicine and solid organ transplant—Update and review of some current issues. *Med J Armed Forces India* 69:162, 2013

Hematopoietic Progenitor Cell Transplantation

HPCs can be obtained from bone marrow, peripheral blood, and cord blood. Diseases treated with HPCs include, but are not limited to, congenital immune deficiencies, aplastic anemia, leukemia, lymphoma, and Hodgkin disease. Table 16.6 is a partial list of diseases treated with HPC transplants.[2] Close allele-level HLA matching between the donor and the recipient of HPC transplants is important to avoid transplant rejection and graft-versus-host disease (GVHD). Preformed HLA antibodies and ABO compatibility are less important in HPC transplants compared with solid-organ transplants.

HPC transplants have become a common medical procedure performed in many tertiary care centers. Hematopoietic cells contain stem cells that are capable of self-renewal. Progenitor cells have the ability to differentiate into committed blood cell lineages. Both cell lines are collectively termed hematopoietic progenitor cells. Progenitor cell transplants can be allogeneic (genetically unrelated), syngeneic (identical twin), or autologous (self). They can be derived from the following:

- Bone marrow—HPC(M)
- Peripheral blood stem cells (PBSC): mononuclear cell fraction separated by apheresis equipment—HPC(A)
- Umbilical cord blood—HPC(C)

The choices for stem cell sources are influenced by availability, optimal HLA matching, patient size, and donor safety. The trends in source transplants are illustrated in Fig. 16.2. HPCs collected by apheresis, also referred to as peripheral progenitor cells, are the most common type of HPC at the present time. HPCs collected by apheresis are used for autologous, **syngeneic**, and allogeneic transplantation. **Colony-stimulating factors** can be given to donors to mobilize sufficient stem cells before apheresis. Collections by apheresis avoid the risk of general anesthesia needed for bone marrow harvest. HPCs derived from cord blood have been successfully used in pediatric patients and, to some extent, adults lacking an HLA-matched adult donor.[1] The decision to use bone marrow over PBSCs is influenced by the type of disease, age of the patient, and risk status of the disease. Comparisons of outcomes related to HPC source consider the speed of engraftment, rate of chronic GVHD, disease relapse, and long-term graft survival. Retrospective reviews have suggested that improved overall survival may be obtained with HPCs collected from bone marrow for pediatric patients with aplastic anemia or acute leukemia.[1] Scan the QR code to read a case report of HPC transplant.

Autologous HPC transplantation is primarily used as a "rescue" in patients who have received myelodepletion therapy (chemotherapy or radiation or both). Patients receive

Syngeneic: possessing an identical genotype, as in monozygotic twins

Colony-stimulating factors: cytokines that promote the expansion and differentiation of bone marrow stem cells and progenitor cells

TABLE 16.6	Therapeutic Uses for Hematopoietic Progenitor Cell Transplantation
Congenital Immune Deficiencies	
Severe combined immunodeficiency disease	
Wiskott-Aldrich syndrome	
Aplastic anemia	
Fanconi anemia	
Hemoglobinopathies	
Thalassemia	
Sickle cell disease	
Malignancy	
Acute leukemia	
Non-Hodgkin and Hodgkin lymphoma	
Myelodysplastic/myeloproliferative disorders	
Multiple myeloma	
Other	
Paroxysmal nocturnal hemoglobinuria	
Multiple sclerosis	

From Fung MK, editor: *Technical manual,* ed 18, Bethesda, MD, 2014, AABB.

Transplants—Distribution of Cell Source

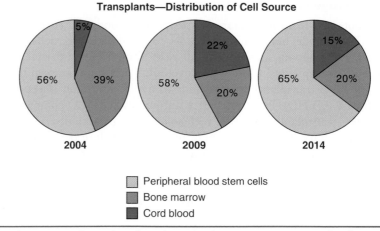

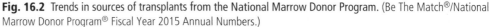

Fig. 16.2 Trends in sources of transplants from the National Marrow Donor Program. (Be The Match®/National Marrow Donor Program® Fiscal Year 2015 Annual Numbers.)

hematopoietic growth factors before collection by leukapheresis, and the HPCs are stored frozen or nonfrozen for later infusion after chemotherapy.

HLA-matched related or unrelated donors provide the source of allogeneic HPCs. HLA class I and class II matching is necessary to reduce the risk of posttransplant GVHD and to achieve successful engraftment. In addition, allogeneic HPCs provide a "graft-versus-leukemia" effect, in which the T cells in the graft attack residual tumor cells. These immune cells also attack the healthy tissues of the patient, however, often causing GVHD. Some studies have shown a decreased incidence of GVHD when transplanting HPCs derived from cord blood, despite the lower HLA-matching requirements of HPC(C).[12]

Graft-versus-Host Disease

In HPC transplantation, the risk of GVHD increases if HLA matching is not close. Allele-level matching is important for optimal graft survival. GVHD occurs when grafted immunocompetent cells from a donor mount an immune response against the host tissue. Because recipients of HPC transplants are often immunosuppressed to allow for donor cell engraftment, this process is more likely to occur. Clinical symptoms include rash, diarrhea, and jaundice, and GVHD can be fatal if left untreated.

GVHD can also occur in immunocompromised patients receiving blood components from related donors. Irradiation of blood components from first-degree relatives is performed to reduce the risk of transfused leukocytes proliferating in the host. Irradiation prevents the viable leukocytes within the blood component from replicating. Leukocyte reduction of the blood components is insufficient to avoid GVHD because even small amounts of leukocytes can proliferate in a susceptible patient. However, in the case of a bone marrow recipient, irradiation of the progenitor cells is contraindicated because viable stem cells that are able to proliferate are essential. Blood products such as platelets and red cells that are often provided to patients after a bone marrow transplant should be irradiated.

Transfusion Support for HPC Transplants

Before transplantation, transfusion support includes leukocyte-reduced blood products to avoid HLA alloimmunization, CMV infection, and febrile reactions. After transplantation, patients usually require extensive platelet and RBC support for about 2 weeks. If the ABO types of the transplant recipient and donor are not matched, careful monitoring by the transfusion service is necessary, and additional RBC support may be necessary if hemolysis occurs.

Because of the immunosuppression of the patients undergoing transplants, the risk of GVHD is serious. Blood products received after transplant should be irradiated. The progenitor cell product must never be irradiated, however, because this would prevent engraftment.[2] CMV infection is another potential problem because of immunosuppression,

| TABLE 16.7 | Example of ABO Component Selection in ABO Unmatched Hematopoietic Progenitor Cell Transplants |

		ABO BLOOD GROUP SELECTION EXAMPLE IN ( )	
TYPE OF INCOMPATIBILITY	TRANSPLANT STAGE	RED BLOOD CELLS COMPATIBLE WITH:	PLASMA/PLATELETS/ CRYOPRECIPITATE COMPATIBLE WITH:
Major (Example: "A" donor to "O" recipient)	Pretransplant	Recipient (O)	Donor (A)
	Transplant	Recipient (O)	Donor (A)
	Recipient antibodies detected (anti-A and anti-B)	Recipient (O)	Donor (A)
	Recipient antibodies no longer detected	Donor (A)	Donor (A)
Minor (Example: "O" donor to "A" recipient)	Pretransplant	Donor (O)	Recipient (A)
	Transplant	Donor (O)	Recipient (A)
	Recipient antibodies detected (anti-A and anti-B)	Donor (O)	Recipient (A)
	Recipient antibodies no longer detected	Donor (O)	Donor (O)
Major and Minor (Example: "B" donor to "A" recipient)	Pretransplant	Group O	Group AB
	Transplant	Group O	Group AB
	Recipient antibodies detected (anti-A and anti-B)	Group O	Group AB
	Recipient antibodies no longer detected	Donor (B)	Donor (B)

Modified from Roback JD, editor: *Technical manual,* ed 17, Bethesda, MD, 2011, AABB.

which can be avoided with leukocyte-reduced or seronegative blood products. The progenitor cell product should never be administered through a leukocyte reduction filter.

Although HLA compatibility is crucial in the successful engraftment of myelosuppressed patients with HPCs, ABO compatibility is not essential. The early committed and uncommitted cells in these transplants do not possess A, B, and H antigens (ABH antigens). Approximately 40% to 50% of HPC transplants are ABO incompatible.[13] Delayed red cell engraftment may occur after a major ABO-incompatible transplant (eg, group "A" HPC donor to group "O" recipient). Hemolysis can be observed after a minor ABO-incompatible transplant (eg, group "O" HPC donor to group "A" recipient). RBC and plasma components transfused after transplant of ABO mismatched grafts must be compatible with the blood type of both the donor and the recipient. An example of the component selected for ABO-incompatible HPC is given in Table 16.7. During the last phase of transplantation, when the forward and reverse typing is consistent with the donor's ABO group, components should be compatible with the donor's type. Scan the QR code for more information about transplants at the National Marrow Donor Program.

Chimerism, or a dual-cell population, may occur if the recipient's hematopoietic cells survive and subsequently coexist with cells produced by the donor's transplanted HPCs.

THERAPEUTIC APHERESIS

Therapeutic apheresis involves the removal of abnormal cells, plasma, or plasma constituents from a patient's blood to achieve a clinical benefit. The replacement fluid varies with the condition and the portion that is removed. The goal may be to:

- Supply an essential substance that is absent
- Reduce the quantity of a particular antibody
- Modify mediators of inflammation
- Clear immune complexes
- Replace cellular elements

This section will summarize a therapeutic plasma exchange (TPE), a red cell exchange, and photopheresis.

A TPE is performed using plasmapheresis and is the most common therapeutic apheresis procedure. The patient's plasma is removed with the return of the cellular components. During the TPE, a large volume of plasma is removed and replaced with a physiologic fluid to maintain the body's normal fluid dynamics. TPE has been a very effective treatment for diseases that involve abnormalities of the immune system such as systemic lupus erythematosus, Guillain-Barré syndrome, and Waldenström macrglobulinemia.[14]

A red cell exchange, or erythrocytapheresis, removes the patient's red cells and returns the patient's plasma and platelets along with compatible allogeneic donor RBCs. The procedure is often used with sickle cell disease to decrease the red cells with hemoglobin S. The reduction of these red cells reduces the complications associated with the disease.[14] Red cell exchange treatment can also be performed in cases of malaria and *Babesia* infections to reduce the parasite load.

Photopheresis is a type of therapeutic apheresis where the buffy coat layer is collected and treated with 8-methoxypsoralen and exposed to ultraviolet (UV) light. The cells are reinfused after treatment. This therapeutic apheresis has been shown to prevent leukocyte replication and to induce apoptosis, or programmed cell death. The application of photopheresis is standard treatment for some forms of cutaneous T-cell lymphoma and is under investigation for conditions such as autoimmune disease, solid-organ transplant rejection, and GVHD after HPC transplantation.[3]

Conditions treated with therapeutic apheresis are listed in Table 16.8. Replacement fluids include crystalloids, albumin, plasma protein fraction, plasma cryoprecipitate reduced, or FFP in the case of a plasma exchange. When exchanges necessitate FFP or RBC support, large quantities are used; this requires adequate planning and communication with the transfusion service. A more comprehensive description of therapeutic apheresis is found in the AABB *Technical Manual*.[2]

ONCOLOGY

A patient undergoing chemotherapy or radiation treatment for cancer relies on the transfusion service for many blood products. Cancers involve the unregulated, uncontrolled growth and division of a clone of cells from an organ or tissue. These clones of

TABLE 16.8	Indications for Therapeutic Apheresis	
PROCEDURE	**INDICATION**	**PURPOSE**
Plasmapheresis	Guillain-Barré syndrome	Remove pathologic autoantibody
	Myasthenia gravis	
	Multiple sclerosis	Remove HLA alloantibody
	Goodpasture syndrome	Remove inhibitor of ADAMTS-13 and large vWF multimers
	Antibody-mediated rejection (kidney)	
	Desensitization before transplant	
	Thrombotic thrombocytopenic purpura	Remove excessive protein or immune complexes
	Cryoglobulinemia	
	Hyperviscosity in monoclonal gammopathies	
Cytapheresis	Sickle cell disease	Reduce hemoglobin S, replace with hemoglobin A
	Hyperleukocytosis	
	Babesiosis, malaria	Remove excessive leukocytes Reduce parasites
Photopheresis	Allograft rejection	Inhibit lymphocyte proliferation and cause induction of apoptosis
	Cutaneous T-cell lymphoma	
	Chronic graft-versus-host disease	

HLA, Human leukocyte antigen; *vWF,* von Willebrand factor.
Modified from Fung MK, editor: *Technical manual,* ed 18, Bethesda, MD, 2014, AABB.

cells may divert the blood supply or crowd out the organ or neighboring organs, causing undesirable effects to the patient. Depending on where the abnormal cell originated, the cells, if left untreated, migrate and take hold in other organ systems in a process known as **metastasis.** The oncology patient in the hospital undergoes a combined treatment regimen of physical (radiation) and chemical therapies (chemotherapy) mostly targeting rapid cellular division. Most chemotherapeutic agents act by slowing down or inhibiting DNA replication or interfering with the DNA translation process to stop cell division.

Metastasis: the spread of a cancer or other disease from one organ or part to another not directly connected with it

Chemotherapeutic agents are not specific for the target cancer or clone of cells. Epithelial cells of the gastrointestinal tract and germinal epithelium of the hair follicles are also particularly affected. In the bone marrow, hematopoietic cells that differentiate into megakaryocytes, erythrocytes, and leukocytes are reduced. As treatment progresses, platelet, leukocyte, hemoglobin, and hematocrit levels decrease. The most common complications are bleeding, anemia, and infection. Careful monitoring of laboratory results and clinical conditions associated with bleeding and anemia is necessary to determine component therapy. Transfusion support with irradiated blood products after intensive chemotherapy and radiation therapy is common. In some patients, multiple platelet transfusions often cause refractoriness or the inability to achieve therapeutic increments.[2] When alloantibodies to HLA antigens cause refractoriness, HLA-matched platelets may become necessary. Colony-stimulating factors are becoming more widely used in preventing infection and bleeding risks associated with chemotherapy (Table 16.9).

CHRONIC RENAL DISEASE

Patients undergoing dialysis have many hematologic complications that necessitate transfusion therapy, usually in the form of RBC support. The high uremic content of the blood leads to altered red cell shapes; this prevents the red cells from traversing the spleen without being removed prematurely by macrophages, which results in hemolytic anemia. The act of dialysis itself causes a shearing of the red cells, which can contribute to hemolysis. These patients fail to produce sufficient levels of erythropoietin because of the nonfunctioning kidney; therefore an erythrocyte production problem adds to the anemic condition.

TABLE 16.9	Alternatives to Transfusion	
FACTOR	**NAMES**	**POTENTIAL USES**
Erythropoietin	EPO rHuEPO (prepared by recombinant technology)	Chronic renal failure Preoperative for orthopedic and cardiac surgery Cancer patients undergoing active myelosuppressive therapy
Colony-stimulating factors (CSFs)	Granulocyte CSF Granulocyte-macrophage CSF Recombinant interleukin-11	Decreased infection in patients undergoing chemotherapy Congenital agranulocytosis Acute leukemia Myelodysplastic syndrome Aplastic anemia in children Autologous and allogeneic bone marrow transplant Cancer patients with thrombocytopenia
DDAVP	Desmopressin	Promotes hemostasis by promoting release of vWF For hemophilia A, von Willebrand disease, and some platelet function disorders

EPO, Erythropoietin; *rHuEPO,* human recombinant erythropoietin; *vWF,* von Willebrand factor.
From Bandarenko N, editor: *Blood transfusion therapy: A physician's handbook,* ed 11, Bethesda, MD, 2014, AABB.

TABLE 16.10	Contributing Factors Associated with Anemia in Chronic Renal Disease
CAUSE	EFFECT
Elevated uremia	Altering of RBC shape, causing their premature removal
Dialysis procedure	Shearing of RBCs
Low erythropoietin level	Low RBC production

RBC, Red blood cell.

Factors contributing to transfusion needs in dialysis patients are summarized in Table 16.10. Careful monitoring of hemoglobin and hematocrit levels that contribute to clinical symptoms determines transfusion therapy. The use of recombinant erythropoietin has significantly reduced the need for transfusion; however, in acute anemia, RBC transfusions are required. Transfusions are usually given while the patient is on dialysis equipment to reduce the need for an additional venipuncture. Leukocyte-poor RBCs are the preferred product to avoid the development of HLA antibodies, which increase the challenge of finding a compatible kidney.

HEMOLYTIC UREMIC SYNDROME AND THROMBOTIC THROMBOCYTOPENIC PURPURA

Hemolytic uremic syndrome (HUS) and thrombotic thrombocytopenic purpura (TTP) are classified together because of the numerous overlaps in clinical symptoms.[15] Clinical symptoms include:
• Thrombocytopenia
• Microangiopathic hemolytic anemia
• Renal dysfunction
• Central nervous system involvement

In both of these disorders, damage to the vessel endothelium has activated and consumed platelets and coagulation proteins, causing microthrombi to become lodged in the kidney. TTP is caused by a deficiency or antibody to a protease (ADAMTS13) that cleaves von Willebrand factor (vWF). Therapeutic plasma exchange removes the inhibitor and large-molecular-weight multimers, while simultaneously replacing the deficient enzyme.[1] HUS usually affects young children, often before their first year. It usually follows a severe viral infection, bacterial gastroenteritis, or treatment with certain cytotoxic drugs. Therapeutic plasma exchange is standard or acceptable supportive treatment for HUS caused by an autoantibody to factor H or complement factor deficiencies.[1]

ANEMIAS REQUIRING TRANSFUSION SUPPORT

Sickle Cell Anemia

Hemoglobinopathy: genetic (inherited) disorder of hemoglobin, the oxygen-carrying protein of the red blood cells

Sickle cell disease (hemoglobin S) is one of the most prevalent **hemoglobinopathy.** The anomaly is a structural variant in the β-chain of the hemoglobin molecule. An amino acid substitution in the sixth position of the polypeptide chain (valine for glutamic acid) on the surface of the molecule alters the solubility of the hemoglobin molecule. The hemoglobin polymerizes under conditions of low oxygen, causing the characteristic sickling of the cell. Blockage of the microvasculature by these sickled cells causes "sickle cell crisis," which results in endothelial damage, thrombosis, and pain. The red cells have a decreased life span, which causes symptomatic and compensated anemia. Serious complications include stroke, acute chest syndrome, and multiorgan failure. The only currently approved treatment with the ability to cure patients with sickle cell disease is hematopoietic stem cell transplantation. The treatment is recommended in patients who have the most severe complications.[16] Scan the QR code to see photographs of sickle cells compared with normal red cells.

TABLE 16.11	Clinical Indications for Transfusion in Patients with Sickle Cell Disease

Acute anemia resulting from:
    Bleeding
    Infection
    Increased hemolysis
    Sequestration of cells in the spleen and liver
Prevention of:
    Stroke—reduce sickling, which blocks blood vessels
    Recurrent pain episodes owing to sickling in joints

From Hillyer CD, Silverstein LF, Ness PM, et al: *Blood banking and transfusion medicine*, ed 2, Philadelphia, 2007, Elsevier.

Hemoglobin and hematocrit values can be low in sickle cell patients before they become symptomatic. Clinical symptoms associated with pulmonary or cardiac insufficiency indicate when RBC transfusions are necessary. In situations of severe pain and crisis, automated RBC exchange is often therapeutic (therapeutic red cell exchange). Indications for transfusion are summarized in Table 16.11.

Because a patient with sickle cell disease requires RBC support throughout most of his or her life, the potential for alloantibody production is high. Of chronically transfused patients with sickle cell disease, 25% to 30% develop red cell alloantibodies.[1] One reason for the high rate of alloantibodies is that the red cell antigens from the predominantly white donor populations are different from the antigens inherited in the black population. To avoid this problem, many hematologists consider partially phenotypically matched (C, E, and K) antigens early in the treatment of sickle cell disease and extend the matching of additional antigens to Fy, Jk, and S once patients develop a red cell antibody to reduce the chance of potentially life-threatening delayed hemolytic transfusion reactions. Encouraging support from black donors in areas where sickle cell disease is common is extremely beneficial for meeting the need for phenotypically matched RBCs. Antigen typing using molecular methods has become more common for transfusion support for sickle cell patients to ensure proper identification of variants or rare phenotypes in both patients and donors.

Iron overload is also a complication of repeated transfusions. A unit of RBCs contains approximately 250 mg of iron. The body can only excrete an average of 1 mg of iron a day. Iron overload can be treated with oral iron chelators, which bind to iron in the body and help remove it. Another way to avoid iron accumulation is red cell exchange therapy.

Iron overload: a delayed nonimmunologic transfusion reaction resulting from multiple transfusions with obligate iron load in transfusion-dependent patients

Thalassemia

Thalassemia is also an inherited syndrome characterized by deficient or abnormal hemoglobin structures. Thalassemia is caused by a deficiency in hemoglobin α-chain or β-chain production that ranges from mild to severe. Total absence of α-chain synthesis is fatal in utero, and absence of the β-chain is classified as thalassemia major. To compensate for the resulting anemia, hematopoietic tissue expands, resulting in bone deformities and liver and spleen enlargement. Transfusion in children is helpful to suppress ineffective erythropoiesis and avoid early complications of the disease.[3] Hemoglobin and hematocrit values are monitored to determine whether transfusion therapy is needed.

With both sickle cell disease and thalassemias, iron chelation therapy must accompany blood transfusions to prevent the iron overload these patients experience because of multiple transfusions.[17] The iron from normal red cell kinetics is neutralized, but the constant addition of cells of varying ages creates the iron excess that becomes stored and detrimental to many tissues.

Immune Hemolytic Anemias

As previously discussed in the textbook, the immune hemolytic anemias belong to a group of disorders characterized by decreased survival of the erythrocyte because of antibody coating the red cell membrane. This sensitization causes red cell removal from the circulation much sooner than the average 120 days. These disorders are summarized for a review:

- *Autoimmune hemolytic anemia:* The antibody is reacting to a self-antigen on the red cell, which results in removal by the spleen and causes anemia. Based on serologic tests, this category is further divided into cold or warm autoantibodies.
- *Drug-induced hemolytic anemia:* Either the drug is adsorbed directly onto the membrane or the drug–antibody combination becomes adsorbed onto the red cell. Some medications can also induce the production of an autoantibody.
- *Alloimmune hemolytic anemia:* This occurs when RBC clearance from alloantibodies is produced against transfused RBCs or against fetal cells in hemolytic disease of the fetus and newborn.

HEMOSTATIC DISORDERS

Hemostatic disorders are characterized in two ways:

- A decrease in or lack of production of one or more of the coagulation proteins
- Normal production but an abnormal structure resulting in a nonfunctioning protein

The most common hereditary bleeding disorder is von Willebrand disease.[18] Quantitative or qualitative abnormalities of vWF cause bleeding. vWF is necessary for platelets to adhere to endothelium. It is also needed for factor VII for correct functioning and maintenance of adequate levels.

Other factor deficiencies are hemophilia A (factor VIII deficiency) and hemophilia B (factor IX deficiency). Factors VIII and IX are needed for the intrinsic pathway of fibrin formation. The clinical characteristics of coagulation deficiencies are prolonged bleeding, bleeding into joints, and subcutaneous bleeds. Most of the hemostatic disorders are treated with factor concentrates or **DDAVP.**

DDAVP: stimulates the release of preformed factor VII and von Willebrand factor from cellular stores; used to treat type 1 von Willebrand disease

Cryoprecipitated AHF is used only in urgent situations when the preferred concentrate is not available.[18] The administration of coagulation factor concentrate has the potential to cause the development of antibodies, or "inhibitors," to one or more of the factors, which can lead to further bleeding episodes.

DIC is an acquired hemostasis disorder in which the patient develops microthrombi, which consume platelets and fibrinogen when the coagulation mechanism is turned on inappropriately, such as during surgery, massive blood loss, or after a snake or insect bite. Strands of fibrin trap platelets. Patients with DIC can spontaneously bleed or form a thrombus. The therapy, as with all other secondary manifestations, is to determine and treat the cause while stabilizing the patient. Scan the QR code for more information on hemotherapy.

SECTION 2
ALTERNATIVES TO TRANSFUSION

Blood is a limited resource and contains risks associated with transfusion-transmitted diseases and adverse reactions. For this reason, ongoing research exists to substitute blood products with safer, more effective, and more readily available products. Tables 16.9, 16.12, and 16.13 summarize three categories of these substitutes for blood, which include hematopoietic growth factors, blood derivatives, and volume expanders. More details regarding these products can be found in *Blood Transfusion Therapy: A Physician's Handbook,* published by the AABB.

Essential components or factors involved in the coagulation cascade, including factor VIII, factor IX, and antithrombin concentrate, are blood derivatives formulated to replace factor deficiencies and overcome the effects of inhibitors. The risk of transmitting viruses has been reduced with the use of heat and detergent treatment. Recombinant technology has eliminated the risk; however, these products are substantially more costly. The factor concentrates are sterile, stable, and lyophilized, which makes administration more convenient than administration of blood components. Each product differs in terms of purity and the method of treatment to inactivate potential viruses. The clotting factor per milligram of protein or specific activity differs and is indicated on the vial.

TABLE 16.12	Alternatives to Transfusion: Factor Concentrates	
DERIVATIVE	**GENERAL INFORMATION**	**INDICATIONS**
Factor VIIa	Recombinant (rFVIIa)	Bleeding episodes in patients with an inhibitor to factor VIII or factor IX and congenital factor VII deficiency
Factor VIII	Produced by recombinant (rFVIII) or fractionation of pooled human plasma (AHF)	Hemophilia A von Willebrand disease
Factor IX	Produced by recombinant and plasma-derived sources	Hemophilia B
Prothrombin Complex Concentrate	Crude preparations of factor IX that contain other vitamin K–dependent factors	Factor II, IX, and X deficiency Warfarin overdose
Antithrombin Concentrate	Inhibitor of coagulation; prepared from pooled plasma	Hereditary antithrombin deficiency
Protein C Concentrate	Inhibitor of coagulation	Congenital protein C deficiency

AHF, Antihemophilic factor.
From Bandarenko N, editor: *Blood transfusion therapy: A physician's handbook,* ed 11, Bethesda, MD, 2014, AABB.

TABLE 16.13	Alternatives to Transfusion: Volume Expanders		
TYPE	**NAME**	**CONTENT**	**USE**
Crystalloids	Normal saline Ringer's lactate	Na^+ and Cl^- ions in water K^+, Ca^{2+} ions, and lactate	Shock from hemorrhage and burns
Colloids	Hydroxyethyl starch (HES)	Synthetic polymer: amylopectin in saline	Prolonged intravascular volume expansion
	Dextran	Polymerized glucose in dextrose or saline	
	PPF: plasma protein fraction (5%)	83% albumin and 17% globulin	
	Albumin (25% or 5%)	96% albumin and 4% globulin	Also used as a replacement fluid for therapeutic plasma exchange

From Bandarenko N, editor: *Blood transfusion therapy: A physician's handbook,* ed 11, Bethesda, MD, 2014, AABB.

Volume expanders include crystalloids and colloids. These products are usually dispensed by the pharmacy rather than the transfusion service and are used with or in place of blood for hypovolemia.

Hematopoietic growth factors stimulate the bone marrow to produce erythrocytes, platelets, and leukocytes for patients with chronic anemia and various conditions causing low cell counts. Their uses for patients undergoing chronic transfusions and renal dialysis and patients undergoing chemotherapy have been well documented.

CHAPTER SUMMARY

Transfusion therapy provides patients with the correct component of critical value for many types of diseases and conditions. Targeted blood component therapy wants to minimize blood exposure and the subsequent risks of adverse transfusion complications. Transfusion support for selected patients discussed in this chapter is summarized in the following table.

SUMMARY OF TRANSFUSION SUPPORT

Disease or Condition	Problem	Transfusion Therapy
Massive transfusion	Risk of hypovolemic shock	Crystalloids, colloids, Plasma, RBCs
Cardiac surgery	Heparin; hypothermia; platelet destruction	RBCs, Platelets, plasma
Premature infant	Iatrogenic blood loss; hemoglobin F; low erythropoietin response	Leukocyte-reduced, CMV antibody negative reduced-risk products irradiated RBCs <7 days old
Liver transplant	Low levels of vitamin K–dependent factors; bleeding	RBCs, FFP, Platelets, Cryoprecipitated AHF
Progenitor cell transplant	Immunosuppression; irradiation of bone marrow	Irradiated and leukocyte-reduced Platelets and RBCs
Oncology	Chemotherapy and irradiation treatment reduce red cell and platelet production	Leukocyte-reduced platelets and RBCs; colony-stimulating factors
Chronic renal disease	Unable to produce erythropoietin; red cell damage from dialysis and increases in uremia	Erythropoietin; leukocyte-reduced RBCs
TTP and HUS	Platelet and coagulation factors are consumed	Therapeutic apheresis, FFP, and RBCs
Sickle cell anemia	Chronic red cell destruction from sickling of cells	RBCs, phenotypically matched to avoid alloantibody production
Hemostatic disorders	Factor deficiencies: von Willebrand disease, hemophilia A and B	Factor derivatives specific for factor that is lacking

RBC, Red blood cell; CMV, cytomegalovirus; FFP, fresh frozen plasma; AHF, antihemophilic factor; TTP, thrombotic thrombocytopenic purpura; HUS, hemolytic uremic syndrome.

CRITICAL THINKING EXERCISES

Exercise 16.1

A trauma patient in the emergency department has received 6 units of group O D-negative RBCs by emergency release. A sample was obtained and sent to the blood bank, and the physician has requested 10 additional units of type-specific RBCs.
1. What are some potential problems in determining an ABO/D type?
2. At what point will the sample from this patient not reflect his own red cells?

Exercise 16.2

A 68-year-old man is undergoing a second cardiac surgery to replace a valve. He has been in surgery 4 hours, and there has been a recent request for platelets, RBCs, and FFP.
1. What are the potential problems that this patient may be experiencing?
2. What factors make this type of surgery a challenge?

Exercise 16.3

A 4-day-old premature infant has been using small aliquots of RBCs. The parents of the infant would like to donate blood for their child.
1. Can the parents be potential donors?
2. What special requirements are necessary for RBC transfusion during the neonatal period?
3. Are crossmatches required?
4. Why is blood from first-degree relatives considered a transfusion risk?
5. What procedure is required to make blood products from family members safer?

Exercise 16.4

A kidney dialysis center requested 2 leukocyte-reduced RBC units stat for a patient with a 7 g/dL hemoglobin. The center is an outpatient clinic, and three other stat orders for preoperative procedures need to be completed before the shift ends. The technologist fills the order, but would like to know why the request did not come earlier.

1. What are the unique transfusion needs of kidney dialysis patients?
2. Why was this transfusion request ordered as a STAT?
3. Does erythropoietin eliminate the need for all RBC transfusions for renal patients?
4. What contributes to the anemia in renal dialysis patients?

Exercise 16.5

The oncology unit has requested that platelets be available for a patient scheduled to undergo chemotherapy for breast cancer. The request for leukocyte-reduced apheresis platelets is common and often extends for a week or more every 2 to 3 days.
1. Why is this product necessary for this patient?
2. What are potential problems associated with platelet transfusions with regard to antibodies?

Exercise 16.6

A sample from a 4-year-old sickle cell patient was sent to the blood bank with a request for 2 units of phenotypically matched RBCs. The patient needs to be phenotyped, and a unit needs to be located.
1. Why are closely matched RBCs important for this child?
2. Will it be difficult to find RBCs for this patient?

STUDY QUESTIONS

1. What disease has been treated effectively using plasmapheresis?
   a. TTP
   b. hemolytic disease of the newborn
   c. sickle cell disease
   d. renal disease

2. Why is it difficult to find compatible blood for patients with autoimmune disease?
   a. potential of underlying alloantibodies
   b. positive DAT
   c. reactive eluate
   d. hemolysis in the serum

3. What infant age period does not require a crossmatch procedure before transfusion?
   a. the first 4 months
   b. the first 6 months
   c. the first year
   d. an indefinite period if a parent's blood is used

4. Select the example of a crystalloid solution used to treat hypovolemia.
   a. PPF
   b. albumin
   c. Ringer's lactate
   d. HES solution

5. How are hemophilia A patients treated for bleeding?
   a. cryoprecipitated AHF
   b. FFP
   c. RBCs
   d. factor VIII

6. Select common complications of chemotherapy from the list.
   a. bleeding
   b. infection
   c. anemia
   d. all of the above

7. Where is erythropoietin produced in the adult for stimulation of red cell proliferation?
   a. bone marrow
   b. liver
   c. kidneys
   d. spleen

8. What factors are compensated for in the transfusion of RBCs to a neonate?
   a. iatrogenic blood loss
   b. hemoglobin F
   c. insufficient erythropoiesis
   d. all of the above

9. ABO-compatible organ transplants are *not* critical in which of the following transplants?
   a. kidneys
   b. liver
   c. heart
   d. bone marrow

10. What colony-stimulating factor can reduce infection while undergoing chemotherapy?
    a. erythrocytes
    b. megakaryocytes
    c. granulocytes
    d. lymphocytes

Answers to Study Questions can be found on page 387.

Ⓔ Additional student resources, including review questions, a laboratory manual, and case studies, can be found on the Evolve website.

REFERENCES

1. Roback JD, editor: *Technical manual*, ed 17, Bethesda, MD, 2011, AABB.
2. Fung MK, editor: *Technical manual*, ed 18, Bethesda, MD, 2014, AABB.
3. Bandarenko N, editor: *Blood transfusion therapy: A physician's handbook*, ed 11, Bethesda, MD, 2014, AABB.
4. Issitt PD, Anstee DJ: *Applied blood group serology*, ed 4, Durham, NC, 1998, Montgomery Scientific.
5. Despotis G, Eby C, Lubin DM: A review of transfusion risks and optimal management of perioperative bleeding with cardiac surgery, *Transfusion* 48:2S, 2008.
6. Sobel M, NcNeill PM: Diagnosis and management of intraoperative and postoperative hemostatic defects. In Rossi EC, Simon TL, Moss GS, editors: *Principles of transfusion medicine*, Baltimore, 1991, Williams & Wilkins.
7. Gross I, Seifert B, Hofmann A, et al.: Patient blood management in cardiac surgery results in fewer transfusions and better outcomes, *Transfusion* 55:1075, 2015.
8. Levitt J: *Standards for blood banks and transfusion services*, ed 29, Bethesda, MD, 2014, AABB.
9. Olcese V, Shapiro R. Transfusion requirements in liver transplantation. http://emedicine.medscape.com/article/431573-overview. Accessed December 2015.
10. Livingston ER, et al.: Increased activation of the coagulation and fibrinolytic systems leads to hemorrhagic complications during left ventricular assist implantation, *Circulation* 94(Suppl 9):II227, 1996.
11. Sarkar RS, Philip J, Yadav P: Transfusion medicine and solid organ transplant—Update and review of some current issues, *Med J Armed Forces India* 69:162, 2013.
12. Laughlin MJ, Eapen M, Rubinstein P, et al.: Outcomes after transplantation of cord blood or bone marrow from unrelated donors in adults with acute leukemia, *N Engl J Med* 351:2276, 2004.
13. Daniel-Johnson J, Schwartz J: How do I approach ABO-incompatible hematopoietic progenitor cell transplantation? *Transfusion* 51(6):1143, 2011.
14. Harmening DM: *Modern blood banking and transfusion practices*, ed 6, Philadelphia, 2012, FA Davis.
15. Hillyer CD, Silverstein LF, Ness PM, et al.: *Blood banking and transfusion medicine*, ed 2, Philadelphia, 2007, Elsevier.
16. Harley MN: Current treatments and prospective therapies to manage sickle cell disease, *Lab Med* 44:e92, 2013.
17. AABB: *Circular of information for the use of human blood and blood components*, 2013. www.aabb.org.
18. McCullough J: *Transfusion medicine*, ed 2, Philadelphia, 2005, Elsevier.

Answers to Study Questions

Chapter 1
1. c   2. d   3. b   4. a   5. c   6. d   7. c   8. a   9. b   10. a   11. c   12. b   13. c   14. b   15. a   16. d   17. d   18. a   19. d   20. b

Chapter 2
1. d   2. a   3. b   4. c   5. d   6. a   7. b   8. a   9. c   10. a   11. a   12. e   13. b   14. c   15. c   16. a   17. b   18. b   19. c   20. c   21. d   22. c   23. b   24. c   25. c

Chapter 3
1. a   2. b   3. a   4. c   5. d   6. c   7. b   8. c   9. a   10. b   11. d   12. a   13. b   14. a   15. c

Chapter 4
1. d   2. b   3. d   4. b   5. a   6. a   7. c   8. a   9. c   10. a   11. d   12. c   13. c   14. b   15. c   16. c   17. b   18. c   19. b   20. d

Chapter 5
1. c   2. d   3. a   4. d   5. a   6. d   7. c   8. c   9. c   10 b   11. c   12. d   13. a   14. d   15. c   16. a   17. b   18. d   19. c   20. b

Chapter 6
1. d   2. a   3. d   4. a   5. a   6, b   7. b   8. d   9. d   10. a   11. a   12. b   13. a   14. c   15. a   16. a   17. b   18. d   19. c   20. b

Chapter 7
1. c   2. c   3. a   4. a   5. d, e, g   6. d   7. d   8. c   9. d   10. c   11. a   12. d   13. a   14. c   15. d   16. a   17. c   18. c   19. b   20. d   21. c   22. b   23. b   24. b   25. d   26. a   27. d   28. b   29. d   30. c

Chapter 8
1. a   2. c   3. d   4. d   5. a   6. c   7. c   8. c   9. b   10. d   11. a   12. c   13. c   14. d   15. c

Chapter 9
1. b   2. c   3. d   4. a   5. b   6. c   7. c   8. b   9. d   10. a   11. c   12. d   13. c   14. c   15. F   16. F   17. F   18. F   19. F   20. F   21. T   22. F   23. F   24. T   25. T

Chapter 10
1. a   2. c   3. c   4. d   5. d   6. c   7. b   8. a   9. d   10. a   11. T   12. T   13. T   14. F   15. T   16. T   17. T

Chapter 11
1. a   2. c   3. d   4. b   5. d   6. c   7. a   8. a   9. c   10. c   11. a   12. b   13. d   14. a   15. b   16. a   17. b   18. b   19. a   20. c   21. d   22. d

Chapter 12
1. c   2. b   3. c   4. c   5. d   6. c   7. a   8. a   9. a   10. c   11. d   12. a   13. b   14. d   15. c   16. c   17. b   18. a   19. a   20. b   21. a   22. a   23. a   24. b   25. c

Chapter 13
1. TD   2. A   3. A   4. TD   5. PD   6. TD   7. A   8. A   9. PD   10. PD   11. PD   12. PD   13. d   14. b   15. c   16. T   17. F   18. F   19. T   20. F

Chapter 14
1. d   2. d   3. d   4. b   5. a   6. b   7. d   8. b   9. a   10. c

Chapter 15
1. d   2. b   3. e   4. f   5. a   6. g   7. c   8. e   9. d   10. b   11. a   12. c   13. f   14. d   15. g   16. a   17. c   18. b   19. d   20. c   21. d   22. d   23. b   24. b   25. b

Chapter 16
1. a   2. a   3. a   4. c   5. d   6. d   7. c   8. d   9. d   10. c

Glossary

AABB professional organization that accredits and provides educational and technical guidance to blood banks and transfusion services

ABO antibodies anti-A, anti-B, and anti-A,B; patients possess the ABO antibody to the ABO antigen lacking on their red cells (eg, group A individuals possess anti-B)

ABO discrepancy occurs when ABO phenotyping of red cells does not agree with expected serum testing results for the particular ABO phenotype

acanthocytosis presence of abnormal red cells with spurlike projections in the circulating blood

acquired agammaglobulinemia absence of gamma globulin and antibodies associated with malignant diseases such as leukemia, myeloma, or lymphoma

acquired hypogammaglobulinemia lower-than-normal levels of gamma globulin in the blood associated with malignant diseases (chronic leukemias and myeloma) and immunosuppressive therapy

acute hemolytic transfusion reaction complication of transfusion associated with intravascular hemolysis, characterized by rapid onset with symptoms of fever, chills, hemoglobinemia, and hypotension; major complications include irreversible shock, renal failure, and disseminated intravascular coagulation

acute reaction reaction occurring within 24 hours of transfusion

adsorption procedure that uses red cells (known antigens) to remove red cell antibodies from a solution (plasma or antisera); group A red cells can remove anti-A from solution

adverse transfusion reaction undesirable response by a patient to the infusion of blood or blood products

affinity strength of the binding between a single antibody and an epitope of an antigen

affinity maturation process of somatic mutations in the immunoglobulin gene causing the formation of variations in the affinity of the antibody to the antigen; B cells with the highest affinity are "selected" for the best fit, and the resulting antibody is stronger

agglutination visible clumping of particulate antigens caused by interaction with a specific antibody

agglutinogen term referring to a group of antigens or factors that are agglutinated by antisera

alleged father man accused of being the biological father; the putative father

alleles alternative forms of a gene at a given locus

alloantibodies antibodies with specificities other than self; stimulated by transfusion or pregnancy

allogeneic cells or tissue from a genetically different individual

allogeneic adsorption use of blood from a genetically different individual, such as reagent or donor cells that have been phenotyped for common red cell antigens to remove alloantibodies and autoantibodies

allogeneic donation donation for use by the general patient population

alternative pathway activation of complement that is initiated by foreign cell-surface constituents

amniocentesis process of withdrawal of amniotic fluid by aspiration for the purpose of analysis

amorphic describes a gene that does not express a detectable product

amplicon short sequence of amplified DNA flanked on either end by the primer

anamnestic response secondary immune response

anaphylatoxins complement split products (C3a, C4a, and C5a) that mediate degranulation of mast cells and basophils, which results in smooth muscle contraction and increased vascular permeability

angioedema rapid swelling of the dermis, subcutaneous tissue, mucosa, and submucosal tissues

antenatal time period before birth

antepartum period between conception and onset of labor, used with reference to the mother

antibody glycoprotein (immunoglobulin) that recognizes a particular epitope on an antigen and facilitates clearance of that antigen

antibody identification procedure that determines the identity of a red cell antibody detected in the antibody screen by reacting serum with commercial panel cells

antibody potentiators reagents or methods that enhance or speed up the antibody–antigen reaction

antibody screen test test to determine the presence of alloantibodies

antigen foreign molecules that bind specifically to an antibody or a T-cell receptor

antigenic determinants sites on an antigen that are recognized and bound by a particular antibody or T-cell receptor (also called epitope)

antigram profile of antigen phenotypes for each donor used in the manufacture of commercially supplied screening and panel cells

antithetical opposite antigens encoded at the same locus

apheresis method of blood collection where whole blood is removed from a donor or patient and separated into components; one or more of the components are retained, and the remainder is returned to the donor or patient

apheresis donation donation of a specific component of the blood; parts of the whole blood that are not retained are returned to the donor

apheresis platelets apheresis procedure in which the platelets are removed from a donor, and the remaining red cells and plasma are returned

audit trail record-keeping system that re-creates every step in the manufacturing process

autoadsorption attachment of the patient's antibodies to the patient's own red cells and subsequent removal from the serum

autoantibodies antibodies to self-antigens

autocontrol testing a person's serum with his or her own red cells to determine whether an autoantibody is present

autoimmune hemolytic anemia immune destruction of autologous (self) red cells

autologous cells or tissue from self

autologous donation donation by a donor reserved for the donor's later use

autosomes chromosomes other than the sex chromosomes

avidity overall strength of reaction between several epitopes and antibodies; depends on the affinity of the antibody, valency, and noncovalent attractive forces

B lymphocytes (B cells) lymphocytes that mature in the bone marrow, differentiate into plasma cells when stimulated by an antigen, and produce antibodies

B(A) phenotype group B individual who acquires reactivity with anti-A reagents in ABO red cell testing; in these individuals, the B gene transfers trace amounts of the immunodominant sugar for the A antigen and the immunodominant sugar for the B antigen

babesiosis microscopic parasites that infect red blood cells and are spread by the bite of infected *Ixodes scapularis* ticks

biphasic hemolysin antibody, such as the Donath-Landsteiner antibody, that requires a period of cold and warm incubations to bind complement with resulting hemolysis

bivalent having a combining power of two

blocking phenomenon D antigen phenotype on cord blood may be falsely negative if the cells are heavily coated with maternal anti-D; usually associated with D-positive cord blood and maternal anti-D

blood bank collects, processes, stores, and transports human blood intended for transfusion

blood group systems groups of antigens on the red cell membrane that share related serologic properties and genetic patterns of inheritance

blood warmer medical device that prewarms donor blood to 37° C before transfusion

Bombay phenotype rare phenotype of an individual who genetically has inherited *h* allele in homozygous manner; individual's red cells lack H and ABO antigens

bradykinin potent vasodilator of the kinin family

calculated panel-reactive antibody (CPRA) estimates the percentage of donors that would be incompatible with a transplant candidate, based on the candidate's antibodies to human leukocyte antigens

carbohydrates simple sugars, such as monosaccharides and starches (polysaccharides)

cation an ion or group of ions with a positive charge

cell separation technique used to separate transfused cells from autologous or patient cells

change control system to plan and implement changes in procedures, equipment, policies, and methods to increase effectiveness and prevent problems

chemokines group of cytokines involved in the activation of white blood cells during migration across the endothelium

chemotactic movement of cells in the direction of the antigenic stimulus

chimerism mixture of donor and recipient cell populations following hematopoietic stem cell transplants

chloroquine diphosphate a reagent that removes IgG antibody from red cells; used when patient has a positive direct antiglobulin test to obtain autologous red cells for phenotype determination

chromosomes structures within the nucleus that contain DNA

chronic granulomatous disease inherited disorder in which the phagocytic white blood cells are able to engulf, but not kill, certain microorganisms

cis two or more genes on the same chromosome of a homologous pair

classical pathway activation of complement that is initiated by antigen–antibody complexes

Clinical Laboratory Improvement Amendment act to ensure that laboratory tests are consistently reliable and of high quality

clinical significance antibodies capable of causing decreased survival of transfused cells as in a transfusion reaction; have been associated with hemolytic disease of the fetus and newborn

clinically insignificant antibody that does not shorten the survival of transfused red cells or has been associated with hemolytic disease of the fetus and newborn

clone family of cells or organisms with genetically identical constitutions

closed system collection of blood in a sterile blood container

Code of Federal Regulations publication from the Food and Drug Administration outlining the legal requirements of blood banking facilities

codominant equal expression of two different inherited alleles

cold alloantibodies red cell antibodies specific for other human red cell antigens that typically react at or below room temperature

cold autoantibodies red cell antibodies specific for autologous antigens that typically react at or below room temperature

cold hemagglutinin disease autoimmune hemolytic anemia produced by an autoantibody that reacts best in colder temperatures (<37° C)

colony-stimulating factors cytokines that promote the expansion and differentiation of bone marrow stem cells and progenitor cells

compatibility testing all steps in the identification and testing of a potential transfusion recipient and donor blood before transfusion in an attempt to provide a blood product that survives in vivo and provides its therapeutic effect in the recipient

competency assessment evaluation of the employee's ability and knowledge to perform a procedure or skill

competitive ELISA enzyme-linked immunosorbent assay (ELISA) technique used to determine the presence or quantity of an antigen or antibody; in this test, a lower absorbance indicates detection of the marker

complement system group of serum proteins that participate in an enzymatic cascade, ultimately generating the membrane attack complex that causes lysis of cellular elements

components parts of whole blood that can be separated by centrifugation; consist of red blood cells, plasma, cryoprecipitated antihemophilic factor, and platelets

compound antigens distinct antigens produced when the same gene encodes two other antigens

congenital agammaglobulinemia genetic disease characterized by the absence of gamma globulin and antibodies in the blood

congenital hypogammaglobulinemia genetic disease characterized by reduced levels of gamma globulin in the blood

constant regions nonvariable portions of the heavy and light chains of an immunoglobulin

cord blood whole blood obtained from the umbilical vein or artery of the fetus

cordocentesis procedure that punctures the umbilical vein at the point of placental insertion and aspirates a sample of fetal blood

corrected count increment relative increase in platelet count adjusted for the number of platelets transfused and the size of the patient

crossing over exchange of genetic material during meiosis between paired chromosomes

crossmatch procedure that combines donor's red cells and patient's serum to determine the serologic compatibility between donor and patient

cryoprecipitate blood component recovered from a controlled thaw of fresh frozen plasma; the cold-insoluble precipitate is rich in coagulation factor VIII, von Willebrand factor, factor XIII, and fibrinogen

cryoprotective solution added to protect against cell damage that occurs at or below freezing temperatures

current Good Manufacturing Practices (cGMPs) methods used in, and the facilities or controls used for, the manufacture, processing, packing, or holding of a drug (including a blood product) to ensure that it meets safety, purity, and potency standards

cytokines secreted proteins that regulate the activity of other cells by binding to specific receptors; they can increase or decrease cell proliferation, antibody production, and inflammation reactions

deacetylating removal of the acetyl group (CH_3CO-)

dengue fever a mosquito-borne viral infection; the infection causes flu-like illness and occasionally develops into a potentially lethal complication called severe dengue

delayed reaction reaction occurring more than 24 hours after transfusion

diastolic blood pressure filling of the heart chamber; the second sound heard while taking a blood pressure

differential adsorption adsorption or attachment of antibodies in the serum to specific known antigens, usually to different aliquots of red cells

differential DAT test that uses monospecific anti-IgG and monospecific anti-C3d/anti-C3b reagents to determine the cause of a positive direct antiglobulin test (DAT) with polyspecific antiglobulin reagents

direct antiglobulin test test used to detect antibody bound to red cells in vivo

direct exclusion exclusion of paternity when a child has a trait that neither parent shows

directed donation donation reserved for use by a specific patient

DNA probe short sequence of DNA complementary to the area being identified and attached to a marker (usually fluorescent) that can be read by an instrument such as a flow cytometer

document control plan for the management of all documents in an organization that addresses the design, responsibility, storage, removal, and revision of all records, forms, and procedures

Dolichos biflorus plant lectin with specificity for the A1 antigen

dominant gene product expressed over another gene

dosage effect stronger agglutination when a red cell antigen is expressed from homozygous genes

DDAVP stimulates the release of preformed factor VII and von Willebrand factor from cellular stores; used to treat type 1 von Willebrand disease

EDTA-glycine acid a reagent that removes IgG antibody from red cells; similar function as chloroquine diphosphate

eluate antibody removed from red cells to be used for antibody identification

elution procedure that dissociates antigen–antibody complexes on red cells; freed IgG antibody is tested for specificity

enhancement media reagents that enhance or speed up the antibody–antigen reaction

epitopes single antigenic determinants; functionally, the parts of the antigen that combine with the antibody

Epstein-Barr virus (EBV) also called human herpesvirus 4 (HHV-4) and is one of eight viruses in the herpes family

erythroblastosis fetalis also called hemolytic disease of the fetus and newborn

extravascular hemolysis red cell destruction by phagocytes residing in the liver and spleen, usually by IgG opsonization

false-negative test result that incorrectly indicates a negative reaction (lack of agglutination); an antigen–antibody reaction has occurred but is not detected

false-positive test result that incorrectly indicates a positive reaction (presence of agglutination or hemolysis); no antigen–antibody reaction occurred

fetomaternal hemorrhage escape of fetal cells into the maternal circulation, usually occurring at the time of delivery

Food and Drug Administration U.S. agency responsible for the regulation of the blood banking industry and other manufacturers of products consumed by humans

fresh frozen plasma (FFP) blood component prepared from whole blood that contains only the plasma portion of whole blood and is frozen after separation to retain labile factors

gene segment of DNA that encodes a particular protein

genetic loci sites of a gene on a chromosome

genotype actual genetic makeup; determined by family studies or molecular typing

glycolipids compounds containing carbohydrate and lipid molecules

glycophorin glycoprotein that projects through the red cell membrane and carries many blood group antigens

glycoproteins compounds containing carbohydrate and protein molecules

glycosyltransferase enzyme that catalyzes the transfer of glycosyl groups (simple carbohydrate units) in biochemical reactions

graft-versus-host disease (GVHD) a disease caused by the reaction of mature T cells in the graft or transfused cells against alloantigens on host cells

granulocyte concentrates blood component collected by cytapheresis; contain a minimum of 1.0×10^{10} granulocytes

Group A with acquired B antigen group A_1 individual with diseases of the lower gastrointestinal tract, cancers of the colon and rectum, intestinal obstruction, or gram-negative septicemia who acquires reactivity with anti-B reagents in ABO red cell testing and appears as group AB

haplotype linked set of genes inherited together because of their close proximity on a chromosome

hapten small-molecular-weight particle that requires a carrier molecule to be recognized by the immune system

haptoglobin plasma protein that binds free hemoglobin and carries the molecule to the hepatocytes for further catabolism

heavy chains larger polypeptides of an antibody molecule composed of a variable and constant region; five major classes of heavy chains determine the isotype of an antibody

hematopoietic progenitor cell (HPC) type of stem cell committed to a blood cell lineage that is collected from marrow, peripheral blood, and cord blood and used to treat certain malignant diseases and congenital immune deficiencies

hematopoietic progenitor cell transplant replacement of hematopoietic stem cells derived from allogeneic bone marrow, peripheral stem cells, or cord blood to treat certain leukemias, immunodeficiencies, and hemoglobinopathies

hemoglobinopathy genetic (inherited) disorder of hemoglobin, the oxygen-carrying protein of the red blood cells

hemolysis lysis or rupture of the red cell membrane

hemolytic disease of the fetus and newborn (HDFN) condition caused by destruction of fetal or neonatal red cells by maternal antibodies

hemorrhage bleeding through ruptured or unruptured blood vessel walls

hemotherapy treatment of a disease or condition by the use of blood or blood derivatives

heterohybridomas hybrid cells formed by the fusion of the lymphocyte of one species with the myeloma cell of a different species

heterozygous two alleles for a given trait are different

hinge region portion of the immunoglobulin heavy chains between the Fc and Fab region; provides flexibility to the molecule to allow two antigen-binding sites to function independently

histamine compound that causes constriction of bronchial smooth muscle, dilation of capillaries, and decrease in blood pressure

homozygous two alleles for a given trait are identical

hybridize to attach a complementary sequence of DNA using the properties of complementary base pair sequencing

hybridomas hybrid cells formed by the fusion of myeloma cells and antibody-producing cells; used in the production of monoclonal antibodies

hydatid cyst fluid fluid obtained from a cyst of the dog tapeworm

hydrops fetalis edema in the fetus

iatrogenic blood loss blood loss caused by treatment, such as the collection of samples for testing

icterus pertaining to or resembling jaundice

ID-NAT individual donation (ID) screening—nucleic acid test (NAT)

idiopathic pertains to a condition without disease or recognizable cause

idiotope variable part of an antibody or T-cell receptor; antigen-binding site

immediate-spin interpretation of agglutination reactions immediately after centrifugation and without incubation

immediate-spin phases source antigen and source antibody used in immunohematologic testing are combined, immediately centrifuged, and observed for agglutination

immune complex complex of one or more antibody molecules bound to an antigen

immune-mediated reaction reactions involving antigen–antibody complexes, cytokine release, or complement activation

immunodominant sugar sugar molecule responsible for specificity

immunogen antigen in its role of eliciting an immune response

immunogenicity ability of an antigen to stimulate an immune response

immunoglobulin antibody; glycoprotein secreted by plasma cells that binds to specific epitopes on antigenic substances

immunohematology study of blood group antigens and antibodies

incompatible crossmatches occur when agglutination or hemolysis is observed in the crossmatch of donor red cells and patient serum, indicating a serologic incompatibility; the donor unit would not be transfused

in vitro reaction in an artificial environment, such as in a test tube, microplate, or column

in vivo reaction within the body

incidence the number of new disease cases that develop in a given period

independent assortment random behavior of genes on separate chromosomes during meiosis that results in a mixture of genetic material in the offspring

independent segregation passing of one gene from each parent to the offspring

indirect antiglobulin test test used to detect antibody bound to red cells in vitro

indirect ELISA enzyme-linked immunosorbent assay (ELISA) technique used to determine the presence or quantity of an antibody; also called EIA

indirect exclusion failure to find an expected marker in a child when the alleged father is apparently homozygous for the gene

intravascular hemolysis red cell hemolysis occurring within the blood vessels, usually by IgM activation of complement

iron overload a delayed nonimmunologic transfusion reaction resulting from multiple transfusions with obligate iron load in transfusion-dependent patients

ISBT 128 International Society of Blood Transfusion (ISBT) recommendations regarding the uniform labeling of blood products for international bar-code recognition by computers

ischemia decreased supply of oxygenated blood to an organ or body part

isotype one of five types of immunoglobulins determined by the heavy chain: IgM, IgG, IgA, IgE, and IgD

kappa chains one of the two types of light chains that make up an immunoglobulin

kinins group of proteins associated with contraction of smooth muscle, vascular permeability, and vasodilation

labile factors factors V and VIII, which are coagulation factors that deteriorate on storage

laboratory information system (LIS) interface allows the direct transfer of test results between the automated test system and an LIS, reducing errors commonly caused by manual transcriptions

lambda chains one of the two types of light chains that makes up an immunoglobulin

Landsteiner's rule rule stating that normal, healthy individuals possess ABO antibodies to the ABO blood group antigens absent from their red cells

lattice formation combination of antibody and a multivalent antigen to form crosslinks and result in visible agglutination

lecithin/sphingomyelin (L/S) ratio ratio of lecithin to sphingomyelin that indicates lung maturity

lectins plant extracts useful as blood banking reagents; they bind to carbohydrate portions of certain red cell antigens and agglutinate the red cells

light chains smaller polypeptides of an antibody molecule composed of a variable and constant region; two major types of light chains exist in humans (kappa and lambda)

Liley graph graph used to predict severity of hemolytic disease of the fetus and newborn during pregnancy by evaluation of the amniotic fluid

linkage disequilibrium occurrence of a set of genes inherited together more often than would be expected by chance

linked when two genes are inherited together by being very close on a chromosome

lipids fatty acids and glycerol compounds

look-back identification of persons who have received seronegative or untested blood from a donor subsequently found to be positive for disease markers

medical directors designated physicians responsible for the medical and technical policies of the blood bank

meiosis cell division in gametes that results in half the number of chromosomes present in somatic cells

membrane attack complex C5 to C9 proteins of the complement system that mediate cell lysis in the target cell

memory B cells B cells produced after the first exposure that remains in the circulation and can recognize and respond to an antigen faster

metastasis the spread of a cancer or other disease from one organ or part to another not directly connected with it

mitosis cell division in somatic cells that results in the same number of chromosomes

mixed-field agglutination agglutination pattern in which a population of the red cells has agglutinated and the remainder of the red cells is unagglutinated

mixed lymphocyte culture (MLC) in vitro reaction of T cells from one individual against major histocompatibility antigens on leukocytes from another individual; the technique measures the response of human leukocyte antigen class II differences between donor and recipient cells, usually through radioactive measurements of DNA synthesis; this test was historically used for compatibility and D (class II) antigen typing

monoclonal antibody made from single clones of B cells that secrete antibodies of the same specificity

mononuclear phagocyte system system of mononuclear phagocytic cells, associated with the liver, spleen, and lymph nodes, that clears microbes and damaged cells

monospecific AHG reagents reagents prepared by separating the specificities of the polyspecific antihuman globulin (AHG) reagents into individual sources of anti-IgG and anti-C3d/anti-C3b

MP-NAT minipools (MP) screening—nucleic acid test (NAT)

multiple myeloma malignant neoplasm of the bone marrow characterized by abnormal proteins in the plasma and urine

neonatal time period within the first 28 days after birth

neonatal alloimmune thrombocytopenia antibody destruction of a newborn's platelets caused by antibodies formed from prior pregnancies and directed to paternal antigens

neutralization blocking antibody sites, causing a negative reaction

non–immune-mediated reaction reactions that may be due to the component transfused, the patient's underlying condition, or the method of infusion

non–red blood cell stimulated immunologic stimulus for antibody production is unrelated to a red cell antigen

nonsecretor individual who inherits the genotype *sese* and does not express H soluble substance in secretions

nucleotide phosphate, sugar, and base that constitute the basic monomer of the nucleic acids DNA and RNA

null phenotypes absences of a particular blood group system from the red cell membrane

obligatory gene gene that should be inherited from the father to prove paternity

Occupational Safety and Health Administration (OSHA) U.S. agency responsible for ensuring safe and healthful working conditions

oligosaccharide chain chemical compound formed by a small number of simple carbohydrate molecules

one-stage enzyme technique antibody identification technique that requires the addition of the enzyme to the cell and serum mixture

open system collection or exposure to air through an open port that would shorten the expiration because of potential bacterial contamination

opsonin substance (antibody or complement protein) that binds to an antigen and enhances phagocytosis

_p_ value probability value; value that provides a confidence limit for a particular event

panagglutination antibody that agglutinates all red cells tested, including autologous red cells

parenterally by routes other than the digestive tract, including needle stick and transfusion

paroxysmal cold hemoglobinuria rare autoimmune disorder characterized by hemolysis and hematuria associated with exposure to cold

partial D D antigen that is missing part of its typical antigenic structure

passively transfused when an antibody is transferred to the recipient from the plasma portion of a blood product during transfusion

perinatal period extends from 28 weeks of gestation to 28 days after delivery

perinatally exposure before, during, or after the time of birth

phagocytic cells cells that engulf microorganisms, other cells, and foreign particles; including neutrophils, macrophages, and monocytes

phenotype observable expression of inherited traits

physiologic saline NaCl prepared in water to a concentration of 0.9%

phototherapy treatment of elevated bilirubin or other conditions with ultraviolet light rays

plasma blood component prepared from whole blood that contains only the plasma portion of whole blood and is frozen after separation

plasma cell antibody-producing B cell that has reached the end of its differentiating pathway

platelets a concentrate of platelets separated from a single unit of whole blood; should contain a minimum of 5.5×10^{10} platelets

plateletpheresis collection of platelets by apheresis

polyagglutination property of the cells that causes them to be agglutinated by naturally occurring antibodies found in most human sera; agglutination occurs regardless of blood type

polyclonal antiserum made from several different clones of B cells that secrete antibodies of different specificities

polymorphic genetic system that expresses two or more alleles at one locus

polyspecific AHG reagent contains both anti-IgG and anti-C3d antibodies and detects both IgG and C3d molecules on red cells

posttransfusion purpura antibody destruction of platelets after transfusion

postzone excess antigen causing a false-negative reaction

potency strength of an Ag-Ab reaction

prenatal time period before birth

prevalence the number of cases of a disease present in a particular population at a given time

preventive maintenance maintenance that maximizes the duration of the equipment or facility, decreases "downtime," and avoids unnecessary costly repairs

prewarming technique patient serum and test cells are prewarmed separately before combining to prevent reactions of cold antibodies binding at room temperature and activating complement

primary immune response immune response induced by initial exposure to the antigen

proteolytic enzymes enzymes that denature certain proteins

prozone excess antibody causing a false-negative reaction

Punnett square square used to display the frequencies of different genotypes and phenotypes among the offspring of a cross

rabbit erythrocyte stroma red cell membranes from rabbits used for adsorption of IgM antibodies such as anti-I

random access system devices or workstations are used for multiple occurrences of a given laboratory operation within the automated procedure

reaction phase observation of agglutination at certain temperatures, after incubation, or after the addition of antihuman globulin

receptors molecules on the cell surface that have a high affinity for a particular molecule, such as antibody, hormone, or drug

recessive trait expressed only when inherited by both parents

recipient patient receiving the transfusion

red cell stroma red cell membrane that remains after hemolysis

refractoriness unresponsiveness to platelet transfusions due to human leukocyte antigen–specific or platelet-specific antibodies or platelet destruction from fever or sepsis; responsiveness is measured by posttransfusion platelet counts

refractory unresponsive to platelet transfusions; responsiveness is measured by posttransfusion platelet counts

regulator gene gene inherited at another locus or chromosome that affects the expression of another gene

respiratory distress syndrome inability to maintain stable pulmonary alveolar structures, caused by low levels of surfactant, lecithin, and other pulmonary lipids in premature infants

reticulocytosis increase in the number of reticulocytes in the circulating blood

Rh immune globulin Rh immune globulin (RhIG) is purified anti-D prepared from immunized donors and is given to D-negative mothers to prevent the formation of anti-D

rigors a sudden feeling of cold with shivering accompanied by a rise in temperature, often with copious sweating, especially at the onset or height of a fever

root-cause analysis investigation and subsequent identification of the factors that contributed to an error

rule of three confirming the presence of an antibody by demonstrating three cells that are positive and three that are negative

rule out to eliminate the possibility that an antibody exists in the serum based on its nonreactivity with a particular antigen

saline replacement technique test to distinguish rouleaux from true agglutination

sanctions penalties or other means of enforcement to provide incentive for obedience with rules and regulations

sandwich ELISA (EIA) enzyme-linked immunosorbent assay (ELISA) technique used to determine the presence or quantity of an antigen

secondary immune response immune response induced after a second exposure to the antigen, which activates the memory lymphocytes for a quicker response

secretor individual who inherits the _Se_ allele and expresses soluble forms of H antigens in secretions

segment sealed piece of integral tubing from the donor unit bag that contains a small aliquot of donor blood; used in the preparation of red cell suspensions for crossmatching

selected cells cells chosen from another panel to confirm or eliminate the possibility of an antibody

sensitization binding of antibody or complement components to a red cell

sensitized immunoglobulin or complement attached to the cells from the immune system (in vivo) or from a test procedure (in vitro)

serotonin potent vasoconstrictor liberated by platelets

serum-to-cell ratio ratio of antigen on the red cell to antibody in the serum

sialic acid constituents of the sugars attached to proteins on red cells that lend a negative charge to the red cell membrane

specificity unique recognition of an antigenic determinant and its corresponding antibody molecule

standard operating procedures written procedures to help ensure the complete understanding of a process and to achieve consistency in performance from one individual to another

standard precautions Centers for Disease Control and Prevention term defining policies of treating all body substances as potentially infectious and applying safety measures to reduce possible exposure; standard precautions incorporate universal precautions and body substance isolation together

Standards for Blood Banks and Transfusion Services AABB publication that outlines the minimal standards of practice in areas relating to transfusion medicine

sulfhydryl reagents reagents that disrupt the disulfide bonds between cysteine amino acid residues in proteins; DTT, 2-ME, and AET function as sulfhydryl reagents

supernatant fluid above cells or particles after centrifugation

suppressor genes genes that suppress the expression of another gene

surrogate markers disease markers such as antibodies or elevations in enzymes that can be used as indicators for other potential infectious diseases; often used when direct testing is not available

syngeneic possessing an identical genotype, as in monozygotic twins

syntenic genetic term referring to genes closely situated on the same chromosome without being linked

systolic blood pressure contraction of the heart; the first sound heard while taking a blood pressure

T lymphocytes (T cells) lymphocytes that mature in the thymus and produce cytokines to activate the immune cells, including the B cell

Technical Manual AABB publication that provides a reference to current acceptable practices in blood banking

thalassemia inherited disorder causing anemia because of a defective production rate of either α-hemoglobin or β-hemoglobin polypeptide

therapeutic apheresis blood is removed from a patient, and the portion that might be contributing to a pathologic condition is retained; the remainder is returned along with a replacement fluid such as colloid or fresh frozen plasma

throughput productivity of a machine, procedure, process, or system over a unit period

titers extent to which an antibody may be diluted before it loses its ability to agglutinate with antigen

Tn-polyagglutinable red cells type of polyagglutination that occurs from a mutation in the hematopoietic tissue, characterized by mixed-field reactions in agglutination testing

trans genes inherited on opposite chromosomes of a homologous pair

transferase class of enzymes that catalyzes the transfer of a chemical group from one molecule to another

transfusion service performs testing and issues blood and blood components for transfusion

two-stage enzyme technique treatment of red cells with an enzyme before the addition of serum

Ulex europaeus plant lectin with specificity for the H antigen

unacceptable antigens antigens that the potential graft recipient is reacting against; antibodies to these antigens could reduce graft survival

universal donors group O donors for red blood cell (RBC) transfusions; these RBCs may be transfused to any ABO phenotype because the cells lack both A and B antigens

universal precautions Occupational Safety and Health Administration term defining policies of treating all body substances as potentially infectious and applying safety measures to reduce possible exposure

universal recipients group AB recipients may receive transfusions of red blood cells from any ABO phenotype; these recipients lack circulating ABO antibodies in plasma

valency the number of antigen-binding sites for any given antibody, or the number of antibody-binding sites for any given antigen

variable regions amino-terminal portions of immunoglobulins and T-cell receptor chains that are highly variable and responsible for the antigenic specificity of these molecules

vasoactive amines products such as histamines released by basophils, mast cells, and platelets that act on the endothelium and smooth muscle of the local vasculature

Waldenström macroglobulinemia overproduction of IgM by the clones of a plasma B cell in response to an antigenic signal; increased viscosity of blood is observed

weak D weak form of the D antigen that requires the indirect antiglobulin test for its detection

western blot test that separates and identifies viral antigens according to molecular weight using viral antibodies in an electrophoretic procedure

Wharton's jelly gelatinous tissue contaminant in cord blood samples that may interfere in immunohematologic tests

whole blood blood collected from a donor before separation into its components

zeta potential electrostatic potential measured between the red cell membrane and the slipping plane of the same cell

zone of equivalence number of binding sites of multivalent antigen and antibody are approximately equal

Index

Pages followed by *b*, *t*, or *f* refer to boxes, tables, or figures, respectively.